Perspectives in Inflammation

Under the Patronage of H.R.H. The Duchess of Kent

Proceedings of an International Meeting on Future Trends in Inflammation
III

Organized by The European Biological Research Association

Under the auspices of

The Arthritis & Rheumatism Council
The British Pharmacological Society
The British Society of Immunology
The European League Against Rheumatism
The Pathological Society of Great Britain & Ireland
The Royal Society of Medicine

Held at the Grosvenor House Hotel, Park Lane, London, February 14th–18th,
1977

Perspectives in Inflammation

Future Trends and Developments

*The Proceedings of the Third International
Meeting on Future Trends in Inflammation
organized by the European Biological
Research Association and held in London,
February 14th–18th, 1977*

Edited by

D. A. Willoughby

*Professor, Department of Experimental Pathology and Rheumatology,
St. Bartholomew's Hospital, London*

J. P. Giroud

*Professor, Department of Pharmacology, Hôpital Côchin,
Paris*

G. P. Velo

*Professor, Department of Pharmacology, Policlinico Borgo,
Rome*

MTP

Published by
MTP Press Limited
PO Box 55, St. Leonard's House
St. Leonardgate, LANCASTER, England

ISBN 978-94-011-7187-8   ISBN 978-94-011-7185-4 (eBook)
DOI 10.1007/978-94-011-7185-4

Contents

v

PERSPECTIVES IN INFLAMMATION

CONTENTS

CONTENTS

ix

PERSPECTIVES IN INFLAMMATION

CONTENTS

Preface

This report on Future Trends in Inflammation III is the record of what is now firmly established as a series of multidisciplinary meetings organized by the European Biological Research Association. The aim of these meetings is to provide a forum for free exchange of information between basic scientists of many disciplines and clinicians to provide better understanding of problems of common interest. The next major meeting will be held in 1980.*

The European Biological Research Association promotes scientific and clinical collaboration among the member countries of the EEC. It encourages exchange of information between scientists and clinicians from centres all over the world. In addition to the major international meetings small workshops are organized on specific problems of common interest.

Once again the Editors have attempted to capture the spirit of the meeting by publishing 'verbatim' the discussion. It can be seen that the discussions were exciting and formed an important part of the meeting.

It is possible that inaccuracies have crept into the discussions; if so we apologize. It was decided that the proceedings of such a meeting had maximum value with rapid publication.

We would like to thank the participants for the enthusiasm and goodwill which persisted throughout the meeting both scientifically and socially.

Above all we wish to thank H.R.H. The Duchess of Kent for acting as Patron of this meeting.

D. A. Willoughby
J. P. Giroud
G. P. Velo

* For further information regarding the 1980 meeting please contact Professor D. A. Willoughby of Department of Experimental Pathology, St. Bartholomew's Hospital, London, EC1A 7BE, England.

List of Contributors

JAN AASETH
Institute of Clinical Biochemistry,
Rikhospitalet. Oslo, 1, Norway

M. ABD-EL-FATTAH
Department of Biochemistry, Faculty of
Science, Ain Sams University, Cairo,
Egypt

T. G. ABRAHAMSEN
Institute of Immunology and
Rheumatology, Rikhospitalet, Oslo 1,
Norway

M. J. P. ADOLFS
Department of Pharmacology, Faculty of
Medicine, Erasmus University,
Rotterdam, The Netherlands

M. ADOLPHE
Laboratory of Cellular Pharmacology,
College for Advanced Studies,
Centre de Recherches de l'Association
Claude Bernard, F-75006 Paris, France

S. YOUSUF ALI
Experimental Pathology Unit, Institute of
Orthopaedics, University of London,
Royal National Orthopaedic Hospital,
Stanmore, Middlesex, HA7 4LP

A. C. ALLISON
MRC Clinical Research Centre,
Harrow, Middlesex, HA1 3UJ

E. ARRIGONI-MARTELLI
Department of Pharmacology,
Leo Pharmaceutical Products,
DK-2750 Ballerup, Denmark

A. AUTERI
Institute of Medical Semeiotics, School of
Medicine, University of Sienna, Italy

Z. M. BACQ
Applied Biochemistry Laboratory,

University of Liege, B-4020 Liege,
Belgium

S. BERGNER-RABINOWITZ
The Department of Oral Biology,
Hadassah School of Medicine,
The Hebrew University, Jerusalem,
Israel

G. BIANCHETTI
Rheumatology Service, L. Sacco Hospital,
Milan, Italy

L. BINDERUP
Department of Pharmacology,
Leo Pharmaceutical Products,
DK-2750 Ballerup, Denmark

D. BLANDELON
Laboratory of Cellular Pharmacology,
College for Advanced Studies, Centre de
Recherches de l'Association Claude
Bernard, F-75006 Paris, France

A. BÖNI
Department of Rheumatology, University
of Zurich, Cantonal Hospital, CH-8091
Zurich, Switzerland

R. J. BONNEY
Merck Institute for Therapeutic Research,
Rahway, New Jersey 07065, USA

L. BONOMO
Institute of Clinical Medicine II,
University of Bari, Policlinico, I-70124,
Bari, Italy

I. L. BONTA
Department of Pharmacology, Faculty
of Medicine, Erasmus University,
Rotterdam, The Netherlands

J. F. BOREL
Biological and Medical Research

Division, Sandoz Ltd., CH-4002 Basel,
Switzerland

J. W. D. BRADFIELD
Department of Experimental Pathology,
St. Mary's Hospital Medical School,
London, W.2

E. BRAMM
Department of Pathology, Leo
Pharmaceutical Products, DK-2750
Ballerup, Denmark

K. BRUNE
University of Basel, CH-4056 Basel,
Switzerland

P. van CANEGHEM
Applied Biochemistry Laboratory,
University of Liege, B-4020 Liege,
Belgium

R. A. CANUTO
Institute of General Pathology,
University of Turin, I-10125 Turin,
Italy

L. CARRATELLI
Merck Sharp and Dohme (Italia) S.p.a.,
I-00191 Rome, Italy

L. CARUSO
Rheumatology Service. L. Sacco
Hospital, Milan, Italy

A. CATS
Department of Rheumatology, University
Hospital, Leiden, The Netherlands

Y.-H. CHANG
Division of Rheumatology, Department
of Medicine, UCLA School of Medicine,
Los Angeles, California 90024, USA

L. DeCHATELET
Department of Biochemistry, The
Bowman Gray School of Medicine,
Wake Forest University, Winston-Salem,
North Carolina 27103, USA

R. COLLINS
Department of Biochemistry, The Bowman
Gray School of Medicine, Wake Forest
University, Winston-Salem, North
Carolina 27103, USA

Ph. CONQUET
MSD-Chibret Research Institute, F-63018
Clermont-Ferrand, France

R. R. A. COOMBS
Division of Immunology, Department of
Pathology, University of Cambridge

P. R. CROCKER
Department of Rheumatology and
Experimental Pathology, St.
Bartholomew's Hospital, London, E.C.1

R. W. CROFTON
Department of Infectious Diseases,
University Hospital, Leiden, The
Netherlands

M. E. DAHLGREN
Merck Institute for Therapeutic Research,
Rahway, New Jersey 07065, USA

P. H.-C. DANG
Diagnostic Data Inc., Mountain View,
California 94043, USA

P. DAVIES
Merck Institute for Therpeutic Research,
Rahway, New Jersey 07065, USA

C. DEBY
Applied Biochemistry Laboratory,
University of Liege, B-4020 Liege,
Belgium

D. A. DEPORTER
Faculty of Dentistry, University of
Toronto, Toronto, Canada

M. DIANZANI
Institute of General Pathology,
University of Turin, I-10125 Turin,
Italy

P. A. DIEPPE
Department of Rheumatology and
Experimental Pathology, St.
Bartholomew's Hospital, London,
E.C.1

M. B. DONATI
Rheumatology Service, L. Sacco Hospital,
Milan, Italy

L. J. DOOREN
Department of Paediatrics, University
Hospital, Leiden, The Netherlands

J. C. LeDOUAREC
MSD-Chibret Research Institute,
F-63018
Clermont-Ferrand, France

Z. DUCHAN
The Department of Oral Biology,
Hadassah School of Medicine, The
Hebrew University, Jerusalem, Israel

R. W. EGAN
Merck Institute for Therapeutic
Research, Rahway, New Jersey 07065,
USA

J. P. FAMAEY
Laboratory of Pharmacology,
Rheumatology Unit, School of Medicine,
University of Brussels, B-1000 Brussels,
Belgium

K. FEHR
Department of Rheumatology, University
of Zurich, Cantonal Hospital, CH-8091
Zurich, Switzerland

F. FEO
Institute of General Pathology,
University of Turin, I-10125 Turin,
Italy

J. FERLUGA
Institute of Medical Microbiology,
Johannes Gutenberg University, D-6500
Mainz, West Germany

M. FERNE
The Department of Oral Biology,
Hadassah Medical School, The Hebrew
University, Jerusalem, Israel

S. H. FERREIRA
Department of Pharmacology, Faculty
of Medicine, University of Sao Paulo,
Sao Paulo, Brazil

CAMILLE FEURER
Biological and Medical Research Division,
Sandoz Ltd., CH-4002 Basel,
Switzerland

J. FONTAGNE
Laboratory of Cellular Pharmacology,
College for Advanced Studies, Centre de
Recherches de l'Association Claude
Bernard, F-75006 Paris, France

J. FONTAINE
Laboratory of Pharmacology,
Rheumatology Unit, School of Medicine,
University of Brussels, B-1000 Brussels,
Belgium

P. FRANCHIMONT
Radioimmunology Laboratory, University
of Liege, B-4000 Liege, Belgium

S. S. FRØHLAND
Institute of Immunology and
Rheumatology, Rikshospitalet, Oslo 1,
Norway

M. FUMGALLI
Rheumatology Service, L. Sacco Hospital,
Milan, Italy

R. van FURTH
Department of Infectious Diseases,
University Hospital, Leiden, The
Netherlands

L. GABRIEL
Institute of General Pathology,
University of Turin, I-10125 Turin,
Italy

M. T. GABRIEL-BROUILLET
Rheumatology Clinic, C.H.U. Tirrone,
Marseilles, France

R. GARCEA
Institute of General Pathology, University
of Turin, I-10125 Turin, Italy

P. GAUTHERON
MSD-Chibret Research Institute, F-63018
Clermont-Ferrand, France

I. GINSBURG
The Department of Oral Biology,
Hadassah School of Medicine, The
Hebrew University, Jerusalem, Israel

J. P. GIROUD
Department of Pharmacology, Hospital
Cochin, Paris 14, France

M. GLATT
Department of Pharmacology, University
of Basel, CH-4056 Basel, Switzerland

L. E. GLYNN
Kennedy Institute of Rheumatology,
Hammersmith, London W6 7DW

P. HAUSER
Laboratory of Physiological Chemistry,
University of Leuven, Leuven, Belgium

F. HAVERKATE
Gaubius Institute, Health Research
Organization TNO, Leiden, The
Netherlands

G. HEYNEN
Radioimmunology Laboratory,
University of Liege, B-4000 Liege,
Belgium

D. A. HOROWITZ
Division of Rheumatology, Department
of Internal Medicine, University of
Virginia School of Medicine,
Charlottesville, Virginia 22901, USA

W. HUBER
Diagnostic Data Inc., Mountain View,
California 94043, USA

E. HULSING-HESSELINK
Department of Infectious Diseases,
University Hospital, Leiden, The
Netherlands

J. L. HUMES
Merck Institute for Therapeutic Research,
Rahway, New Jersey 07065, USA

E. C. HUSKISSON
St. Bartholomew's Hospital, London

G. HUYBRECHT-GODIN
Laboratory of Physiological Chemistry,
University of Leuven, Leuven, Belguim

Y. JEANDEL
Rheumatology Clinic, C.H.U. Tirrone,
Marseilles, France

E. JELLUM
Institute of Clinical Biochemistry,
Rikshospitalet, Oslo 1, Norway

G. KATONA
Rheumatology Service, General Hospital,
Mexico City, Mexico, D. F.

J. KAUFMANN
Department of Biochemistry, The Bowman
Gray School of Medicine, Wake Forest
University, Winston-Salem, North
Carolina 27103, USA

C. KLUFT
Department of Rheumatology, University
Hospital, Leiden, The Netherlands

D. KRUZE
Department of Rheumatology, University
of Zurich, Cantonal Hospital, CH-8091
Zurich, Switzerland

F. A. KUEHL, Jr.
Merck Institute for Therapeutic Research,
Rahway, New Jersey 07065, USA

P. LALLOUETTE
41, rue Camille Pelletan, F-92305
Levallois-Perret, France

R. LATINI
Rheumatology Service, L. Sacco Hospital,
Milan, Italy

P. LECHAT
Laboratory of Cellular Pharmacology,
College for Advanced Studies, Centre
de Recherches de l'Association Claude
Bernard, F-75006 Paris, France

J. LEFORT
Centre de Recherches Merrell International
F-67084 Strasbourg, France

G. P. LEWIS
Department of Pharmacology, Royal
College of Surgeons of England,
London, WC2A 3PN

G. LOEWI
MRC Clinical Research Centre, Harrow,
Middlesex, HA1 3UJ

BERENICE B. LORENZETTI
Department of Pharmacology, Faculty
of Medicine, University of Sao Paulo,
Sao Paulo, Brazil

M. P. LORIA
Institute of Clinical Medicine II,
University of Bari, Policlinico, I-70124,
Bari, Italy

E. LUCKHURST
Lister Institute of Preventive Medicine,
Elstree, Herts

W. H. LYLE
Dista Products Limited, Speke, Liverpool,
L24 9LN

H. MASHBURN
Department of Biochemistry, The Bowman
Gray School of Medicine, Wake Forest
University, Winston-Salem, North
Carolina 27103, USA

K. B. MENANDER-HUBER
Diagnostic Data Inc., Mountain View,
California 94043, USA

P. MERCIER
Transfusion Centre, Marseilles, France

H. MIELANTS
Section of Rheumatology, University
Hospital, B-9000 Ghent, Belgium

N. MOKHTAR
Department of Pathology, St.
Bartholomew's Hospital Medical College,
London

J. L. MOLENAAR
Central Laboratory of the Netherlands'
Red Cross Blood Transfusion Service,
Amsterdam, The Netherlands

F. MONTRONE
Rheumatology Service, L. Sacco Hospital,
Milan, Italy

E. MUNTHE
Oslo Rheumatism Hospital, Oslo 1,
Norway

J. B. NATVIG
Oslo Rheumatism Hospital, Oslo 1,
Norway

V. NOORDHOEK HEGT
Gabius Institute, Health Research
Organization TNO, Leiden, The
Netherlands

S. NORMANN
Department of Pathology, College of
Medicine, University of Florida,
Gainesville, Florida 32610, USA

R. NUMO
Rheumatology Service, University of
Bari, Policlinico, I-70124 Bari, Italy

D. A. A. OWEN
Department of Pharmacology, The
Research Institute, Smith Kline and
French Laboratories Ltd., Welwyn
Garden City, Herts

J. PAHLE
Oslo Rheumatism Hospital, Oslo 1,
Norway

W. E. PARISH
Unilever Research, Colworth House,
Sharnbrook, Bedford

N. E. PARKER
University College Hospital Medical
School, London

M. J. PARNHAM
Department of Pharmacology, Faculty
of Medicine, Erasmus University,
Rotterdam, The Netherlands

F. LAGHI PASINI
Institute of Medical Semeiotics, School
of Medicine, University of Sienna,
Sienna, Italy

C. M. PEARSON
Division of Rheumatology, Department
of Medicine, UCLA School of Medicine,
Los Angeles, California, USA

C. PEETERS-JORIS
Laboratory of Physiological Chemistry,
University of Leuven, Leuven, Belgium

M. PELLETIER
Laboratory of Cellular Pharmacology,
College for Advanced Studies, Centre de
Recherches de l'Association Claude
Bernard, F-75006 Paris, France

L. PELUS
Merck Institute for Therapeutic Research,
Rahway, New Jersey 07065, USA

T. Di PERRI
Institute of Medical Semeiotics, School
of Medicine, University of Sienna,
Sienna, Italy

P. J. PIPER
Department of Pharmacology, Royal
College of Surgeons of England,
London, WC2A 3PN

V. PIPITONE
Rheumatology Service, University of
Bari, Policlinico, I-70124 Bari, Italy

A. R. POOLE
Joint Diseases Laboratory,
Shriners Hospital for Crippled Children,
Montreal, Quebec, H3G 1A6, Canada

L. B. A. van de PUTTE
Department of Rheumatology, University
Hospital, Leiden, The Netherlands

J. REUSSE
Laboratory of Pharmacology,
Rheumatology Unit, School of Medicine,
University of Brussels, B-1000 Brussels,
Belgium

D. ROOS
Central Laboratory of the Netherlands'
Red Cross Blood Transfusion Service,
Amsterdam, The Netherlands

H. ROUX
Rheumatology Clinic, C.H.U. Tirrone,
Marseilles, France

G. RUHENSTROTH-BAUER
Max-Planck-Institute for Biochemistry,
D-8032 Martinsried bei München, West
Germany

M. G. P. SAIFER
Diagnostic Data Inc., Mountain View,
California 94043, USA

A. SEGAL
MRC Clinical Research Centre, Harrow,
Middlesex, HA1 3UJ

R. SCHERER
Max-Planck-Institute for Biochemistry,
D-8032 Martinsried bei München, West
Germany

H. U. SCHORLEMMER
Institute for Medical Microbiology,
Johannes Gutenburg University, D-6500
Mainz, West Germany

R. K. B. SCHUURMAN
Sophia Children's Hospital, Rotterdam,
The Netherlands

A. SCHWARTZ
41, rue Camille Pelleton, F-92305
Levallois-Perret, France

A. SCHWEITZER
Department of Biopharmaceutics,
Sandoz AG, CH-4002 Basel,
Switzerland

A. SEGAL
MRC Clinical Research Centre, Harrow
Middlesex, HA1 3UJ

G. SERRATRICE
Rheumatology Clinic, C.H.U. Tirrone,
Marseilles, France

J. SONDERGAARD
Department of Dermatology, Hvidovre
Hospital, Hvidovre, Denmark

E. SORKIN
Department of Medicine, Swiss Research
Institute, CH-7270 Davos, Switzerland

R. L. SOUHAMI
University College Hospital Medical
School, London

G. SPECCHIA
Institute of Clinical Medicine II,
University of Bari Medical School,
I-70124 Bari, Italy

W. G. SPECTOR
Department of Pathology, St.
Bartholomew's Medical College, London

LIESBETH STRICKER
Central Laboratory of the Netherlands'
Red Cross Blood Transfusion Service,
Amsterdam, The Netherlands

NANNA SVARTZ
King Gustav V Research Institute, S-10
401 Stockholm, Sweden

J. SYMOENS
Department of Clinical Research,
Janssen Pharmaceutica Research
Laboratories, B-2340 Beerse, Belgium

P. TOOTH
MRC Clinical Research Centre, Harrow,
Middlesex, HA1 3UJ

M. V. TORRIELLI
Institute of General Pathology,
University of Turin, I-10125 Turin, Italy

J. L. TURK
Department of Pathology, Royal College
of Surgeons of England, London,
WC2A 3PN

R. TURNER
Department of Medicine, The Bowman
Gray School of Medicine, Wake Forest
University, Winston-Salem, North
Carolina 27103, USA

A. TURSI
Institute of Clinical Medicine II,
University of Bari Medical School,
I-70124 Bari, Italy

LIST OF CONTRIBUTORS

B. VARGAFTIG
Centre de Recherche Merrell International,
F-67084 Strasbourg, France

G. VAES
Laboratory of Physiological Chemistry,
University of Leuven, Leuven, Belgium

G. P. VELO
Department of Pharmacology,
Policlinico Borgo Roma, I-37100 Verona,
Italy

E. M. VEYS
Rheumatology Section, University
Hospital, B-9000 Ghent, Belgium

T. L. VISCHER
Department of Rheumatology,
University of Geneva, Hôpital Cantonal
CH-1211 Geneva, Switzerland

L. van VLIET
Department of Pharmacology, Faculty
of Medicine, Erasmus University,
Rotterdam, The Netherlands

G. A. VOISIN
Centre of Immuno-Pathology and
Experimental Immunology,
l'Association Claude Bernard, Hôpital
Saint-Antoine, F-75012 Paris, France

D. van WAARDE
Department of Infectious Diseases,
University Hospital, Leiden, The
Netherlands

KÄTHY WAGNER
Department of Pharmacology, University
of Basel, CH-4056 Basel, Switzerland

R. S. WEENING
Central Laboratory of the Netherlands'
Red Cross Blood Transfusion Service,
Amsterdam, The Netherlands

G. WIJNGAARDS
Gaubius Institute, Health Research
Organization TNO, Leiden, The
Netherlands

P. C. WILKINSON
Bacteriology and Immunology
Department, University of Glasgow,
Western Infirmary, Glasgow, G11 6NT

D. A. WILLOUGHBY
Department of Rheumatology and
Experimental Pathology, St.
Bartholomew's Hospital, London,
E.C.1

D. F. WOODWARD
Department of Pathology, The Research
Institute, Smith Kline and French
Laboratories Limited, Welwyn Garden
City, Herts

MARIA TERESINHA ZANIN
Department of Pharmacology, Faculty
of Medicine, University of Sao Paulo,
Sao Paulo, Brazil

Section I
Immunological Aspects of Inflammation

CHAIRMAN: J. L. Turk

CO-CHAIRMAN: G. A. Voisin

Co-Chairman's Introductory Remarks—Immunostimulation and immunosuppression of what?*

GUY ANDRE VOISIN (France)

It is usual to speak of immunostimulatory and immunosuppressive substances without referring to the part of the immune reaction that is altered by them.

This is not satisfactory since an immunosuppressor of one aspect can be an immunostimulant of the other.

As a consequence, we must first analyse the immune reaction, its stages, its different agents, types and consequences, each one of these stages, agents and types being a potential target for a drug that might increase or decrease it.

I STAGES OF THE IMMUNE REACTION

They are best expressed in the immune cycle.

1 Immune cycle (Figure 1). It begins with an antigen-bearing target which induces an immune reaction and shall undergo the consequences of it. Then an afferent arc brings the antigenic information to the immunological centres. These react and build the immune agents of the specific reaction. An efferent arc brings these agents to the target where they accomplish their task.

2 The significant steps of this cycle are:
  (a) Recognition of the antigen.
  (b) Induction of the reactive cells.
  (c) Maturation of the reacting cells with:
      —differentiation, DNA synthesis and multiplication;
      —production of the immune agents, with RNA and protein syntheses.
  (d) Triggering of built-in regulatory mechanisms.
  (e) Effector mechanisms which include release of various active substances or activation of enzymatic systems.
  (f) Inflammatory consequences usually follow.

* Work partially supported by DGRST and the Fondation pour la Recherche Médicale Française.

3

THE IMMUNE REACTION CYCLE

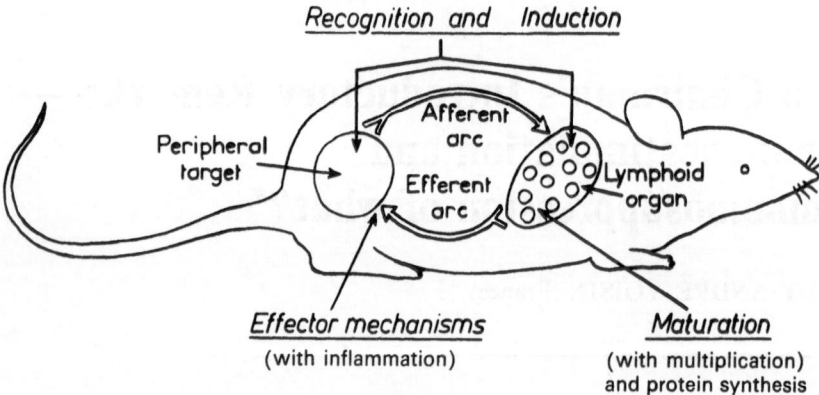

Figure 1

   These stages are an element of complexity when trying to understand the mechanism of action of an immuno-modificatory drug.
   Another factor of complexity is the number of immune agents involved in the immune reaction.

II IMMUNE AGENTS

These are of three categories and are endowed with various, sometimes opposed, properties.

1 Antibodies. Specific for the corresponding antigen through the variable (and mainly hypervariable) part of their Fab portion, they differ in their biological properties through their Fc part (μ, γ, a, ε, δ) responsible for their IgM, IgG, IgA, IgE and IgD class. Subclasses multiply the variety. To give an example, IgG 1 guinea pig antibodies directed against sheep red blood cells can protect them against *in vitro* destruction through complement and IgG 2 antibodies of same specificity[1]. Because of these different properties, it would be important to possess drugs capable to enhance or suppress selectively the synthesis of one or another class of antibodies.

2 Antigen-specific sensitized cells. These are or derive from lymphocytes: B-lymphocytes independent from the thymus, T-lymphocytes dependent of it. Subpopulations of these two series differentiate before or after contact with the antigen for which they have the adequate receptors. B-cells differentiate

4

into antibody-producing plasma cells of different classes and specificities, while several subpopulations (at least seven: see Waksman[2]) of T-cells with different surface markers play various roles:

(a) T-helper cells (Ly 1), helping B-cells to make antibodies against T-dependent antigens and other T-cells to become killers.

(b) T-suppressor (specific) cells (Ly 2–3, Ia +), inhibitory for B- cells and some T (Ly 1) cells.

(c) T-suppressor (non-specific) cells (Ly 1, Ly 2–3) inhibitory for various cells.

(d) T-amplifier cells (Ly 1, Ly 2–3) able to amplify the action of T-helper or T-suppressor cells.

(e) T MLR (Ly 1) responsible for the mixed lymphocyte reaction.

(f) T CMI (Ly 1) responsible for cell mediated immunity and delayed hypersensitivity.

(g) T-killer (Ly 2) responsible for the direct killing of the antigen-bearing target cells without the help of antibodies or complement.

Here again it is highly desirable to be able to alter selectively the production of this or that type of lymphocytes; not merely B or T.

3 Non-specific cells. Several other types of cells, non-specific for the antigen (although sometimes rendered so by antibodies fixed on their Fc receptors), are also agents of the immune reaction. This is the case for the following ones:

(a) Macrophages first with their Fc receptors for IgG 2 (mouse and guinea pig) are of prime importance in the afferent (antigen captation and processing), central (processed antigen presentation and cell cooperation) and efferent (target phagocytosis and killing) parts of the immune reaction. They are necessary for most if not all immune defence reactions, as well as for delayed hypersensitivity.

(b) K cells (Ig −, θ−, Fc receptor +) able to kill antigen-bearing target cells covered with the corresponding antibodies. But are these K cells 'nul' lymphocytes or macrophages?

(c) Mast cells and basophils with their Fc receptors for IgE (receptors on which anaphylactic IgG are also active) releasing their histamine, serotonine, heparine, ECFA, SRSA (?) containing granules upon challenge with the antigen. They are also present at the sites of delayed hypersensitivity reactions and more so at the sites of Jones-Mote reactions.

(d) Eosinophils, less well known but playing a certain role in serum-mediated hypersensitivity inflammatory reactions.

(e) Polymorphonuclears, with their potent lysosomal enzymes, are chemotactically attracted at the sites where immune complexes have activated C chemotactic factors. They phagocytose these immune complexes after immune adherence has taken place.

To increase or decrease the immuno-physiological activity of each one of these categories of cells would also be of great interest.

5

III REGROUPMENT OF THE IMMUNE AGENTS IN TWO MAIN TYPES OF REACTIONS

The preceding immune agents can be grouped in two sets acting in two opposite directions: rejection and facilitation (prevention of and protection against rejection)[3].

A Rejection reaction

This reaction has been selected and perfected during evolution in view of its protective value against intrusion and proliferation of foreign invaders. Its main immune agents are sensitized T-cells (CMI and killer), complement-fixing antibodies (IgM and rodent IgG 2) plus complement, leading to lysis or opsonization and K-cells activated by antibodies fixed on the target. Would this rejection reaction be the only one, it would threaten alloantigen-bearing fetuses and auto-antigen bearing organs to say the least. Actually, it is moderated or even counteracted by an opposite reaction.

B Facilitation reaction

This reaction protects the antigen-bearing target by preventing it from inducing or undergoing a rejection reaction. At a moderate level it is the expression of a homeostatic regulatory mechanism; at an extreme level its consequences

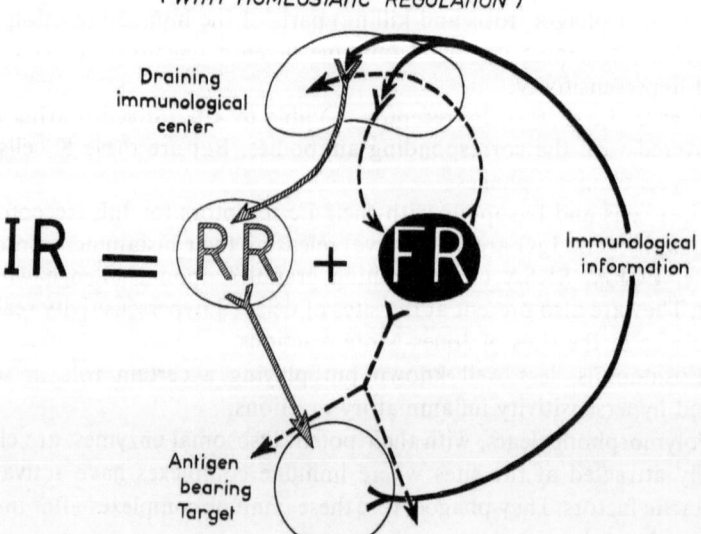

Figure 2

are indistinguishable from that of immunological tolerance. Its immune agents are IgG antibodies (IgG 1 and, at low concentrations, IgG 2) and suppressor cells. One may add that antibodies act on the target as free antibodies (peripheral effect) and on the specific lymphocytes as immune complexes (central effect). These two types of reactions almost invariably coexist as we have shown. One may therefore represent the immune reaction according to the equation of Figure 2; which means that what is usually observed in an immune reaction is what is left of the rejection reaction after the intervention of the facilitation reaction.

C   By-products of these reactions

At the effector level, the actions of these immune agents on the corresponding target are not without consequence on the surrounding tissues. The consequences, inflammatory in nature, are helpful to a certain extent, to complete a rejection reaction; but they may lead to immunopathological consequences through hypersensitivity reactions.

D   The implications

The implications are first that an 'immunosuppressor' of the facilitation reaction would have effects comparable to that of an immuno-stimulant of the rejection reaction.

As a matter of fact, cyclophosphamide, the well known immunosuppressor, when administered 3 days before sensitization of a guinea pig or a mouse, will increase sensitivity reactions to the sensitizing antigen (i.e. contact sensitivity to oxazolone or to DNFB or Jones-Mote sensitivity to ovalbumine).

Concomitantly (and it is not too dangerous a bet to say causally) the

Table 1   Target-structures and type of predominant reaction

Antigen-bearing target-structure (cell, tissue or other)	Predominant elements of the immune reaction	
	In normal physiological situation	In pathological or experimental situation
I—Allografted cells Bacteria Viruses Fungi Parasites Tumour cells	REJECTION	FACILITATION
II—Fetus (paternal alloantigen carrier)	FACILITATION	REJECTION
Autoantigen bearing organ		

7

production of IgG 1 anti-oxazolone antibodies is decreased and the level of a B population of suppressive cells is also decreased[4].

Conversely, an immunostimulation of the facilitation reaction would result in a suppression of the rejection reaction. This seems to have been seen for 2 classical immunostimulants: *B. pertussis*, which may increase the survival time of dog renal allografts (J. Corman, 1976, personal communication) and BCG which at high or repeated doses in guinea pig may decrease cell-mediated immunity with development of suppressive cells (G. Lamoureux, 1976, personal communication).

The importance of a selective action on the rejection reaction or the facilitation reaction becomes even more striking when one looks at the possible targets for rejection and facilitation. Under normal physiological conditions, and under some experimental or pathological conditions, the balance between the facilitation and the rejection reactions can be reversed (Table 1).

IV SPECIFICITY

Last but not least is the problem of specificity.

To knock down the whole capacity of immune reactions of an organism in order to suppress a reaction directed against one or a few antigens (in organ transplantation or autoimmune diseases, for instance) is too heavy a toll to be paid. It is like killing a fly on a glass with a hammer, and results in disarming the body in its fight against invading bacteria, viruses, mycetes and possibly cancer. Each of these possibilities unfortunately has been substantiated.

Conversely, to globally increase the immune reactivity of an organism might lead to autoimmune diseases and to immunopathological disorders as can be seen in experimental animals.

Since no drug has the capacity, by itself, to limit its effects to a given antigen, research should be pursued in 2 theoretical directions.

One is to administer the antigen in a certain time sequence with the drug in order for the latter to act on the specific cells when these are in the proper state of metabolic activity and differentiation to be a selective target for the drug.

The other is to conjugate the antigen to a substance so as to make this antigen play the role of a carrier or of a hapten. This should induce a reaction of a cellular or humoral type respectively against the antigen. This procedure, associated with a drug acting in a given direction on the immune system, might result in a further increase—or a decrease—of a given type of reactivity against this antigen.

Obviously, these kinds of procedures necessitate knowing and preparing the responsible antigens, which may not be possible. Even then, one may imagine that certain schedules and sites of administration of a drug could help.

CONCLUSIONS

A   Theoretical

There are three requirements to progress in the fields of immunosuppression and immunostimulation:

(1) *Selectivity*: the drug must be able, either by its intrinsic properties or by its administration schedule, to act on a restricted compartment of the immune reaction (stage and type of cell).

(2) *Specificity* for the considered antigen(s) that usually necessitates the knowledge of the antigen.

(3) *Better knowledge of the immune reaction*, especially its main stages, the cell subpopulations involved, the mechanisms of the interactions between the cells and molecules involved and their peripheral effects.

B   Practical

It is clear that each drug assayed for immunosuppressor or immunostimulant (and to a lesser extent for anti-inflammatory) capacities should be studied not only as for their action on the number of plaque forming cells, delayed hypersensitivity and tumour graft survival for instance, but one should be able to answer the questions concerning:

(1) *The site (or sites) of action on the immune cycle*: recognition, induction, differentiation and/or DNA synthesis, RNA and protein synthesis, peripheral expression (transfer experiments), activation of various enzymatic systems.

(2) *The immune agents concerned by the suppression or stimulation*: B-cells and antibody production and of what class(es), T-cells and what sub-population(s) (among several possible ones), macrophages, polymorpho-nuclears, or even, conceivably, some other type of cells involved in the immune reaction.

(3) *The possibility to restrict the action to a given antigen or sets of antigens*, by simultaneous or time-sequenced administration, injection schedule and site, chemical coupling.

(4) *The overall results in several experimental situations* including auto-immune syndromes, allogenic and isogenic tumour grafts, graft-versus-host reactions, infections with cocci and with mycobacteria or viruses.

When, and only when, these questions will have been answered, for a given substance, we shall be able to answer the question: immunostimulant or immunodepressor of what?

9

References

1. Kourilsky, F. M., Bloch, K. J, Benacerraf, B. and Ovary, Z. (1963). Properties of guinea pig 7S antibodies. V. Inhibition by guinea pig γ_1-antibodies of passive immune lysis provoked by γ_2-antibodies. *J. exp. Med.*, **118**, 699.
2. Waksman, B. H. (1977). Les divers types de cellules suppressives. *Ann. Immunol. (Inst. Pasteur)*, **128**, 427.
3. Voisin, G. A. (1971). Immunity and tolerance: a unified concept. *Cell. Immunol.* **2**, 670.
4. Turk, J. L., Polak, L. and Parker, D. (1976). Control mechanisms in delayed-type hypersensitivity. *Br. Med. Bull.*, **32**, 165.

1

The rationale of using levamisole in the treatment of rheumatoid arthritis

J. SYMOENS (Belgium)

Abbreviations used: RA: rheumatoid arthritis
RF: rheumatoid factor
Ig: immunoglobulin

INTRODUCTION

IMMUNOLOGICAL CHARACTERISTICS OF RHEUMATOID ARTHRITIS

It cannot be denied that the rheumatic joint is the site of an intense immunological activity[1]. The joint is heavily populated by lymphocytes, macrophages and polymorphonuclear cells[2]. B-cells are hyperactive and produce large amounts of antibodies, some of which are directed against the patient's own immunoglobulins[3-5]. There is increased complement consumption[6] and formation of immune complexes[2,7]. But the most outstanding clinical feature of rheumatoid arthritis is the formation and persistence of chronic granulomata within the joints and other tissues[8]. The predominant infiltrating lymphocyte is the T-cell[9]. This T-cell seems to be functionally active since lymphokines are produced in the rheumatic joint[10] and since patients with rheumatoid arthritis possess cell-mediated immunity to autologous IgG and to antigens present in the rheumatoid synovium[11,12].

Tissue damage is thought to be caused by the products released during these immune responses and during the ensuing inflammatory reactions (rheumatoid factor, immune complexes, lysosomal enzymes and chemical mediators of inflammation)[2,13].

The trigger of these chronic hyperimmune phenomena could be a persisting antigen or a self-perpetuating autoimmune process[14,15]. This explanation, however, is not satisfactory. Why does the immune process fail to effectively

11

eliminate the (hypothetical) pathogen, or why should the auto-immune process be self-perpetuating?

A selective defect of cell-mediated immunity has been incriminated. Cell-mediated immunity is essentially aimed to eliminate unwanted antigens. After having recognized the antigen, T-cells secrete soluble mediators that attract polymorphonuclear cells, macrophages and other T-cells to the target area, immobilize them, and activate them to eliminate the pathogen. If one of these multiple mechanisms fails to function—either by an inherent defect or by secondary immunosuppression—the pathogen may persist and cause chronic B-cell stimulation and inflammation. Alternatively, but not mutually exclusive, a selective defect of suppressor T-cells may produce the same pathology[16]. Suppressor T-cells have been shown to exert a feed-back control on B-cells and to play a crucial role in tolerance to self and non-self antigens[17,18]. A loss of suppressor T-cell function, and a loss of tolerance, can thus cause chronic antigenic stimulation of B-cells and chronic inflammation. Such a mechanism is held responsible for the initiation and perpetuation of certain autoimmune diseases in animals[17,18].

In short, both a failure of cell-mediated immunity to eliminate a pathogen, and a failure of suppressor T-cells to regulate the immune response, could explain the B-cell hyperactivity and the chronic inflammation of patients with rheumatoid arthritis (Figure 1.1).

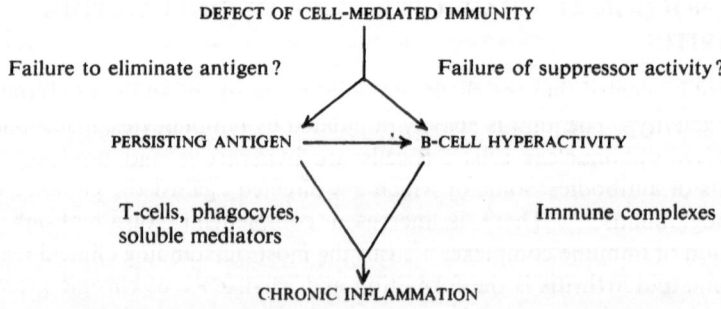

Figure 1.1 Hypothetical pathogenesis of rheumatoid arthritis

There is some evidence that patients with rheumatoid arthritis have a defect of cell-mediated immunity[14,19]. A number of reports have described reduced delayed skin hypersensitivity to sensitizing and recall antigens[20,21], reduced lymphocyte responsiveness to antigenic or mitogenic stimulation[22-24], reduced E-rosette formation[25,26], and reduced chemotaxis[27,28]. A high percentage of null cells was seen in some patients and not in others[25]. As a group, however, RA patients seem not to have dramatically reduced cell-mediated immune responses in the test systems studied. RA patients appear to cluster in two groups—one with values within the normal range and a second showing low values[20,25,26]. Low values tended to correlate with disease activity[20,22,23,25,26] and may well be secondary to the disease. Indeed, serum factors, synovial fluid, rheumatoid factor and RF-Ig complexes have been shown to depress certain functions of intrinsically normal lymphocytes and phagocytes in RA patients[23,28-33].

In conclusion, cell-mediated immune defects do exist in RA patients. The most consistent finding was reduced delayed skin hypersensitivity. Since this response is the end result of a chain of cell-mediated immune reactions, the available methods may have failed so far to demonstrate the specific immune defect that is responsible for the disease.

THE TREATMENT OF RHEUMATOID ARTHRITIS

The objective of therapy in rheumatoid arthritis is to control the basic destructive process of the disease (disintegration of cartilage, bone, connective tissue) and to prevent the possible ankylosis of joints.

None of the symptomatic agents (analgesics, corticosteroids or non-steroid anti-inflammatory drugs) significantly inhibits progression of the disease. The non-steroid anti-inflammatory drugs inhibit chemical mediators of inflammation but have no effect on erythrocyte sedimentation rate, acute phase protein, complement-mediated immune complex reactions or production and function of lymphokines[34,35]. Glucocorticosteroids have a marked effect on acute phase proteins and sedimentation[35], but joint damage may progress despite an almost complete suppression of symptoms[36].

In contrast, a number of drugs and procedures which seem to influence the course of the disease, reduce chronic inflammation (erythrocyte sedimentation rate, acute phase proteins, fibrinogen levels), reduce B-cell hyperactivity (rheumatoid factor, immune complexes, plasma immunoglobulin levels) and control other extra-articular features of the disease (nodules, vasculitis)[37-45]. Some of them retard radiological joint deterioration[36,40].

Unlike the symptomatic agents, which are clinically characterized by a quick onset (within days), and an immediate flare up of disease symptoms upon discontinuation of treatment, drugs that seem to influence the course of the disease act slowly (they may take months to achieve their maximal effect) and are able to induce long-term remission beyond the scope of conventional anti-inflammatory drugs. Their therapeutic response, when it occurs, is often very complete.

For three of such drugs—gold, d-penicillamine and antimalarials—the mode of action remains inadequately explained[39,43,46,47]. The immunosuppressive agents, such as cyclophosphamide and azathioprine, are thought to reduce chronic inflammatory and immunological responses[48,49]. They act differently from classical anti-inflammatory drugs. They do not inhibit prostaglandin synthesis[34], and strongly retard joint destruction[36,40]. With thoracic duct drainage, essentially T-lymphocytes are removed[50]. Since the

13

cellularity of the synovial membrane decreases after thoracic duct drainage, the therapeutic benefit of this measure is thought to derive from depletion of synovial cells that are inducing and continuing and propagating the inflammatory response[8,51].

Transfer factor, BCG and levamisole present the opposite approach. They probably act by improving cell-mediated immune mechanisms. Transfer factor and BCG have been evaluated in pilot studies only[52-54]. Levamisole has been more thoroughly investigated[26,44,45,55-70,91].

Levamisole very much resembles gold and d-penicillamine in its effects. It takes approximately 6 weeks before the patient improves and its maximal effect is reached after 3 to 6 months only. After discontinuation of treatment, long-term remissions of more than a year have been observed.

Some patients respond dramatically, others more moderately and some do not respond at all. In responders, an overall improvement of symptoms is seen, such as the number of affected joints, joint swelling and tenderness, grip strength, walking time, pain and morning stiffness (Table 1.1).

Table 1.1   Clinical effects of levamisole in R.A. patients
(References: 44*, 59, 62, 63, 65*, 68*, 69)

Objective	Subjective
Swollen joints ✓	Morning stiffness ✓
PIP ✓	Joint tenderness ✓
Walking time ✓	Total pain ✓
Grip strength ↗	
Technetium index ✓	

*Controlled study

The signs of chronic inflammation, such as elevated erythrocyte sedimentation rate and acute phase protein, fibrinogen and complement levels improve strikingly. Rheumatoid factor and immune complex titres decrease or become negative and elevated immunoglobulin levels return to normal (Table 1.2).

Table 1.2   Biological effects of levamisole in R.A.
patients

	References
ESR ✓	44, 62, 63, 68, 69, 70
CRP ✓	68, 91
Haptoglobin ✓	91
Fibrinogen ✓	91
CH_{50} ✓	70
Rheumatoid factor ✓	44, 59, 69, 70
Immune complexes ✓	45, 91
IgG ✓	44, 61, 70

Table 1.3 Immunological effects of levamisole in R.A. patients

	References
Delayed skin hypersensitivity ↗	44, 59, 61, 63, 91
E-rosettes ↗	26, 63, 70, 91
Null cells ↙	60
PHA stimulation (↗)	63, 66
Leukocyte migration inhibition ↗	44

When cell-mediated immune responses are low they are often, but not always, restored (Table 1.3). This restoration does not correlate with clinical responsiveness.

THE IMMUNOLOGICAL PROFILE OF LEVAMISOLE

The effects of levamisole in rheumatoid arthritis cannot be explained by a direct effect on invading organisms—if they exist— nor by an anti-inflammatory or an immunosuppressive effect. All available evidence suggests that levamisole acts by restoring a defective cell-mediated immune mechanism[71].

Studies on isolated phagocytes—polymorphonuclear cells or macrophages —have shown that levamisole restores each of the major functions of these cells, this is to say movement to the target area, phagocytosis and killing[71].

Levamisole has similar restorative effects on the functions of T-lymphocytes[71]. The drug increases to normal E-rosette formation in patients with reduced T-cell numbers, and decreases excessive B- or null-cell numbers in such patients. It can boost nucleic acid or protein synthesis by T-cells in response to antigenic stimulation. It increases antigen-induced lymphokine production. It stimulates suppressor activity, cytotoxicity and lysosomal activity. Plaque cell formation is enhanced in some instances and not in others.

In vivo studies confirm the selective restorative effect on cell-mediated immunity[71]. As a rule, levamisole does not increase antibody production, nor does it elevate serum immune globulin levels. Levamisole restores or boosts skin delayed hypersensitivity to antigens in anergic patients, increases graft-versus-host reactions and enhances blood clearance of colloidal particles in animals or subjects with a deficient phagocyte system. It increases macrophage concentration on subcutaneous coverslips in mice[72].

Levamisole does not stimulate cellular immunity above normal level: it does not shorten skin graft rejection time in mice[73,74] and does not induce adjuvant arthritis[72,75,76] or experimental allergic encephalomyelitis[77,78] when used instead of Freund's adjuvant. It however potentiates the adjuvant effects[72,75–77].

Levamisole has no anti-inflammatory effect comparable to that of the usual anti-inflammatory agents. It does not reduce the primary lesions of adjuvant arthritis[72,75,76], or carrageenan induced pleurisy[72].

Levamisole has a favourable effect on the course of spontaneous immune deficiency diseases in animals. It tempers the evolution of auto-immune nephritis in NZB/NZW mice[79-81], and of aleutian disease in mink[82].

Levamisole has been shown to be of clinical benefit in a whole range of apparently unrelated diseases of man, including recurrent and chronic infections, rheumatic diseases and cancer[71]. Many of the responding diseases are characterized by a reduced cellular immune responsiveness, antigenic persistence, chronic inflammation and B-cell hyperactivity. The effect of levamisole in these diseases is most likely due to restoration of the particular cellular immune defect that is responsible for the disease. The nature of the defect may be different for each disease entity. For instance, children with hypergammaglobulinaemia E and recurrent staphylococcal infections have a selective defect of chemotaxis, and this defect is restored by levamisole (Weening, this symposium).

In rheumatoid arthritis, one can only speculate on the mechanism that is influenced by levamisole. The drug may activate immune cells to respond to and eliminate the persisting antigen, and so control B-cell hyperactivity. Alternatively, but not mutually exclusive, levamisole may activate suppressor T-cells and possibly induce tolerance to the persisting antigen.

CONCLUSION

Present knowledge permits to conclude that the clinical and immunological effects of levamisole in rheumatoid arthritis are not unique to this disease. Levamisole behaves very similarly in other chronic inflammatory diseases with T-B-imbalance such as systemic lupus erythematosus, Crohn's disease, immunoblastic lymphadenopathy and lepromatous leprosy[26,83-90], and in many other diseases with known or suspected defects of cell mediated immunity. This broad spectrum of activity of levamisole gives strong support to the concept that rheumatoid arthritis is an immune deficiency disease.

References

1. Ziff, M. (1973). Pathophysiology of rheumatoid arthritis. *Fed. Proc.*, **32**, 131
2. Zvaifler, N. J. (1973). The immunopathology of joint inflammation in rheumatoid arthritis. In F. J. Dixon and H. G. Kunkel (eds.) *Advances in Immunology*, **16**, pp. 265–336. (New York and London: Academic Press)
3. Vaughan, J. H. and Chihara, T. (1975). Lymphocyte function in rheumatic disorders. *Arch. Intern. Med.*, **135**, 1324
4. Smiley, J. D., Sachs, C. and Ziff, M. (1968). In vitro synthesis of immunoglobulin by rheumatoid synovial membrane. *J. Clin. Invest.*, **47**, 624
5. Johnson, P. M. and Page Faulk, W. (1976). Rheumatoid factor: its nature, specificity, and production in rheumatoid arthritis. *Clin. Immunol. Immunopathol.*, **6**, 414
6. Ruddy, S. and Austen K. F. (1973). Activation of the complement system in rheumatoid synovitis. *Fed. Proc.*, **32**, 134

7. Luthra, H. S., McDuffie, F. C., Hunder, G. G. and Samayoa, E. A. (1975). Immune complexes in sera and synovial fluids of patients with rheumatoid arthritis. *J. Clin. Invest.*, **56**, 458

8. Pearson, C. M., Paulus, H. E. and Machleder, H. I. (1975). The role of the lymphocyte and its products in the propagation of joint disease. In R. J. Perper (ed.) *Mechanisms of Tissue Injury with Reference to Rheumatoid Arthritis*, **256**, pp. 150–168. *Ann. New York Acad. Sci.*

9. Van Boxel, J. A. and Paget, S. A. (1975). Predominantly T-cell infiltrate in rheumatoid synovial membranes. *N. Engl. J. Med.*, **293**, 517

10. Stastny, P., Rosenthal, M., Andreis, M., Cooke, D. and Ziff, M. (1975). Lymphokines in rheumatoid synovitis. In R. J. Perper (ed.) *Mechanisms of Tissue Injury with Reference to Rheumatoid Arthritis*, **256**, pp. 117–131. *Ann. New York Acad. Sci.*

11. Bacon, P. A., Bluestone, R., Cracchiolo, A. and Goldberg, L. S. (1973). Cell-mediated immunity to synovial antigens in rheumatoid arthritis. *Lancet*, **ii**, 699

12. Weisbart, R. H., Bluestone, R. and Goldberg, L. S. (1975). Cellular immunity to autologous IgG in rheumatoid arthritis and rheumatoid-like disorders. *Clin. Exp. Immunol.*, **20**, 409

13. Hirschhorn, R. (1975). The blind men and the rheumatoid elephant. *N. Engl. J. Med.*, **293**, 554

14. Yu, D. T. Y. and Peter, J. B. (1974). Cellular immunological aspects of rheumatoid arthritis. *Semin. Arthritis Rheum.*, **4**, 25

15. Fudenberg, H. H. (1971). Genetically determined immune deficiency as the predisposing cause of 'autoimmunity' and lymphoid neoplasia. *Am. J. Med.*, **51**, 295

16. Fudenberg, H. H. and Wells, J. V. (1976). The paradox of immunosuppression: T-cell deficiency as the cause of autoimmunity. In D. C. Dumonde (ed.) *Infection and Immunology in the Rheumatic Diseases*, pp. 549–562. (Oxford, London, Edinburgh, Melbourne: Blackwell Scientific Publications)

17. Allison, A. C., Denman, A. M. and Barnes, R. D. (1971). Cooperating and controlling functions of thymus-derived lymphocytes in relation to autoimmunity. *Lancet*, **ii**, 135

18. Pierce, C. W., Peavy, D. L. and Tadakuma, T. (1975). Suppressor T-cells as regulators of lymphocyte functions. In R. J. Perper (ed.) *Mechanisms of Tissue Injury with Reference to Rheumatoid Arthritis*, **256**, pp. 365–374. *Ann. New York Acad. Sci.*

19. Lockshin, M. D. (1976). Immunological status of patients with rheumatic disease. In D. C. Dumonde (ed.) *Infection and Immunology in the Rheumatic Diseases*, pp. 541–547. (Oxford, London, Edinburgh, Melbourne: Blackwell Scientific Publications)

20. Waxman, J., Lockshin, M. D., Schnapp, J. J. and Doneson, I. N. (1973). Cellular immunity in rheumatic diseases. I. Rheumatoid arthritis. *Arthritis Rheum.*, **16**, 499

21. Toh, B. H., Roberts-Thomson, I. C., Mathews, J. D., Whittingham, S. and Mackay, I. R. (1973). Depression of cell-mediated immunity in old age and the immunopathic diseases, lupus erythematosus, chronic hepatitis and rheumatoid arthritis. *Clin. Exp. Immunol.*, **14**, 193

22. Lance, E. M. and Knight, S. C. (1974). Immunologic reactivity in rheumatoid arthritis. Response to mitogens. *Arthritis Rheum.*, **17**, 513

23. Keystone, E. C., Gladman, D. D., Urowitz, M. B., Clarke, D. A., Falk, J. A., Osoba, D. and Gordon, D. A. (1976). Mixed leukocyte reaction in rheumatoid arthritis. *Arthritis Rheum.*, **19**, 532

24. Griswold, W. R. and McIntosh, R. M. (1973). Lymphocyte responses to phytohemagglutinin in rheumatoid arthritis and glomerulonephritis and the effects of immunosuppression. *Experientia*, **29**, 606

25. Williams, R. C., DeBoard, J. R., Mellbye, O. J., Messner, R. P. and Lindström, F. D. (1973). Studies of T- and B-lymphocytes in patients with connective tissue diseases. *J. Clin. Invest.*, **52**, 283

26. Verhaegen, H., De Cree, J., De Cock, W. and Verbruggen, F. (1977). Restoration, by levamisole, of low E-rosette forming cells in patients suffering from various diseases. *Clin. Exp. Immunol.*, **27**, 313

27. Mowat, A. G. and Baum, J. (1971). Chemotaxis of polymorphonuclear leukocytes from patients with rheumatoid arthritis. *J. Clin. Invest.*, **50**, 2541

28. Beeuwkes, H. and Bijlsma, A. (1974). Reduced chemotaxis of polymorphonuclear

leukocytes in sera from patients with rheumatoid arthritis. *Antonie van Leeuwenhoek*, **40**, 233

29. Turner, R. A., Schumacher, H. R. and Myers, A. R. (1973). Phagocytic function of polymorphonuclear leukocytes in rheumatic diseases. *J. Clin. Invest.*, **52**, 1632

30. Ward, P. A. and Zvaifler, N. J. (1973). Quantitative phagocytosis by neutrophils. II. Release of the C5-cleaving enzyme and inhibition of phagocytosis by rheumatoid factor. *J. Immunol.*, **111**, 1777

31. Sheldon, P. J., Papamichail, M. and Holborow, E. J. (1974). Studies on synovial fluid lymphocytes in rheumatoid arthritis. *Ann. Rheum. Dis.*, **33**, 509

32. Roberts-Thomson, P. J., Hazleman, B. L., Barnett, I. G., MacLennan, I. C. M. and Mowat, A. G. (1976). Factors relating to circulating immune complexes in rheumatoid arthritis. *Ann. Rheum. Dis.*, **35**, 314

33. Holt, P. J. L. and Popovic, M. (1976). Alteration of T-cell function by serum factors in rheumatoid arthritis and systemic lupus erythematosus. In D. C. Dumonde (ed.) *Infection and Immunology in the Rheumatic Diseases*, pp. 467–470. (Oxford, London, Edinburgh, Melbourne: Blackwell Scientific Publications)

34. Ferreira, S. H. and Vane, J. R. (1974). New aspects of the mode of action of nonsteroid anti-inflammatory drugs. *Annu. Rev. Pharmacol.*, **14**, 57

35. McConkey, B., Crockson, R. A., Crockson, A. P. and Wilkinson, A. R. (1973). The effects of some anti-inflammatory drugs on the acute-phase proteins in rheumatoid arthritis. *Q. J. Med.*, **42**, 785

36. Cooperating Clinics Committee of the American Rheumatism Association (1970). A controlled trial of cyclophosphamide in rheumatoid arthritis. *N. Engl. J. Med.*, **283**, 883

37. Huskisson, E. C., Gibson, T. J., Balme, H. W., Berry, H., Burry, H. C., Grahame, R., Dudley Hart, F., Henderson, D. R. F. and Woftulenski, J. A. (1974). Trial comparing d-penicillamine and gold in rheumatoid arthritis. *Ann. Rheum. Dis.*, **33**, 532

38. Multicentre Trial Group (1973). Controlled trial of d(-)penicillamine in severe rheumatoid arthritis. *Lancet*, **i**, 275

39. Zvaifler, N. J. (1968). Antimalarial treatment of rheumatoid arthritis. *Med. Clin. N. Am.*, **52**, 759

40. Currey, H. L. F., Harris, J., Mason, R. M., Woodland, J., Beveridge, T., Roberts, C. J., Vere, D. W., Dixon, A. St. J., Davies, J. and Owen-Smith, B. (1974). Comparison of azathioprine, cyclophosphamide and gold in treatment of rheumatoid arthritis. *Br. Med. J.*, **3**, 763

41. The Research Sub-Committee of the Empire Rheumatism Council (1960). Gold therapy in rheumatoid arthritis. Report of a multi-centre controlled trial. *Ann. Rheum. Dis.*, **19**, 95

42. Jaffe, I. A. (1975). Penicillamine treatment of rheumatoid arthritis: effect on immune complexes. Part VI. Prospectives on possible therapy for prevention of joint destruction in rheumatoid arthritis. In R. J. Perper (ed.) *Mechanisms of Tissue Injury with Reference to Rheumatoid Arthritis*, **256**, pp. 330–337. *Ann. New York Acad. Sci.*

43. Huskisson, E. C. and Berry, H. (1974). Some immunological changes in rheumatoid arthritis among patients receiving penicillamine and gold. *Postgrad. Med. J.*, 59–61

44. Huskisson, E. C., Dieppe, P. A., Scott, J., Trapnell, G., Balme, H. W. and Willoughby, D. A. (1976). Immunostimulant therapy with levamisole for rheumatoid arthritis. *Lancet*, **i**, 393

45. Rosenthal, M., Graf, U. and Müller, W. (1977). Der Effekt der Therapie auf Immunkomplexe bei der chronischen Polyarthritis. *Dtsch. Med. Wochenschr.*, **102**, 415

46. Walz, D. T., Dimartino, M. J. and Sutton, B. M. (1974). Design and laboratory evaluation of gold compounds as antiinflammatory agents. In R. A. Scherrer and M. W. Whitehouse (eds.), *Antiinflammatory Agents, Chemistry and Pharmacology*, **1**, pp. 209–244. (New York, San Francisco, London: Academic Press)

47. Shen, T. Y. (1974). IV. Clinical antirheumatic studies. In R. A. Scherrer and M. W. Whitehouse (eds.), *Antiinflammatory Agents, Chemistry and Pharmacology*, **1**, pp. 203–207. (New York, San Francisco, London: Academic Press)

48. Kaplan, S. R. and Calabresi, P. (1973). Immunosuppressive agents (first of two parts). *N. Engl. J. Med.*, **289**, 952

49. Goebel, K. M., Janzen, R., Joseph, K. and Börngen, U. (1976). Disparity between

clinical and immune responses in a controlled trial of azathioprine in rheumatoid arthritis. *Eur. J. Clin. Pharmacol.*, **9**, 405

50. Yu, D. T. Y., Peter, J. B., Stratton, J. A., Paulus, H. E. and Machleder, H. I. (1973). Lymphocyte dynamics: change in density profiles and response to phytohemagglutinin of human lymphocytes during prolonged thoracic duct drainage. *Clin. Immunol. Immunopathol.*, **1**, 456

51. Pearson, C. M. (1976). Lymphocyte depletion in patients with rheumatoid arthritis. *Agents Actions*, **6**, 28

52. Fröland, S. S., Natvig, J. B., Höyeraal, H. M. and Kass, E. (1974). The principle of immunopotentiation in treatment of rheumatoid arthritis: effect of transfer factor. *Scand. J. Immunol.*, **3**, 223

53. Maini, R. N., Scott, J. T., Roffe, L. M., Hamblin, A. S. and Dumonde, D. C. (1976). Preliminary experience of transfer factor in rheumatoid arthritis: clinical and immunological studies. In D. C. Dumonde (ed.) *Infection and Immunology in the Rheumatic Diseases*, pp. 579–589. (Oxford, London, Edinburgh, Melbourne: Blackwell Scientific Publications)

54. Rewald, E. (1974). B.C.G. in rheumatoid arthritis. *Lancet*, **ii**, 785

55. Dinai, Y. and Pras, M. (1975). Levamisole in rheumatoid arthritis. *Lancet*, **ii**, 556

56. Leca, A. P., Crouzet, J., Prier, A. and Camus, J. P. (1976). Vingt cas de polyarthrite rhumatoide traités par le lévamisole. *Nouv. Presse Méd.*, **5**, 89

57. Lequesne, M. and Floquet, J. (1976). Les effets secondaires au cours des traitements prolongés par le lévamisole notamment dans les polyarthrites. *Nouv. Presse Méd.*, **5**, 358

58. McGill, P. E. (1976). Levamisole in rheumatoid arthritis. *Lancet*, **i**, 149

59. Rosenthal, M., Trabert, U. and Müller, W. (1976), Immunotherapy with levamisole in rheumatic diseases. *Scand. J. Rheumatol.*, **5**, 216

60. Rosenthal, M., Trabert, U. and Müller, W. (1976). The effect of levamisole on peripheral blood lymphocyte subpopulations in patients with rheumatoid arthritis and ankylosing spondylitis. *Clin. Exp. Immunol.*, **25**, 493

61. Szpilman, H., Luft, S., Glinska-Urban, D., Fischer, W. and Plachecka, M. (1976). Levamisole and cell-mediated immunity and serum-immunoglobulins in rheumatoid arthritis. *Lancet*, **ii**, 208

62. Veys, E. M., Mielants, H., De Bussere, A., Decrans, L. and Gabriels, P. (1976). Levamisole in rheumatoid arthritis. *Lancet*, **i**, 808

63. Basch, C. M., Spitler, L. E., Engleman, E. P. and Engleman, E. (1976). Cellular immune reactivity in patients with rheumatoid arthritis and effect of levamisole on immunologic reactivity. Unpublished Report, May

64. Basch, C., Spitler, L. E., Engleman, E. G., and Engleman, E. P. (1976). Cellular immune reactivity in patients with rheumatoid arthritis following continuous or intermittent therapy with levamisole (abstract). Presented at the *National Scientific Meeting of the American Rheumatism Association*, December, Miami, Florida

65. Franchimont, P., Berghs, H., Remans, J. and Vroninks, Ph. (1976). Double-blind placebo-controlled evaluation of levamisole in chronic rheumatoid arthritis. Unpublished Report, August

66. Levy, J. and Miller, B. (1976). Deficient cell mediated immune responses in rheumatoid arthritis and reversal with levamisole. Presented at the *American Rheumatism Association Annual Scientific Meeting*, June 1976, Chicago, Illinois

67. Nelson, H. G. (1976). The use of levamisole in rheumatoid arthritis in comparison with gold therapy. Unpublished Data, February

68. Runge, L. A., Pinals, R. S. and Lourie, S. N. (1976). Treatment of rheumatoid arthritis (R.A.) with low-dose levamisole. Double-blind study (abstract). Presented at the *American Rheumatism Association National Scientific Meeting*, December, Miami, Florida

69. Schuermans, Y., De Cree, J., Symoens, J. and Verhaegen, H. (1976). Le traitement de la polyarthrite rhumatoide par le lévamisole. *Rev. Rhum.*, **43**, 437

70. Verhaegen, H., De Cree, J., De Cock, W., Schuermans, Y., Engels, M. and Sonck, W. (1977). Immunologic evaluation of rheumatoid arthritis and therapy with levamisole. *Biomedicine*. (In press)

71. Symoens, J. and Rosenthal, M. (1977). Levamisole in the modulation of the immune

19

response—The current experimental and clinical state. *J. Reticuloendothel. Soc.*, **21**, 175

72. Dieppe, P. A., Willoughby, D. A., Stevens, C., Kirby, J. D., and Huskisson, E. C. (1976). Specific therapy in new and conventional animal models. *Rheumatol. Rehabil.*, **15**, 201

73. Flannery, G. R., Rolland, J. M. and Nairn, R. C. (1975). Levamisole. *Lancet*, **i**, 750

74. Benazet, F., Guy-Loe, H., Maral, R., Werner, G., Berteaux, S, and Godard, C. (1973). Bilan actuel des résultats obtenus au cours de l'étude de l'action immunostimulante du tétramisole (16535 R.P.) et du lévamisole (20605 R.P.). Unpublished Report, March

75. Trabert, U., Rosenthal, M. and Müller, W. (1976). The effect of levamisole on adjuvant arthritis in the rat. *J. Rheumatol.*, **3**, 166

76. Hirayama, T. and Ohta, S. (1975). Antiinflammatory effect of levamisole. Unpublished Report, November

77. Spreafico, F., Vecchi, A., Mantovani, A., Poggi, A., Franchi, G., Anaclerio, A. and Garattini, S. (1975). Characterization of the immunostimulants levamisole and tetramisole. *Eur. J. Cancer.*, **11**, 555

78. Hierholzer, E. and Kuwert, E. (1975). Immunologische Wirksamkeit von Levamisol unter Verwendung des Versuchmodells der 'experimentellen allergischen Encephalomyelitis (Immunoencephalomyelitis)' am Kaninchen. Unpublished Report, April

79. Klassen, L. W., Budman, D. R., Williams, D. R., Williams, G. W., Steinberg, A. D. and Gerber, N. L. (1977). Ribavirin: efficacy in the treatment of murine autoimmune disease. *Science*, **195**, 787

80. Russell, A. S. (1976). Therapeutic trials with levamisole and other agents in NZB/W mice. *J. Rheumatol.*, **3**, 380

81. Vogler, C,. Morris, A. D., Mierzwa, P. and Moeschberger, M. (1976). Immunostimulation therapy of lupus erythematosus (SLE): effect of levamisole on NZB/NZW nephritis. Presented at the *Annual Meeting of the Midwest Section of the AFCR Immunology-Rheumatology Section*, November

82. Kenyon, A. J., Kassel, R., Notani, G. and Hahn, E. C. (1976). Separation of aleutian disease antibody response from induction of gammapathy with levamisole (abstract). *Fed. Proc.*, **35**, 569

83. Gordon, B. L. and Keenan, J. P. (1975). The treatment of systemic lupus erythematosus (SLE) with the T-cell immunostimulant drug levamisole: a case report. *Ann. Allergy*, **35**, 343

84. Gordon, B. L. and Yanagihara, R. (1977). Treatment of systemic lupus erythematosus with the T-cell immunopotentiator levamisole: a follow-up report of sixteen cases under treatment for a minimum period of 4 months. Unpublished Report, May

85. Bertrand, J., Renoux, G., Renoux, M. and Palat, A. (1974). Maladie de Crohn et lévamisole. *Nouv. Presse. Méd.*, **3**, 2265

86. Bensa, J.-Cl., Faure, J., Martin, H., Sotto, J.-J. and Schaerer, R. (1976). Levamisole in angio-immunoblastic lymphadenopathy. *Lancet*, **i**, 1081

87. Ellegaard, J. and Boesen, A. M. (1976). Restoration of defective cellular immunity by levamisole in a patient with immunoblastic lymphadenopathy. *Scand. J. Haematol.*, **17**, 36

88. Martinez, D., Zaias, N. (1976). Levamisole as adjunct to dapsone in leprosy. *Lancet*, **ii**, 209

89. Saint-André, P. and Louvet, M. (1976). Stimulation de l'immunité cellulaire dans la lèpre lépromateuse par lévamisole. *Med. Armées*, **4**, 223

90. Nelson, K. E., Pagels, G. A., Batt, M. D. and Vithaysai, V. (1977). Studies of levamisole in lepromatous leprosy (abstract). *Clin. Res.* (In press.)

91. Franchimont, P., Hauwaert, C., Betz-Rigaux, C. and Heynen, G. (1976). Efficacy, tolerance and mode of action of levamisole in rheumatoid arthritis. Unpublished Report, November

2
Immunostimulation, levamisole and rheumatoid arthritis

E. C. HUSKISSON (UK)

Levamisole is interesting not only as yet another anti-rheumatic drug, but also because it is capable of enhancing cell-mediated immune responses. If enhancement of cell-mediated immunity proved to be the mode of action of the drug, we might learn something about the disease itself as well as providing a new approach to its treatment.

WHAT KIND OF DRUG IS LEVAMISOLE IN RHEUMATOID ARTHRITIS?

Available evidence supports the view that levamisole has an action described as 'specific' in rheumatoid arthritis[1]. Drugs with this type of action work more slowly than anti-inflammatory drugs. They take 4–6 months to achieve their maximum effect, whereas most anti-inflammatory drugs work within a few days. 'Specific' drugs affect extra-articular features of rheumatoid arthritis as well as the joints themselves and produce reductions in ESR and rheumatoid factor titre. Some are capable of altering the outcome of the disease, as shown by progression of radiological changes. Penicillamine, for example, halts radiological progression in patients able to continue treatment[2]. Drugs of this type are effective in rheumatoid arthritis, but not in all types of inflammatory arthritis.

Levamisole has been shown to have a number of these properties[3,4]. It produces its beneficial effects slowly, and the effect on joints is accompanied by reduction of ESR and rheumatoid factor titre. Clinical experience with the drug suggests that like penicillamine, it is capable of producing a reduction in the number and size of subcutaneous nodules and promoting the disappearance of vasculitic skin lesions. The duration of treatment has not yet

21

been sufficient to expect changes in radiological progression of the disease, but present clinical evidence certainly suggests that levamisole will be a useful addition to the group of 'specific' drugs. It has so far been compared only with penicillamine and the two drugs were found to be equivalent and both were superior to placebo[3]. These findings have since been confirmed in larger numbers of patients.

Two different dosage regimes have been used in rheumatoid arthritis. Levamisole has been given in a continuous dosage of 50 mg three times daily[3]. There is some reason to think that intermittent dosage might be just as effective or even more effective. Veys et al.[5] used 50 mg three times daily on four consecutive days of each week, showed significant improvement and regarded their results as comparable to those of other investigators who had used continuous therapy. Direct comparison of continuous and intermittent therapy (50 mg three times daily on three days of each week) in our department has shown the two regimes to be equivalent.

Formal studies have not been completed in diseases other than rheumatoid arthritis but Rosenthal et al.[4] reported improvement in 7 of 13 patients with ankylosing spondylitis and one with Reiter's disease. Studies are in progress in systemic lupus erythematosus and psoriatic arthropathy.

Most of the 'specific' drugs for rheumatoid arthritis, like gold and penicillamine, have serious side effects which limit the number of patients able to continue treatment and therefore diminish the usefulness of the drug. This type of treatment is designed to suppress the disease and prevent progression and is of little value if it cannot be continued. Levamisole causes a number of side effects including rashes, loss of taste, neutropenia, nausea, vomiting, and mouth ulcers[3,4]. Delayed healing of a varicose ulcer has also been reported[6].

Nausea and occasionally vomiting are early problems which can be almost eliminated by the use of a slowly increasing dosage schedule. Our current practice is to give 50 mg daily for the first 2 weeks, then 100 mg daily for 2 weeks, then 150 mg daily. Rashes are of several different types, the commonest being erythematous with an urticarial component. This type of rash disappears rapidly when the drug is withdrawn. Treatment can usually be restarted, either at a lower dose or using an intermittent regime. Some more serious rashes have occurred, with skin lesions resembling those of systemic lupus erythematosus and accompanied by histological evidence of vasculitis. Taste abnormalities have been mild and transient and nothing like the disturbance which occurs in patients receiving penicillamine.

Neutropenia appears to be the most serious problem in patients receiving levamisole. Some depression of neutrophil counts is common in patients receiving the drug but this shows no correlation with clinical improvement. Occasional patients show falls to serious levels, below 1000 neutrophils per mm^3. This is often but not always predictable—in many instances the counts show a progressive decline. It has occurred on both continuous and intermittent therapy and at any time up to 2 years after the start of treatment. Bone marrow may show agranulocytosis. Recovery is usually rapid when the drug is withdrawn but there have been reported fatalities particularly, it seems, in patients receiving steroids or other dangerous drugs. This complication appears to be particularly hazardous for patients receiving steroids for their arthritis. Antibiotics may be required to treat infections but other drugs should be avoided while recovery is awaited. Patients should be advised to report at once to the physician supervising their treatment if they become ill in any way. Full blood counts should be carried out at least monthly during treatment. Neutropenia and various other complications appear to be much commoner in rheumatoid arthritis than in other conditions for which levamisole is given, perhaps a reflection of the immunological status of the rheumatoid patient.

Mouth ulcers have been an occasional problem as with other drugs of this type. Many patients with neutropenia have mouth ulcers but not all patients with mouth ulcers have neutropenia.

MODELS AND MECHANISMS

Levamisole is not an anti-inflammatory drug and it is not therefore surprising that it is inactive in models of inflammation such as carrageenan-induced pleurisy or the primary lesions of adjuvant arthritis. Levamisole has been shown to enhance the secondary lesions of adjuvant arthritis in rats and also the inflammatory reaction induced by pertussis vaccine in previously sensitized animals[3,7,8]. These effects demonstrate levamisole's ability to enhance a cell-mediated immune reaction as well as providing a potentially useful model for screening drugs of this type. There is a large amount of evidence in other experimental systems for the ability of levamisole to enhance various types of cell-mediated phenomena[9].

Elucidation of the mechanism of action of levamisole in man is not so easy. There is some evidence for enhancement of cellular immunity. Huskisson et al.[3] showed a trend (not statistically significant) towards enhancement of tuberculin skin reactions and leukocyte migration inhibition in the presence of PPD. There was a significant correlation between clinical response and these measurements. Rosenthal et al.[4] showed increased skin sensitivity using five antigens in 9 of 23 patients tested. Recent work in this department by Dr. K. Wynn has examined the effect of levamisole on phagocytosis of latex particles. Enhancement of phagocytosis was demonstrated in both polymorphs and neutrophils from the blood of patients treated with levamisole but not in cells from synovial fluid. This effect occurred within a short time of starting treatment, long before clinical improvement was demonstrable and there was no correlation between changes in phagocytic activity and clinical responses.

The similarities between levamisole and penicillamine deserve emphasis.

23

No-one would suggest that all drugs with a 'specific' action in rheumatoid arthritis were the same or worked in the same way. But similarities between drugs of this type may provide clues to their mode of action. Levamisole does not chelate copper and penicillamine does not kill worms, and similarities between the drugs are likely to be more important than differences such as these. Both drugs have the same type of action in rheumatoid arthritis. Both are capable of enhancing cell-mediated immune reactions as judged by their effect in models such as adjuvant arthritis and pertussis vaccine oedema or pleurisy[3,8-10]. It would be nice to believe that such drugs act by increasing phagocytosis. Rheumatoid arthritis might be a chronic inflammatory reaction maintained by a persistent foreign antigen which occurs only in subjects whose ability to remove or conceal the antigen is deficient. Levamisole might restore the ability of their cell-mediated mechanisms to process the antigen, though there is no direct evidence for this. An alternative view is that it acts on lymphocytes and an effect on suppressor T-cells would readily explain these and almost any other phenomena.

References

1. Huskisson, E. C. (1976). Specific therapy for rheumatoid arthritis. *Rheumatol. Rehabil.*, **15**, 133
2. Gibson, T., Huskisson, E. C., Woftulenski, J. A., Scott, P. J., Balme, H. W., Burry, H. C., Grahame, R. and Hart, F. D. (1976). Evidence that D-penicillamine alters the course of rheumatoid arthritis. *Rheumatol. Rehabil.*, **15**, 211
3. Huskisson, E. C., Dieppe, P. A., Scott, P. J., Trapnell, J., Balme, H. W. and Willoughby, D. A. (1976). Immunostimulant therapy with levamisole for rheumatoid arthritis. *Lancet*, i, 393
4. Rosenthal, M., Trabert, U. and Müller, W. (1976). Immunotherapy with levamisole in rheumatic diseases. *Scand. J. Rheumatol.*, **5**, 216
5. Veys, E. M., Mielants, H., de Bussere, A., Cecrans, L. and Gabriel, P. (1976). Levamisole in rheumatoid arthritis. *Lancet*, i, 808
6. El-Ghobarey, A. F., Mavrikakis, M., Morgan, I. and Mathieu, J. P. (1977). Delayed healing of varicose ulcer with levamisole. *Br. Med. J.*, **1**, 616
7. Arrigoni-Martelli, E., Bramm, E., Huskisson, E. C., Willoughby, D. A. and Dieppe, P. A. (1976). Pertussis vaccine oedema: an experimental model for the action of penicillamine-like drugs. *Agents Actions*, **6**, 613
8. Dieppe, P. A., Willoughby, D. A., Huskisson, E. C. and Arrigoni-Martelli, E. (1976). Pertussis vaccine pleurisy: a model of delayed hypersensitivity. *Agents Actions*, **6**, 618
9. *Lancet*, i, 151 (1975). Levamisole
10. Arrigoni-Martelli, E. and Bramm, E. (1975). Investigations on the influence of cyclophosphamide, gold sodium thiomalate and D-penicillamine on nystation oedema and adjuvant arthritis. *Agents Actions*, **5**, 264

Discussion 2

G. Loewi:
(UK)

Dr. Symoens says the polymorph chemotaxis is low. In our hands at least this was entirely normal.

Many of the other features which are commonly ascribed to rheumatoid arthritis, such as impaired T-cell functions are probably non-specific.

My last point concerns the work of Scott and Maini who to my knowledge treated very few patients. The transfer factor did not affect noticeably the course of rheumatoid arthritis.

G. Velo:
(Italy)

Were the side effects which were noted dependent effects?

Huskisson:

No.

Velo:

Were they independent effects?

Huskisson:

I do not know.

Velo:

How long after commencing treatment would one start to find side effects?

Huskisson:

I did not mention dosage. I should have done so.

Most of our work has been done with continuous doses of 150 mg/day, but we have recently completed a study in which we compared this with intermittent therapy and there is some experimental justification for thinking we may have more immunostimulant effect. We found this equally effective with the continuous therapy, with a slight reduction in the overall incidence of side effects. It is certainly sometimes possible to treat patients with lower doses and to alleviate the side effects, but this varies.

J. Abeles:
(USA)

The spectrum of activity described by Dr. Huskisson for levamisole is very similar to penicillamine. This begs the question of whether, like penicillamine, levamisole, which is an imidazole compound, has the ability to chelate copper and gold.

R. Turner:
(USA)

Dr. Huskisson mentioned that phagocytosis was affected by treatment with levamisole in rheumatoid arthritics. Did he compare phagocytosis other than rheumatoid arthritis neutrophils with controls, and also the phagocytosis of the synovial fluid neutrophils in these patients?

Huskisson:

The baseline was too variable to compare between patients. We did not have measurements in rheumatoids and controls, but the variation between people is such that it would be impossible to make a comparison.

We looked at synovial fluid cells as well and they did not show enhancement by levamisole.

M. Jasani:
(UK)

I should like to address the same question to both speakers although only one showed a slide of the effect of levamisole on adjuvant arthritis. We all know that this is the test model which has been widely used in the past ten years to represent compounds which are at least widely held to be useful in rheumatoid arthritis. When the speakers found that levamisole was effective in this particular model of arthritis

25

	what was their first reaction—surprise, disappointment, or what? Following on that first reaction, was any hypothesis put forward to explain this remarkable effect on one model, as opposed to the clinical model in which we are interested?
Symoens:	We were surprised because we had expected no effect. Levamisole does not augment cellular immune responses in normals and the surprise here was that it seemed to decrease the effect of the tumour. This is still unexplained.
	The major effect of levamisole that we have observed is that for certain immune responses in T-cells, polymorphs and macrophages, when one of their functions is decreased, it may be restored to normal by levamisole. But it is extremely rare to see responses in excess of normal; hence my surprise.
Jasani:	I agree with that interpretation of the observations although it does not answer the important question which we must all face in the light of Dr. Symoens's findings. Is there some suggestion that in future drugs which augment adjuvant reaction, e.g. levamisole, might be more useful than drugs which depress adjuvant reaction?
Symoens:	I am not sure.
D. A. Willoughby: (UK)	Some unpublished work by Michael Whitehouse in Australia shows that if a mild adjuvant arthritis was produced in immune-deficient animals that were then treated with levamisole, he managed to get a suppression. This might be extremely relevant to the discussion.
Symoens:	I have no knowledge of that particular work.
S. Wong: (USA)	I wish to address the question of levamisole activity in adjuvant arthritis. Our own experience is that levamisole is active in the adjuvant arthritis model. It depends on how the animal is treated. Levamisole administered for three to four days or four to five days subsequent to the administration of interplantar mycobacterium is more active than continuous treatment with levamisole over a long period of time. Investigators will have to take care as to what the dosage regimen is before they get activity: the dosage relative to periods of treatment and non-treatment is very important.
	There is no doubt that levamisole is active in adjuvant arthritis.
D. Freed: (UK)	What proportion of rheumatoid arthritis patients respond to levamisole?
Huskisson:	Probably 80%.
Freed:	Is anything known of the effects of levamisole on the secretory antibodies?
Huskisson:	Not by me.
E. Munthe: (Norway)	Are there any reports of treatment of arthritis in patients with immune deficiencies with levamisole?
Symoens:	I do not know of any.
D. Sofia: (USA)	Dr. Huskisson mentioned neutropenia among the side effects. Has he also seen a thrombocytopenia?
	Secondly, was there any correlation between activity and achieved blood levels with levamisole?
Huskisson:	The blood changes are really nothing. Only one of the six cases had a thrombocytopenia and neutropenia appears to be the main feature.
	I have not yet managed to do blood levels.
J. L. Turk: (UK)	Does anyone have any comment to make on a recent report of increased lymphocyte production following treatment with levamisole?
Symoens:	Lymphocyte production has been shown to increase after levamisole in patients with some sort of deficiency in their cellular immunity and at least one attempt has been made to increase their production in normal cells.
Abeles:	Concern has been expressed in the USA with regard to metronidazole, otherwise known as Flagyl, which was shown to be mutagenic in certain biological tests. There has been some suspicion of animal

26

carcinogenicity following high doses.

Due to the resemblance here with imidazole has anyone any information on the long-term animal toxicity or carcinogenicity?

Symoens: The kinds of drugs to which Dr. Abeles has referred are not likely to prove useful.

Levamisole is primarily a veterinary drug and for it to be accepted in countries such as the USA it has been necessary to prove lack of toxicity etc. and that it does not produce carcinogenicity if used in medically approved doses.

I. L. Bonta: I was wondering about lymphokine production and the influence of
(The Netherlands) levamisole. What kind of lymphokine activity was measured? Lymphokines consist of several substances each with a different kind of pharmacological activity. What kind of lymphokine was in fact measured?

Symoens: It was essentially MIF.

M. Jayson: Have Dr. Huskisson or Dr. Symoens any information about the value
(UK) of levamisole on systemic lupus? The evidence is, if anything, even greater than in rheumatoid arthritis.

Huskisson: A small number of patients have been treated in double-blind trials but so far I have not been impressed that there has been any dramatic alteration.

Symoens: I have seen published results (Dr. Gordon of Hawaii) relating to one case of SLE treated with levamisole. The same author is now treating 15 or 16 patients with systemic lupus, using low-level doses.

K. Fehr: How many rheumatoid vasculitis patients have been treated and how
(Switzerland) many have responded?

Secondly, how many 'Felty syndromes' with leukopenia have been treated and how did the leukocytes respond to that treatment?

Huskisson: I have only had one vasculitis case, and I showed it. Had I had more I would have shown them.

I have not yet treated any patients with 'Felty syndrome'.

3

The effect of cytotoxic drugs on the formation of mononuclear phagocytes

R. L. SOUHAMI, J. W. B. BRADFIELD AND N. E. PARKER (UK)

Cytotoxic drugs and X-rays appear to have little direct effect on the phago-cytic activity of the mononuclear phagocyte system *in vivo* as judged by clearance studies[1]. These tests measure the functional activity of existing cells as a result of treatment but not the formation of new cells. Chronic inflam-matory lesions on the other hand are maintained by an influx of newly formed mononuclear phagocytes and cytotoxic drugs would be expected to impair the formation of these cells and therefore the ability of the organism to replace macrophages in the tissues. When considering the use of cytotoxic drugs in chronic inflammatory diseases, possible effects of these agents on mononuclear phagocyte formation are clearly of importance, and the dose and timing of administration of the drugs may be critical in inhibiting pro-duction of these cells.

No simple screening test has existed previously which enables the investi-gator to determine the effect of these drugs on the reproductive integrity of the macrophage precursors in the bone marrow. The present communication describes a method for measuring the effect of cytotoxic drugs easily and quantitatively *in vivo*. Information obtained by this method can be used in experiments on suppression of chronic inflammatory responses.

The test rests on the observation that the intravenous injection of a colloidal compound profoundly diminishes the ability of the liver to phagocytose a labelled particle such as sheep red blood cells (SRBC). In normal mice injected i.v. with 2×10^7 SRBC labelled with ^{51}Cr, after 2 h 80% of radioactivity was recovered from the liver and 2–3% from the spleen. Following the injection of 5 mg of colloidal carbon, before the SRBC, there was a profound de-pression of liver uptake of the labelled cells, reaching a maximum between 2 and 6 h. Associated with the depressed hepatic uptake was an increased uptake by the spleen which we have shown leads to an increase in the immune response.[2] Over the next 4 days the liver recovered and by 4 days the liver uptake of labelled cells returned to normal.

We have shown[3] that this recovery process is associated with repopulation of the liver by bone marrow derived mononuclear phagocytes. The evidence leading to this conclusion is as follows. Firstly the process was arrested by 600 rads irradiation to the whole animal, given *before* the blockading injection and this effect of irradiation on recovery can be prevented if the bone marrow was partly shielded during the irradiation (Table 3.1). Secondly, in experiments when animals were treated with vinblastine sulphate during the

Table 3.1 The protective effect of bone marrow shielding on the recovery of hepatic phagocytosis in irradiated mice

Blockade	Irradiation	Liver uptake ($\% \pm SE$)
No	No	84 ± 3.8
Yes	No	76 ± 3.3
Yes	Total body	11.3 ± 3.3
Yes	Total body with bone marrow shielded	80 ± 2.7

Groups of 8 mice. 600 rads DXR given 4 days before 5 mg of carbon i.v. 4 days later 2×10^8 ^{51}Cr labelled SRBC were injected i.v. and the mice killed after 2 h.

recovery process, very few mitoses were seen in the Kupffer cells, suggesting that local division of Kupffer cells was not occurring. Lastly *in vivo* labelling with [³H]thymidine during the recovery period showed large numbers of labelled Kupffer cells (Table 3.2).

Table 3.2. Percentage of labelled Kupffer cells during recovery of hepatic phagocytosis after silica blockade

Blockade	% Labelled cells Individual values	Mean
No	2.0, 1.8, 2.1	2.0
Yes	11.8, 9.0, 27.3	16.0

5 mg of silica i.v. given as blockade. 25 μCi[³H]thymidine given i.p. 8 and 16 h after blockade.

The recovery process following administration was shown by Benacerraf and others[4] to be inhibited by nitrogen mustard as judged by the return of normal rates of clearance of colloidal carbon. We have used the recovery of

THE EFFECT OF CYTOTOXIC DRUGS

hepatic phagocytosis of sheep RBC after blockade with dextran sulphate (MW 900 000) as a measure of formation of monocytes in the bone marrow.

The Figure 3.1 shows the effect of a single subcutaneous injection of 5 fluorouracil (5FU) on the recovery process. In each case the blockading injection was given at day 0 and recovery was judged by the uptake of ^{51}Cr labelled SRBC at day 4. The maximum effect of the drug in preventing recovery was seen if it was given on day -2 and -3, that is *before* the blockading injection. This indicates that the drug is acting on a population of cells

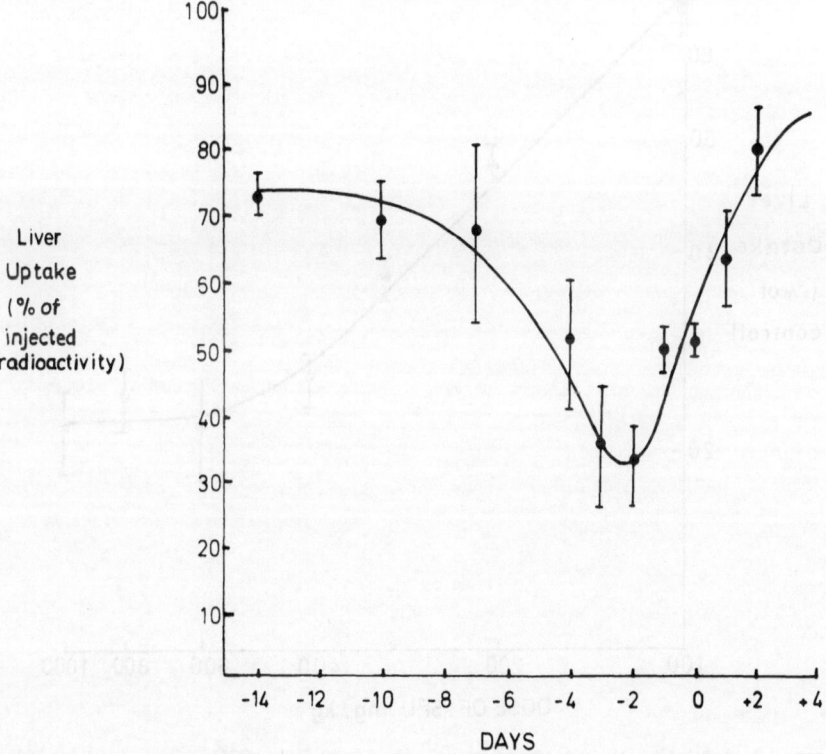

Figure 3.1 The effect of 5FU on recovery of hepatic phagocytosis of sheep RBC, 4 days after blockade with dextran sulphate (500 µg i.v.). 5FU (300 mg/kg) was given at varying times before or after blockade. Standard errors as shown

which is already rapidly proliferating and this demonstrates the bone marrow origin of the new cells. Control animals given 5FU without blockade never showed any depression of uptake of SRBC.

A dose response relationship was found between degree of recovery at day 4 and dose of 5FU given on day -3 (Figure 3.2). On a log/log plot the curve was linear over the range 100 mg/kg to 500 mg/kg. No further suppression was seen if the dose was increased beyond 500 mg/kg, but if injections of 300 mg/kg were given on day -3 and day -2 then recovery was

31

reduced to 11 % of injected radioactivity on day 4, indicating that no recovery has taken place at all at this time.

If recovery was prevented by 300 mg/kg 5FU given on day −3, but the animals were then tested for recovery over the following week the recovery process began after a delay of 5 days (Figure 3.3). When recovery occurred it proceeded at the same rate as recovery in normal mice. This implies that the effect of the 5FU was to deplete monocyte precursors to an extent where

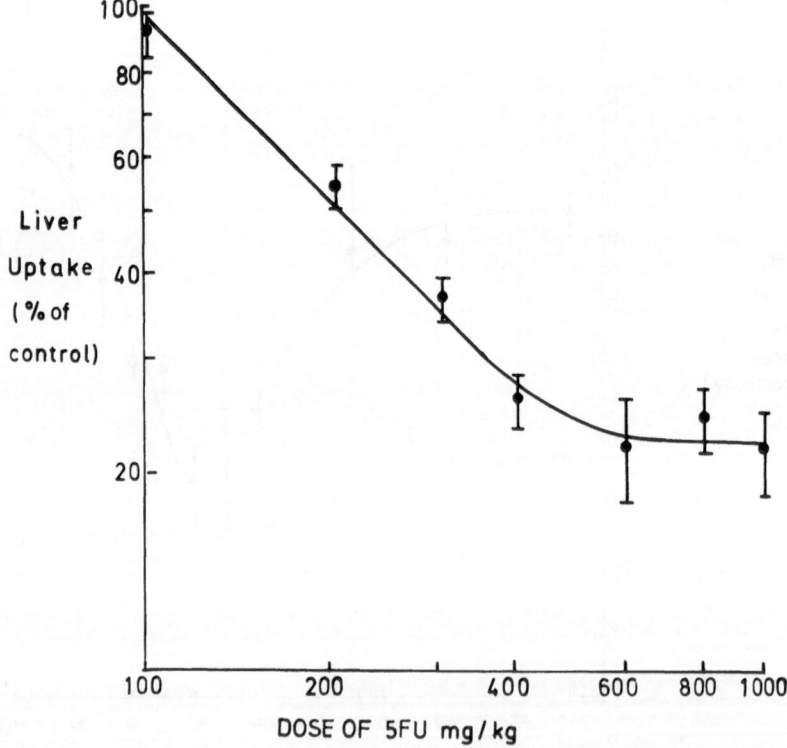

Figure 3.2 Inhibition of recovery of hepatic phagocytosis by 5FU given subcutaneously on day −2. Liver uptake is expressed as a percentage of recovery of blockade mice not treated with 5FU. Standard errors are shown

5 days elapsed before sufficient numbers had accumulated to allow recovery to be detected.

The effect of 5FU on Kupffer cell formation was also shown by auto-radiographic experiments in which mice were injected with tritiated thymidine throughout the recovery period after dextran sulphate blockade (Table 3.3). Small doses of dextran sulphate, insufficient to cause blockade as judged by suppression of sheep red cell uptake, were none the less associated with a great increase in numbers of labelled Kupffer cells compared with control non-blockaded mice. 5FU injected on day −2 and −3 not only prevented the

Table 3.3 Percentage of labelled Kupffer cells following dextran sulphate administration

Dose of dextran sulphate	%Labelled cells (±SE)
50 µg	33.6 ± 1.8
250 µg	53.4 ± 6.1
500 µg	49.3 ± 5.2
Normal	5.7 ± 2.8
500 µg + 5FU	0.44 ± 0.2*

*$p = <0.05$ against normal
25 µCi[^{3}H]thymidine given 8-hourly for 72 h following dextran sulphate

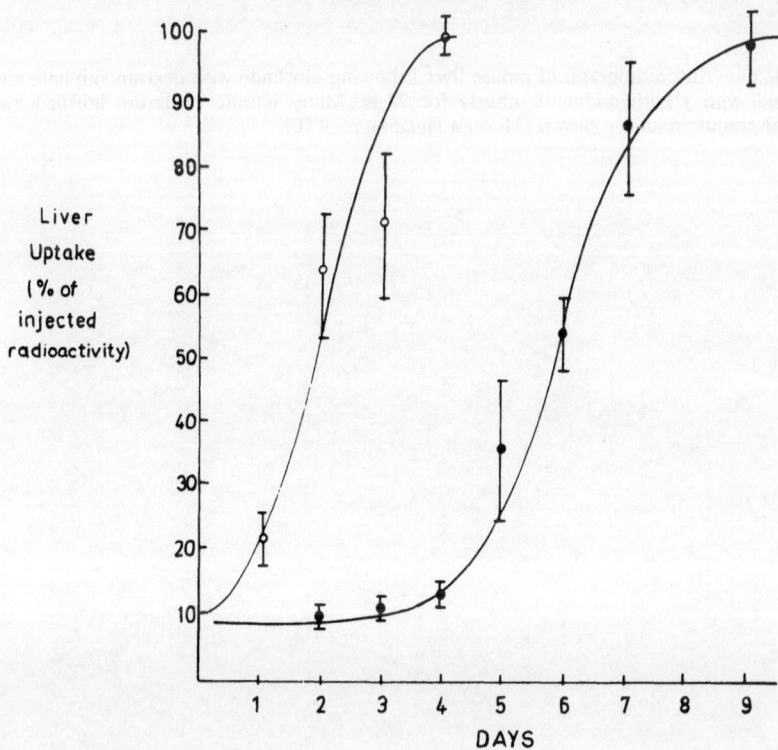

Figure 3.3 Recovery of hepatic phagocytosis after blockade with dextran sulphate on day 0. Closed circles are animals treated with 300 mg/kg 5FU on day −3. Open circles are untreated animals recovering normally. Standard errors are shown

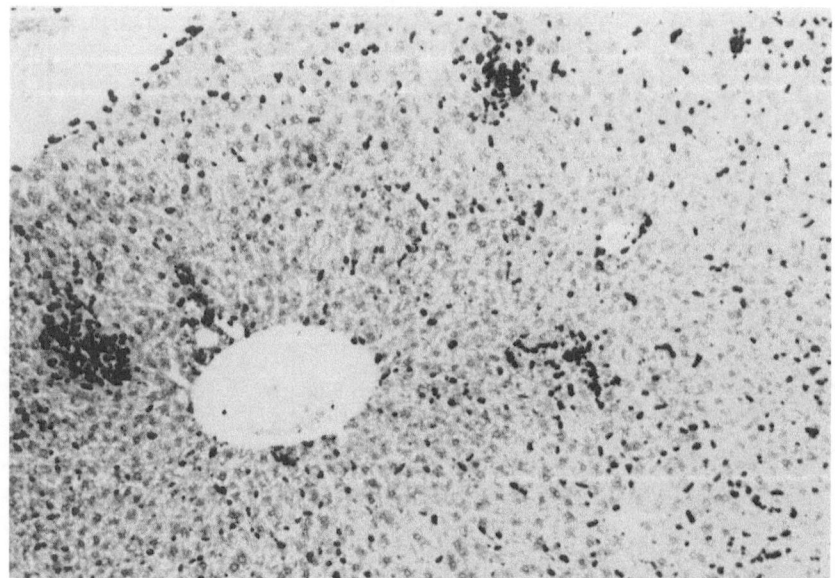

Figure 3.4 Autoradiograph of mouse liver following blockade with dextran sulphate and labelled with [^{3}H]thymidine 8 hourly for 72 h. Many Kupffer cells are labelled and several granulomata are shown (Meyer's Haemalum × 80)

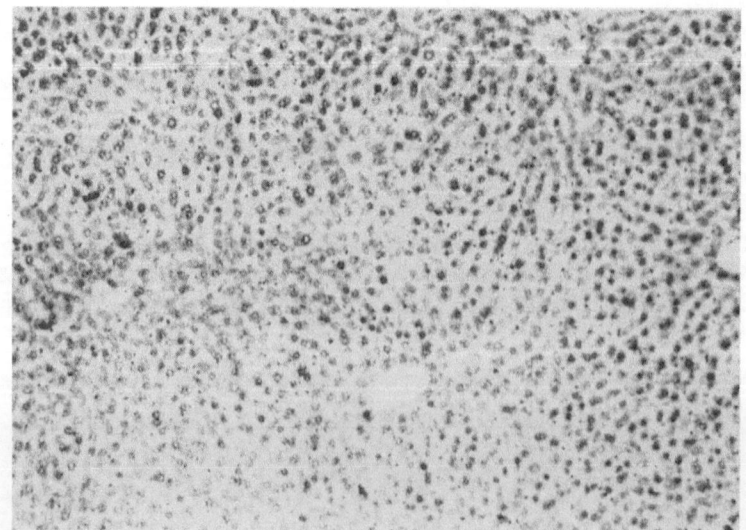

Figure 3.5 Autoradiograph of mouse liver. Animal treated as in Figure 3.4 but 300 mg/kg 5FU given subcutaneously on day −3 and −2. Labelling of Kupffer cells is inhibited and no granulomata are seen (Meyer's Haemalum × 100)

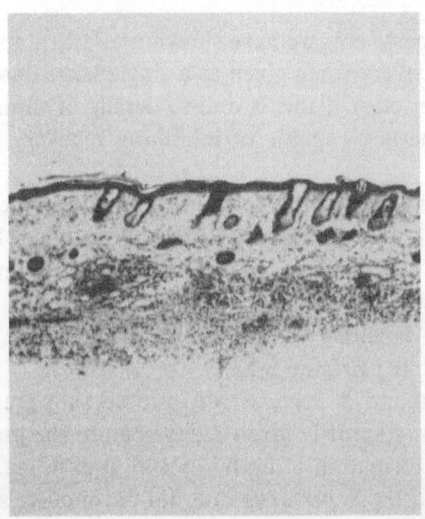

Figure 3.6 Mouse skin. Carageenan injected 4 days previously. A dense cellular infiltrate is present in the dermis and subcutaneously (H & E ×40)

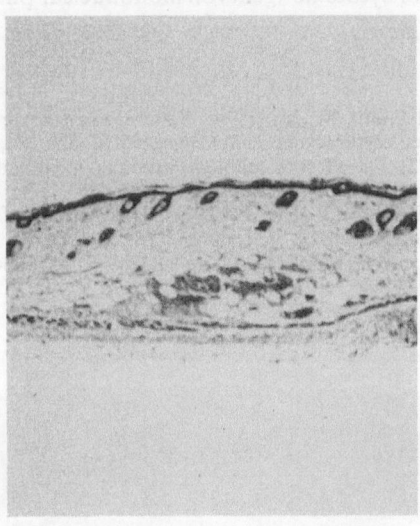

Figure 3.7 Mouse skin as in Figure 3.6, but 5FU 300 mg/kg given on day −3 and −2 (H & E ×40)

labelling associated with blockade but also inhibited the labelling found in *normal* mice.

In preliminary experiments we have shown that azathioprine does not have any effect on the recovery when given as a single large dose at the same time as 5FU. It is not yet clear if this is due to details of timing and dosage, or whether azathioprine is incapable of inhibiting recovery in any dose or at any time.

This simple experimental model may allow one to predict which drugs and in which dose will inhibit granuloma formation in mice. Following dextran sulphate numerous granulomata appear in the liver. Figure 3.4 shows the appearance of these granulomata in autoradiographic experiments; and following 5FU, the labelling of both Kupffer cells and the formation of granulomata is inhibited (Figure 3.5).

Using carrageenan and *B. pertussis* we induced skin granulomata in mice. We found that 300 mg/kg 5FU given 2 days before the granuloma inducing agent prevented the formation of both types of granuloma. Figure 3.6 shows a granuloma induced by *B. pertussis* in a normal mouse, and Figure 3.7 the effect of 5FU subcutaneously 2 days previously on the formation of the granuloma.

Further experiments are now in progress to relate the details of timing and administration which have been developed in the experiments on recovery from blockade to the inhibition of granuloma formation. We believe that recovery from blockade provides a simple and quantitative means for measuring the effect of cytotoxic agents on mononuclear phagocyte formation.

References

1. Atkinson, J. P. and Frank, M. M. (1974). Failure of cytotoxic agents to inhibit the clearance of sensitised erythrocytes. *J. Reticuloendothel. Soc.*, **16**, 122
2. Souhami, R. L. (1972). The effect of colloidal carbon on the organ distribution of sheep red cells and the immune response. *Immunology*, **22**, 685
3. Souhami, R. L. and Bradfield, J. W. E. (1974). The recovery of hepatic phagocytosis after blockade of Kupffer cells. *J. Reticuloendothel. Soc.*, **16**, 75
4. Benacerraf, B., Halpern, B. N., Biozzi, G. and Benos, S. A. (1954). Quantitative study of the granulopectic activity of the RES

Discussion 3

R. van Furth:
(The Netherlands)

This very nice study supplements the contribution which I shall make tomorrow.

Has Dr. Souhami looked at the number of monocytes in the circulation. If his hypothesis is true, and I believe that it is, it should be possible to predict whether there will be any increase or decrease following treatment with the drug.

Secondly, what was the dose of azothiaprine? Was it only a single dose. A single dose does not affect the number of monocytes and there might be no decrease of these cells.

Souhami:

We have not yet looked in detail at the circulating number of monocytes, but we are doing it at the moment for exactly the reason advanced by Professor van Furth. I would predict that they would fall, and at the time which one would expect.

I am aware of the question of timing in the administration of azothiaprine. It is interesting that if the same thing is done with two different antimetabolites—the same thing to the animal—one sees entirely different effects.

The point that I wanted to make was that details of dosage and timing are obviously extremely important.

J. L. Turk:
(UK)

Could I ask about other alkylating agents?

Souhami:

I have done studies with cyclophosphamide and again the results are preliminary.

Cyclophosphamide, even in what is a conventional immuno-suppressive dose, a single dose (250 mg/kg in mice), no matter when it is given in relationship with the blockading agent does not affect the recovery.

van Furth:

A suggestion. If corticosteroids are used, I would expect to find a very sharp decrease in uptake of any substances, and that might make a nice study.

4

Rheumatoid factor–immunoglobulin G complex precipitation and neutrophil stimulation: an *in vitro* model for rheumatoid inflammation

R. TURNER, H. MASHBURN, R. COLLINS, L. DECHATELET
AND J. KAUFMANN (USA)

INTRODUCTION

The inflammatory process occurring in the joints of patients with rheumatoid arthritis is usually characterized by synovial effusions involving moderate to large numbers of neutrophils and soluble and/or insoluble immunoglobulin G complexes[1,2]. Our studies utilize $^{51}CrCl_3$ labelled and unlabelled complexes to determine immunoglobulin G complex interactions with rheumatoid factor and neutrophils and a radiolabelled glucose assay of neutrophil hexose monophosphate shunt activity to further explore these interactions which may be an important contributor to the inflammatory process occurring in the joints of patients with rheumatoid arthritis[1].

MATERIALS AND METHODS

Preparation of sera and neutrophils

Rheumatoid serum was obtained with informed consent from patients with definite or classical rheumatoid arthritis and rheumatoid factor titres were determined utilizing a commercial latex globulin reagent (RA-Test, Biological Corporation of America, Port Reading, NJ). Normal serum was obtained from healthy volunteers whose neutrophils were also used in these studies. All sera was centrifuged at $10\,000 \times g$ for 15 min and any precipitate removed prior to use in each test system. In experiments involving radiolabelled complexes, non-radioactive $CrCl^3$ was added to all sera to a final concentration of 1.3×10^{-5} M before centrifugation.

Normal human neutrophils were isolated as previously described[3] with cell preparations containing 80–90% neutrophils. They were suspended at a concentration of 5×10^6 neutrophils/ml in either 0.9% NaCl for the Cr-labelling studies or in 20% fresh serum for the hexose monophosphate shunt studies. In some experiments, neutrophils were killed by placing them in boiling water for 3 min, after which time more than 98% failed to exclude trypan blue dye.

Preparation of complexes

Insoluble complexes were prepared utilizing a 1 g/100 ml solution of human gamma-globulin (Cohn Fraction II—US Biochemical Corporation, Cleveland, Ohio) in 0.9% NaCl. This solution contained IgG, IgM, and IgA in a ratio of 104:2:1 as determined by radial immunodiffusion (Behring, Marburg, Germany). For radiolabelling experiments, the IgG solution was incubated with $^{51}CrCl_3$ (New England Nuclear, Boston, Mass.) for 1 h at 25 °C. This yielded approximately 1×10^6 c.p.m./ml of the solution. The IgG was heated at 63 °C for 45 min as previously described[4]. The resulting precipitate was washed twice and resuspended in 0.9% NaCl at a protein concentration of 2.4 mg/ml. In some experiments this insoluble IgG suspension was incubated with normal and/or rheumatoid serum for 1 h at 25 °C as previously described[5]. After centrifugation the precipitate was washed and resuspended in the same fashion as above.

Soluble complexes were prepared as previously described[5] utilizing the same procedures as described for insoluble complexes except that unbound chromium was removed by passing the solution through a Sephadex G-10 column and the IgG solution was incubated at 63 °C for 7 min instead of 45 min. The resulting solution was chromatographed on a Sephadex G-200 column and found to contain 50% soluble IgG complexes with the remainder of the IgG in its native form. This solution was diluted with 0.9% NaCl to contain soluble complexes at a concentration of 2.4 mg/ml. Immunoglobulin G–rheumatoid factor (IgG–RF) precipitate complexes were prepared by combining the soluble preparation with rheumatoid sera in a ratio of 1:5. After incubating at 25 °C for 1 h the suspensions were centrifuged at 10 000 × g for 15 min and the precipitates washed twice and resuspended in 0.9% NaCl at a protein concentration of 2.4 mg/ml.

Neutrophil–complex interactions and data analysis

Neutrophils were exposed to various IgG complexes over a 60 min period and hexose monophosphate shunt activity was assayed utilizing methods previously described[6] measuring the release of $^{14}CO_2$ from glucose-1-^{14}C. For

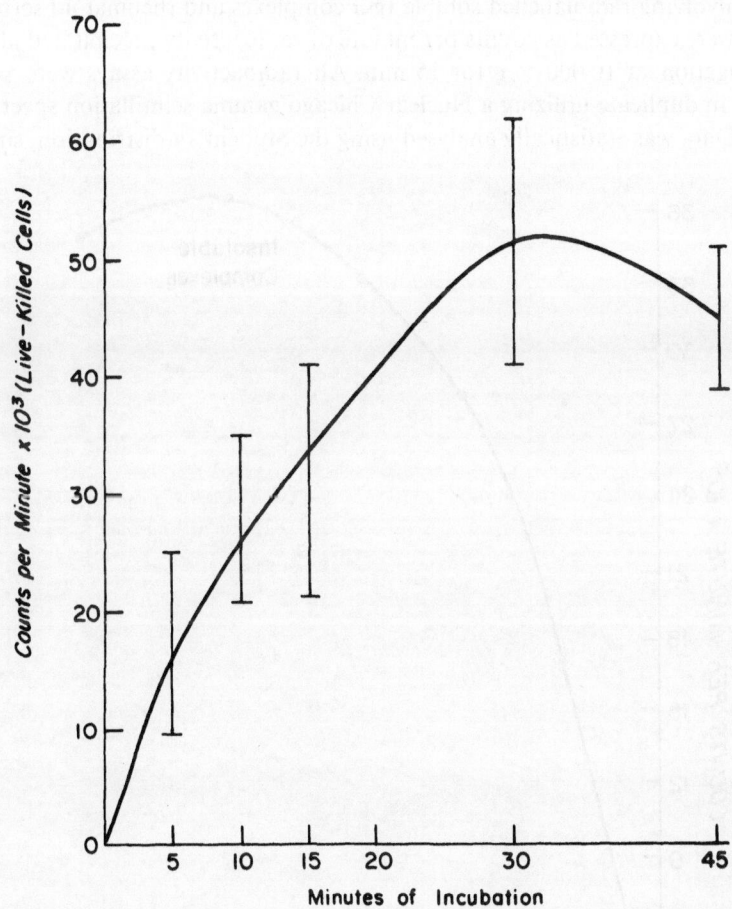

Figure 4.1 Time curve of neutrophil uptake of insoluble heat aggregated radioactive immunoglobulin G complexes ($n = 5$; $\bar{x} \pm$ SEM). Uptake is shown to increase with time to 30 min at which time significantly ($p < 0.05$) more uptake is shown by live cells than dead cells

uptake studies, equal volumes of neutrophils and radiolabelled insoluble IgG complexes were incubated at 37 °C for varying time intervals. Uptake of the radioactive complex by neutrophils was expressed as counts per minute remaining in the cell pellet after two saline washes minus the counts per minute in tubes containing control killed neutrophils. In precipitation experiments involving radiolabelled soluble IgG complexes and rheumatoid serum, results were expressed as counts per minute of radioactivity precipitated after centrifugation at 10 000 $\times$ g for 15 min. All radioactivity assays were performed in duplicate utilizing a Nuclear Chicago gamma scintillation spectrometer. Data was statistically analysed using the Student's t-distribution, since

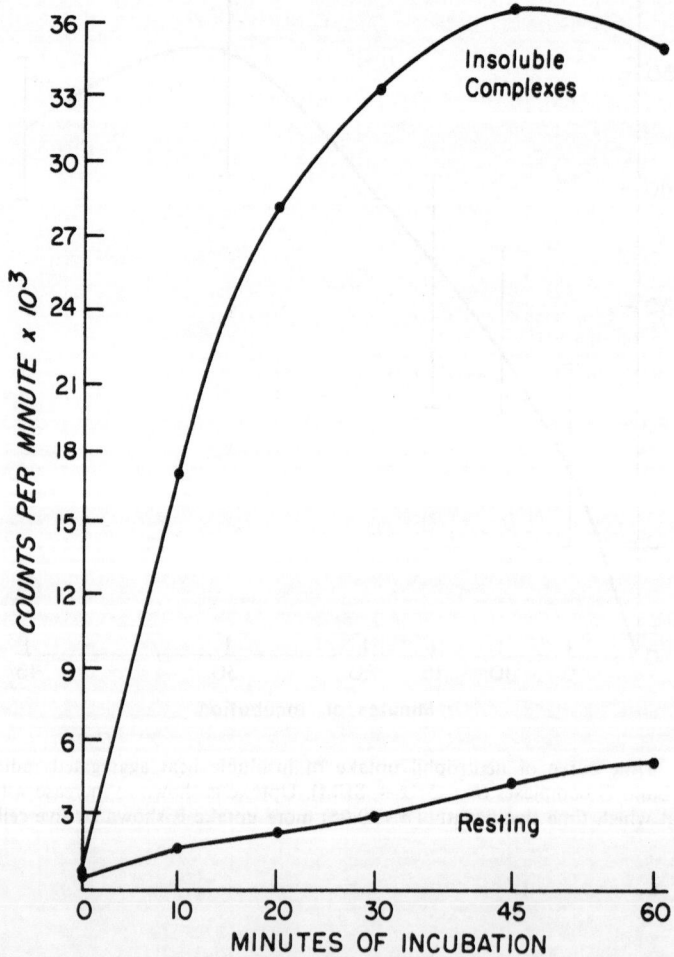

Figure 4.2 Neutrophil hexose monophosphate shunt activity on exposure to insoluble complexes. Shunt activity was measured as the counts per minute of $^{14}CO_2$ released from glucose-1-^{14}C by test minus resting cells at the time intervals shown. Each point is the mean of closely agreeing duplicate determinations

sample sizes were comparatively small in most of the experiments. Two tail Student's *t*-tests were performed on all groups and differences between these groups were considered to reach statistical significance when values of $p < 0.05$ were obtained.

RESULTS

Incubation of neutrophils on five occasions with insoluble immunoglobulin G complexes over a time period of 45 min produced a time curve of radio complex uptake shown in Figure 4.1. Although there were wide variations in the individual determinations, maximum uptake was apparent at 30 min, live cells = 136 442 $\pm$ 19 080 ($\bar{x} \pm$ SEM) c.p.m. and killed cells = 85 137 $\pm$ 11 326 c.p.m., with differences significant at the 0.05 level.

Neutrophils were then exposed over a 60-min period to insoluble complexes and hexose monophosphate shunt activity measured by determination of

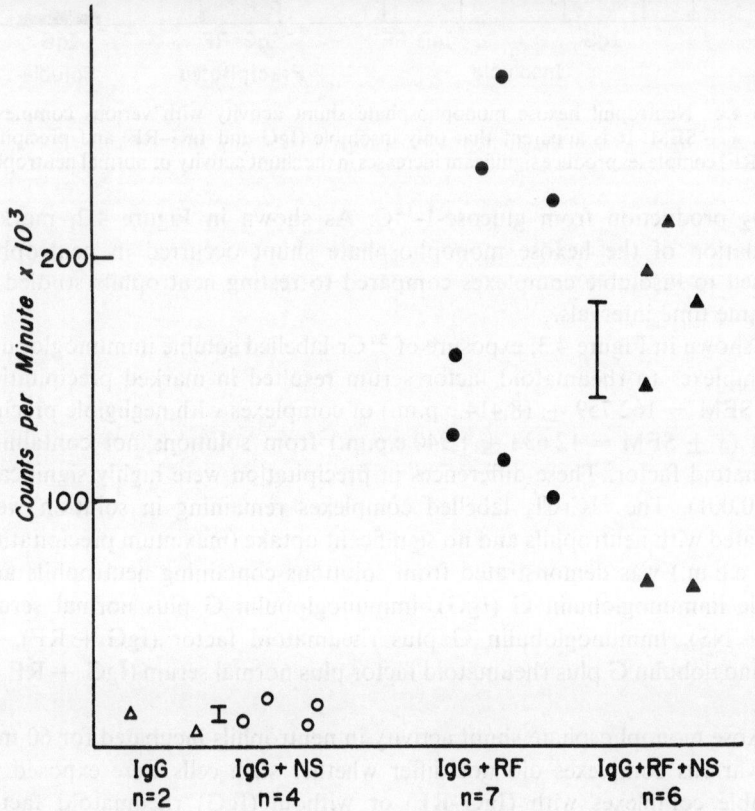

Figure 4.3 Precipitation from soluble immunoglobulin G complex solutions. Mean $\pm$ SEM shown without rheumatoid factor (RF) ○ △ and with RF ● ▲. It is apparent that while normal serum (NS) has no effect on the system, RF induces marked precipitation of complexes

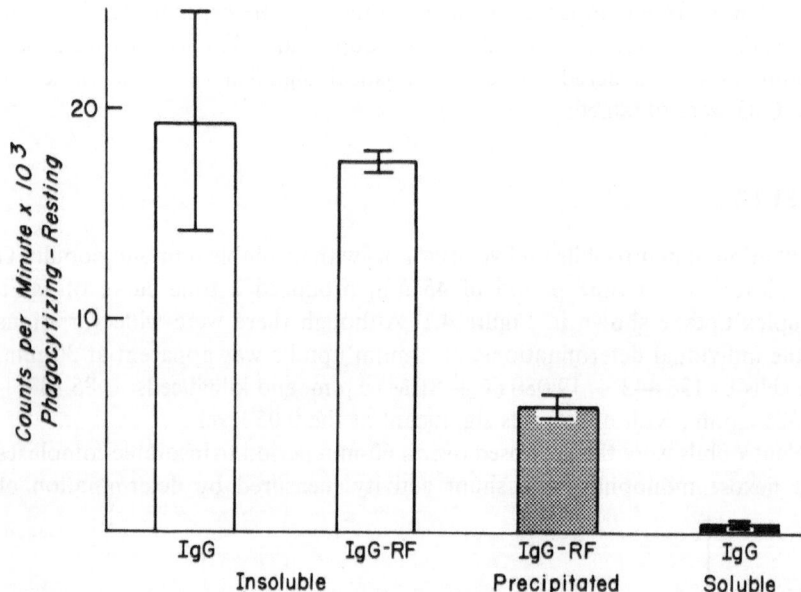

Figure 4.4 Neutrophil hexose monophosphate shunt activity with various complexes, $n = 3$, $\bar{x} \pm$ SEM. It is apparent that only insoluble (IgG and IgG–RF) and precipitate (IgG–RF) complexes produce significant increases in the shunt activity of normal neutrophils

$^{14}CO_2$ production from glucose-1-^{14}C. As shown in Figure 4.2, marked stimulation of the hexose monophosphate shunt occurred in neutrophils exposed to insoluble complexes compared to resting neutrophils studied at the same time intervals.

As shown in Figure 4.3, exposure of ^{51}Cr-labelled soluble immunoglobulin G complexes to rheumatoid factor serum resulted in marked precipitation ($\bar{x} \pm$ SEM $= 162\ 759 \pm 18\ 414$ c.p.m.) of complexes with negligible precipitation ($\bar{x} \pm$ SEM $= 12\ 633 \pm 1\ 940$ c.p.m.) from solutions not containing rheumatoid factor. These differences in precipitation were highly significant ($p < 0.001$). The $^{51}CrCl_3$ labelled complexes remaining in solution were incubated with neutrophils and no significant uptake (maximum precipitation 1 234 c.p.m.) was demonstrated from solutions containing neutrophils and soluble immunoglobulin G (IgG), immunoglobulin G plus normal serum IgG + NS), immunoglobulin G plus rheumatoid factor (IgG + RF), or immunoglobulin G plus rheumatoid factor plus normal serum (IgG + RF + NS).

Hexose monophosphate shunt activity in neutrophils incubated for 60 min with various complexes did not differ whether such cells were exposed to insoluble complexes with (IgG–RF) or without (IgG) rheumatoid factor (Figure 4.4, first two boxes). These insoluble complexes and immunoglobulin G–rheumatoid factor (IgG–RF) precipitate complexes (Figure 4.4, box 3) produced significantly ($p < 0.05$) more shunt stimulation than did soluble

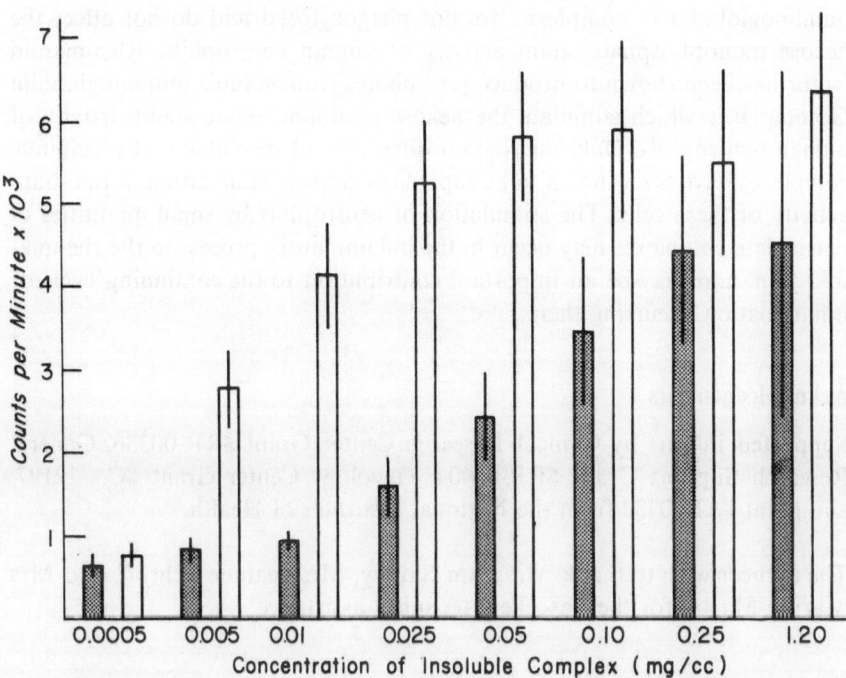

Figure 4.5 Neutrophil hexose monophosphate shunt activity with varying complex doses. Dotted strips = soluble immunoglobulin G–rheumatoid factor (IgG–RF) precipitate complexes. White strips = insoluble immunoglobulin G (IgG) complexes; $n = 3$, $\bar{x} \pm$ SEM. It is apparent that microgram doses of these complexes produce significant ($p < 0.05$) shunt stimulation

immunoglobulin G complexes (Figure 4.4, box 4). Soluble complexes produced no increase in shunt activity compared to that demonstrated by normal resting control neutrophils.

Neutrophils exposed to varying amounts of complexes (Figure 4.5) demonstrated significant ($p < 0.05$) stimulation with (IgG–RF) precipitate complexes at a concentration of 50 μg/ml and insoluble (IgG) complexes at a concentration of 5 μg/ml. Differences in the stimulatory capacity of the two types of complexes became significant at the 5 μg/ml dose level and remained so throughout most of the study. It was apparent, however, that these differences became less marked at higher complex concentrations.

CONCLUSIONS

These studies have shown that insoluble radio-labelled immunoglobulin G and immunoglobulin G–rheumatoid factor complexes are phagocytosed by normal human neutrophils and stimulate the hexose monophosphate shunt activity of these cells. These studies have also shown that radiolabelled soluble immunoglobulin G complexes are not phagocytosed and do not affect the hexose monophosphate shunt activity of human neutrophils. Rheumatoid factor has been shown to produce precipitates from soluble immunoglobulin G complexes which stimulate the hexose monophosphate shunt activity of human neutrophils. Only microgram quantities of insoluble and precipitate complexes have been shown to be capable of causing stimulation of the shunt activity of these cells. The stimulation of neutrophils by small quantities of particulate complexes may occur in the inflammatory process in the rheumatoid joint and may be an important contribution to the continuing cycle of inflammation occurring there.

Acknowledgements

Supported in part by Clinical Research Center Grant #RR-00336, General Research Support Grant #RR-05404, Oncology Center Grant #CA-12197, and grant #AI-10732 from the National Institutes of Health.

The authors wish to thank Mrs Pam Shirley, Mrs Jeannie Schroff, and Mrs Martha Martin for their excellent technical assistance.

References

1. Hollander, J. L., McCarty, D. J. and Astorga, G., et al. (1965). Studies on the pathogenesis of rheumatoid joint inflammation. Ann. Int. Med., 62, 271
2. Winchester, R. J. (1975). Characterisation of IgG complexes in patients with rheumatoid arthritis. Ann. N.Y. Acad. Sci., 256, 73
3. Turner, R. A., Collins, R. L. and Browner, S., et al. (1976). Neutrophil and rheumatoid factor immunoglobulin G insoluble complex interactions: phagocytosis and sequelae. J. Rheum., 3, 109
4. Turner, R. A., Schumacher, H. R. and Myers, A. R. (1973). Phagocytic function of polymorphonuclear leukocytes in rheumatic diseases. J. Clin. Invest., 52, 1632
5. Turner, R. A., Collins, R. L. and Stott, K., et al. (19—). Immunoglobulin G complex interactions with rheumatoid factor and neutrophils: $^{51}CrCl_3$ labelling and $^{14}CO_2$ hexose monophosphate shunt studies. J. Rheum. (In press.)
6. DeChatelet, L. R., Cooper, M. R. and McCall, C. E. (1971). Disassociation by colchicine of hexose monophosphate shunt activation from the bactericidal activity of the leukocyte. Infect. Immun., 3, 66

Discussion 4

J. L. Turk: **(UK)**	It is an important subject—the role of soluble complexes, particularly the role of rheumatoid factor in relationship to them, because we are faced always with the question of the relative roles of immune complexes and cell mediated immunity in rheumatoid arthritis and in chronic inflammatory disease. To what extent do immune complexes play a role in these diseases, and to what extent do cell-mediated immune mechanisms?
D. Roos: **(The Netherlands)**	Has Dr. Turner measured the uptake of the soluble complexes which he bound with his rheumatoid factor, or has he only measured the shunt activity induced in the cells?
Turner:	As I pointed out in the slide, we looked at the uptake of soluble complexes in two ways in this study. We looked at them in other ways in subsequent studies. In this study we looked at them with the chromium tag system and with the hexose monophosphate shunt and it did not produce stimulation of the shunt, nor were the soluble complexes taken up.
Roos:	I meant the complexes that were precipitated with the rheumatoid factor.
Turner:	We only looked at them with the shunt, and it did stimulate the shunt, as the slides showed.
Roos:	It is well known that shunt stimulation may be induced by adherence only. Uptake is not needed for shunt stimulation.
Turner:	We have subsequently looked at this in other ways, for example, looking at the cells by electron microscopy, and we have found the finely granular material in the cytoplasm. We have looked at it with EM and we have looked at it with the shunt, and these precipitated complexes stimulate in both ways. We have not looked at it with the chromium system. That may be where the confusion arises.
R. L. Souhami: **(UK)**	Have the group looked to see whether there is a release of enzymes from the cells into the supernatant from the neutrophils as a result of phagocytosis?
Turner:	We have. Dr. Collins reported this. We found release of β-glucuronidase, but not release of the cytoplasmic enzyme LDH, with the precipitated or the insoluble complexes, but not with the soluble complexes.
G. A. Voisin: **(France)**	Is this activation complement-dependent?
Turner:	All of our studies were done in the presence of serum. We have not specifically addressed that question in a reportable way to date.
Voisin:	That would explain the difference between precipitated and soluble complexes, and even the curve that was shown.
Turner:	The reaction itself between the soluble complexes? The soluble complexes will bind complement. The insoluble complexes bind complement also. All of this is done in the presence of serum.

47

Voisin: But the soluble complexes will bind the complement less according to the proportion.

Turner: But we are using maxi amounts; 2.4 mg/ml is well over the minimum amount that it takes.

Turk: Have cryoglobulins been studied at all in this system?

Turner: No.

Turk: There is a whole range of interesting cryoglobulins that might have a similar effect to rheumatoid factor.

Chairman's Summing-up and Future Trends—Immunological aspects of inflammation—the network of interactions

J. L. TURK (UK)

In this session we have been discussing particularly the role of drugs that can affect chronic inflammatory disease by their action on immunological pathways. In the past we have approached the study of inflammatory conditions of immunological origin by studying the various mechanisms in isolation. Over the past 20 years this approach has borne fruit by devising models of delayed hypersensitivity contaminated with only a minor degree of humoral antibody production. The various pathways involved in cell-mediated immune hypersensitivity reactions have been worked out and it is possible to differentiate this pathway from that produced by immune complex tissue damage. We can now separate the proliferation and differentiation of T-lymphocytes in the lymph node paracortical areas from that of B-lymphocytes in the lymph follicles germinal centres and cortico-medullary junction. We can confidently assign one pharmacological pathway, the lymphokine system, to cell-mediated immunity, and another, the complement cascade, to immune complex activation. We can associate granulocyte activation with complement and immune complexes, while we associate the macrophage particularly with lymphokine activation and cell-mediated immunity. It has only been possible to make such clear cut definitions by a strict process of dissection. However all of us remember hearing papers on lymphocyte proliferation in what we now know as the paracortical areas—in fact T-lymphocytes—associated with antibody production, and papers on the effect of anti-complement sera on delayed hypersensitivity reactions. In the past we have had to discard data of this type to get a clear view of the primary processes involved in the two forms of hypersensitivity reactions—immediate and delayed—that underlie the development of immunological inflammatory reactions. This dogmatic and somewhat naive approach has served its purpose. We can understand the basic mechanisms far more clearly. It is now the turn of a more integrated approach to the study of immunological inflammatory reactions.

The first point that must be accepted is that in any situation where there is a full complement of T- and B-lymphocytes both populations will be stimulated by antigen to some degree. Secondly antigen stimulated cells of one population will influence the response of the second population of lymphocytes. Thirdly the inflammatory reaction produced in the periphery will be the resultant of the two types of inflammatory reaction, that produced

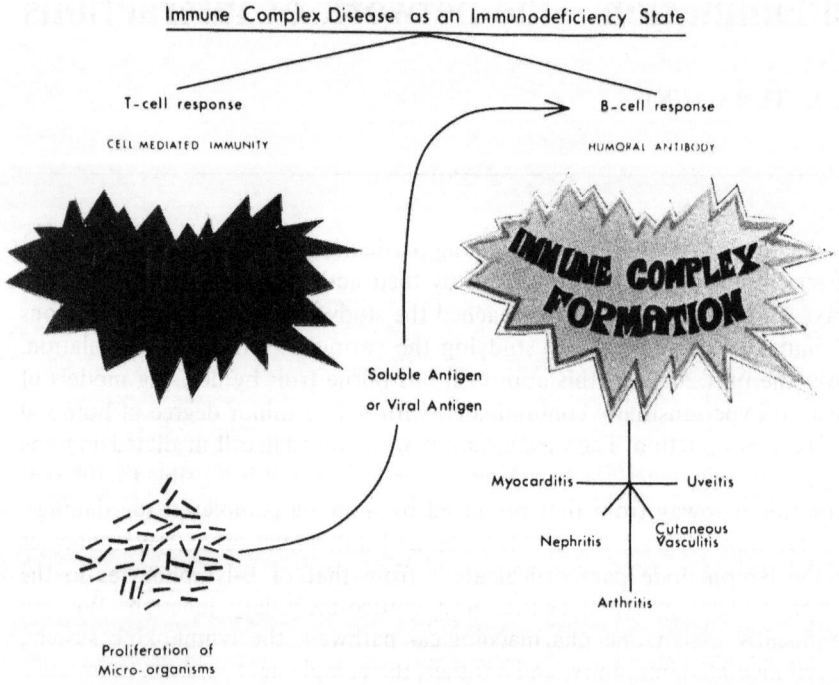

Figure 1 Immune complex disease as an immunodeficiency state

by humoral antibody and that produced by cell-mediated immunity. In addition it should be remembered that we are rarely dealing with the response to a single antigen. We tend to forget that when an animal is injected with a specific antigen in Freund's complete adjuvant it is responding to a heavy bombardment by mycobacterial antigens as well as the specific antigen that is mixed up in the adjuvant. Before discussing how some of the anti-inflammatory drugs work that act on immunological mechanisms, it might be useful to look at some of these interactions, as newer drugs such as levamisole may be working through one of these pathways.

1. THE INFLUENCE OF T-LYMPHOCYTES AND CELL-MEDIATED IMMUNE MECHANISMS ON INFLAMMATORY REACTIONS DUE TO HUMORAL ANTIBODY

The effect of simultaneous stimulation of T-lymphocytes on humoral antibody production by B-lymphocytes has been a fruitful field for research over the past ten years since the demonstration that there was reduced antibody production to certain antigens in neonatally thymectomized mice and rats, and the demonstration of the phenomenon of T–B cooperation. Cooperation may occur as a result of the action of specific or non-specific mechanisms. T-lymphocytes have been envisaged as having specific receptors on their surface that concentrate antigen directly on the B-cell surface. Another mechanism demonstrated by Feldmann[1] was that cell cooperation was mediated by a soluble specific factor derived from specifically sensitized T-lymphocytes. This soluble factor was found to be cytophilic for macrophages and it was the macrophage rather than the T-cell that focused the antigen directly on the B-cell surface. Other workers[2] have described a T-dependent non-specific enhancement of B-cells which is also mediated by soluble factors that could be synthesized by macrophages.

T-cells can also depress B-cell activation. This is a function of T-suppressor cells which has now been demonstrated in a wide range of immunological reactions including the immune response to sheep red cells[3] and accounts for increased levels of antibodies to polysaccharide and other 'T-independent' antigens following thymectomy.

2. THE INFLUENCE OF B-LYMPHOCYTES AND HUMORAL ANTIBODIES ON INFLAMMATORY REACTIONS CAUSED BY DELAYED HYPERSENSITIVITY MECHANISMS

The increased intensity of tuberculin type delayed hypersensitivity at 24 h in animals sensitized with antigen in Freund's complete adjuvant can be accounted for partly by the overlay of an Arthus reaction. This reaction can be increased with some antigens such as ovalbumin by boosting B-cell reactivity by antigen given intravenously, and can be reduced by giving cyclophosphamide (CY) 3 days before sensitization to reduce B-cells[4].

In contrast other T-cell systems can also be modulated by B-cell function. The classical example of this is the phenomenon of immunological enhancement in which humoral antibody blocks tumour immunity produced by cell-mediated immunity. This process, which allows increased tumour growth, is part of a wider biological process that Dr. Voisin has called 'immunological facilitation'. In addition to modulation of CMI by antibody, B-cells can interact directly with T-cells, modulating their ability to produce a delayed hypersensitivity reaction. Chemical contact sensitivity and the Jones-Mote type of delayed hypersensitivity induced by immunization of animals with antigen in Freund's incomplete adjuvant are examples of this situation. Jones-Mote reactions occur only transiently between 7 and 10 days after immunization. They are of maximum intensity 24 h after skin testing but resolve by 48 h. If animals are pretreated with CY to reduce the number of B-cells, the intensity of these reactions increases to that found with tuberculin type reactions at 48 and 72 h after skin testing[5]. Moreover delayed hypersensitivity reactions can be induced 14 days after sensitization at a time when in normal sensitized animals this type of reactivity is suppressed. Delayed hypersensitivity can also be inhibited by specific suppressor T-cells as has been demonstrated in certain models of immunological tolerance in the mouse, such as chemical contact sensitivity[6].

3. NON-SPECIFIC CHANGES IN MACROPHAGE REACTIVITY BY SPECIFIC IMMUNOLOGICAL REACTIONS

A further field that needs investigation in the future concerns the reactivity of immune and other inflammatory processes as a result of the simultaneous or sequential reactions with a series of different antigens. We know that in real life immunological reactions do not occur in isolation. We are beset continuously with wide range of different antigens. Response to one antigen will affect the response to another. An obvious example of this is the use of bacteria such as mycobacteria or *H. pertussis* that result in a T-cell or B-cell response respectively. A further example of this in the other direction is the observation that infection with a malaria parasite 7 days previously will result in a decreased immune response to sheep erythrocytes[7] and an increased incidence of Moloney sarcoma following the injection of an oncogenic virus.

These changes may arise from interaction at the level of the responding lymphocytes. However changes can also develop at the level of the macrophage. The intravenous injection of an antigen such as horse cytochrome c (Cyt. c.) into guinea pigs sensitized 14 days previously with this antigen can result in a temporary state of desensitization. However in addition to the failure of response to specific antigen *in vivo* and *in vitro*, the macrophages of these animals show a temporary refractoriness to lymphokine *in vitro* and fail to show the normal inhibition of migration[8]. A similar state of macrophage refractoriness can be observed in guinea pigs 2 weeks after infection with the protozoan *Leishmania enriettii*, at a time when the site of intradermal infection is beginning to show evidence of local inflammation[9]. If animals are reinfected with the same organism they develop a delayed hypersensitivity reaction at the site of infection. Their macrophages then show a rapid development of refractoriness to lymphokine, which reaches its greatest intensity 3 days after infection. Such a state of macrophage anergy could be prolonged during certain chronic inflammatory diseases of infective origin. This might result in a need for a higher concentration of lymphokine to cause normal activation of macrophages. In this way a rationale might be provided for the action of drugs such as levamisole which augment delayed hypersensitivity and cause an increased lymphokine release in certain chronic inflammatory diseases[10].

CHRONIC INFLAMMATORY DISEASE AS AN ASSOCIATION OF IMMUNODEFICIENCY

The concept of chronic inflammatory disease resulting from a state of immunodeficiency has arisen partly from a study of leprosy[11]. In the lepromatous form of this disease there is a specific deficiency of CMI with a failure of lymphocyte responsiveness. However when treated with sulphone drugs these patients develop skin lesions resembling Arthus reactions (erythema nodosum leprosum) and other conditions suggestive of immune complex disease. These include especially arthritis and uveitis. In some cases the lesions resemble those of rheumatoid arthritis. A proposed mechanism for this is shown in Figure 1. Failure of CMI results in increased proliferation of the organism or release of soluble antigen. If there is normal B-cell function antibody will be released and immune complexes formed in antibody excess. Moreover it could be postulated that the specific failure of T-cell function in such a condition was also related to increased B-cell activity. This could be the result of either the production of high levels of circulating antibody leading to a 'facilitation' phenomenon, or to the formation of circulating complexes which have also been demonstrated as underlying certain forms of immunological 'enhancement'. Another possibility is that B-cells might be acting either centrally or peripherally to suppress the T-cell response.

Such a model could explain the action of both cyclophosphamide and levamisole in rheumatoid arthritis. One has to postulate that the disease is due to an infective agent such as a virus that needs cell-mediated immunity for its elimination in the same way as *Mycobacterium leprae*. Under these conditions CY could act in two ways by having a selective effect on B-cell function. It could release T-cells from the effect of suppressor B-cells or 'facilitating' antibody, allowing an increased elimination of the organism and a reduction in the circulating antigen load. At the same time it could reduce the level of circulating antibody, thus preventing immune complex formation. Levamisole has been shown to act by increasing cell-mediated immunity. It both increases delayed hypersensitivity in anergic patients and augments the production of soluble mediators by normal stimulated lymphocytes. Thus it would be able to allow the stimulation of macrophages whose threshold of reactivity had been increased in some non-specific way. The final effect of levamisole as a T-cell adjuvant would be the same as that of cyclophosphamide as a B-cell suppressor, but without the latter compound's toxic side effects.

THE INTERACTION OF DELAYED HYPERSENSITIVITY AND IMMUNE COMPLEXES IN CHRONIC INFLAMMATORY DISEASE

However then can we account for the known therapeutic efficacy of chronic thoracic duct drainage on rheumatoid arthritis? Having suggested that the arthritis is a B-cell phenomenon due to circulating immune complexes, one has to admit that the arthritis of rheumatoid disease is very different from typical immune complex arthritis as seen in chronic serum sickness or the infectious arthritides. This could be the result of the overlay of chronic inflammatory disease due to delayed hypersensitivity reaction.

Histologically the lesions seen are those of a chronic granuloma, the main feature of which is the accumulation of macrophages. These cells first take on the appearance of activated macrophages and then epithelioid cells, finally forming giant cells. In addition the lymphocytes may form germinal centres or differentiate into plasma cells. The early stages of chronic granuloma formation have recently been studied during the development of an animal model of allergic granuloma formation to sodium zirconium lactate in the guinea pig[12]. In these studies it was found that guinea pigs, when maximally sensitized to NaZrL, first developed a typical delayed hypersensitivity skin reaction. However after 48 h the skin lesion instead of resolving, developed further, increasing in size to a nodular granuloma which reached peak intensity 7–8 days after skin testing. Histologically the lesion at 24–48 h showed more polymorphs than mononuclear cells. The lesion at 8 days showed activated macrophages and giant cells typical of a granuloma. However at this stage there were considerable numbers of polymorphs also present. The persistence of a polymorphonuclear leukocyte infiltration as late as 8 days would appear to indicate that there was a considerable persistent overlay of immune complex deposition in addition to the basic delayed hypersensitivity reaction. It would appear likely that most chronic inflammatory lesions of immunological basis involve humoral antibody as well as delayed hypersensitivity. In some situations either one or the other reaction may be directed against the instigating mechanism, possibly an infecting organism. However in addition there will be the overlay of auto-immune process either against normally unexposed antigen such as those of the immunoglobulin molecule as in rheumatoid arthritis, or against 'endogenous antigen'.

Thus it will be possible to maintain improvement in conditions of this type if either limb of the immune response is blocked. However it is important to determine whether the improvement is long lasting. Only if long lasting improvement can be maintained, can one be sure that the fundamental process has been attacked.

In summary, outside specific experimental models, inflammatory reactions are generally the resultant of an interacting network of effector and suppressor elements. Some of these are immunologically specific, others are non-specific. The mechanisms frequently involve both T-cell and B-cell products as well as a wide range of pharmacological agents. Therefore the therapeutic effect of a particular drug or combination of drugs may be due to action at a large number of different points within this network of inter-actions. This might account for the paradoxical situation in which two drugs or regimes which superficially have antagonistic effects in experimental models, have the same therapeutic effect in a clinical disease situation.

References

1. Feldmann, M. (1972). Cell interactions in the immune response *in vitro*. V. Specific collaboration via complexes of antigen and thymus derived cell immunoglobulin. *J. exp. Med.*, **136**, 737
2. Waldmann, H. and Munro, A. J. (1975). The interrelationships of antigenic structure, thymus independence and adjuvanticity. *Immunology*, **28**, 509
3. Gershon, R. K. (1975). A disquisition on suppressor T cells. *Transplant. Rev.*, **26**, 170
4. Scheper, R. J., Parker, D., Noble B. and Turk, J. L. (1977). The relation of immune depression and B-cell stimulation during the development of delayed hypersensitivity to soluble antigens. *Immunology*, **32**, 265
5. Turk, J. L., Polak, L. and Parker, D. (1976). Control mechanisms in delayed hyper-sensitivity. *Brit. med. Bull.*, **32**, 165
6. Zembala, M. and Asherson, G. L. (1973). Depression of the T-cell phenomenon of contact sensitivity by T-cells from unresponsive mice. *Nature*, **244**, 227
7. Salaman, M. H., Wedderburn, N. and Bruce-Chwatt, J. L. (1969). The immuno-depressive effect of murine plasmodium and its interaction with murine oncogenic viruses. *J. gen. Microbiol.*, **59**, 383
8. Poulter, L. W. and Turk, J. L. (1976). Changes in macrophages *in vivo* induced by desensitization. *Cell. Immunol.*, **23**, 171
9. Poulter, L. W. (1976). Changes in macrophage status *in vivo* during infection with and immunity to *Leishmania enriettii*. *Cell. Immunol.*, **27**, 17
10. Whitcomb, M. E., Merluzzi, V. J. and Cooperband, S. R. (1976). The effect of levami-sole on human lymphocyte mediator production *in vitro*. *Cell. Immunol.*, **21**, 272
11. Turk, J. L. and Bryceson, A. D. M. (1971). Immunological phenomena in leprosy and related diseases. *Adv. Immun.*, **13**, 209
12. Turk, J. L. and Parker, D. (1977). Sensitization with Cr, Ni and Zr salts and allergic-type granuloma formation in the guinea pig. *J. invest. Derm.* (In press.)

General Discussion

Chairman: J. L. Turk (UK)

G. Loewi: (UK)	Professor Turk is to be thanked for an excellent exposé, which I am sure everybody enjoyed.
	My question may not be fair. Professor Turk has discussed chronic stimulation, chronic inflammation, and the accompaniment, especially Leishmaniasis which he mentioned, is so often amyloid. Has he any thought which he would be prepared to air on how this connection works?
Turk: (UK)	The connection with amyloid! It is a fascinating subject because we nowadays know much more about amyloid than we did sometime ago. The soluble serum amyloid factor is in the serum of all people, but it is increased in certain chronic inflammatory diseases. That really must indicate that all of us have the potential to produce amyloid circulating in us at any time.

I was interested in the work of Keith Macadam on amyloid disease. Keith visited us before he went to New Guinea, where he studied it, and he found high levels of SAA in lepromatous leprosy and even higher levels in erythema nodosum leprosum—the immune complex disease. This would indicate that amyloid probably does not have much relation to the cell mediated immune aspects of the immune reaction because these were patients where cell-mediated immunity, in both its hypersensitivity and host-resistance effects was depressed.

So, the first indication is that one is dealing with a disease that is stimulated in situations of chronic immune complex disease. This is the clinical observation as well—that where there is a chronic infection, with evidence of chronic immune complex disease, one would expect to find evidence of amyloid.

I should like to see whether the patients who have developed amyloid following tuberculosis are those who have other stigmata of immune complex disease, and I should like people to go back to the other associations—to patients with, say, rheumatoid arthritis, and to find out whether there are other clinical stigmata particularly associated with amyloid; whether perhaps the vasculitis is associated with amyloid.

I remember when Jeff Green was working with us—he worked on cryoglobulins which are another aspect of chronic immune complex disease—he found that acute vasculitis patients did not develop cryoglobulins, but he always found cryoglobulins in the serum of patients with chronic, long-standing cutaneous vasculitis. Perhaps there could be an association with cryoglobulins again. It is unfortunate that the SAA activity really just parallels several other factors, e.g. C-reactive protein and so forth. But that does not stop us using it to investigate the mechanisms.

D. Horwitz:
(USA)

I should like to offer a clinical observation on β-lymphocytes and cyclophosphamide. Some years ago we were interested in monitoring cyclophosphamide therapy in patients with systemic lupus erythematosus and rheumatoid arthritis with immunological methods. We learnt that the Ig bearing—i.e. the β-lymphocytes—were more sensitive to cyclophosphamide than T-cells, and we conducted a study to use this as a way of titrating cyclophosphamide. We learnt that in patients with both SLE and rheumatoid arthritis a dose of cyclophosphamide could be given which would maintain patients' B-cells at a very low level and T-cells at very close to normal levels, and induce remission. These patients received full courses of cyclophosphamide to begin with, but then the dose was tapered so that the B-cells remained low and the T-cells came back to normal. With this we were able to induce remission in both SLE and RA—and the studies have been published.

There is now a long-term follow up which I should like to summarize. Of the series of six or seven lupus patients that were treated (some have now been going on for three to four years) that went into remission, and have stayed in remission, none have relapsed. The story with rheumatoid arthritis was much different. After we stopped Cytoxan therapy they all relapsed, and in going back and re-treating we found that we had to use larger and larger doses of Cytoxan in that the schedule of titrating β-lymphocytes really did not work after one or two treatment schedules. In some patients the Cytoxan had to be stopped because the lymphocytes fell and they did not respond.

Interestingly, many of these patients have now been treated with levamisole, and that drug has been helpful in this group.

Turk:

It is fascinating to hear of a long-term effect on systemic lupus which is probably a pure B-cell disease, whereas I would postulate that in the case of rheumatoid arthritis, one is dealing not only with an immune complex disease—as in systemic lupus—but also with the added delayed hypersensitivity disease, which is why cyclophosphamide had only a temporary effect. This is another example of what I was saying. Drugs must be sought that have a long-term effect. Two drug regimes may have to be used in parallel in the long term, at one stage hitting at the B-cell disease and at another stage hitting at the T-cell disease. It may be that in some severely-ill people these regimes will have to be alternated.

A. Mackenzie:
(UK)

I should like to comment on some experiments we have done on adjuvant arthritis which demonstrate the kind of interaction that Professor Turk described between the human immune system and delayed hypersensitivity. We have been able to show that rats that have been pretreated with cyclophosphamide and then injected with adjuvant fail to develop adjuvant arthritis. Animals treated in the same way, however, still develop a delayed hypersensitivity response to PPD. In fact, those responses are enhanced and much longer lasting.

We have also been able to show that the response to developed adjuvant arthritis can be reconstituted in those animals by the transfer of immune serum—which demonstrates clearly that we are dealing with an immune complex situation and delayed hypersensitivity—mediated pathogenesis.

D. A. Willoughby:
(UK)

Might I comment on skin reactivity, of rheumatoid patients treated with levamisole, to PPD. It is relevant to the last contribution.

Although the patients who were treated improved markedly, their skin response to PPD was enhanced, and also lymphocyte transformation to PPD. Skin responses sequentially to PPD is a very dangerous operation because the patients are being sensitized. But if the lymphocytes were taken out and transformations were done, this also was elevated as the patients showed improvement in their clinical condition rheumatoid arthritis.

57

C. M. Pearson:
(USA)

Professor Turk talked about T-cells, B-cells, and their interactivity, and productions or products of T-cells, macrophages, and the like, and leprosy, and he then briefly mentioned something about infection of one type or another in rheumatoid arthritis, and maybe in some of the models too. A great deal of work has been done on diphtheroids, on viruses, on mycoplasma and the like. Could he perhaps speculate some more about where we stand today as regards the potential of infection in humans in rheumatoid arthritis.

Turk:

The hypothesis of the role of infection in a disease such as rheumatoid arthritis really stems from the clinical observations that so many acute infectious diseases of viral and bacterial origin are associated with an acute arthritis—examples being the arthritis of Shigella, associated with gonococcal infection, associated with mumps—the typical immune complex disease, the chronic serum sickness where there is arthritis. In these conditions there is a defined antigen that in some cases can be demonstrated in the joints. Dr. Greenwood demonstrated a meningococcal antigen in meningococcal arthritis.

There is the hypothesis that immune complex disease causes arthritis, and one does see the arthritis in diseases such as erythema nodosum leprosum where there is association with the cutaneous vasculitis where immunoglobulin and complement have been demonstrated in the skin lesion. This is one aspect of the thought process.

These arthritides generally show a polymorphonuclear leukocyte infiltrate and are fairly typical of those seen in an immune complex disease in an experimental system.

The books tell me that the nearest disease to human rheumatoid arthritis of infective origin is a mycoplasma disease of pigs—Hierrhinus—where there is a lesion and a chronicity, more approaching that of rheumatoid arthritis in man. These are the only solid observations that go towards an infective origin of rheumatoid arthritis.

There have been a number of reports of the role of diphtheroids in rheumatoid arthritis, the role of mycoplasma in rheumatoid arthritis. We would all like to see an infectious origin. We believe that there is. However, with so many beliefs evidence is frequently lacking for the present. We feel that the final lesion, as seen in rheumatoid arthritis, has so many of the features of a chronic disease of this type that one would expect with a chronic infectious process leading on to a chronic inflammatory state. There are two possibilities that always come to mind.

First, this (RA) may be instigated by an infectious process and the infection has been lost; but, the damage has been done—either the production of endogenous antigen, or auto-antigen, the role of rheumatoid factor in producing immune complexes where the antibody is damaged immunoglobulin or affected immunoglobulin.

So, how does one finally bring these all together? One has to say that we are very much in the same situation with rheumatoid arthritis as we are with multiple sclerosis. The pointers are there, but the organism has not been demonstrated with any degree of surety.

With multiple sclerosis one hopes that one is dealing with an infective agent. We are thinking still along the lines that we were led to think along by our masters in the 19th century. They made such advances in medicine along the 'infective pathway' that we know that we shall only have a magic bullet if we can find a magic organism. There still is enough data to indicate that we should still go on looking for that organism.

But we should always remember the mathematician who made his name by proving that the particular mathematical phenomenon that he was investigating did not exist!

J.-P. Giroud:
(France)

I should like to ask Dr. Symoens about levamisole and about its metabolism after long administration. We know something about the short administration of levamisole, but do we know anything about long-term administration?

J. Symoens: (Belgium)

We know its metabolism after acute administration. So far we have not tested the metabolism of levamisole after very prolonged administration. We have a lot of experience of prolonged administration clinically, but we have no similar experience with metabolism. One reason why this has not been done is that there is no evidence at all that the metabolism or the blood curves are anywhere related to the effects. For instance, after a single dose of levamisole there may be a prolonged immunological effect over weeks or months. Work in Israel with 'Hodgkin' patients has shown that after three days of treatment with levamisole the E-rosettes are restored, and remain restored, for at least 2 months, and delayed skin hypersensitivity remains restored for at least six months following a three-day course of levamisole—so we cannot see any relation between metabolism, blood curves, and long-term effects. It is apparently an acute effect that persists.

Willoughby:

I am sure that we all agree that the immunostimulants can be made immuno-suppressive, given certain circumstances. Also, the immuno-suppressives can be made immunostimulant, given certain circumstances. Would Professor Turk give us a typical 'Turkism' and introduce a new terminology? Obviously, if we are to discuss immunostimulants under those circumstances where they are acting as immunosuppressant, or vice versa, it becomes meaningless.

Could the Meeting decide on a new form of terminology. We are using very loose terms at the moment.

Chairman:

The precision should be given of what is stimulated. By beginning with 'immuno' the whole immune system is implied. This might have had some value at the time when nothing was known of the whole immune system, but now more and more is known about the cells, about the physiology. The terms immunostimulants and immunosuppressives might well be dropped and we might then simply say what the drugs are doing to what, and when.

Turk:

I start my lecture to the primary FRCS students at the Royal College of Surgeons by telling them that immunology could have been written by Lewis Carroll. A negative is always a positive and a positive is always a negative. We use words like enhancement—meaning un-responsiveness, and there is a positive Wassermann test which is a failure of lysis of red cells.

With these thoughts in mind I dare anyone to understand immunology!

D. Sofia: (USA)

One more point on the metabolism of levamisole. Is there any indication that any particular tissue has an affinity for levamisole? For example, using radio-tagged levamisole is there a pattern of distribution?

Symoens:

We have made studies of the distribution of levamisole using radio-labelled material, but these studies were aimed at finding out the excretion rate in animals, and they were relatively rough studies. We have not looked at the affinity of levamisole for macrophages or lymphocytes. We have only looked at the distribution in the body, and it is equally-distributed in all tissues, but that does not exclude the possibility of a higher affinity for these cells.

I have one point on terminology. The term immunostimulant for levamisole is wrong. Levamisole restores energy and it has been suggested that compounds of this kind be named anti-anergic compounds.

Turk:

Back to the question of nomenclature. The answer really is that one should not be using words like immunosuppressants or immuno-stimulators. One should define what one is doing in each situation.

PERSPECTIVES IN INFLAMMATION

From now on we should stop saying that cyclophosphamide is an immunosuppressive drug. It can be immunosuppressive if used in some ways, and it can be stimulating if used in other ways. These are drugs that modify the immune response, and then there are other drugs that modify the immune reactions without modifying the immune response. We should talk about immuno-modifiers, or immuno-modulators, and include levamisole and cyclophosphamide in this process. Even Dr. Pearson's chronic thoracic duct drainage should be talked of as an immuno-modulating regime.

By using terms such as suppression and stimulation we are only getting halfway to what we should be talking about.

At present we do not know how levamisole works, so it would be wrong to say that it is stimulating. It may not be stimulating at all. It may be unlocking, or restoring. It may be an immuno-restorer.

Let us just talk about these things as immuno-modifiers, or immuno-modulators.

C. da Rocha-Afodu: We should strike at the base of the problem. In fact we have always
(Italy) used the terms antigens and antibodies. In 1973 I coined two words: I call an antigen an *immunin* and an antibody an *anti-immunin*.

If we speak of suppressors, what are we suppressing? We are suppressing the anti-immunin, and a suppressor is therefore an *anti-anti-immunin*.

To put it another way, we are in the missile age!

Chairman: That would seem to be a proper conclusion to the session, but let me pose a question. Immunostimulation and immunosuppression of what?

60

Section II
Chronic Inflammation: Cellular Events

CHAIRMAN: A. C. Allison

CO-CHAIRMAN: P. C. Wilkinson

Co-Chairman's Introductory Remarks— Cellular mechanisms in chronic inflammation

P. C. WILKINSON (UK)

The functions and interrelationships of cells in chronic inflammation are so complex that there is no obvious single model that can be taken as a paradigm. This means that the introduction to a session on cellular mechanisms cannot do more than select one or two topics which may be pertinent. Forty years ago, there would have been much said in such a session about tuberculosis, which was, and in many ways still is, the best model for posing, if not answering, important questions about chronic inflammation. Nowadays rheumatoid arthritis is the disease at centre-stage, and, there too, there are still more questions than answers. The presence of lymphocytes in the lesions of these diseases and the immune responses which they mediate have long been recognized as of central importance. There is still not much known about how and why lymphocytes migrate into sites of inflammation. I want to mention briefly some recent studies of chemically directed lymphocyte locomotion *in vitro* and some factors which may attract them into inflammatory sites *in vivo*. We must also consider the role of macrophages as carriers of antigenic information, as cooperators with lymphocytes and as effector cells. Macrophages and neutrophils are both efficient phagocytes but neutrophils do not live long and do not differentiate, and present-day dogma has it that they do not play the type of role that macrophages do in cooperating with lymphocytes in the induction of immune responses. Perhaps it is fortunate that neutrophils do not pass on messages to lymphocytes about the antigens in the effete tissue cells which they presumably scavenge under physiological conditions, otherwise autoimmunity might be commoner than it is. Mononuclear phagocytes, like neutrophils, are stimulated immediately by contact with inflammatory agents to perform short-term functions which require a metabolic burst and which mobilize the contractile machinery of the cell, i.e. chemotaxis, phagocytosis, lysosome–phagosome fusion. However, unlike neutrophils, they are also 'activated' in the longer term inasmuch as over a period of days they show enhanced DNA and protein synthesis, increase their content of hydrolases and become more efficient as killers of microorganisms such as *Listeria monocytogenes* than the blood monocytes from which they were derived.

There are now a number of chemical mediators which are known to initiate macrophage activation. However, the cell biology of this activation is still poorly understood and there is nothing like the information available that there is about, for instance, lymphocyte activation by polyclonal activators. The isolation and definition of soluble factors which determine cell–cell interactions of this type will, one hopes, in time, open the door to an exploration of chronic inflammation at the molecular level. This is certain to present problems due to the complexity of the phenomena under study. Some of these problems might be exemplified by some difficulties we have recently encountered in defining the macrophage stimulating activity of the anaerobic coryneform bacteria (*Corynebacterium parvum*).

IMMUNOPOTENTIATING EFFECTS OF CORYNEFORM BACTERIA: PROBLEMS IN CHARACTERIZATION

The anaerobic coryneform bacteria, best known under the inaccurate designation *Corynebacterium parvum*, can easily be shown to stimulatevarious functions of mononuclear phagocytes *in vivo* and *in vitro*. They have chemotactic activity, they enhance carbon clearance, they have immunopotentiating effects on antibody synthesis *in vivo* and they may cause tumour regression, perhaps through an enhancing effect on the ability of macrophages to kill tumour cells. The anaerobic coryneforms are notoriously changeable organisms and the same batch may give excellent results in these assays on one occasion, then fail completely on the next. Since no-one had tried to relate activity to the growth and morphological characteristics of the organisms, R. J. Russell in our laboratory set out to do this using the simple macrophage chemotaxis assay as his basic measure of activity. On culturing and filming sample batches of fifteen or so strains of anaerobic coryneforms at intervals, he found that the bacteria which were most active possessed, at the stage of growth when biological activity was present, a thick coat of what resembled capsular material which was loosely attached to the bacterial body and which later sloughed off into the medium[1]. This coat consisted of polysaccharide and some lipid. Bacteria which possessed it had biological activity as stimulators of macrophage function. The material was lost into the culture fluid during the logarithmic phase of growth, and then strong activity was found in this fluid after centrifuging out the bacteria. The active material was found not only to stimulate chemotaxis, but also, when injected into mice it enhanced carbon clearance, and, when injected directly into a tumour, it caused regression. It was clearly of interest to try to isolate the active substance.

Chloroform–methanol–water extraction showed that a chloroform-soluble lipid fraction possessed chemotactic and clearance-enhancing activity[1]. However, problems came when this material was further separated by thin-layer chromatography and other methods. Several fractions possessed activity and no single fraction was nearly as active as the crude material or the whole organisms. Furthermore, it was shown by Dawes, Tuach and McBride[2] that the antigenic moiety which stimulated immune responses when injected into animals resided in the polysaccharide fraction rather than in the lipid. Otu, Russell and White[3], showed that the lipid fraction injected into mice gave some enhancement of carbon clearance during the day or two after injection. However, the whole bacteria, but not lipid alone, gave a second peak of much more efficient carbon clearance, maximal 14 days after injection. This delayed enhancement of clearance may have resulted from lymphocyte-induced activation of the mononuclear phagocyte system resulting from an immune response to the bacterial polysaccharide antigen. Thus in this series of experiments, attempts to isolate activity in pure fractions led to loss of full activity, partly because different enhancing functions are mediated by different moieties of the bacterial surface. Simple molecules may be cleared from the site of administration more easily than whole bacteria and possibly the chronic inflammatory stimulus therefore does not persist when purified fractions are used as it does when whole organisms are injected. It seems possible that, in such bacteria, multiple factors are necessary to mediate biological effects. These need to be dissected apart to understand their behaviour as molecules but then recombined to attain maximal effects in the whole animal.

CHEMOTAXIS OF LYMPHOCYTES

I want also to discuss in brief the chemotactic locomotion of lymphocytes and the mechanisms by which lymphocytes reach inflammatory lesions. Lymphocytes are motile cells but for many years workers were unable to show that they responded to chemotactic stimuli and they were placed in a special category as non-chemotactic cells whose emigration in inflammation was controlled by obscure mechanisms different from those which controlled phagocyte emigration. However, it was observations of chronic inflammation *in vivo* which provided one of the vital clues for demonstrating lymphocyte chemotaxis *in vitro*. Several workers[4-6] reported that blast-transformed lymphocytes, which were very motile cells, preferentially migrated from the blood into sites of inflammation. We, therefore, decided to study, not the lymphocytes present in normal blood which we had previously used unsuccessfully, but purified lymphoblast populations. The first populations we studied were cultured human B-lymphoblasts which had been maintained *in vitro* for long periods. These showed vigorous and easily reproducible chemotactic responses to a number of agents which were already known to attract phagocytic cells. They included endotoxin-activated plasma, casein, *Corynebacterium parvum* and denatured serum albumin[7,8]. We also studied mouse lymphoblasts from the lymph nodes draining the site of contact sensitization with oxazolone. These cells migrated vigorously in the presence of chemotactic agents, but the migration was random, not directional. The factors induced a chemokinetic reaction in the cells, i.e. they increased their *rate* of locomotion, but did not control the *direction* of locomotion, i.e. induce a chemotactic reaction. Chemokinetic locomotion of lymphocytes has, in subsequent experiments, proved to be very important. The concentration of serum albumin in which the cells are suspended controls their rate of loco-motion, that is to say, it acts as a chemokinetic factor and this chemokinetic stimulation is necessary for lymphocytes to show chemotaxis to certain factors. Cells suspended in the absence of serum albumin may fail to move at all to chemotactic factors[9].

In subsequent experiments we have examined the locomotion of the lymphocytes of normal human blood after culture *in vitro* for 2–3 days in the presence of polyclonal activators (e.g. mitogens such as PHA)[10]. Cultured lymphocytes show good chemotactic reactions to inflammatory stimuli. We have shown that they migrate towards endotoxin-activated serum, and towards purified peptides (probably C5-derived) from activated serum, towards casein, alkali-denatured HSA, certain fatty acids and formyl methionyl peptides, all of which are also attractants for neutrophils. Even more interestingly such lymphocytes can be induced to migrate towards polyvalent ligands. Two of these have been studied, PHA and staphylococcal protein A[10]. PHA is chemotactic for cultured blood lymphocytes provided it is used at a concentration of a hundred-fold to a thousand-fold lower than the mitogenic dose. Similarly protein A, which binds to immunoglobulin, presumptively on the lymphocyte surface, is chemotactic at concentrations round 10^{-8}–10^{-9}M. From observation of the cells from cultured populations which migrate into filters, it is obvious that not only the large blast-like cells respond but also many smaller cells including typical small lymphocytes. We now no longer believe that the phenomenon of chemotaxis of lymphocytes is confined to blast forms, but that small cells can also show it. A period of culture *in vitro* or activation *in vitro* or *in vivo*, seems to facilitate the response of these cells (O'Neill and Parrott, in preparation). Since most of the lympho-cytes in inflammatory sites are small, it seems reasonable that these small cells have migrated by a similar mechanism to macrophages and other inflam-matory cells.

Our most recent experiments have been studies of the role of antigen in lymphocyte chemotaxis[9]. Lymphocytes migrate towards protein antigens such as serum albumins. Some of this locomotion is chemokinetic and is shown by unprimed cells. However, in mice primed with serum albumin, then challenged with the same antigen, a population of cells can be found in the draining lymph nodes 3–10 days later which migrate chemotactically towards the antigen. Ovalbumin-sensitized lymphocytes suspended in serum albumin migrated chemotactically in response to nanogram concentrations of ovalbumin. The specificity of this antigen-sensitive response remains to be defined precisely.

It is plausible to suggest that the lymphocytes in chronic inflammatory lesions are attracted there by chemotactic factors. Whether locomotion to antigen has anything at all to do with migration into inflammatory sites is debatable since most of the cells which reach the lesion are not reactive against the inducing antigen. It may be that antigen-specific chemotaxis is of greater physiological importance in the organization of antigen-sensitive cells within lymphoid tissue and in facilitating cooperation between them by providing a mechanism for them to home onto antigen and onto each other. However, the observation that lymphocytes respond chemotactically to defined factors such as complement and other inflammatory mediators makes good sense to the student of inflammation since *in vivo* the time course of their ingress into inflammatory sites is very similar to that of mononuclear phagocytes which have been known for some time to respond to similar factors. The demonstration that lymphocyte chemotaxis *in vitro* is not essentially different from the chemotaxis of the much better-understood phagocytes, and also that lymphocytes in lymph nodes after all migrate out of vessels between and not through endothelial cells[11] suggests that lymphocytes are not specially exotic, at least in their locomotor behaviour, and allows a rational basis for future studies of their migration in chronic inflammation.

References

1. Russell, R. J., McInroy, R. J., Wilkinson, P. C. and White, R. G. (1976). A lipid chemotactic factor from anaerobic coryneform bacteria including *Corynebacterium parvum* with activity for macrophages and monocytes. *Immunology*, 30, 935
2. Dawes, J., Tuach, S. J. and McBride, W. H. (1974). Properties of an antigenic polysaccharide from *Corynebacterium parvum*. *J. Bact.*, 120, 24
3. Otu, A. A., Russell, R. J. and White, R. G. (1977). Biphasic pattern of activation of the reticuloendothelial system by anaerobic coryneforms in mice. *Immunology*, 32, in press
4. Moore, A. R. and Hall, J. G. (1973). Non-specific entry of thoracic duct immunoblasts into intradermal foci of antigens. *Cell. Immun.*, 8, 112
5. Asherson, G. L., Allwood, G. G. and Mayhew, B. (1973). Contact sensitivity in the mouse. XI. Movement of T-blasts in the draining lymph nodes to sites of inflammation. *Immunology*, 25, 485
6. McGregor, D. D. and Logie, P. S. (1974). The mediator of cellular immunity. VII. Localization of sensitized lymphocytes in inflammatory exudates. *J. Exp. Med.*, 139, 1415
7. Russell, R. J., Wilkinson, P. C., Sless, F. and Parrott, D. M. V. (1975). Chemotaxis of lymphoblasts. *Nature*, 256, 646
8. Wilkinson, P. C., Russell, R. J., Pumphrey, R. S. H., Sless, F. and Parrott, D. M. V. (1976). Studies of chemotaxis of lymphocytes. *Agents Actions*, 6, 243
9. Wilkinson, P. C., Parrott, D. M. V., Russell, R. J. and Sless, F. (1977). Antigen-induced locomotor responses in lymphocytes. *J. Exp. Med.* (In press.)
10. Wilkinson, P. C., Roberts, J. A., Russell, R. J. and McLoughlin, M. (1976). Chemotaxis of mitogen-activated human lymphocytes and the effects of membrane-active enzymes. *Clin. Exp. Immunol.*, 25, 280
11. Anderson, A. O. and Anderson, N. D. (1976). Lymphocyte emigration from high endothelial venules in rat lymph nodes. *Immunology* 31, 731

5

A model for assessing effects of drugs on granulocyte emigration *in vivo*

J. F. BOREL AND CAMILLE FEURER (Switzerland)

A method for quantification of *in vivo* leukocytic emigration in experimental animals has been developed[1]. This involved mainly adaptation to the rabbit ear of the window-box of Gowland[2] or the skin chamber of Senn *et al.*[3] used on the human forearm. This technique was called localized leukocyte mobilization (LLM).

The ear collection chamber was made of polyacetylene caps of 24 mm diameter with an edge of 6 mm width to ensure tight adhesion to the ear surface. Its capacity was about 0.8 ml. An aperture on top to be closed by a plastic press-button allowed filling and emptying of the chamber. The lesion itself was produced by repeatedly sticking firmly onto the skin and tearing off a piece of plaster until the epidermis was removed and the lesion appeared exuding and pink. By this procedure the basal cell layer was more or less removed, but the underlying corium and capillary network remained intact. A sterile chamber was placed over the lesion, glued to the ear and firmly fixed with wide strips of tape. The chamber was then filled with test fluid and the aperture closed. Gey's solution was used for negative controls and undiluted, fresh, homologous, normal rabbit serum (NRS) for the positive controls. The collection of the emigrated leukocytes was routinely performed after 6 h of *in situ* incubation and the cells counted in a haemocytometer.

One possible disadvantage of the collection chamber technique lies in its failure to promote the escape of mononuclear cells. Histological sections taken through the reaction site of rabbit ears on which chambers containing Gey's solution or fresh NRS had been placed 6 or 24 h before, indicated the presence of only few mononuclear cells scattered randomly within the tissues (Figures 5.1 and 5.2). However, massive emigration of neutrophils from the venules into the perivascular tissues towards the skin abrasion was observed with fresh NRS.

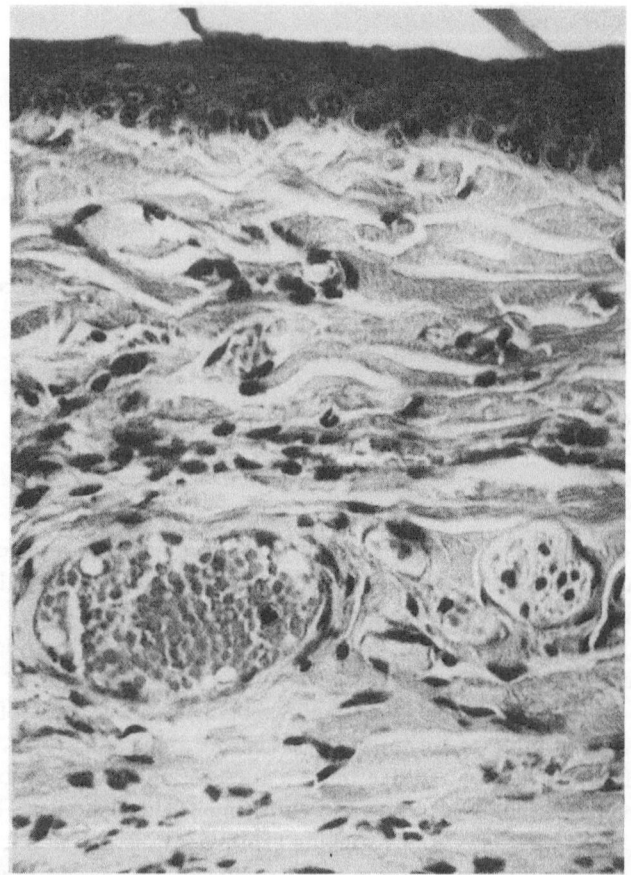

Figure 5.1 Histological section taken through a rabbit ear underneath the abraded skin (visible at top of the section) on which a chamber containing Gey's solution had been placed for 24 h. Very few leukocytes are seen. Magnification 320 ×

Results obtained by this method, which allows a quantitative assessment of leukocyte emigration *in vivo*, were related to those obtained *in vitro* with the Boyden chamber technique[4]. There is good evidence that the *in vitro* test performed in the Boyden chamber measures chemotactic migration. It has not yet been conclusively demonstrated that cellular migration, as it occurs in the local mobilization test, is truly chemotactic and not a random phenomenon. However, a comparison between the *in vivo* and the *in vitro* results supports the concept that *in vivo* leukocyte migration is directional[1]. Since heat-inactivated NRS induces extremely weak chemotactic migration both *in vivo* and *in vitro* and fresh NRS was highly active in the ear chamber, a heat-labile component reacting with the damaged skin tissue and thus forming a potent cytotaxin was presumed to be present in fresh NRS. The abraded skin did not by itself promote chemotactic activity, for Gey's solution was ineffective.

In conclusion, the LLM provides a simple and valuable method for quantitating the migration of granulocytes, but not of other cell types. Its major advantages over other methods consist in the induction of a physiological, strictly localized, acute type inflammatory lesion mediated through the interaction of fresh homologous serum with abraded skin tissue. A quantification of the invading polymorphonuclear leukocytes is feasible at any time and without interrupting the assay. Both experimental and control values may be obtained from a single animal and an experiment can also be repeated within the same rabbit. This method appears, therefore, suitable for the assessment of substances inhibiting granulocyte emigration *in vivo* after either systemic or topical application.

Table 5.1 Estimation of the ED-50 of active compounds after oral administration to rabbits. Results derived from dose-response curves using non-toxic doses (LLM assay)

Active compounds	Oral ED-50 (mg/kg)
Anti-inflammatory drugs	
Dexamethasone	0.6
Indomethacin	7
Phenylbutazone	65
Proquazone	140
Acetylsalicylic acid	50
Sodium-salicylate	310
D-Penicillamine	2×240
Cytostatic agents	
Cyclophosphamide	43
Colchicine	3.2

The following schedule was used for the assessment of drugs after oral administration to rabbits. A positive control assay (chamber filled with fresh NRS) was performed first on the untreated animals. Two to 3 days later the rabbits were given the drug to be tested by gastric intubation and 1 h later the plastic chamber containing fresh NRS was placed on the ear. Those compounds which were administered twice were given first 16 h and again 1 h before fixation of the ear chamber. A second positive control was carried out about 3 weeks after the treatment with drug. The inhibition rate was calculated in percentage of the average value of the positive controls. Each dose of a compound was assessed at least in three different animals. Counts of emigrated cell per mm^3 obtained under treatment with effective drugs were clearly and reproducibly much lower than the corresponding control values without drug treatment, although the latter counts may often vary within the

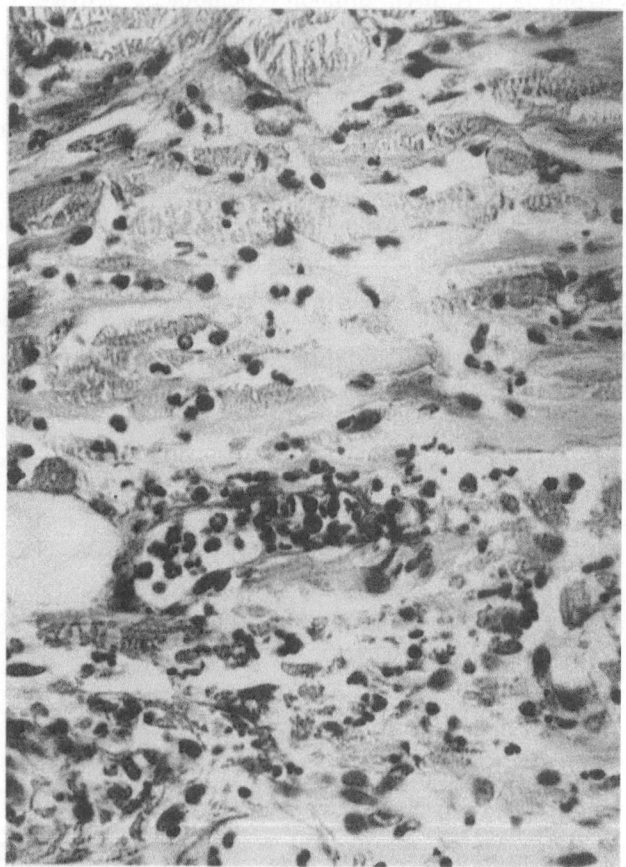

Figure 5.2 Section similar to that in previous figure, except that a chamber containing fresh NRS had been fixed for 24 h. Note the presence of numerous polymorphonuclear leukocytes both in the capillary vessel and surrounding tissues. (×320)

same animal. Occasional failure of an animal to respond was encountered with most inhibitory agents.

With the exceptions of hydrocortisone and naproxen, all anti-inflammatory drugs were effective in significantly reducing the LLM following a single or two oral doses (Table 5.1). Among the cytostatic agents, cyclophosphamide and colchicine produced an inhibitory effect within a therapeutic dose range. Agents exerting other pharmacological effects, showed no inhibition in non-toxic doses. The effective oral doses used with all anti-inflammatory compounds never elicited any short- or long-term toxic side effects. Although some ED-50 values seem relatively high on a mg/kg basis compared to the corresponding values in the adjuvant arthritis in rats, a direct comparison may be misleading, since in arthritis treatment the compounds are usually given daily for 2 weeks, since one model is concerned with acute and the other with chronic inflammation and since there is a species difference. Moreover, this particular component of granulocyte migration inhibition might, in respect to the different drugs, represent a more or less important aspect of their anti-inflammatory spectrum.

A list of all agents tested in this LLM assay is given in Table 5.2. The results indicated that only compounds with some degree of anti-inflammatory activity, though not all of them, were effective in this model. Furthermore, the topical application of a restricted number of compounds produced results correlating closely with those after systemic administration. However, the *in vivo* results obtained with the LLM assay widely differed from those

Table 5.2 List of all compounds tested in the LLM assay in rabbits. Results obtained after oral administration and for some compounds also after topical application (in brackets). Inhibition of granulocyte emigration is indicated by +, moderate effect by ±, and no effect by 0

Anti-inflammatory drugs			Cytostatic agents		
Hydrocortisone	0	(0)	Cyclophosphamide	+	
Dexamethasone	+	(+)	Azathioprine	0	
Indomethacin	+		Amethopterin	0	
Phenylbutazone	+	(+)	Colchicine	+	(+)
Naproxen	0	(0)			
Proquazone	+		*Miscellaneous agents*		
Acetylsalicylic acid	+		Cytochalasin B	0	(+)
Na-salicylate	±		Histamine	0	(0)
D-penicillamine	+		Clemastine	0	
			Chlordiazepoxide	0	
			Chlorpromazine	0	
			Pindolol	0	

observed in the *in vitro* Boyden chamber technique. All antiphlogistics tested with the latter method exerted no effect on granulocyte chemotaxis, except some slightly inhibitory, but inconsistent results with sodium salicylate and colchicine[5]. Therefore, it was concluded that these compounds were not primarily interfering with cell migration *in vitro*. It is obvious that this much more complex *in vivo* model includes a number of steps which are absent from the *in vitro* system; in particular regulation of microcirculation, whereby the supply of leukocytes, their adhesion to the vascular endothelium and cell deformability are controlled. It still remains a matter of conjecture, at which level and by which mechanisms the different drugs affect granulocyte emigration in the *in vivo* system.

References

1. Feurer, Camille and Borel, J. F. (1974). Localised leukocyte mobilisation in the rabbit ear. In E. Sorkin (ed.) Chemotaxis: Its biology and biochemistry. *Antibiot. Chemotherap.*, **19**, p. 161

2. Gowland, E. (1964). Studies on the emigration of polymorphonuclear leucocytes from skin lesions in man. *J. Path. Bact.*, **87**, 347
3. Senn, H. J. and Jungi, F. (1975). Neutrophil migration in health and disease. In J. R. Humbert, P. A. Miescher and E. R. Jaffé (eds.) *Neutrophil Physiology Pathology*, pp. 25–43. (New York: Grune & Stratton.)
4. Boyden, S. (1962). The chemotactic effect of mixtures of antibody and antigen on polymorphonuclear leucocytes. *J. Exp. Med.*, **115**, 453
5. Borel, J. F. (1973). Effects of some drugs on the chemotaxis of rabbit neutrophils in vitro. *Experientia*, **29**, 676

6

A polymorph abnormality in Crohn's disease

G. LOEWI, A. SEGAL AND P. TOOTH (UK)

In a previous communication[1] we have reported diminished arrival of polymorphs in skin window studies on patients suffering from Crohn's disease. We have now increased the number of observations and confirmed our earlier finding. We have also undertaken experiments *in vitro*, and found that here also there is diminished polymorph migration when cells or skin window fluid from patients suffering from Crohn's disease are tested.

METHODS

The method has been described previously[1] and follows in general that used by Senn[2] and the modification thereof described by Borel and Feurer in this volume (chapter 5). Briefly, the skin of the flexor aspect of the forearm is lightly abraded and a small plastic cup, volume 0.6 ml, attached.* This is filled with the patient's serum. After 5 h the serum is withdrawn, the cup is washed with a similar volume of tissue culture medium, and the total number of polymorphs is counted in a counting chamber using phase contrast illumination.

In vitro experiments were carried out in two different ways. The first of these was an adaptation of the migration inhibition method widely used for mononuclear cells; the capillaries were filled with polymorphs which were allowed to migrate overnight in medium RPMI with 10% fetal calf serum.

Migration was measured with a planimeter on a photograph. The second method consisted of migration under agarose, as described by Nelson, Quie and Simmons[3]. The chemotactic agent was skin window fluid from Crohn's or control patients. For this purpose, the skin-adherent cups were filled with

* The procedure was explained to the patients and their agreement, as well as that of the Ethical Committee obtained

tissue culture medium without protein and left *in situ* for 18 h. The area covered by polymorphs was measured by planimetry.

RESULTS

The distribution of polymorph numbers, compared with sick and healthy controls is shown in a histogram (Figure 6.1). It is clear that the number of cells produced by patients with Crohn's disease was significantly less than those of sick or healthy controls. The sick controls consisted of patients with ulcerative colitis, tuberculous enteritis, rheumatoid arthritis, duodenal and

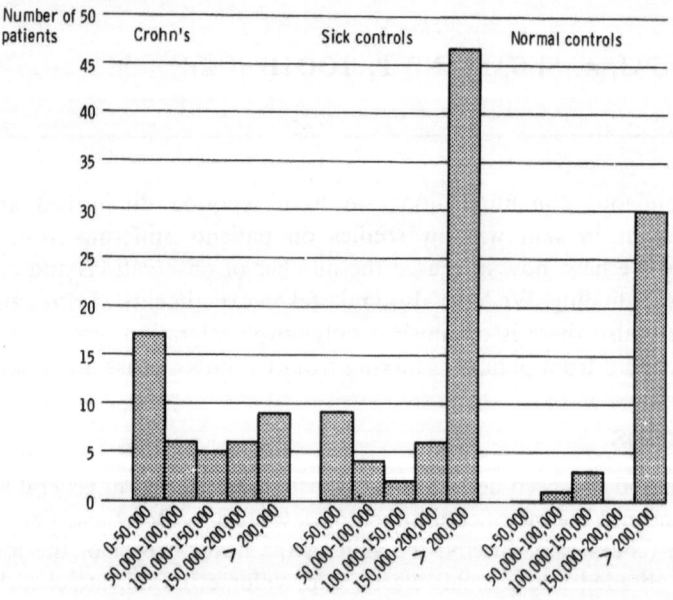

Figure 6.1 The distribution of the numbers of polymorphs in skin windows of patients with Crohn's disease and sick and normal controls. Skin windows were in position for 5 h

gastric ulcers, liver disease, Behcet's disease and immune deficiency. The normal controls were laboratory and hospital staff.

Polymorph migration tests from capillary tubes similarly showed a difference between Crohn's patients and sick controls. Each experiment included a set of normals which were regarded as having given 100% migration. From this, the percentage migration of Crohn's and sick controls was determined. Crohn's showed appreciably less migration than sick controls, the significance of the difference giving a p value of <0.01.

Migration of normal polymorphs under agar towards the skin window fluid of a normal control showed streaming of the polymorphs towards the fluid well. On the other hand, the cells failed to move towards fluid obtained from patients with Crohn's disease.

Chemotaxis performed with a modified Boyden chamber and a double filter (12 μm and 0.45 μm) with casein, endotoxin-activated serum and plasma as chemo-attractants produced abnormally low values in two of the Crohn's patients who had given very low skin window responses, but was normal in 10 others.

CONCLUSION

The failure of polymorphs to migrate into the skin chamber may be due to an abnormality in the serum, in mediators from the abraded skin, or to a chemotactic abnormality on the part of the cell. In a few patients, normal serum (known to be Australia antigen negative) was applied in a second chamber; this produced a figure in Crohn's patients which was comparable in number of cells to that given by autologous serum. A serum factor is therefore unlikely. In the migration experiments, Crohn's polymorphs failed to migrate normally from capillaries, suggesting an abnormality on the part of the cell. On the other hand, when tissue culture medium was left in contact with the skin for 18 h, this became chemotactic for polymorphs *in vitro*, though not *in vivo*, whereas, with very few exceptions, similar medium from Crohn's patients failed to stimulate *in vitro* chemotaxis. This might indicate the presence of an inhibitor which we would postulate also to be present on the polymorph surface. The alternative would be a failure of Crohn's patients to produce an activating principle from the skin, but this would fail to explain the *in vitro* migration behaviour of Crohn's polymorphs. More work on the unravelling of these questions is in progress.

SUMMARY

The migration of polymorphs into skin windows is greatly reduced in Crohn's disease, compared with sick and normal controls. This defect is mirrored in *in vitro* experiments, measuring polymorph migration. Tissue culture fluid which had been in contact with abraded skin of normal controls for 18 h was chemotactic for polymorphs, while such material obtained from Crohn's disease patients failed to attract normal polymorphs.

Acknowledgements

We thank Dr J. F. Borel of Sandoz, Basel, for a supply of plastic skin window cups.

References

1. Segal, A. and Loewi, G. (1976). Neutrophil dysfunction in Crohn's disease. *Lancet*, **ii**, 219
2. Senn, H. (1972). Infehtabwehr Hämoblastosen, (Berlin, Springer)
3. Nelson, R. D., Quie, P. G. and Simmons, R. L. (1975). Chemotaxis under agarose: a new and simple method for measuring chemeotaxis and spontaneous migration of human polymorphonuclear leukocytes and monocytes. *J. Immunol.*, **115**, 1650

Discussion 6

G. Loewi: The work which I shall report briefly was done by Mr. Tony Segal, Mr. Tooth and myself at the Clinical Research Centre, Northwick Park. I need not describe the chamber since Mr. Borel has already discussed it. We used the identical chamber. We left it on for 5 h, because that is a convenient time for patients, and removed the total and washed it out once. Then we counted the cells in the usual way in the haemocytometer.

The abrasion is made with a little carborundum wheel, with great care, so as not to cause bleeding. If bleeding occurs, I would go to another site and make another abrasion with the little wheel. On the whole patients say that it is quite painless.

I shall be talking about Crohn's Disease. *Slide 1* is taken from the large intestine of a patient with the disease. The section is taken through the whole of the large intestine. The surface is somewhat flattened. There are the typical fissures of Crohn's Disease. Inflammation pervades the whole of the tissue down to the serosa. There are abnormally large numbers of lymphoid follicles and a little granuloma.

Slide 2 shows the numbers of polymorphs. I must stress, as did Mr. Borel, that polymorphs appear with only very few mononuclear cells or monocytes. That only amounts to about 5%. Nevertheless, if a coverslip is put on to the skin lesion after the cup has been put on to it the usual number of monocytic cells can be produced.

The *third slide* shows the frequency distribution in a series of patients. In Crohn's Disease many patients produce no cells at all, and in the majority of patients it is 0–50 000. In the other ranges there are also some producers. The controls will be more fully discussed. They made a response where the majority of the responders were above 200 000 cells in the whole chamber. In effect there were many. It was quite frequent to find people with 1 million, 2 million, and even 3 million cells accumulating in 5 h.

Lastly the column of normals, where most people behaved by producing a large number of cells. Crohn's is entirely different from both sick controls and normals.

Slide 4 shows the diseases chosen as controls: ulcerative colitis; tuberculous colitis; duodenal ulcer; gastric ulcer; immune deficiency of various sorts; Behcet's; sarcoid; cirrhosis of the liver; asthma, and a large number of patients with rheumatoid arthritis.

There is a relationship of these numbers to chemotaxis but so far it has not been a relationship which is easily analysed. Some people showed a similar diminution in the double-membrane modified Boyden chamber; others did not. I cannot go into this further at the moment, but we are working on it.

Slide 5 shows what happened when we put the polymorphs of people with Crohn's Disease, and of normal people, into a capillary tube and we let them emigrate from the end of the capillary. There is no doubt that the normals show by far the greater area of emigration.

Slide 6 shows the numerical appearance which this gave. In Crohn's it was considerably lower than in the sick controls. Since then we have done even more controls but even here the P value was less than 0.01.

Slide 7 shows what happens when the polymorphs—i.e. normal polymorphs—are put into an agar plate and allowed to migrate under the agar. On one side, emigration occurs towards *E-coli* endotoxin, which is placed near the rim of the Petri dish. On the other side there is normal skin window fluid; that is to say fluid obtained not in the presence of serum but in the presence only of RPMI culture medium which is applied in a similar way in the chamber and taken off after 18 h. That is clearly chemotactic for these polymorphs in the conditions of the experiment.

Slide 8 shows what happens when Crohn's chamber fluid is taken. On one side normal chamber fluid has been taken, and on the other side there are three Crohn's fluids. There is practically no emigration of polymorphs towards the medium which comes from the chambers. In other words, there is still a great deal to be worked out, but at present it is fair to say that somehow the polymorphs are not sensitive to the usual stimuli, and that there seems to be a serum factor which presumably covers the polymorph *in vivo*, and which can also be demonstrated *in vitro*. So far there is no evidence that this is an antibody, but I have looked at it only by fluorescence which is not a sensitive enough test. We propose to do other types of test.

R. van Furth:
(The Netherlands)
Is there any explanation for the different behaviour of emigration in the chambers and in the classical Rebuck technique, where a glass-adherent population of cells is used?

Loewi:
I am sorry, but the answer is no. We cannot give a good answer at the moment. We do not know the answer. We do not get mononuclear cells in these windows, other than to the tune of about 5%, and yet when the ordinary coverslip is put on we get the usual number. We have no good explanation to offer.

M. Jasani:
(UK)
Has any difference been noticed between the response of the polymorphs in the ear chamber technique when there is an immunological stimulus in the chamber, as opposed to free emigration of cells? Has this been tried?

Borel:
We have done some tests and we have not found any differences. The serum can be activated by immune complexes or by endotoxins that can be put into the chamber. It would be heat-inactivated first, to be sure that one is not activating the serum with the skin tissues, and there is no difference.

Jasani:
Has the effect of lymphokines been tried—with respect to lymphokines in the chamber?

Borel:
No.

7

The origin and kinetics of liver macrophages during steady state and inflammation *(Abstract)*

R. VAN FURTH AND R. W. CROFTON (Netherlands)

Ed: Unfortunately the complete manuscript was not received in time for publication.

The general concept is now accepted that macrophages in the tissues derive from monocytes in the circulation which in turn derive from promonocytes in the bone marrow. Promonocytes are proliferating cells that divide only once and are descendants of the monoblasts, which derive from the (committed) stem cell.

Until recently macrophages in the peritoneal or pleural cavity were taken as examples of tissue macrophages, since these cells are easy to collect. Since a method has been developed to isolate macrophages from the liver in suspension, it is now possible to study these tissue macrophages in more detail.

Morphological, cytochemical and functional analyses of liver macrophages obtained from normal mice have shown that these macrophages are very similar to peritoneal macrophages. *In vitro* labelling with ^{3}H thymidine has shown that liver macrophages do not divide.

In vivo labelling indicated that liver macrophages derive from blood monocytes. Proof of the monocytic origin of liver macrophages was obtained with labelling experiments in animals treated with hydrocortisone, which causes a monocytopenia so that no circulating cells are available to migrate into the tissues, and in animals x-irradiated with hind-limb shielding.

Following an inflammatory stimulus, (e.g. zymosan intravenously) the number of macrophages in the liver increases. Labelling experiments have shown that these cells are recently recruited from the bone marrow; there was no indication that so-called resident macrophages can be stimulated to proliferate locally.

Discussion 7

G. Velo: (Italy)	There is a very large percentage of monocytes; 56%. How long does it take for these monocytes to become liver macrophages. Is there a short gap between the two times or is it something of a continuous cycle?
van Furth:	The question is not easily answered. Probably as soon as the monocytes are in the tissue compartments they will change their function and they will change their behaviour. However, that is an assumption. No one has done the experiments to find out whether the circulating cells, the biochemical differences in the tissues, are really different immediately. From the labelling experiment, because there is a more or less homogeneous population of cells, one must say that as soon as they come to the liver they are called liver macrophages, and that the transition is very rapid.
S. Normann: (USA)	I should like to refer to work published in 1976 (Volkmann) relating to the peritoneal macrophage. Parabiosed rats were used and little evidence was found to support the bone marrow origin of those cells in a resting, normal condition. Because this may relate to studies being done with Kupffer cells, would Professor van Furth comment on that work? I believe that it has a bearing on this issue.
van Furth:	It is not completely fair, since Dr. Normann is not a part of that group, for me to criticize those experiments. I have read them very carefully and there is something wrong with the experiment because it is not a real parabiosis. If the number of cells in one animal is compared with the number in another animal, then the number of labelled cells in the non-labelled animal is much smaller. Further, it was not a real steady state situation. There can be inflammation in one animal or in the other because the levels of cells were also not the same. The number of animals was small, 13, but this is always so with parabiotic animals.

Reading the experiments carefully one could come to another conclusion. |
Normann:	What was the per cent yield of Professor van Furth's cells that he harvested from the liver?
van Furth:	It is hard to estimate numbers of non-parenchymal cells in the normal liver, but between 85 and 90% of the cells are alive. About 95% of the Kupffer cells which we had in our suspension are recovered on the glass. Probably a small number of the Kupffer cells will die, because of the pronase treatment, and a small percentage of the other parenchymal cells will die off.
G. MacPherson: (UK)	If one cannulates an hepatic afferent lymphatic in sheep's liver one can find a large traffic of mononuclear phagocytes through the liver. A lot of these have the characteristics of monocytes and I wonder whether Professor van Furth has any idea of what proportion of his recently-labelled cells would not be replacing Kupffer cells, but would

be forming a part of the normal circulation of mononuclear phagocytes through the liver?

van Furth: Dr. Macpherson is saying that there is a population of cells that will travel through the liver and come out into the afferent lymph—which we call Kupffer cells. I therefore try to avoid the name Kupffer cells—because that is another anatomical site, and I call them liver macrophages.

If that is true, then the turnover time of the cells would be much faster. In my calculations I always calculated that the labelled cells are just a part of the normal population. There would be a very fast turnover of cells in the liver, and one would have to really set down whether that would account for the influx of cells.

Macpherson: It would be interesting to look in the lymph, e.g. after zymosan injection, to see whether there is this enormous increase.

It could be a very productive field. One report which we found suggests that if a small amount of endotoxin is injected intravenously into a sheep, then the afferent lymph becomes absolutely full of cells which look like Kupffer cells; mature macrophages.

P. C. Wilkinson: (UK) Professor van Furth has looked at several of the properties of these liver macrophages after putting them through his *in vitro* treatment. But has he looked to see if they are locomotor cells? I think that they are.

Do they locomote?

van Furth: We have not looked.

K. Brune: (Switzerland) We find the zymosan experiments attractive since they have a bearing on our own experiments.

We were wondering. *In vitro*, zymosan causes decay of macrophages, to some extent at least. It is not only a trigger to activate these cells, but some of them also die. Could there be dead macrophages *in vivo* in the liver which then cause increased release and turnover of new macrophages?

van Furth: That might well be. I do not know. We have looked at the liver cells in suspension which have eaten the zymosan. The zymosan can be seen in these cells for a long period of time, and they look quite healthy. We have no indication of an increased 'dead' percentage, but we have never really done a trypan blue exclusion comparison of normal cells and zymosan. We should perhaps do it to check, but we have not done it.

On the next point that was made in one of Monday's papers—if zymosan is injected intravenously, there is uptake and stimulation of new cells which come from the bone marrow, and I would think, although we have not studied it, that after zymosan there is the same type of blockade as was demonstrated in this work. That might be because cells are blocked because they have eaten so much, or it might be because some of the cells die off.

8

Lymphocyte-mediated eosinophilia in guinea pigs with delayed hypersensitivity to a chemical

W. E. PARISH AND E. LUCKHURST (UK)

INTRODUCTION

Eosinophilia is a common feature of anaphylactic reactions. There is no certain knowledge of the stimuli eliciting increased numbers of eosinophils in the blood and tissues, but more is known of the lymphocyte-mediated proliferation of eosinophils in the bone marrow, and increased numbers in the blood.

Passive transfer of eosinophilia by lymphocytes from sensitized to normal inbred or irradiated rats or mice showed conclusively that T or thymus-dependent lymphocytes mediate increased numbers of eosinophils in the blood[1-5]. Treatment of the recipients with antilymphocyte sera or immuno-suppressive drugs before transfer of the sensitized lymphocytes[6], or treatment of the lymphocytes with anti-theta sera[5] which inhibit T-cell activity, also abolishes the stimulus to eosinophilia transferred by the sensitized cells.

We have reported that citraconic anhydride induces delayed hypersensitivity, and eosinophilia of the blood and bone marrow; sensitized lymphocytes adoptively transfer all these phenomena to normal syngeneic recipients, and treatment of the lymphocytes with antilymphocyte (thymocyte) globulin or puromycin destroys their ability to transfer delayed hypersensitivity and eosinophilia (Reference 7 and below).

Furthermore the sites of delayed hypersensitivity skin responses on challenge with citraconic anhydride become infiltrated by eosinophils. Excision of these sites at 6 h, before they contain eosinophils, and implantation of the skin in the peritoneal cavity of normal guinea pigs results in increased numbers in the peritoneum of the recipient 24 h later.

85

MATERIALS AND METHODS

Guinea pigs

The Lister colony inbred from Porton stock since 1956. Guinea pigs from a commercial source (Tuck & Son, Rayleigh, Essex) and strain XIII guinea pigs, some bought, others bred.

Eosinophil counts

Blood eosinophils were counted as before using Eosin Y[8], and in bone marrow preparations[7].

Anti-guinea pig lymphocyte globulin

This material from rabbits immunized with guinea pig thymocytes was described previously[7].

Hapten–protein conjugates

The DNP guinea pig albumin was a conjugate of 2,4-dinitrofluorobenzene and guinea pig albumin prepared in cold alkali. Citraconic anhydride was either conjugated directly with guinea pig albumin and precipitated with N HCl, or with albumin oxidized by performic acid[7]. The conjugated antigens were used in the skin tests of the recipients sensitized by passive transfer of lymphocytes, and for peripheral blood leukocyte migration inhibition tests.

Sensitization of guinea pigs

Guinea pigs sensitized to 2,4-dinitrochlorobenzene (DNCB) and to citraconic anhydride (CA) in the tests reported in Table 8.2 were injected thrice with 1% of the antigen in olive oil at 7-day intervals. On each occasion two injections of 0.05 ml were made intradermally. On the 14th day after the last injection the animals were challenged by topical application of 0.05% DNCB in acetone, or CA in dioxane.

Guinea pigs sensitized as donors of peritoneal lymphocytes (Table 8.4) were immunized as above, but 0.1 ml was injected at each site, which was followed by topical application on the last injection sites, and on three further sites at 3-day intervals when 0.1% antigen was applied. All showed strong reactions. They were injected intraperitoneally with 10 ml paraffin oil at the time of the last antigenic stimulation and killed 3 days later to harvest the peritoneal exudate cells.

86

Separation and treatment of lymphocytes for transfer

The preparation of DNCB and CA sensitized lymphocytes from the peritoneal exudate cells for passive transfer to normal recipients has been described in detail[7].

The lymphocytes were separated from other peritoneal cells on nylon wool columns, to prepare pools, one sensitized to DNCB, one to CA. The results of the pool sensitized to CA are presented. This was divided into four samples: (1) untreated (Eagle's with 10% normal guinea pig serum), (2) treated with medium containing 1/1000 normal globulin (NG), (3) with medium containing 1/1000 antilymphocyte globulin (ALG), and (4) with medium containing 5 μg puromycin/ml cell suspension[7].

Recipients (Table 8.3) received 5 to 7 × 10[7] cells intravenously and the residuum, about 2 × 10[8] intraperitoneally, donor:recipient ratio 4.2:1, four recipients per group, total 24.

Implantation of skin with delayed hypersensitivity

Guinea pigs strongly sensitized to DNCB which elicited delayed hypersensitivity without eosinophilia, and CA which elicited delayed hypersensitivity with eosinophilia, were challenged over a large area of shaved skin with 0.05% DNCB in acetone or 0.05% CA in dioxane as appropriate. Six hours later the animals were killed, the treated skin excised, pinned out, and the stratum corneum and much of the epidermis removed by a knife with the action of a dermatome. This removed all the outer squames, which probably bound most of the antigen applied. The subcutaneous surface was then gently scarified, to facilitate release of any soluble substances. The skin was then cut in portions and 2 g implanted in the peritoneal cavity of normal strain XIII anaesthetized recipients, as described previously[9]. Peripheral blood eosinophil counts were made on the day before and the day after implantation. Peritoneal lavage to determine the number of eosinophils in the peritoneal cavity was done on the freshly killed animals by injecting 10 ml physiological saline containing 20 IU heparin/ml[8]. For this test it was considered that one post-test examination to be compared with the nonimplanted controls was more appropriate than doing pre-implantation counts on each animal, which reduces the number of eosinophils[8].

RESULTS

Antigens eliciting eosinophilia at sites of delayed hypersensitivity responses (summary and findings)

During studies on properties of activated lymphocytes and on tissue changes in delayed hypersensitivity, it was observed that the challenge skin responses induced by some antigens were frequently infiltrated by or surrounded by eosinophils. The skin responses elicited by other antigens were not, or were rarely infiltrated by eosinophils. A summary of these incidental findings is presented in Table 8.1.

Table 8.1 Antigens which did or did not elicit local eosinophilia when inducing delayed hypersensitivity skin responses

Antigens	Sensitization		Challenge		Eos. lesion
	Inj.	Top.	Inj.	Top.	
Tuberculoprotein (PPD)	+	−	+	−	−
Bovine gamma-globulin aggregated (BGG)	+	−	+	−	−
Potassium dichromate (K$_2$Cr$_2$O$_7$)	+	−	+	−	−
Ascaris	+	−	+	−	+
Dinitrochlorobenzene (DNCB)	+	&/or +	−	+	−
Citraconic anhydride (CA)	+	&/or +	−	+	+
Phthalic anhydride (PA)	+	&/or +	−	+	+

Inj.: injection.   Top.: topical application.   Eos.: eosinophils entering the challenge site.

All the antigens were tested on various numbers from 12 to more than 200 of the Dunkin–Hartley closed colony of guinea pigs at the Lister Institute. When the PPD, BGG, DNCB and CA antigens were tested on guinea pigs obtained from a commercial source, there was more individual variation in the degree of sensitivity induced by the same regimens of immunization as used for the Lister Institute animals. Nevertheless, when comparing the results of groups of the commercial animals, rather than of individuals, eosinophils were seen in significant numbers only in the animals sensitized to CA.

Evidence of delayed hypersensitivity was confirmed in nearly all the animals by histology of the skin challenge sites and by macrophage migration inhibition tests. Further indirect evidence in tests on some animals, including lymphocyte transformation, macrophage aggregation, and macrophage surface adhesion, confirmed that the animals had delayed sensitivity to the appropriate antigen.

The amount and physical state of the antigen influences the response of the immunized animals. Tuberculoprotein in 10 μg amounts in complete Freund's adjuvant, or bound to latex particles, or in alum, or in solution, induced delayed hypersensitivity; the greatest responses in adjuvant treated animals, less in animals with other antigens, and almost none in animals injected with soluble antigen. There were variable amounts of agglutinins, and increasing amounts of IgGl anaphylactic antibodies especially in animals treated with antigen in alum or in solution. There was a very slight increase of eosinophils in the blood of the guinea pigs receiving antigen in alum, otherwise no eosinophilia occurred in the blood or skin test sites after these regimens of sensitization.

A freeze-press soluble total extract of Ascaris, also injected in 10 μg amounts by the same procedures, induced delayed hypersensitivity as for the tuberculoprotein; none being elicited when soluble antigen without adjuvant was injected. There were greater amounts of IgGl antibodies than in animals sensitized to tuberculoprotein, and some IgE antibodies, especially in the group sensitized with Ascaris in alum. Eosinophilia was elicited in the blood and at the skin test sites of guinea pigs in all groups except that receiving antigen in Freund's adjuvant.

Eosinophilia elicited in animals sensitized to *Ascaria* antigen cannot be attributed to any special property of the antigen, because the response could have been conditioned by previous exposure of the animals to helminth parasites with antigens in common with Ascaris.

This would not apply in animals sensitized to chemical haptens.

Eosinophilia induced concomitantly with delayed hypersensitivity to a chemical hapten

Strain XIII guinea pigs required for compatible cell transfer tests, were compared with those of the Lister colony for their susceptibility to delayed hypersensitivity, and to eosinophilia of the blood and bone marrow after sensitization to DNCB and to CA by three courses of injection.

Both CA and DNCB induced delayed hypersensitivity as seen in the skin responses to topical challenge on the 14th day after sensitization, which was confirmed by blood leukocyte migration inhibition tests when the animals were killed one day later. The DNCB induced greater sensitivity, as judged by both tests, than CA.

Sensitization by CA elicited increased numbers of eosinophils in the blood of Lister colony and strain XIII guinea pigs; the greatest number appearing on the 3rd day after the third sensitizing injection (Table 8.2) and decreasing by the 13th day post sensitization. The details are published elsewhere[7]. Sensitization to DNCB did not elicit eosinophilia.

Changes in the percentage of eosinophils in the bone marrow reflected the changes in the numbers appearing in the blood. Three days after the last antigen sensitization to CA there was a mean of 12.2% in the bone marrow of the Lister animals, and 10.3% in the marrow of strain XIII animals. The increased number of eosinophils remained above that of the presensitization observations and of the controls. There was no increase in eosinophils in the bone marrow of animals sensitized to DNCB (Table 8.2).

Eosinophils infiltrated the delayed hypersensitivity reaction sites of the skin of animals sensitized to, and challenged topically by, CA when the skin was examined 24 h after challenge, but not to sites challenged by DNCB in animals sensitized to that antigen. In animals from the Lister colony sensitized to CA the mean number of eosinophils per 12×40 fields at CA challenged sites was 21, and at the nonspecific DNCB antigen site on the contralateral

Table 8.2 Change in number of eosinophils in blood and bone marrow on 3rd day after sensitization, compared to pre-sensitization results, related to leukocyte migration inhibition at end of test

| Guinea pigs | Sensitizing antigen | No./group | Change eos. 3rd day post sens.[2] | | Blood LMI[3] (% migration) |
			Blood (no/mm³)	Bone Marrow (%)	
Lister colony	DNCB	6	+31	−1.4	38
	CA	6	+191	+8.2	46
	Nil	28	+5	−0.2	112 (DNCB)
Strain XIII	DNCB	6	+9	−0.6	58
	CA	6	+99	+7.4	50
	Nil	8	−1	−0.7	97 (CA)

[1] DNCB: dinitrochlorobenzene.   CA: citraconic anhydride

[2] Difference in number eosinophils/mm³ blood and % in bone marrow on 3rd day after 3rd antigen injection compared to pretest results

[3] % mean inhibition of migration of buffy coat leukocytes. Cells from each animal tested with antigen were compared with cells from the same animal without antigen, in triplicate. Lister nil group tested with the DNCB–albumin conjugate, and the strain XIII nil group with CA–albumin conjugate, demonstrating that the antigens were not toxic

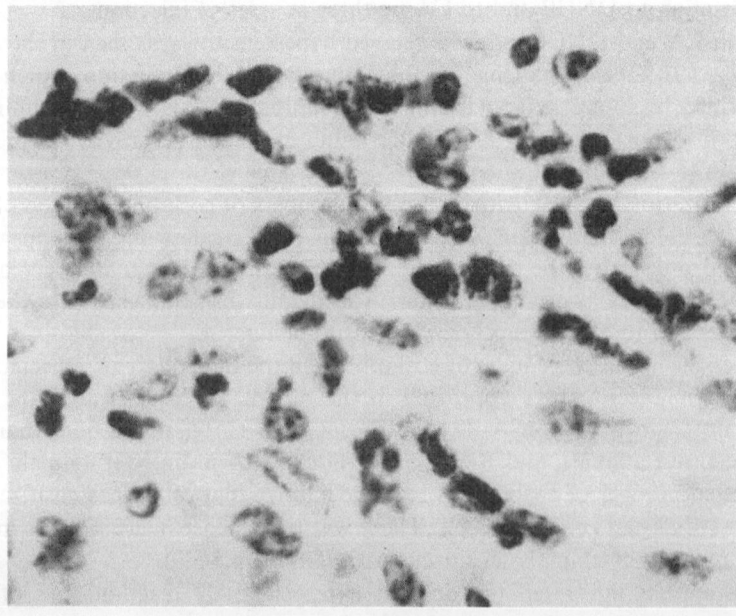

Figure 8.1 Numerous eosinophils (the dark cells) infiltrating the periphery of a delayed hypersensitivity skin response to topical application of citraconic anhydride. The eosinophils tend to accumulate round large, basophilic, mononuclear cells. Stained Chromotrope 2R, ×1040

side, 9. Similarly in strain XIII guinea pigs there were mean of 14 eosinophils per field at the CA challenged site, and 5 at the DNCB challenged site.

The eosinophils at the skin reaction sites tended to accumulate round the edge of the perivascular accumulations of mononuclear cells, being more evident near vessels with small numbers of mononuclear cells rather than greatly infiltrated areas (Figure 8.1). There was also a tendency for the eosinophils to cluster round large strongly basophilic mononuclear cells, particularly groups of them, and not in the areas which contained predominantly small lymphocytes.

Transfer of stimulus to blood and bone marrow eosinophilia to normal animals by peritoneal exudate lymphocytes

Strain XIII guinea pigs were exquisitely sensitized to DNCB or to CA (Methods). Peritoneal leukocytes were obtained three days after the last antigenic stimulation, and passed through columns of nylon wool to prepare two pools, one from donors, sensitized to DNCB, and one from those sensitized to CA. Table 8.3 shows the outline of the test. Samples of each pool

Table 8.3 Outline of procedure and results of transferring to normal recipients, lymphocytes from donor syngeneic guinea pigs sensitized to dinitrochlorobenzene (DNCB) or to citraconic anhydride (CA)

	DNCB		CA	
DONORS	delayed hypersensitivity		delayed hypersensitivity	
	no eosinophilia		with eosinophilia	
	peritoneal lymphocytes		peritoneal lymphocytes	
	untreated	ALG or	untreated	ALG or
	or NG	puromycin	or NF	puromycin
	Inject into normal recipients			
RECIPIENTS	DH	nil	DH	nil
	no eosinophilia		with eosinophilia	

DH: delayed hypersensitivity.   NG: normal globulin.   ALG: antilymphocyte (thymocyte) globulin

were untreated, or treated with normal rabbit globulin (control), rabbit anti-guinea pig lymphocyte (thymocyte) globulin or with puromycin. Only the results of treating the CA sensitized animals are presented here in detail.

Recipients injected intravenously and intraperitoneally with DNCB-sensitized lymphocytes which were untreated showed specific delayed hypersensitivity but no eosinophilia. Lymphocytes from CA-sensitized donors, untreated, or treated with normal globulin, passively transferred delayed hypersensitivity, and induced eosinophilia of the blood and of the bone marrow. Antilymphocyte globulin and puromycin destroyed these activities of the lymphocytes (Table 8.4 from Reference 7).

Table 8.4 Eosinophilia and delayed hypersensitivity on transferring peritoneal lymphocytes untreated or after treatment with antilymphocyte globulin or puromycin, from sensitized to normal strain XIII guinea pigs

Donor		Recipients					
Sensitization	Treatment[1] lymphocytes	No. eos. blood[2] −1d	+6d	% eos. marrow[3] −1d	+6d	DH (mm), +7d[4] DNCB	CA
DNCB	nil	32	19	2.8	3.1	14	4
CA	nil	35	146	3.4	7.1	3	11
	NG	31	127	3.1	6.2	2	10
	ALG	28	21	3.5	3.0	4	5
	puromycin	33	42	2.6	3.1	2	2
Nil	nil	38	44	2.9	2.5	nd	nd

Reprinted from *Clin. Exp. Immunol.*[7]

[1] Treatment of lymphocytes before transfer with NG, normal rabbit globulin; ALG, rabbit antilymphocyte globulin
[2] Mean number of eosinophils/mm^3 blood at −1d, 1 day before; and +6d, 6 days after injection of lymphocytes
[3] Mean % eosinophils of nucleated cells in bone marrow at 1 day before and 6 days after injection of lymphocytes
[4] Mean size (mm) of erythematous induration of delayed hypersensitivity skin test response. All animals showed some response to the appropriate antigen
Four recipients per group; total 24

The sensitized lymphocytes transferred to the recipients a stimulus to increased maturation of eosinophils in the bone marrow, and a stimulus to release them into the circulation spontaneously, without antigenic challenge.

The transfer of the large numbers of lymphocytes made the skin of the recipients slightly susceptible to antigen nonspecific irritation, so that the control nonspecific antigen elicited reactions of 2–5 mm size 24 h after the skin test (Table 8.4). This did not occur when smaller numbers of lymphocytes were transferred in other groups of recipients tested with the same antigens in the same manner[7].

Failure of sera from sensitized animals to elicit eosinophilia

Sera of the strain XIII guinea pigs sensitized to DNCB and to CA failed to elicit eosinophilia of the blood or bone marrow when injected intravenously into normal commercial-bred guinea pigs (Reference 7 and to be published). There was a slight increase in the number of eosinophils in the blood, which was considered too small to be significant, following injection of sera of guinea pigs sensitized by multiple antigenic stimulators of CA and obtained 3 days after the last.

Peritoneal eosinophilia following implantation of skin with delayed hypersensitivity and eosinophilia

Fresh anaphylactic lung implanted in the peritoneal cavity of normal guinea pigs elicits eosinophilia in the blood and in the peritoneal cavity of the recipient within 24 h[9,10]. Implantation of normal lung rarely does so; it usually reduces the number of circulating eosinophils[9]. We therefore took skin of the sensitized animals 6 h after topical challenge with the chemical hapten to detect any substance in the test sites that could elicit eosinophilia in the normal recipients.

Normal guinea pigs had a mean of 246 eosinophils/mm³ peritoneal lavage fluid, which is consistent with previous tests[8]. Implantation of normal skin reduced the number of circulating eosinophils, and the mean number in the peritoneal fluid to 88 (Table 8.5).

The delayed hypersensitivity skin responses in animals sensitized to, and challenged with, DNCB were not infiltrated by eosinophils. When skin so treated was implanted in the peritoneal cavity of the normal recipients, the number of circulating eosinophils was reduced, and the number recovered from the peritoneal cavity was less than found in the control, nonimplanted animals. These results apply to skin of DNCB-sensitized animals tested with CA, or CA-sensitized animals tested with DNCB.

When the 6-h skin reaction sites of CA-sensitized animals, challenged with CA, were implanted, the number of circulating eosinophils was decreased, but the number recovered from the peritoneal cavity was nearly twice that of the normal, nonimplanted control animals (Table 8.5).

Table 8.5 Number of eosinophils per mm³ in peripheral blood or peritoneal fluid after implantation of skin from animals with delayed hypersensitivity to DNCB or to CA, or skin of PCA sites

Implantation sensitization with challenge ag.	Number recipients	Number eosinophils in	Pre-test −1 day	Post-test +1 day
Nil	5	Blood	28	26
		Peritoneum	246	
Normal skin	3	Blood	34	12
		Peritoneum		88
DNCB with DNCB	4	Blood	31	14
		Peritoneum		91
DNCB with CA	3	Blood	38	13
		Peritoneum		82
CA with CA	4	Blood	28	19
		Peritoneum		483
CA with DNCB	3	Blood	34	16
		Peritoneum		94
PCA with CA	3	Blood	29	14
		Peritoneum		79
PCA with BPA	4	Blood	32	21
		Peritoneum		98

Implantation. DNCB, dinitrochlorobenzene. CA, citraconic anhydride. BPA, bovine plasma albumin. PCA, passive cutaneous anaphylaxis

Skin of animals sensitized to the first antigen and challenged with the second. Otherwise skin sensitized by serum for PCA

Number of eosinophils reported on day before implantation, and the day after

Though few eosinophils infiltrate these delayed hypersensitivity sites at 6 h, compared to the large number at 24 h after challenge, it was necessary to determine if the increase in eosinophils in the recipients was due to attraction of the recipients' eosinophils, or release of eosinophils of the donor that had infiltrated the skin site before excision. To examine this possibility, skin was taken from sites of passive cutaneous anaphylaxis 18 h after challenge, when there are the greatest number of eosinophils infiltrating the site in animals with 100 or more circulating eosinophils/mm^3 blood. Implantation of these skin samples containing many more eosinophils than present in the 6-h delayed hypersensitivity responses, did not result in eosinophilia of the blood or peritoneum of the recipients (Table 8.5).

At 18 h after passive cutaneous anaphylaxis challenge, any mast cell anaphylactic eosinophil-attracting substance would be dissipated or inactivated. Nevertheless, samples of the implanted skin were recovered after the test and examined histologically. Though some eosinophils, and monocytes, adhered to the fibrin laid down over the pieces of skin, there was no significant penetration by eosinophils. Therefore the reduction in number in the peritoneal cavity was not due to eosinophils infiltrating the implanted skin.

An incidental observation of the histology of the implanted skin, was that most of the implanted tissue was still living.

Procedures inhibiting the activity of skin eliciting peritoneal eosinophilia

It was not possible to show that a soluble, diffusible substance mediated the eosinophilia of the peritoneum of guinea pigs implanted with skin from the early, 6-h, phase of the delayed hypersensitivity response to CA. Skin enclosed in Millipore filters reduced the number of eosinophils in the peritoneum and in the blood (Table 8.6), as seen previously in tests with anaphylactic lung in chambers[9].

Killing the tissue cells by freezing and thawing, or by incubating the skin

Table 8.6 Inhibition of peritoneal eosinophilia induced by citraconic anhydride-challenged skin. Effects of Millipore chambers, freezing, or treating with puromycin

Implantation and treatment of skin	Number eosinophils in	Pre-test −1 day	Post-test +1 day
Challenge skin	Blood	19	4
	Peritoneum		398
Challenge skin in chambers,	Blood	24	2
1.0 μm pore size	Peritoneum		111
Challenge skin frozen and thawed	Blood	17	0
	Peritoneum		68
Challenge skin puromycin treated	Blood	23	11
	Peritoneum		98

Three recipients in each test
Number of eosinophils on day before implantation, and the day after

in medium containing puromycin also destroyed the ability of the skin to attract eosinophils into the peritoneal cavity, indicating that actively synthesizing cells are necessary for this phenomenon.

DISCUSSION

Adoptive transfer of blood and bone marrow eosinophilia

It was shown that blood eosinophilia can be induced in normal guinea pigs by transfer of lymphocytes from compatible inbred sensitized donors, as has been demonstrated in rats[1] and mice[3,4]. It was further shown that the transferred lymphocytes induced increased eosinopoiesis in the bone marrow. This had previously been shown to occur when rats were actively sensitized[11].

The lymphocytes adoptively transferring the stimulus to eosinopoiesis and eosinophilia were almost certainly T-cells, because peritoneal exudate cells of sensitized animals contain many more T- than B-cells. One passage of cells down a nylon wool column removed most B-cells, and the antilymphocyte globulin we used was prepared from guinea pig thymocytes[7]. The treatments of the lymphocytes that abolished the transfer of delayed hypersensitivity, which is T-cell mediated, also abolished the stimulus to eosinophilia in the recipients.

The stimulus to eosinophilia, though occurring concomitantly with delayed hypersensitivity, appears to be an independent phenomenon and may be mediated by different clones of T-cells. Delayed hypersensitivity without eosinophilia was induced by DNCB, and in the CA-sensitized individuals the magnitude of the delayed hypersensitivity skin responses and of the inhibition of migration of blood leukocytes was not related to the number of circulating eosinophils or their proportion of the bone marrow cells. Observations in tests with several antigens indicated that some antigens are more potent than others in mediating eosinophilia with delayed hypersensitivity (Table 8.1). Those that were the more potent in mediating eosinophilia were also more potent at stimulating formation of anaphylactic antibodies. This applies also to the two chemicals used to sensitize the guinea pigs in this study. CA readily stimulates formation of anaphylactic antibodies[12,13], whereas DNCB is a weaker stimulant to formation of antibody[12].

The sera of the sensitized animals did not induce a significant eosinophilia of the blood, and passive cutaneous anaphylaxis does not induce a significant increase in the bone marrow (Reference 7 and to be published). Furthermore, experimentally eosinophilia occurs before, or when, the first antibody is detected, and there may be fewer eosinophils when an animal forms larger amounts of antibody. IgE tends to be an early response to stimulation by some antigens, and to disappear quickly.

We have postulated[7] that T-helper cells, possibly carrier-specific for haptens, activate B-cell precursors, particularly those that will later mature to synthesize IgE. The activated B-cell precursors synthesize a substance that mediates eosinophilia. If this does occur the stimulus to increased eosinopoiesis is either an indirect effect following excessive mobilization of eosinophils into the circulation, or a direct effect on the marrow stem cells. Once formed, the increased number of eosinophils in the marrow remains a reserve of mature cells for any future anaphylactic reaction.

In vivo eosinophil-attracting activity of allergic skin

Peritoneal implantation of skin from animals sensitized to, and challenged by CA, a chemical which elicits both delayed hypersensitivity and eosinophilia, results in increased numbers of eosinophils in the peritoneum 24 h later.

Animals implanted with nonallergic skin, or skin not active for eosinophils, had reduced numbers of eosinophils in the blood and peritoneum 24 h later. The cause of the decrease in number was not fully examined in this investigation as not being strictly relevant to the phenomenon studied. However, previous experience showed that the decrease in the number in the blood was associated with increased numbers in the lungs and spleen of the recipient, where they are thought to accumulate due to increased adhesiveness generated by a transient generalized inflammatory response to the implantation of excised living tissue. Skin is particularly active in this respect. The decrease in number in the peritoneum was not due to eosinophils infiltrating the implanted skin, which was examined histologically. Some cells became enmeshed in the fibrin film covering the pieces of skin, but more eosinophils were seen on the skin that was 'eosinophil-activating' than 'eosinophil-inactive'. Many other eosinophils probably degenerated during the inflammatory response for 24 h after implantation.

It is concluded that the decrease in number of peritoneal eosinophils following the implantation of normal, or 'eosinophil-inactive' skin is due to degeneration of the existing cells during the inflammatory response. The increase in number following implantation of the 'eosinophil-active' skin reflects an attraction of cells in greater number than necessary to replace those that have degenerated.

The origin and nature of the substance attracting the eosinophils is not known, but its presence seems to depend upon living, actively synthesizing cells, because killing the tissue by freezing, or treating it with puromycin, inhibited the activity.

We believe that the eosinophil-attracting properties of the CA-sensitized and challenged skin result from stimulation of B-lymphocyte precursors that would eventually mediate formation of antibody, particularly IgE anaphylactic antibody. T-helper cells appear necessary to activate the B-cell precursors[14,15]. In the CA-induced delayed hypersensitivity responses, T-helper cells activate the B-cell precursors, which during their transformation to B-cells, synthesize an eosinophil-promoting substance in the site. This probably resembles their activity on bone marrow stem cells.

Evidence for this contention is based on:

(i) Intraperitoneal challenge of sensitized animals results in clusters or rosettes of eosinophils round large, sometimes binucleate mononuclear cells[16-18]. They also adhere to similar cells in the milk spots of anaphylactic mesentery[19], or in human asthmatic peribronchial connective tissue[18].

(ii) Granulomata induced by intravenous injection of particles of Ascaris become surrounded by eosinophils[19]. Subsequent examination showed these granulomata to contain cells synthesizing immunoglobulin. Peritoneal granulomata that become infiltrated by eosinophils contain blast cells and plasma cells[20], presumably synthesizing antibody.

(iii) Re-injection of antigen into a site of delayed hypersensitivity leads to eosinophil infiltration of the site[21]. Furthermore, lymphocytes from animals with delayed hypersensitivity release a substance which when incubated with antigen–antibody complexes formed of the same antigen inducing the hypersensitivity, results in selective attraction of eosinophils[22].

These findings are consistent with our evidence reported above and previously[7] that sites of delayed hypersensitivity mediated by a substance, CA, that readily induces formation of antibody, become infiltrated by eosinophils, whereas sites of delayed hypersensitivity mediated by a weaker antibody-inducing antigen are not so infiltrated.

Many tests show that eosinophilia associated with formation of granulomata precedes antibody formation. Therefore the active substance is likely to be synthesized by B precursor cells, possibly the large basophilic mononuclear cells that attract eosinophils in the peritoneum or milk spots.

References

1. Basten, A. and Beeson, P. B. (1970). Mechanism of eosinophilia. II. Role of the lymphocyte. *J. Exp. Med.*, **131**, 1288
2. Spry, C. J. F. (1972). The origin, kinetics and distribution of large lymphocytes from the thoracic duct of rats with trichinosis. *Immunology*, **22**, 663
3. McGarry, M. P., Speirs, R. S., Jenkins, V. K. and Trentin, J. J. (1971). Lymphoid cell dependence of eosinophil response to antigen. *J. Exp. Med.*, **134**, 801
4. Speirs, R. S., Gallagher, M. T., Rauchwerger, J., Heim, L. R. and Trentin, J. J. (1973). Lymphoid cell dependence of eosinophil response to antigen. II. Location of memory cells and their dependence upon thymic influence. *Exp. Hematol.*, **1**, 150
5. Ponzio, N. M. and Speirs, R. S. (1975). Lymphoid cell dependence of eosinophil response to antigen. VI. The effect of selective removal of T or B lymphocytes on the capacity of primed spleen cells to adoptively transferred-immunity to tetanus toxoid. *Immunology*, **28**, 243
6. Boyer, M. H., Basten, A. and Beeson, P. B. (1970). Mechanism of eosinophilia. III. Suppression of eosinophilia by agents known to modify immune responses. *Blood*, **36**, 458
7. Parish, W. E., Luckhurst, E. and Cowan, S. I. (1977). Eosinophilia V. Delayed hypersensitivity, blood and bone marrow eosinophilia, induced in normal guinea-pigs by

adoptive transfer of lymphocytes from syngeneic donors. *Clin. Exp. Immunol.* **28,** (In the press.)

8. Parish, W. E. (1972). Eosinophilia. I. Eosinophilia in guinea-pigs mediated by passive anaphylaxis and by antigen–antibody complexes containing homologous IgGla and IgGlb. *Immunology,* **22,** 1087

9. Parish, W. E. and Coombs, R. R. A. (1968). Peripheral blood eosinophilia in guinea-pigs following implantation of anaphylactic guinea-pig and human lung. *Brit. J. Haematol.* **14,** 425

10. Litt, L. (1960). Studies in experimental eosinophilia. II. Induction of peritoneal eosinophilia by the transfer of tissues and tissue extracts. *Blood,* **16,** 1330

11. Spry, C. J. F. (1971). Mechanism of eosinophilia. V. Kinetics of normal and accelerated eosinopoiesis. *Cell Tissue Kinet.,* **4,** 351

12. Chase, M. W. (1947). Studies on the sensitization of animals with simple chemical compounds. X. Antibodies inducing immediate-type skin reactions. *J. Exp. Med.,* **86,** 489

13. Hunziker, N. (1964). Experimental eczema. Passive transfer of guinea-pig's hypersensitivity to citraconic anhydride. *Dermatologica,* **129,** 475

14. Tada, T. and Okumura, K. (1971). Regulation of homocytotropic antibody formation in the rat. V. Cell cooperation in the anti-hapten homocytotropic antibody response. *J. Immunol.,* **107,** 1137

15. Hamaoka, T., Katz, D. H. and Benacerraf, B. (1973). Hapten-specific IgE antibody responses in mice. II. Cooperative interactions between adoptively transferred T and B lymphocytes in the development of IgE response. *J. Exp. Med.,* **138,** 538

16. Speirs, R. S. (1963). Antigenic material: persistence in hypersensitive cells. *Science,* **140,** 71

17. Speirs, R. S. (1964). The action of antigen upon hypersensitive cells. *Ann. N.Y. Acad. Sci.,* **113,** 819

18. Parish, W. E. (1974). Substances that attract eosinophils *in vitro* and *in vivo* and that elicit blood eosinophilia. In: *Antibiotics and Chemotherapy,* vol. 19, Chemotaxis: its biology and biochemistry. Basel: Karger, p. 233

19. Parish, W. E. (1970). Investigations on eosinophilia. The influence of histamine, antigen–antibody complexes containing γ_1 or γ_2 globulins, foreign bodies (phagocytosis) and disrupted mast cells. *Br. J. Dermatol.,* **82,** 42

20. Athanassiades, T. J. and Speirs, R. S. (1972). Granuloma induction in the peritoneal cavity. A model for the study of inflammation and plasma-cytopoiesis in nonlymphatic organs. *Res. J. Reticuloendothel. Soc.,* **11,** 60

21. Arnason, B. G. and Waksman, B. H. (1963). The retest reaction in delayed sensibility. *Lab. Invest.,* **12,** 737

22. Cohen, S. and Ward, P. A. (1971). *In vitro* and *in vivo* activity of a lymphocyte and immune complex-dependent chemotactic factor for eosinophils. *J. Exp. Med.,* **133,** 133

Discussion 8

<table>
<tr>
<td>J. L. Turk:
(UK)</td>
<td>Citraconic anhydride is the contact agent that was used in one of the earliest transfer studies, in about 1947 (Merrill Chase), which reported passive transfer with serum of a contact sensitivity. However, when picryl chloride was used there was no passive transfer with serum of contact sensitivity. As far as I remember, to do this test with the citraconic anhydride the skin was scratched.

Citraconic anhydride was shown to be a compound that had produced a lot of circulating basophils; more than the other contact agents.

There is something special about this contact agent. It appears to produce antibody, homocytotropic antibody, at an earlier stage than other sensitizers, and a considerable amount of the reaction appears to be produced by antibody.

Mr. Parish has said that he could not transfer the eosinophilia with serum in his experiment, but if he had transferred with B-cells he might have got local production of antibody. I know that he says that he got rid of B-cells, or he talks about pure T-cells, by passing through a nylon wool column, but is he absolutely sure that he got rid of all his B-cells?</td>
</tr>
<tr>
<td>Parish:</td>
<td>No. But I still think it holds. Professor Turk's grasp of the literature is, as usual, fantastic. In that early work these were divided up—citraconic anhydride was one—into chemicals of high reactivity, and substances like DNCB of medium reactivity.

What seems to be happening is that the B-cell precursor, which is activated by T-cells, is related to IgE antibody, and there are many numerous references of the degree of eosinophilia correlated with the amount of IgE in man.

May I take my thesis one step further. What is happening is that T-cells are involved where they are acting directly with the B-cell precursor, but, by stimulating the eosinophilia at the very beginning of the stimulation, by the time there is antibody and the individual is anaphylactically sensitive, if there should be an anaphylactic event in that person, then there are a large number of mature eosinophils in the bone marrow ready to be mobilized, to be released into the blood to carry out any beneficial function that eosinophils have in anaphylaxis.</td>
</tr>
<tr>
<td>H. Hahn:
(West Germany)</td>
<td>I am most enthusiastic about Mr. Parish's paper. When we used sheep red blood cells as an antigen, and using the regimen of cyclophosphamide before sensitization we induced delayed hypersensitivity against sheep red cells. The lesions which we could elicit in the donor animals, the sensitized animals—mice—were very much as those which Mr. Parish has described. There were quite a number of eosinophils in them. When that reaction of peritoneal exudate cells was transferred, the same thing happened, namely eosinophilic infiltration of the recipient animals after antigen challenge.</td>
</tr>
</table>

We tried to use these peritoneal T-lymphocytes—presumably T-lymphocytes are anti-θ sensitive—and to assess their 'helper' cell function for IgG production, and they were completely negative.

There may be a difference in these T-cells as to 'helper' cell function, and their mediating delayed hypersensitivity, but they certainly elicit eosinophilic histology in mice.

Parish: I started thinking that it was a function of T-cells together but I think that there is definitely a sub-clone or sub-line of T-cells mediating delayed hypersensitivity and preparing an animal for an eosinophil stimulus.

Chairman: It is an interesting and important point which does not seem to be settled. There are other stimuli of delayed hypersensitivity which are thought to be extremely efficient, and which, so far as I know, also do not elicit eosinophilia.

There is something peculiar about those stimuli that do it, in terms of ordinary contact hypersensitivity. This then brings up the possibility of a helper function of a rather special kind, presumably in making, or the formation of, a special class or a subclass of antibody which may be involved in recruiting the eosinophils.

It is interesting because the original experiments of Bastin, Beeson, and others carried with them the implication that this was just another T-cell function. There was nothing special about it.

M. Jasani: The question arises out of the observation of the effect of ALG on the
(UK) peritoneal exudate cells. I am not too happy to accept that ALG would affect sensitized lymphocytes. Is there any possibility that when the challenging substance is injected into the peritoneal cavity, non-sensitized T-cells could be exuding, more because of the inflammatory reaction set up by the antigen. ALG would then utilize those 'helper' function cells rather than sensitized T-lymphocytes.

Parish: We only injected paraffin oil into the peritoneal cavity—no antigen in that—in order to get the peritoneal exudate cells.

It is known that such a peritoneal exudate is rich in cells able to transfer delayed hypersensitivity, which is why we did it.

We transferred the activity by draining-lymph node cells also.

P. C. Wilkinson: It looks as though the eosinophils are really moving towards the blast
(UK) cells—whatever they were. Were they B-cells?
Parish: I do not know. That is my one line for what happens. I have found these large cells. I like to think of them as B-cell precursors. I do not know what they are.

Wilkinson: Whatever they are, is it possible to demonstrate that eosinophils really do chemotax towards such a cell. It might be difficult in a chamber, but I am sure that it could be done with a time-lapse film.

Parish: It would be interesting to try.

9

A role for L-lymphocytes in chronic inflammation

DAVID A. HORWITZ (USA)

There is a large body of evidence that lymphocyte-mediated immune responses perpetuate certain chronic inflammatory reactions. Under conditions when T-lymphocytes become sensitized to host antigens, they develop the capacity to kill host cells and can produce mediators which activate macrophages to cause tissue destruction. Further, appropriately sensitized T-lymphocytes can induce B-cells to produce autoantibodies which may result in tissue injury by other mechanisms. In the synovitis of rheumatoid arthritis, T- and B-lymphocytes are present in abundant numbers[1].

This report deals with a newly described population of human blood lymphocytes that possess an especially avid receptor for the Fc fragment of IgG. This population was first described by Frøland and Natvig who reported that Fc receptor lymphocytes which bound human erythrocytes coated with Ripley anti-Rh IgG lacked other T- and B-cell markers. These Fc receptor lymphocytes were effective mediators of antibody-dependent lymphocyte cytotoxicity[2].

At that time there was a considerable controversy about normal values for B-lymphocytes in normal human subjects as detected by immunofluorescence techniques[3]. This controversy was resolved by Dr. Peter Lobo in my laboratory. He found that there was not one, but two populations of lymphocytes bearing easily detectable surface immunoglobulin. The first, B-cells, had membrane-incorporated, surface-stable Ig determinants. A second equally numerous population lacked membrane-incorporated determinants, but had surface-labile determinants[4]. They were named L-lymphocytes because of the surface-labile IgG determinants and are defined in Table 9.1. This population appears to be the same as the one described by Frøland and Natvig[2] and reports from the laboratories of Grey[5], Winchester[6] and Nussenweig[7] have also confirmed their existence.

Table 9.1 Definition of L-lymphocytes

---

1. Have membrane-labile immunoglobulin determinants
2. Reversibly bind small aggregates of IgG found in normal human serum (bound at 4° C and eluted at 37° C)
3. Comprise 10–20% of the total lymphocyte population

In this report methods to quantitate L-lymphocytes will be described, the surface properties which distinguish L-lymphocytes from B-lymphocytes will be reviewed, and the functional properties of L-lymphocytes will be summarized. Finally a model for a possible role of L-lymphocytes in chronic inflammation will be proposed.

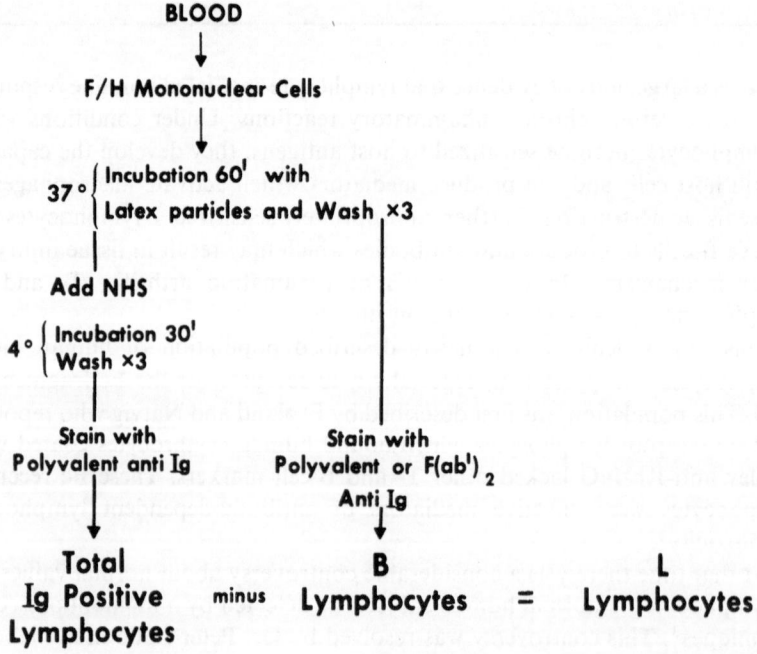

Figure 9.1 Procedure to quantitate B-cells and L-cells by immunofluorescence

Figure 9.1 illustrates the method to quantitate B-cells and L-cells by immunofluorescence. Lymphocytes are first incubated at 37 °C in the presence of latex particles. This procedure elutes small aggregates of IgG from the cell membrane and also labels phagocytic monocytes. After the cells are extensively washed at 37 °C they are divided into two portions. The first is stained with a polyvalent goat antihuman serum. This procedure stains the number of B-cells, those with surface-stable Ig determinants. In our experience these values are identical with the use of $F(ab')_2$ antibodies to stain cells. The second tube is incubated at 4 °C with purified IgG or with normal human serum as a source of IgG. After washing, the cells are then stained. This pro-

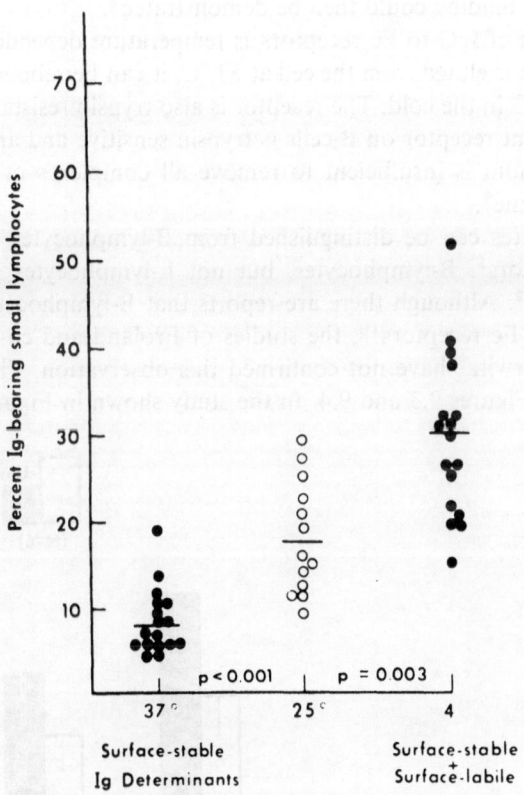

Figure 9.2 Per cent Ig-bearing lymphocytes found in normal adults. Cells were pre-incubated at the temperatures indicated before staining

cedure gives the total number of Ig-bearing cells. The number of L-lympho-cytes is calculated by subtracting the number of B-cells from the total stained.

Figure 9.2 demonstrates the two populations of Ig-bearing lymphocytes in healthy hospital personnel. When lymphocytes were first pre-incubated and washed at 37 °C, 8% of the cells were positive. After the cells were incubated with normal human serum at 4 °C, an additional 10–20% became Ig positive.

If lymphocytes were prepared and stained at room temperature, an inter-mediate value was observed.

Further studies revealed that only IgG was passively bound to the cells. Purified IgM or IgG did not fix to the cell surface[4]. Moreover, only aggregated IgG could attach to the cell membrane. Studies with agarose chromatography revealed that monomeric IgG was not bound. It should be emphasized, however, that within hours after fractionation aggregation occurred spon-taneously and binding could then be demonstrated[8].

The fixation of IgG to Fc receptors is temperature dependent and revers-ible. After IgG is eluted from the cell at 37 °C, it can be rebound by exposing the cells to IgG in the cold. The receptor is also trypsin resistant. In contrast, the complement receptor on B-cells is trypsin sensitive and an incubation at 37 °C for 30 min is insufficient to remove all complexes of IgG from the B-cell membrane[9].

L-lymphocytes can be distinguished from B-lymphocytes by three other surface receptors[1]. B-lymphocytes, but not L-lymphocytes have receptors for mouse C3[2]. Although there are reports that B-lymphocytes bind aggre-gated IgG by Fc receptors[10], the studies of Frøland and co-workers[11] and Lobo and Horwitz[9] have not confirmed this observation. These points are illustrated in Figures 9.3 and 9.4. In the study shown in Figure 9.3, comple-

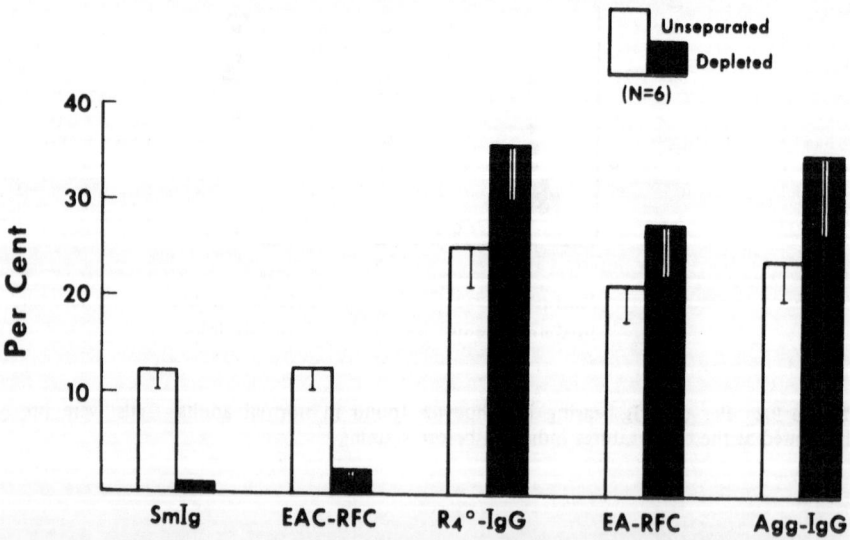

Figure 9.3 The effect of depleting complement receptor lymphocytes on Ig positive and Fc positive lymphocytes

Abbreviations: SmIg—membrane-incorporated Ig; EAC—sheep erythrocytes coated with IgM antibody and mouse complement; R4°–IgG—a receptor binding serum IgG at 4° C; Agg–IgG, aggregated guinea pig IgG detected by indirect immunofluorescence; EA— human erythrocytes coated with Ripley anti CD IgG

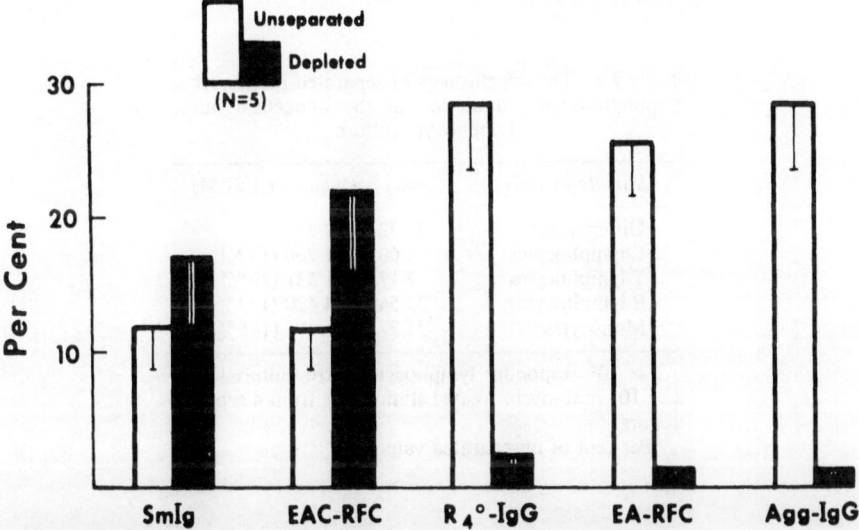

Figure 9.4 The effect of depleting lymphocytes forming Ripley rosettes on B-cells and Fc positive lymphocytes as detected by other methods. Abbreviations are the same as Figure 9.3

ment receptor (EAC rosette forming) lymphocytes were removed from other cells by density gradient centrifugation and the effect of the procedure on numbers of lymphocytes with surface-stable Ig (B-cells) and Fc receptor lymphocytes was examined. Three methods were used to detect Fc receptors: (1) binding of serum IgG, (2) binding of aggregated guinea pig IgG (measured by indirect immunofluorescence) and (3) the formation of EA Ripley rosettes. C3b and C3d rosettes were formed by mixing lymphocytes with sheep erythrocytes sensitized with 19S antibody and mouse complement. It can be seen that depletion of C3 receptor cells also depleted B-cells, but increased Fc receptor cells as measured by all methods.

In the study shown in Figure 9.4, depletion of lymphocytes forming Ripley (EA) rosettes also removed Fc receptor cells detected by other methods. This procedure, however, increased the number of Ig positive and C3 positive lymphocytes.

Studies with double-label immunofluorescence further substantiated these findings. When lymphocytes were pretreated to remove all exogenous Ig and then incubated with aggregated guinea pig IgG, lymphocytes staining for both membrane-incorporated Ig and Fc receptors were rare.

The mixed lymphocyte culture has revealed the third important difference in surface markers on L- and B-lymphocytes. B-cells, but not L-cells, are effective stimulators of allogeneic lymphocytes (Table 9.2). L-lymphocytes, then, lack Ia-like surface antigens that are present on B-cells[12].

Table 9.3 summarizes the surface markers found on the four major mononuclear populations. L-lymphocytes and monocytes have high avidity Fc

Table 9.2 The effectiveness of separated mononuclear populations as stimulators in the allogeneic mixed lymphocyte culture

Stimulator cells	Counts per minute ($\pm$SEM)
Unseparated	24 324 $\pm$ 5 850
L-lymphocytes	3 605 $\pm$ 1 266 (15%)*
T-lymphocytes	7 173 $\pm$ 1 531 (29%)
B-lymphocytes	33 549 $\pm$ 4 420 (137%)
Monocytes	35 271 (145%)

2×10^5 responder lymphocytes were cultured with 2×10^5 mitomycin-treated stimulators from 4 separate donors
*Per cent of unseparated value

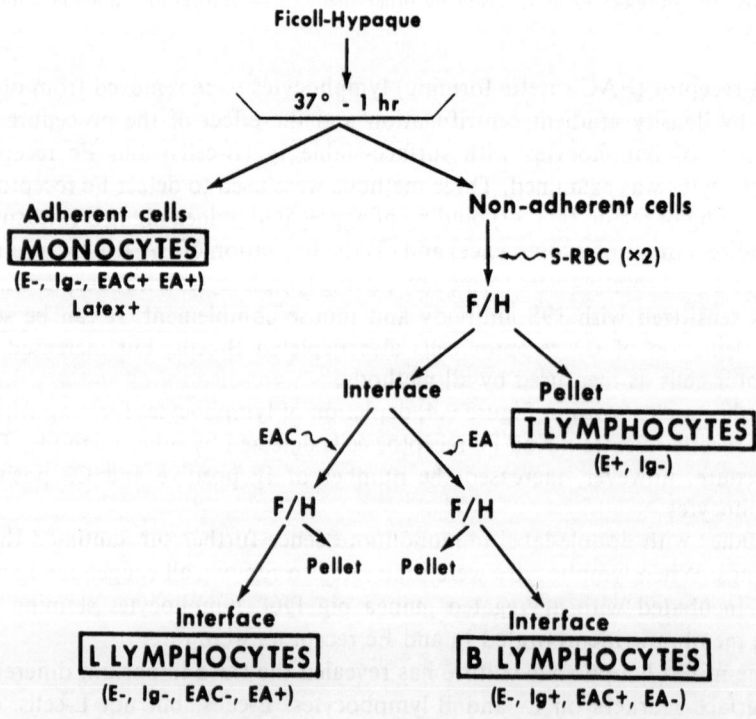

Figure 9.5 Procedure for separating four human mononuclear cell populations

receptors which bind serum IgG. The monocyte Fc receptor differs from the L-lymphocyte receptor in the reversibility of binding IgG. This immuno-globulin is not readily eluted from the monocyte membrane after a short elution at 37 °C. Unlike L-lymphocytes both B-lymphocytes and monocytes have C3 receptors and are excellent stimulators in the mixed lymphocyte culture. Therefore, when lymphocytes from healthy subjects are examined each of these mononuclear populations has a characteristic profile.

Table 9.3 Surface markers on mononuclear populations

	L-lymphocyte	B-lymphocyte	T-lymphocyte	Monocyte
Sheep RBC (E) rosette	0	0	+	0
Membrane-incorporated immunoglobulin	0	+	0	0
High avidity Fc receptor for IgG	+	0	0	+
C3 receptor (EAC$_{mo}$ rosette)	0	+	0	+
Strong stimulator in mixed lymphocyte culture	0	+	0	+

It has been possible to isolate each of these four populations and examine their functional properties. Figure 9.5 shows the method employed. Mono-cytes are first removed from the populations by allowing them to adhere to petri dishes. Next, E rosette-forming T-cells are removed from non-T-cells by pelleting them through Ficoll-Hypaque. B- and L-lymphocytes are then prepared by negative selection by taking advantage of the fact that L-lymphocytes do not form complement rosettes and B-cells do not form Ripley rosettes.

The possibility was considered that L-lymphocytes were monocyte pre-cursors. Purified L-lymphocytes, however, did not develop phagocytic capa-city after 3 days of culture, they were non-specific esterase negative and could not replace monocytes in helping T-lymphocytes respond to polyclonal mitogens[12].

The possibility was considered that L-lymphocytes were B-cell precursors. Others have reported that E rosette negative, surface Ig negative lymphocytes

Table 9.4 Functional properties of the lymphocyte populations

	L-lymphocyte	B-lymphocyte	T-lymphocyte
Develop into Ig synthesizing cells	0	+	0
Proliferate in mixed lymphocyte culture	0	0(+)	+
Proliferate in response to polyclonal mitogens	0	0(+)	+
Effector in antibody-dependent lymphocyte cytotoxicity	+	0	0(+)

Parentheses indicate secondarily activated cells

isolated by another method become Ig positive in culture[13]. We have been unable to confirm this observation. L-lymphocytes do not develop surface immunoglobulin after 3 days of culture. Moreover, unlike B-lymphocytes, they cannot be induced to form cytoplasmic Ig by pokeweed mitogen[12].

The possibility was also considered that L-lymphocytes were an E rosette negative T-cell or T-cell precursor. L-lymphocytes were unable to proliferate in response to polyclonal mitogens or antigens, and were unable to function as responders in mixed lymphocyte culture (Table 9.4). These findings do not exclude the possibility that L-lymphocytes may be a subset of regulatory T-cells. This possibility, however, is unlikely.

Purified L-lymphocytes, B-lymphocytes, T-lymphocytes and monocytes were examined for cytotoxic effects on human lymphocytes sensitized with IgG alloantibodies or heterologous antilymphocyte serum. Only L-lymphocytes were effective mediators of ADCC (Figure 9.6). Although the precise relationship of L-lymphocytes to T- and B-cells is not known, Table 9.4 clearly

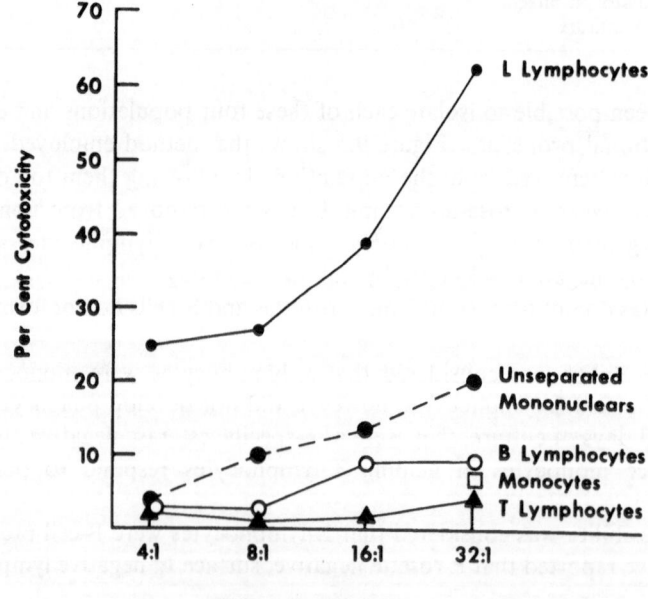

Figure 9.6 The effectiveness of three lymphocyte populations and monocytes in antibody-dependent cellular cytotoxicity. Unstimulated ^{51}Cr labelled lymphocytes coated with IgG antibody served as the target cells

indicates that the functional profile of L-lymphocytes is unlike that of the other lymphocyte populations.

Perlmann has operationally defined lymphocytes that mediated ADCC as K-cells. Although L-lymphocytes have K-cell activity, the terms should not be considered synonymous. B-lymphocytes obtained by positive selection[14] (which may be partially activated) and antigen-activated T-cells[15] have K-cell activity. An emerging picture, then, is that non-activated L-lymphocytes and activated T- and perhaps B-cells may each have K-cell activity.

The role of L-lymphocytes in the immune response is not known. Besides their cytotoxic potential they may modulate the activities of other lymphocyte populations. Ryan and Henkart have recently shown that immobilized immune complexes inhibit B-lymphocyte mitogenesis[16] and that this effect was dependent on intact Fc fragments. Although the immune complexes were thought to be acting directly on B-cells, an alternative possibility is that they induced L-lymphocytes to inhibit B-cell proliferation. L-lymphocytes, then, may become suppressor cells under the appropriate conditions.

L-lymphocytes may also perpetuate inflammatory reactions by their cytotoxic capacity. A possible role for L-lymphocytes in the cycle of chronic inflammation is schematically shown in Figure 9.7. There are three major

L lymphocytes in chronic inflammation

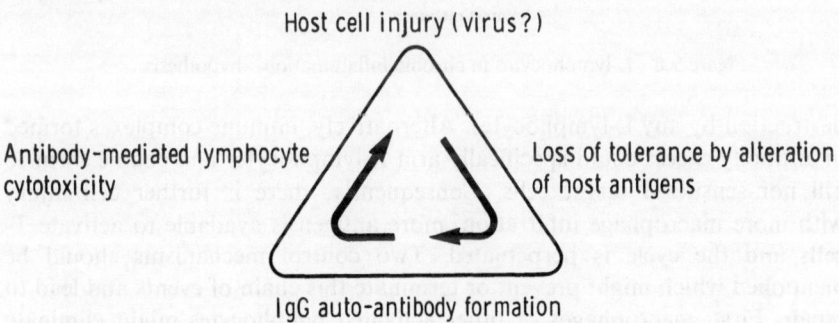

Figure 9.7 A possible role for L-lymphocytes in chronic inflammation

components to this model. (1) In line with the current concepts of immune tolerance as developed by Allison[17] and Weigle[18], host antigens are altered by poorly defined trigger factors, such as viruses, in a manner which can now activate host T-lymphocytes. (2) B-lymphocytes then produce IgG autoantibodies with specificities against host-cell surface components. (3) The IgG antibodies allow L-lymphocytes to combine with host target cells and kill them.

The model is presented in more detail in Figure 9.8. Host antigens could be directly altered by virus, or macrophage degradation of virus-killed cells could secondarily alter host antigens. (2) Antigen-activated T-cells in cooperation with macrophages produce a soluble factor which stimulates B-cells to produce IgG autoantibodies. (3) IgG autoantibodies then enable L-lymphocytes to kill target cells by non-specific and specific mechanisms. IgG antibodies could either fix to cell surface antigens and prime these cells for

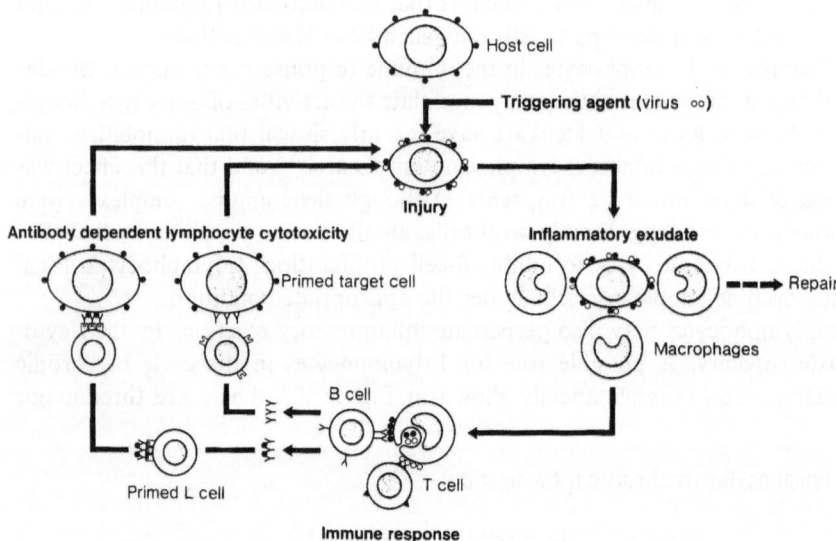

Figure 9.8 L-lymphocytes in chronic inflammation—hypothesis

destruction by any L-lymphocytes. Alternatively, immune complexes formed in antibody excess could specifically arm L-lymphocytes and enable them to kill non-sensitized target cells. Consequently, there is further cell injury with more macrophage infiltration, more antigen is available to activate T-cells and the cycle is perpetuated. Two control mechanisms should be mentioned which might prevent or terminate this chain of events and lead to repair. First, macrophages or other activated lymphocytes might eliminate the triggering agent. Secondly, L-lymphocytes or other suppressor mechanisms might prevent autoantibody production by B-cells before sufficient antibody becomes available for a vigorous autoimmune hypersensitivity reaction.

It is apparent that L-lymphocytes may play a major role in the normal regulation of immune responses as well as participate in pathological responses. Further studies of this intriguing population are clearly needed.

Acknowledgements

Supported by Grants from The John A. Hartford Foundation Grant #74466 USPHS Grant #AM 11766. Dr. Horwitz is a recipient of The Clinical Scholar Award from The Arthritis Foundation.

References

1. Ziff, M. (1974). Relation of cellular infiltration of rheumatoid synovial membrane to its immune response. *Arthr. Rheum.*, **17**, 313

2. Frøland, S. S. and Natvig, J. B. (1973). Identification of three different human lymphocyte populations by surface markers. *Transplant. Rev.*, **16**, 144
3. Warner, N. L. (1974). Membrane immunoglobulins and antigen receptors on B and T lymphocytes. *Adv. Immunol.*, **19**, 67
4. Lobo, P. I., Westervelt, F. B. and Horwitz, D. A. (1975). Identification of two populations of immunoglobulin-bearing lymphocytes in man. *J. Immunol.*, **114**, 116
5. Kurnick, J. T. and Grey, H. M. (1975). Relationship between immunoglobulin bearing lymphocytes and cells reacting with sensitized human erythrocytes. *J. Immunol.*, **115**, 305
6. Winchester, R. J., Fu, S. M., Hoffman, T. and Kunkel, H. G. (1975). IgG on lymphocyte surfaces; technical problems and the significance of a third cell population. *J. Immunol.*, **114**, 1210
7. Ehlenberger, A. G., McWilliams, M., Phillips-Quagliata, J. M., Lamm, M. E. and Nussenweig, V. (1975). Immunoglobulin-bearing and complement-receptor lymphocytes constitute the same population in human peripheral blood. *J. Clin. Invest.*, **57**, 53
8. Horwitz, D. A. and Lobo, P. I. (1975). Characterization of two populations of human lymphocytes bearing easily detectable surface immunoglobulin. *J. Clin. Invest.*, **56**, 1464
9. Lobo, P. L. and Horwitz, D. A. (1976). An appraisal of Fc receptors on human blood, B and L lymphocytes. *J. Immunol.*, **117**, 939
10. Dickler, H. B. and Kunkel, H. G. (1972). Interaction of aggregated γ-globulin with B lymphocytes. *J. Exp. Med.*, **136**, 191
11. Frøland, S. S., Natvig, J. B. and Michaelson, T. E. (1974). Binding of aggregated IgG by human B lymphocytes independent of Fc receptors. *Scand. J. Immunol.*, **3**, 375
12. Horwitz, D. A. and Garrett, M. A. (1977). Distinctive functional properties of human blood L lymphocytes; a comparison with T lymphocytes, B lymphocytes and monocytes. *J. Immunol.*, **118**, 1712
13. Chess, L., Levine, H., MacDermott, R. P. and Schlossman, S. F. (1975). Immunologic functions of isolated human lymphocyte populations. VI. Further characterization of the surface Ig negative, E-rosette negative, (Null cell) subset. *J. Immunol.*, **115**, 1483
14. Brier, A. M., Chess, L. and Schlossman, S. F. (1975). Human antibody dependent cellular cytotoxicity: isolation and identification of a sub-population of peripheral blood lymphocytes which kill antibody coated autologous target cells. *J. Clin. Invest.*, **56**, 1580
15. Saal, J. G., Rieber, E. P., Hadam, M. and Riethmuller, G. (1977). Lymphocytes with T cell markers cooperate with IgG antibodies in the lysis of human tumour cells. *Nature*, **265**, 158
16. Ryan, J. L. and Henkart, P. A. (1976). Fc receptor-mediated inhibition of murine B lymphocyte activation. *J. Exp. Med.*, **144**, 768
17. Allison, A. C., Denman, A. M. and Barnes, R. D. (1971). Cooperating and controlling functions of thymus-derived lymphocytes in relation to autoimmunity. *Lancet*, **ii**, 135
18. Weigle, W. O. (1971). Immunological unresponsiveness and autoimmunity. *Clin. Exp. Immunol.*, **9**, 437

Discussion 9

G. Loewi: (UK)	I enjoyed this very much and it was plainly explained. I have three brief questions. Has Dr. Horwitz looked at a lymphocytic leukaemia? What sort of targets have been used, and how widespread is the target effect? Is the L-cell permissive for viral replication?
Horwitz:	I do not know the answer to the last question. In answer to the second question, the only targets that we have looked at have been non-activated, non-stimulated human lymphocytes, and we have not looked at chronic lymphatic leukaemia. There is a whole series of experiments under investigation right now and these will confirm that they will kill other targets. Other lymphocyte populations may also kill different targets.
O. Voisin: (France)	May we have some information or comment on the killer activity of T- and B-cells in the AMCC phenomenon—the one that Dr. Horowitz said made his slide out of date?
Horwitz:	The experiment with which I am familiar was reported in the last *Leucocyte Culture Conference* (from Peter Perlman's Laboratory). Those involved had been able to look at individual K-cells by a plaque technique and there is evidence that both T- and B-cells are able to have killer capacity. Dr. Allison recently visited that laboratory and may have other comments.
Chairman:	They have a plaque system where they can identify individual lytic cells in the centre of large numbers of target cells. The majority of these do not have either T- or B-characteristics of the usual kind, but some do. It would be very nice to think of the L-cell as being the only antibody-dependent cytotoxic effector cell, or K-cell, but this appears to be an oversimplification. There are certain things we know. For example, that monocytes will kill erythrocytes very well, but not other target cells. But it looks as though both subpopulations of B- and T-cells have some antibody-independent cytolytic activity (according to Perlman—others have made similar observations).
Horwitz:	As more of this evidence becomes available, there will be two important factors: the target cells selected for study and the state of activation of the cell. Unactivated L-cells have K-cell activity. Partially or completely activated B- and T-cells may acquire K-cell activity.
S. Normann: (USA)	I am curious to know if there is any relationship between this cell and the recently-described natural killer cells that are also presumed to be a subpopulation of lymphocytes. More specifically, do the L-cells require antibody for their killing? Are they only active in an antibody-dependent killing mode, or can they also exhibit killing in the absence of antibody, as has been attributed to the K-cell.

Horwitz:	That is an excellent question. These studies are now under really active process and I have no further information at this time.
D. Freed: (UK)	Is Dr. Horwitz saying that there is a degree of auto-immunity every time one gets a virus infection?
Horwitz:	There may be. Certainly with virus infections like measles and infectious mononucleosis, if one looks carefully one may find rheumatoid factor, and one can find DNA anti-nuclear factor antibodies which appear transiently and then go away.

I am not aware of this being a general phenomenon for all viral infections, but for many viruses certain auto-immune phenomena have been demonstrated.

Freed:	It would make a nice overall picture to fit auto-immunity into the overall scheme of things. But what then gives rise to a long-term auto-immune disease with chronic progression? A failure of some sort of suppressor?
Horwitz:	I would say a failure of some type of control mechanism, whether it is elimination of the agent, or of turning out or turning off the cells which can make auto-antibodies.
P. C. Wilkinson: (UK)	Those cells which mediate antibody-mediated cytotoxicity—what part do they play in parasitic infestations? I am thinking of some kind of a defence model, rather than an auto-immune model, for explaining what the cells do.

May I also ask what 'L' stands for? What are L-lymphocytes?

Horwitz:	It comes from the way that we describe these cells. These have membrane labile IgG determinants. They are capable of picking up IgG in serum at 4 °C, and if treated to 37 °C it goes away.
Chairman:	May I answer the other point?

On parasites: Cryptococcus is killed by antibody and K-cells. There was a Paper in the *Journal of Immunology* recently. Leishmania, trypanosomes, and some other parasites are also killed by this mechanism. Malaria parasites apparently not, as far as we know.

What is interesting is that for certain helminths (i.e. schistosoma), the very small forms that come in from the skin, the effector mechanism there appears to be via eosinophils. In other words, in the presence of antibody eosinophils will kill those cells. It looks as though in the same way as different cell types are killed by different effector cells, so are different parasites. Eosinophils are not good at killing those that we have been discussing, but they are very good at killing schistosoma. Cryptococcus, and some others, are quite sensitive to the K-cell type system in the presence of antibody and K-cells.

K. Fehr: (Switzerland)	I believe that Dr. Horwitz has data about human disease. Could he elaborate on the findings in rheumatoid arthritis and in lupus? There are many null cells in synovial fluid. Are these those L-cells described here?
Horwitz:	We have not fooked at synovial fluid, but in rheumatoid arthritis and systemic lupus erythematosus 98% of blood lymphocytes can be classified by these techniques. Null cells, cells which lack any marker, are rare in my experience. We found in essence that in SLE, RA and scleroderma there is a non-selective decrease in T-, B- and L-lymphocytes.

Our control groups were infections: tuberculosis, viral infections and pneumonia. In the infections, the T- and the B-cells were down, but the L-cells were normal or increased.

10

Cartilage degradation by macrophages, fibroblasts and synovial cells in culture. An *in vitro* model suitable for studies on rheumatoid arthritis

G. VAES, P. HAUSER, G. HUYBRECHT-GODIN AND
C. PEETERS-JORIS (Belgium)

INTRODUCTION

The progressive destruction of the connective tissues that comprise the joint, and particularly of cartilage, is one of the most serious consequences of chronic rheumatoid arthritis. The present evidence indicates that articular cartilage is destroyed mainly by contact with diseased synovial membrane[1] at the interface between the cells of the advancing pannus and the area of cartilage undergoing resorption[2]. Although some experimental studies suggest that the chondrocytes themselves can degrade the surrounding matrix under some circumstances[3,4], there is apparently no clear evidence in rheumatoid arthritis for the active involvement of the chondrocytes in the lysis of cartilage. The major cause of rheumatoid cartilage erosion appears to be a lysis of the cartilage matrix by infiltrating effector cells, mainly macrophages and possibly also fibroblasts[5]. The associated presence, in close contact with these cells, of abundant T- and B-lymphocytes[6] suggests that these immuno-competent cells are controlling the activity of the effector cells, possibly through the action of extravascular immune complexes[7,8] or through the secretion of lymphokines[9,10]. Under proper stimulation, the effector cells would then exert their lytic action by secreting hydrolytic enzymes able to degrade the proteoglycans and the collagen of the cartilage matrix[11-13].

To investigate the biochemical and the cytological mechanisms underlying these phenomena and to study possible direct pharmacological interference with them, we developed *in vitro* models in which either the synovial cells or the presumed main effector cells present within the synovium, namely macrophages and fibroblasts, are cultivated in contact with dead ^{35}S-labelled cartilage. The degradation of the proteoglycans and of the collagen of the cartilage matrix was followed by the release of soluble ^{35}S-labelled material and of hydroxyproline.

In this communication, an overall preliminary view of our results is presented (see also Reference 14). Their detailed description, as well as that of the methods used, will be published elsewhere.

MATERIALS AND METHODS

The cartilage substrate

Discs (± 10 mg each) of rabbit ear cartilage, biosynthetically labelled in their proteoglycans with ^{35}S, were prepared as done by Ignarro et al.[15]. The cartilage cells were killed by repeated freezing and thawing and the cartilage was washed extensively before the cultures or the enzyme assays.

The degradation of the proteoglycans was measured by the release of soluble ^{35}S-material in the medium. Under either trypsin or neutral protease (from macrophage conditioned media) digestion, the release of ^{35}S and of uronic acid (both expressed as a percentage of the total amount initially present) were similar up to about 50% degradation of the discs. As shown in Figure 10.1A and 10.1B (curves ◯), autolysis of the cartilage proteoglycans was important under the cell culture conditions but it was considerably reduced by heating the cartilage for 30 min at 60 °C.

The degradation of the collagen was measured by the loss of hydroxyproline from the cartilage over the culture period. There was no significant autolysis of the cartilage collagen over 5 days culture; this collagen was also resistant to trypsin treatment (25 μg/ml/4 days). After heating the cartilage for 30 min at 60 °C, 20–40% of the total hydroxyproline of the tissue could be released into soluble form by trypsin (see Figures 10.4 and 10.5), indicating that part of the collagen had been denatured. Therefore, degradation of native collagen was considered to occur only when the amount of hydroxyproline lost from the heat-treated cartilage during the cultures or during the assays was in excess of the maximum amount solubilized by trypsin.

Cell cultures

Mononuclear phagocytes were obtained from cultures of rabbit bone marrow in a serum-containing medium. After 6–8 days of culture, suspensions of differentiated monocytes (mononuclear cells with typical nucleus on Giemsa staining, having Fc receptors and capable of rapid phagocytosis of latex beads) were obtained which further differentiated into macrophages and adhered to the plastic wall of the culture vessel at a later stage (after 8–10 days).

116

Synovial cells were obtained following the method of Dayer *et al.*[16] from either human rheumatoid synovia or from the synovia of rabbits having an experimental Dumonde and Glynn's[17] type of immune arthritis[18]. Fibroblasts were obtained from outgrowths of rabbit skin or synovial explants in culture or directly from the carcass of rabbit embryos. Whenever necessary great care was taken in the cultures of either synovial cells or fibroblasts to eliminate possible residual activities of the trypsin or (for the synovial cell cultures) of the bacterial collagenase used to disperse the cells. This was achieved by repeated washings with excess medium containing serum. Further washings were done with normal medium to eliminate remnants of serum. Controls for residual activities of either trypsin or collagenase were run by incubating either cell lysates or samples of the last washing medium with ^{35}S-labelled cartilage; this resulted only in a minimal amount of cartilage degradation. Also cartilage degradation by living cells did usually not occur in the presence of cycloheximide (1 or 2 μg/ml).

RESULTS AND DISCUSSION

Macrophages

Non-adherent phagocytes were first cultivated during several days in the presence of the cartilage discs in a medium devoid of serum (Figure 10.1).

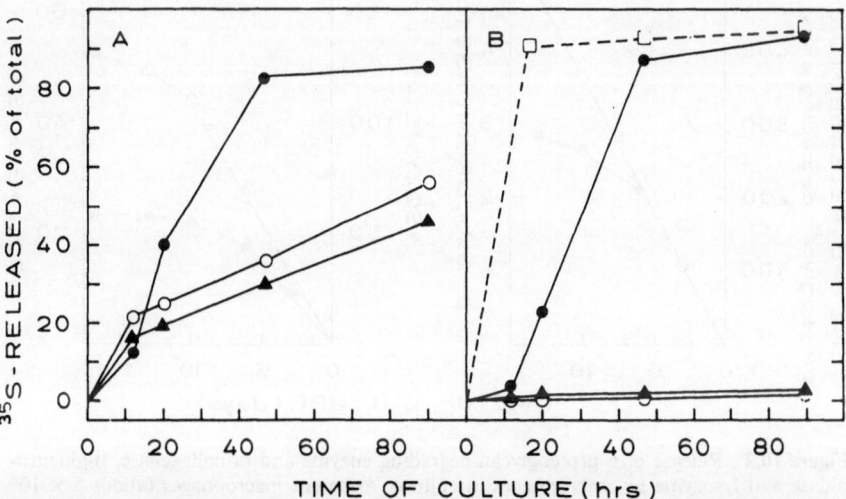

Figure 10.1 Digestion of cartilage proteoglycans by mononuclear phagocytes. Non-adherent phagocytes (5×10^5 cells), either living (●) or killed by repeated freezing and thawing (▲) were cultivated for the time indicated in 0.5 ml of a modified Dulbecco's medium, together with a disc of ^{35}S-labelled 'killed' cartilage used either as such (A) or after heat inactivation (B). Controls involved ^{35}S-cartilage incubated either without cells to evaluate autolysis (○) or with 5 μg trypsin (□). The release of ^{35}S-soluble material is expressed in percentage of the total ^{35}S-label present in the cultures. Each point is the mean of three cultures. (From Reference 14.)

In the presence of living phagocytes, an almost complete degradation of the
^{35}S-proteoglycans (but not of collagen) occurred over 2–3 days culture after
a short initial lag-phase. This effect was suppressed either by freezing and
thawing the phagocytes or by the addition of cycloheximide (1 μg/ml) to the
cultures suggesting that it depended on a protein synthesis by the cells. It
was half-inhibited by the addition of 9% (v/v) heat-inactivated fetal calf
serum to the cultures.

A search was then made for a proteoglycan-degrading enzyme in conditioned media surrounding adherent macrophages in culture by studying the
property of these cell-free media to release soluble ^{35}S-material from the
cartilage discs (Figure 10.2). Such an enzyme was indeed released by the
macrophages in an almost linear manner during the first 6 days of culture;
its release levelled off thereafter. The rate of its secretion was similar to that
of collagenase while that of lysozyme went on linearly for 10 days and that
of β-glucuronidase, for at least 14 days. After 4 days culture, insignificant
amounts of proteoglycan-degrading enzyme and of collagenase were found
within the macrophages; the whole activity was in the culture fluid. This
contrasted with the distribution of β-glucuronidase between cells (50%) and
medium (50%). Lysozyme was for 95% in the medium.

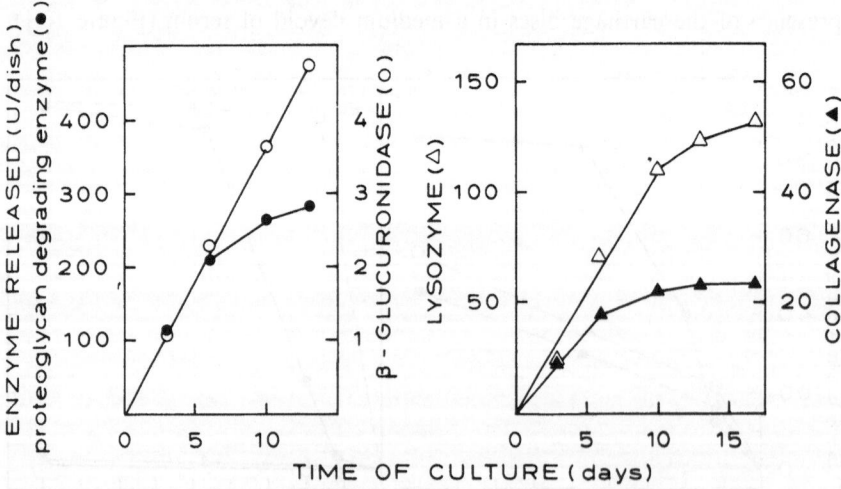

Figure 10.2   Release of a proteoglycan-degrading enzyme and of collagenase, β-glucuro-
nidase and lysozyme by macrophages in culture. Adherent macrophages (about 5×10^6
cells), obtained after 12 days culture of bone marrow cells, were further cultivated in 10 ml
of modified Dulbecco's medium. The results of the enzyme assays, done on conditioned
media obtained at the times indicated, are presented in a cumulative manner. One unit of
proteoglycan-degrading enzyme ($\bullet$) releases 1% of the total ^{35}S present in standard-
sized ^{35}S-labelled cartilage discs/h. One unit of neutral collagenase ($\blacktriangle$) degrades 1 μg of
soluble native collagen/min at 25° C[29]. One unit of β-glucuronidase ($\bigcirc$) decomposes
1 μmole of phenolphthalein glucuronidase/min under optimal conditions. Lysozyme,
assayed by measuring the initial rate of lysis of *Micrococcus lysodeikticus*, is expressed in
μg by comparison with a standard of pure egg white lysozyme ($\triangle$). (From Reference 14.)

The proteoglycan-degrading enzyme had its optimal activity on ^{35}S-cartilage around pH 7.0–7.5. EDTA (0.1 mM), cysteine (2 mM) and fetal calf serum (5%) inhibited almost completely the enzyme while azocoll (40 mg/ml) and casein (10 mg/ml) caused a 75% inhibition. Diisopropyl phosphofluoridate (2 mM), tosyl lysine chloromethyl ketone (0.5 mM), Trasylol® (50 μg/ml), soybean trypsin inhibitor (5 mg/ml) or p-chloromercuribenzoate (0.2 mM) had no effects. The ^{35}S-labelled cartilage degradation products released by the enzyme chromatographed on a Sepharose 6-B column at a position intermediate between the void volume and the ^{35}S-labelled material released by papain. Conditioned media also decreased the viscosity of solutions of proteoglycan subunits purified from bovine nasal cartilage according to Hascall and Sajdera[19]; this effect was also optimal around pH 7.0 and blocked by EDTA or cysteine.

It is thus clear that macrophages in culture are able to secrete a proteoglycan-degrading enzyme together with other enzymes whose secretion had already been demonstrated by others (for a review, see Reference 20): neutral collagenase, lysozyme and lysosomal enzymes (β-glucuronidase). The proteoglycan-degrading enzyme is not stored within the cells. Its secretion is dependent on a protein-synthesis by living cells and occurs spontaneously in our conditions over several days of culture. Its exact nature is still under investigation. However, our data suggest strongly that it is a neutral metal-dependent proteinase, that splits the protein-core of the proteoglycan subunits, releasing into soluble form intact glycosaminoglycan chains bound to peptide fragments. This proteinase appears to be distinct from other neutral proteinases secreted by macrophages under some circumstances: indeed plasminogen activator[21] and elastase[22] are both inhibited by diisopropylphosphofluoridate while collagenase[23,24] is not significantly inhibited by casein (Vaes, unpublished) and its secretion does not necessarily accompany that of the proteoglycan-degrading protease in our experience.

It is to be expected that such a proteoglycan-degrading enzyme could play an important role in the degradation of connective tissues, particularly of cartilage, under chronic inflammatory situations, such as in rheumatoid arthritis. Its role could be complementary to that played in acute inflammation by the polymorphonuclear leukocyte proteases that degrade cartilage proteoglycans[25–27]. The regulation of its secretion is under study as well as the conditions under which the cartilage collagen is being degraded by the collagenase that is secreted by the adherent macrophages.

Fibroblasts

Rabbit fibroblasts from various origins (carcass or skin from fetus; synovium or skin from young animals) were cultivated for various lengths of time and with various numbers of subculture passages before being put into culture in the presence of dead cartilage discs in a medium devoid of serum.

In some cultures, the fibroblasts slowly degraded over several days the cartilage proteoglycans (Figure 10.3A, B and C). This effect was abolished by the addition of cycloheximide (2 μg/ml). It was linked to the secretion into the surrounding medium of an enzyme that released ^{35}S-soluble material from the cartilage discs when cell-free conditioned media from these cultures were incubated together with the discs. This enzyme has its optimal activity around pH 7.0. It is completely inhibited by EDTA (10 mM) or o-phenanthroline (1 mM) while serum (0.5%) caused a 60% and cysteine (2 mM) a 35% inhibition of its activity. It may thus be similar to the proteoglycan-degrading

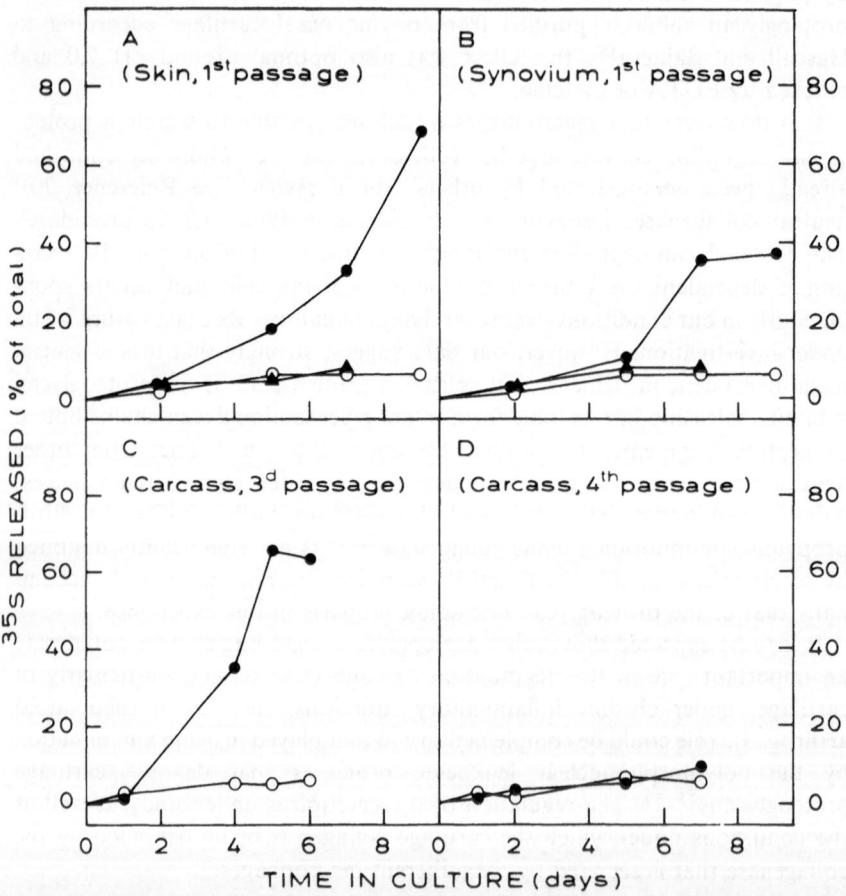

Figure 10.3 Digestion of cartilage proteoglycans by rabbit fibroblasts. Fibroblasts, obtained from outgrowths of skin (A) or synovium (B) of young rabbits or after direct trypsinization of rabbit embryo carcasses (C and D), were cultivated for the time indicated in 0.2 ml of a modified Dulbecco's medium together with a disc of ^{35}S-labelled heat-inactivated cartilage (●). Controls included heat inactivated ^{35}S-cartilage incubated either without cells to evaluate autolysis (○) or with cells in the presence of 2 μg cycloheximide/ml (▲). The release of ^{35}S-soluble material is expressed as in Figure 10.1. Each point is the mean of three cultures

proteinase secreted by the rabbit macrophages in culture; its characterization is in progress. It may be identical with a neutral metal-dependent proteinase active on azocoll, gelatin or azocasein whose secretion by rabbit synovial fibroblasts was stimulated by endocytosis[28].

However, the attack of the cartilage proteoglycans by the fibroblasts was not constantly observed. Indeed several cultures or subcultures of fibroblasts did not degrade the cartilage and did not secrete the proteoglycan-degrading enzyme over 7–10 days culture. The reasons for these differences are unknown. In some cases, it was observed that a cell line that degraded the proteoglycans after the first passages lost that property thereafter (compare C and D in Figure 10.3), indicating the possible influence of some 'ageing' processes. Attempts to stimulate the secretion of the enzyme by endocytosis of latex particles or by other means were so far unsuccessful.

Fibroblasts that degraded the cartilage proteoglycans did not degrade its collagen over 7–9 days of culture. However, cells that did attack the proteoglycans usually also secreted a neutral collagenase into their surrounding fluids but most of that collagenase was found in a latent trypsin-activatable form. Trypsin-activatable latent collagenase, first found by us in the medium surrounding bone explants in culture[29-32], was later found in the culture fluids of several types of tissues or cells, including fibroblasts[33-36]. It is tempting to speculate that the resistance of the cartilage collagen to the degradation by the fibroblasts over the first 7–9 days of culture in our experiments is due to a lack of activation of the latent collagenase released by the cells. We observed indeed that the cartilage collagen was degraded when the cartilage discs were incubated with conditioned cell-free media containing active collagenase.

Synovial cells

Synovial cells obtained from either arthritic rabbits (Figure 10.4) or rheumatoid human patients (Fig. 10.5) were put into culture together with dead cartilage discs in a medium without serum or in a medium supplemented with 0.5% heat-inactivated fetal calf serum. Primocultures of these cells digested both the proteoglycans and the collagen of the cartilage; this digestion varied from one culture to the other but it was often rapid and important as shown on Figures 10.4 and 10.5. Collagen degradation, measured by the loss of hydroxyproline from the discs, seemed usually to lag slightly behind the degradation of the proteoglycan as evaluated by the release of ^{35}S-soluble material. The degradation of the cartilage did however no longer occur when the cells were obtained after the first subculture passage. Low concentrations of serum in the culture medium inhibited slightly the degradation of both proteoglycans and collagen which proceeded then more slowly at the beginning of the cultures (Figures 10.4 and 10.5). The enzymes responsible for these phenomena as well as their source are presently under investigation.

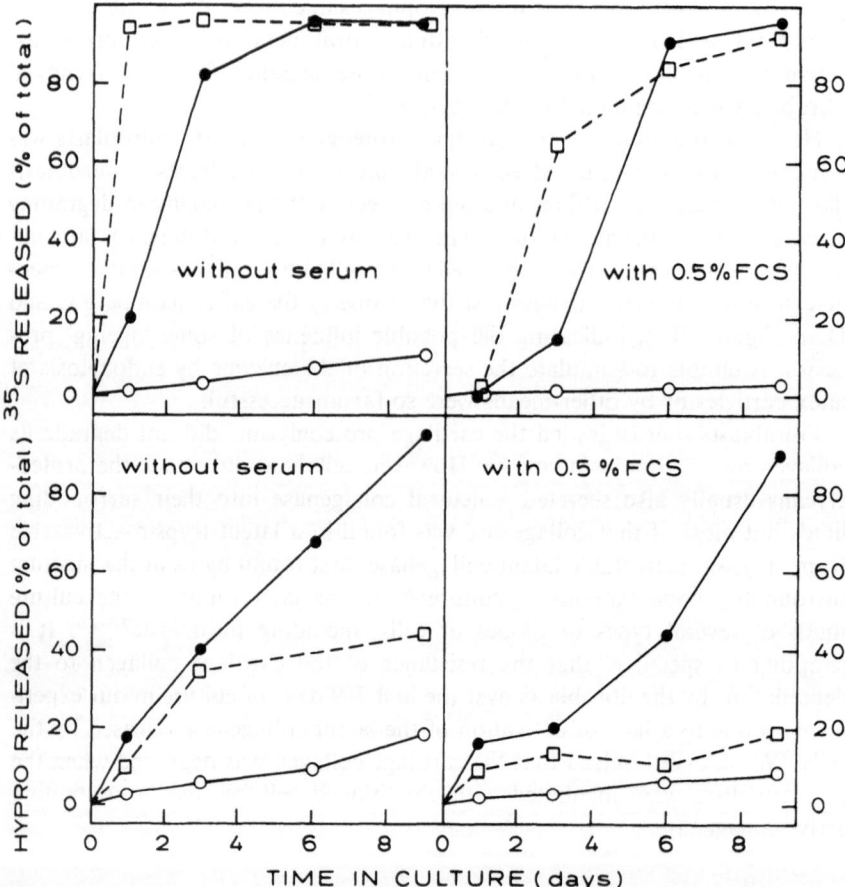

Figure 10.4 Digestion of the cartilage matrix components (collagen and proteoglycans) by synovial cells from rabbits with an experimental immune arthritis (primocultures). The cells were cultivated for the time indicated in 0.2 ml of a modified Dulbecco's medium together with one heat-inactivated ^{35}S-labelled cartilage disc (●) either in the absence of serum (left graphs) or in the presence of 0.5% fetal calf serum (right graphs). The release of ^{35}S-soluble material (upper graphs) or of hydroxyproline (lower graphs) are expressed in per cent of the total ^{35}S or hydroxyproline present in the cultures. Controls involved heat-inactivated ^{35}S-cartilage incubated either without cells (○) or in the presence of 25 μg trypsin/ml (□). Each point is the mean of three cultures

It is of interest to compare these observations with those of others who have cultivated living cartilage together with synovial cells in a similar attempt to study *in vitro* the degradation of the cartilage matrix. Hamerman *et al.*[37] added articular cartilage fragments to monolayers of rheumatoid synovial membrane cells grown in tissue culture for many generations and observed histologically after 3 weeks of incubation a loss of proteoglycans in the cartilage that did not occur with cells from normal synovia. Our experience

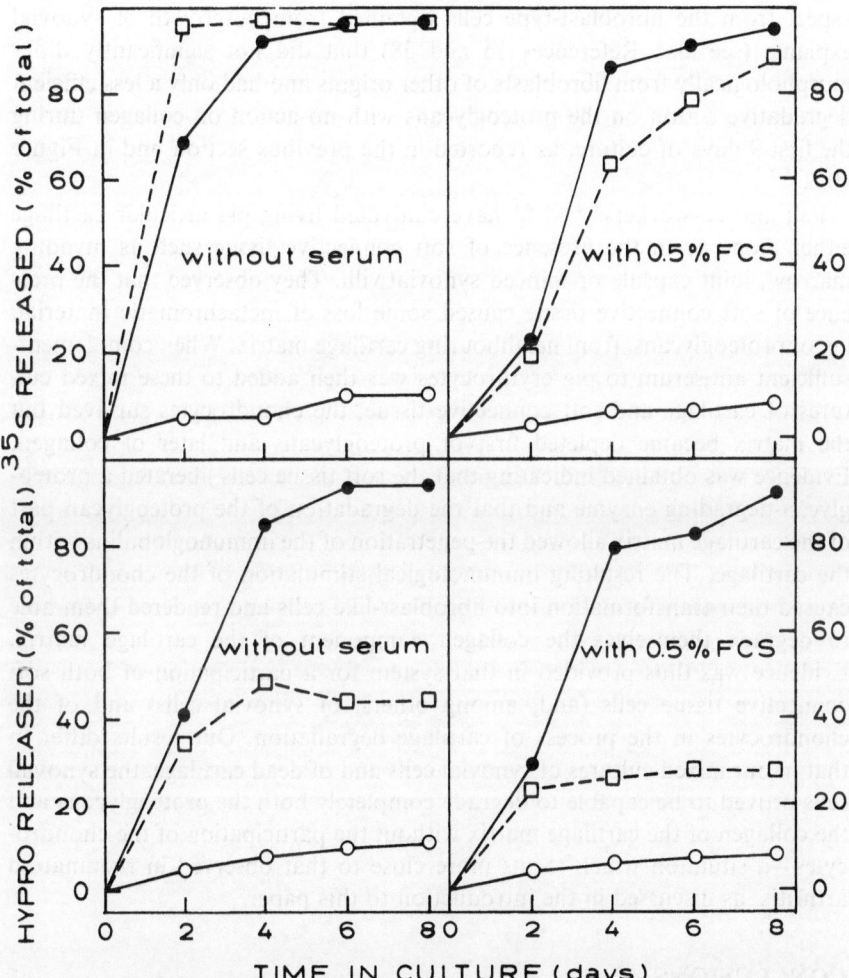

Figure 10.5 Digestion of the cartilage matrix components (collagen and proteoglycans) by human rheumatoid synovial cells in primoculture. The experimental conditions and the expression of the results are the same as indicated in Figure 10.4. Each point is the mean of three cultures containing either cells (0.5×10^6/well) and heat-inactivated cartilage (●) or heat-inactivated cartilage cultivated alone (○) or with 25 μg/ml trypsin (□)

with normal synovia is still too limited to be conclusive. However, we observed regularly the degradation of both the main components (collagen and proteoglycans) of the cartilage only during the primocultures of the synovial cells. When viewed at low power under phase contrast microscopy, the cell population at that time was much more heterogeneous than the cell population viewed later after a few subculture passages, at a time when cartilage degradation was no longer observed. Moreover, it was very different in its

123

aspect from the fibroblast-type cells obtained from outgrowth of synovial explants (see also References 16 and 38) that did not significantly differ morphologically from fibroblasts of other origins and had only a less efficient degradative action on the proteoglycans with no action on collagen during the first 9 days of culture, as reported in the previous section and in Figure 10.3.

Fell and co-workers[3,4,39–41] have cultivated living pig articular cartilage either alone or in the presence of soft connective tissue such as invading marrow, joint capsule or minced synovial villi. They observed that the presence of soft connective tissue caused some loss of metachromatic material, i.e. of proteoglycans, from neighbouring cartilage matrix. When complement-sufficient antiserum to pig erythrocytes was then added to these mixed cultures of cartilage and soft connective tissue, the chondrocytes survived but the matrix became depleted first of proteoglycans and later of collagen. Evidence was obtained indicating that the soft tissue cells liberated a proteoglycan-degrading enzyme and that the degradation of the proteoglycan part of the cartilage matrix allowed the penetration of the immunoglobulins within the cartilage. The resulting immunological stimulation of the chondrocytes caused their transformation into fibroblast-like cells and rendered them able to degrade themselves the collagen component of the cartilage matrix. Evidence was thus provided in that system for a participation of both soft connective tissue cells (and, among others, of synovial cells) and of the chondrocytes in the process of cartilage degradation. Our results differ in that in our mixed cultures of synovial cells and of dead cartilage, the synovial cells proved to be capable to degrade completely both the proteoglycans and the collagen of the cartilage matrix without the participation of the chondrocytes—a situation which seems more close to that observed in rheumatoid arthritis, as discussed in the introduction to this paper.

CONCLUSIONS

This work is only in its initial phase. However, it is apparent that it provides model systems that will prove useful for further *in vitro* studies on the cellular pathophysiology and biochemistry of joint erosion in rheumatoid arthritis as well as on possible pharmacological interactions with these processes. Indeed, it renders possible the study of the cartilage degradative processes under a variety of situations, either under the global action of the various cell types present in the diseased synovia or under the specific action of macrophages or fibroblasts, i.e. the cell types that are generally believed to be the direct source of the lytic enzymes that degrade rheumatoid cartilage matrix. Control mechanisms governing the cellular release and the extracellular actions of these enzymes are being studied as well as possible interactions between these and other cell types in the processes that lead to cartilage destruction.

Acknowledgements

This work is supported by grants from Société Rhône-Poulenc, Paris, and from the Belgian Fonds de la Recherche Scientifique Médicale. We thank Drs. P. De Nayer, Chr. Rombouts-Tindemans, J. J. Rombouts and A. Vincent who kindly supplied the human synovia for our studies.

References

1. Chaplin, D. M. (1971). The pattern of bone and cartilage damage in the rheumatoid knee. *J. Bone Joint Surg.*, **53B**, 711
2. Krane, S. M. (1974). Joint erosion in rheumatoid arthritis. *Arthritis and Rheumatism*, **17**, 306
3. Dingle, J. T., Horsfield, P., Fell, H. B. and Barratt, M. E. J. (1975). Breakdown of proteoglycan and collagen induced in pig articular cartilage in organ culture. *Ann. Rheum. Dis.*, **34**, 303
4. Fell, H. B., Barratt, M. E. J., Welland, H. and Green, R. (1976). The capacity of pig articular cartilage in organ culture to regenerate after breakdown induced by complement-sufficient antiserum to pig erythrocytes. *Calcif. Tiss. Res.*, **20**, 3
5. Kobayashi, I. and Ziff, M. (1975). Electron microscopic studies of the cartilage–pannus junction in rheumatoid arthritis. *Arthritis and Rheumatism*, **18**, 475
6. Ishikawa, H. and Ziff, M. (1976). Electron microscopic observations of immuno-reactive cells in the rheumatoid synovial membrane. *Arthritis and Rheumatism*, **19**, 1
7. Ziff, M. (1973). Pathophysiology of rheumatoid arthritis. *Federat. Proceed.*, **32**, 131
8. Zvaifler, N. J. (1974). Rheumatoid synovitis. An extravascular immune complex disease. *Arthritis and Rheumatism*, **17**, 297
9. Ziff, M. (1974). Relation of cellular infiltration of rheumatoid synovial membrane to its immune response. *Arthritis and Rheumatism*, **17**, 313
10. Stastny, P., Rosenthal, M., Andreis, M. and Ziff, M. (1975). Lymphokines in the rheumatoid joint. *Arthritis and Rheumatism*, **18**, 237
11. Barrett, A. J. (1975). The enzymatic degradation of cartilage matrix. In P. M. C. Burleigh and A. R. Poole (eds.), *Dynamics of Connective Tissue Macromolecules*, pp. 189–226. (Amsterdam: North-Holland Publ. Co.)
12. Harris, Jr., E. D. (1976). Recent insights into the pathogenesis of the proliferative lesion in rheumatoid arthritis. *Arthritis and Rheumatism*, **19**, 68
13. Vaes, G. (1977). Lysosomal enzymes and connective tissue damage of immunological origin. In T. E. W. Feltkamp (ed.), *Non-articular Forms of Rheumatoid Arthritis*. (Leiden: Stafleu.) pp. 72–76
14. Hauser, P. and Vaes, G. (1977). Synthesis and secretion by rabbit bone marrow macrophages of a neutral protease that degrades cartilage proteoglycans. *Biochem. Soc. Transact.* (In press.)
15. Ignarro, L. J., Oronsky, A. L. and Perper, R. J. (1973). Breakdown of noncollagenous chondromucoprotein matrix by leukocyte lysosome granule lysates from guinea pig, rabbit and human. *Clin. Immunol. Immunopathol.*, **2**, 36
16. Dayer, J. M., Krane, S. M., Russell, R. G. G. and Robinson, D. R. (1976). Production of collagenase and prostaglandins by isolated adherent rheumatoid synovial cells. *Proc. Natl Acad. Sci. U.S.A.*, **73**, 945
17. Dumonde, D. C. and Glynn, L. E. (1962). The production of arthritis in rabbits by an immunological reaction to fibrin. *Brit. J. Exptl Pathol.*, **43**, 373
18. Cooke, T. D. and Jasin, H. E. (1972). The pathogenesis of chronic inflammation in experimental antigen-induced arthritis. I. The role of antigen on the local immune response. *Arthritis and Rheumatism*, **15**, 327
19. Hascall, V. C. and Sajdera, S. W. (1969). Proteinpolysaccharide complex from bovine nasal cartilage. The function of glycoprotein in the formation of aggregates. *J. Biol. Chem.*, **244**, 2384
20. Davies, P. and Allison, A. C. (1976). Secretion of macrophage enzymes in relation to the pathogenesis of chronic inflammation. In: D. S. Nelson (ed.) *Immunobiology of the Macrophage*, pp. 427–461. (New York: Academic Press.)

21. Unkeless, J. C., Gordon, S. and Reich, E. (1974). Secretion of plasminogen activator by stimulated macrophages. *J. Exptl Med.*, **139**, 834

22. Werb., Z. and Gordon, S. (1975a). Elastase secretion by stimulated macrophages. *J. Exptl Med.*, **142**, 361

23. Wahl, L. M., Wahl, S. M., Mergenhagen, S. E. and Martin, G. R. (1974). Collagenase production by endotoxin-activated macrophages. *Proc. Natl Acad. Sci. U.S.A.*, **71**, 3598

24. Werb, Z. and Gordon, S. (1975b). Secretion of a specific collagenase by stimulated macrophages. *J. Exptl Med.*, **142**, 346

25. Oronsky, A., Ignarro, L. and Perper, R. (1973). Release of cartilage mucopolysaccharide-degrading neutral protease from human leukocytes. *J. Exptl Med.*, **138**, 461

26. Janoff, A., Feinstein, G., Malemud, C. J. and Elias, J. M. (1976). Degradation of cartilage proteoglycan by human leukocyte granule neutral proteases—A model of joint injury. I. Penetration of enzyme into rabbit articular cartilage and release of $^{35}SO_4$-labelled material from the tissue. *J. Clin. Invest.*, **57**, 615

27. Keiser, H., Greenwald, R. A., Feinstein, G. and Janoff, A. (1976). Degradation of cartilage proteoglycan by human leukocyte granule neutral proteases—A model of joint injury. II. Degradation of isolated bovine nasal cartilage proteoglycan. *J. Clin. Invest.*, **57**, 625

28. Werb, Z. and Reynolds, J. J. (1974). Stimulation by endocytosis of the secretion of collagenase and neutral proteinase from rabbit synovial fibroblasts. *J. Exptl Med.*, **140**, 1482

29. Vaes, G. (1972). The release of collagenase as an inactive proenzyme by bone explants in culture. *Biochem. J.*, **126**, 275

30. Vaes, G. and Eeckhout, Y. (1975). Procollagenase and its activation. In P. M. C. Burleigh and A. R. Poole (eds.), *Dynamics of Connective Tissue Macromolecules*, pp. 129–146. (Amsterdam: North-Holland Publ. Co.)

31. Gillet, Ch., Eeckhout, Y. and Vaes, G. (1977). Purification of procollagenase and collagenase by affinity chromatography on Sepharose-collagen. *FEBS Letters*, **74**, 126

32. Eeckhout, Y. and Vaes, G. (1977). Further studies on the activation of procollagenase, the latent precursor of bone collagenase. Effects of lysosomal cathepsin B, plasmin and kallikrein and spontaneous activation. *Biochem. J.*, **164**. (In press.)

33. Hook, R. M., Hook, C. W. and Brown, S. I. (1973). Fibroblast collagenase partial purification and characterization. *Invest. Ophthalmol.*, **12**, 771

34. Bauer, E. A., Stricklin, G. P., Jeffrey, J. J. and Eisen, A. Z. (1975). Collagenase production by human skin fibroblasts. *Biochem. Biophys. Res. Commun.*, **64**, 232

35. Harris, Jr., E. D., Reynolds, J. J. and Werb, Z. (1975). Cytochalasin B increases collagenase production by cells *in vitro*. *Nature*, **257**, 243

36. Birkedal-Hansen, H., Cobb, C. M., Taylor, R. E. and Fullmer, H. M. (1976). Synthesis and release of procollagenase by cultured fibroblasts. *J. Biol. Chem.*, **251**, 3162

37. Hamerman, D., Janis, R. and Smith, C. (1967). Cartilage matrix depletion by rheumatoid synovial cells in tissue culture. *J. Exptl Med.*, **126**, 1005

38. Krey, P. R., Scheinberg, M. A. and Cohen, A. S. (1976). Fine structural analysis of rabbit synovial cells. II. Fine structure and rosette-forming cells of explant and monolayer cultures. *Arthritis and Rheumatism*, **19**, 581

39. Fell, H. B. and Barratt, M. E. J. (1973). The role of soft connective tissue in the breakdown of pig articular cartilage cultivated in the presence of complement-sufficient antiserum to pig erythrocytes. I. Histological changes. *Int. Arch. Allergy*, **44**, 441

40. Poole, A. R., Barratt, M. E. J. and Fell, H. B. (1973). The role of soft connective tissue in the breakdown of pig articular cartilage cultivated in the presence of complement-sufficient antiserum to pig erythrocytes. II. Distribution of immunoglobulin G (IgG). *Int. Arch. Allergy*, **44**, 469

41. Fell, H. B. and Jubb, R. W. (1977). The destructive action of synovial tissue on articular cartilage in organ culture. In J. L. Gordon and B. L. Hazleman (Eds.). *Rheumatoid Arthritis: Cellular Pathology and Pharmacology*, pp. 193–197. (ASP Biological and Medical Press.), 193-197

Discussion 10

<table>
<tr><td>Chairman:</td><td>What does Professor Vaes think about the role of polymorphs in degradation of cartilage? This is a view which is espoused by our American colleagues in particular, and I should like to know what he thinks about it.</td></tr>
<tr><td>Vaes:</td><td>Two different things must be considered: the area of the cartilage covered by the pannus and the area of the cartilage not covered by synovium, which is merely basted by the synovial fluid. I am no pathologist, but from a careful study of the literature, and from conversations with competent pathologists, the main erosion of cartilage seems to occur under the pannus at the junction between the cell and the pannus. This is not the only site of erosion. There may be some attack, particularly of proteoglycans, where there are no synovial cells. But, apparently, this is not the main site of action. Where this occurs I would suspect that this comes from diffusion of proteases from polymorphonuclear leukocytes that are abundant in the synovial fluid, but they are not abundant in the pannus, and this could explain that part of the phenomenon.</td></tr>
<tr><td>K. Fehr:
(Switzerland)</td><td>In my own laboratory another assay with cartilage has been devised using purified neutral protease from, probably, mainly human peripheral blood leukocytes: polymorphs. It is not Professor Vaes's protease. It is distinctly distinguished from that protease. This protease degrades. One microgram of this protease degrades 170 μg of proteoglycan in the assay per minute, that is 170 times more than the enzyme per minute. There was some difficulty in studying with this assay. Bovine nasal cartilage was used, without heating it. It was lyophilized and pulverized, but not heated. The cartilage was extracted to get rid of the enzymes, it was lyophilized again and washed again, then there was a blank of the digestion at 20% which levelled completely at 20 min and stayed level there, and the enzyme activity could be measured in nanograms of enzyme activity.</td></tr>
</table>

It was difficult to do it with human articular cartilage.

Has Professor Vaes done any studies, in his very nice assay system, with human articular cartilage?

<table>
<tr><td>Vaes:</td><td>So far we have done nothing with human articular cartilage, although we have plans.</td></tr>
</table>

We heat the cartilage, as I showed, to 60 °C for 30 minutes, very exactly. If one overdoes it, one denatures the collagen far too much. It is not a requirement for the action of the enzyme. I can show the action of the macrophage enzyme on non-heated cartilage. It is important because it means that absolutely native proteoglycan—we do not know how native it is after heat treatment—is degraded.

We have a further proof which I did not mention. We have another assay of this enzyme, a viscosometric assay which we set up using proteoglycan subunits from bovine nasal cartilage. It worked just as well. We had the same pH activity curve and the same pattern of inhibition.

The enzyme from these macrophages is absolutely distinct from that from the leukocytes so far as I know.

Honor Fell: I should like to congratulate Professor Vaes and his colleagues on this
(UK) extremely interesting paper.

Recently in Cambridge we have done some experiments on another organ culture model which has given complementary results to those presented by Professor Vaes. We have compared the effects of synovial tissue on living and dead cartilage. We have used the articular tissues of normal pigs, obtained from pigs' trotters, and we have killed our cartilage by freezing and thawing rather than by heating. We have found by comparing the effects of the synovial tissue on the living and the dead, that in our system the synovium has two apparently distinct mechanisms causing breakdown. If the cartilage is put into direct contact with the synovium, there may be a complete disappearance of the matrix in the living cartilage, but there will be a severe depletion in the dead. But, never in our hands does the matrix of the dead cartilage disintegrate to the extent that it does in the living cartilage.

We then tried placing the cartilage at a distance from the synovium. We put our explants on a millipore filter substrate. We found that whereas the living cartilage underwent a similar breakdown, the dead cartilage was unaffected, so this suggested to us that the synovium had a direct enzymatic effect when it was in direct contact with the cartilage, and also that it had some indirect effect—the nature of which we do not understand—which was mediated through the chondrocytes.

I have a number of slides which will illustrate these points.

The *first slide* shows an isolated piece of articular cartilage which has been in culture for 14 days. The two little purple patches underneath represent regenerated new cartilage beneath the old. Otherwise no particular change.

The *second slide* shows the effect of growing such a piece of cartilage on top of synovial tissue. One is stained with toluidine blue and shows the disappearance of proteoglycan, which has been confirmed by chemical observations on the medium. Below is the same specimen stained by van Gieson to show the collagen. The depletion of the collagen round the periphery and underneath the synovial tissue can be seen.

Slide 3 is the extreme form of the effect. All the matrix has gone out of the cartilage and the cells appear to be perfectly healthy. The cartilage cells are almost indistinguishable from fibroblasts in appearance and often are actively mitosing.

Slide 4 shows dead cartilage on top of living synovium, and the complete depletion of the proteoglycan is similar to what Professor Vaes has described.

Slide 5 shows the same specimen stained with van Gieson. Some depletion of the collagen can be seen in the general depletion in the explant. Small bays are seen in the cartilage. These are formed by invading cells from the underlying synovium. In our system, and during our culture period, this is the maximum effect obtained with dead cartilage.

Slide 6: The two pieces of cartilage shown were grown on the same millipores of the synovium, but separated from it so that there was no cellular contact between them. The top piece has been frozen and thawed and remains unchanged. The lower piece is living and is almost completely depleted of proteoglycan.

We feel that these results demonstrate quite clearly that there are in our system—whether this applies *in vivo* we do not yet know—there are these two effects; one directly on the matrix, and the other mediated

128

through living chondrocytes. It also shows what complete degradation of the cartilage can be found without any inflammatory cells being present.

Vaes: I should like to take the opportunity to pay tribute to Dame Honor Fell, whose work has been a constant source of inspiration to us in the course of our own work.

It was a nice study and what she showed was very evident and very clear. We have done some work with living cartilage, but we did not concentrate on it. We wanted to have a more simplistic system on the one hand, and on the other hand by looking through the literature, and with no personal experience, we have the feeling that most people would agree that in rheumatoid arthritis—which was the field in which we were really interested—the chondrocytes were apparently not among the affected cells in the destruction of the cartilage matrix. But, this could be a false impression from a superficial view of the data.

11

Adjuvant arthritis: immune responses and effects of Tilorone or interferon in partially suppressing the disease

CARL M. PEARSON AND YI-HAN CHANG (USA)

The injection of complete Freund's adjuvant into rats induces a chronic arthritis which resembles human rheumatoid arthritis or Reiter's syndrome in many respects[1,2]. The pathogenesis of adjuvant-induced arthritis has not yet been clearly established. It is generally believed to be the result of a delayed hypersensitivity response to bacilli on their components[3], such as peptidoglycans[4] which resist degradation by mammalian lysosomal enzymes[5] and may remain in macrophages to serve as a persistent source of immunogen[6]. Alternatively, the disease has been speculated to result from the development of autoantibodies and/or specifically sensitized lymphocytes acting against the animals' own tissue (i.e. in autoimmune phenomenon)[7,8]. There is a third possibility, namely, that adjuvant arthritis may involve the activation of latent virus by a yet undefined hypersensitivity reaction of the host[9]. Similar suggestions have also come from the work of Kupusta and his associates[10,11], who observed that the interferon-inducers (anti-viral) such as statolon and Pyran copolymer provide a degree of suppression of the otherwise induced state.

While we have been actively engaged during the past several years in the isolation and identification of chemical moieties in the bacterial cell wall which seem to be responsible for the induction of adjuvant arthritis[4], we have at the same time been investigating possible virus involvement as a step in the sequential generation of this experimental disease. This discussion summarizes our findings into the immune mechanisms involved in a modified model of adjuvant arthritis and of studies relative to a possible viral aetiology of the disease.

A MODIFIED MODEL OF ADJUVANT ARTHRITIS

The experimental system used for the studies to be described is shown schematically in Figure 11.1. A suspension of EL_4 cells (2×10^7 cells) was

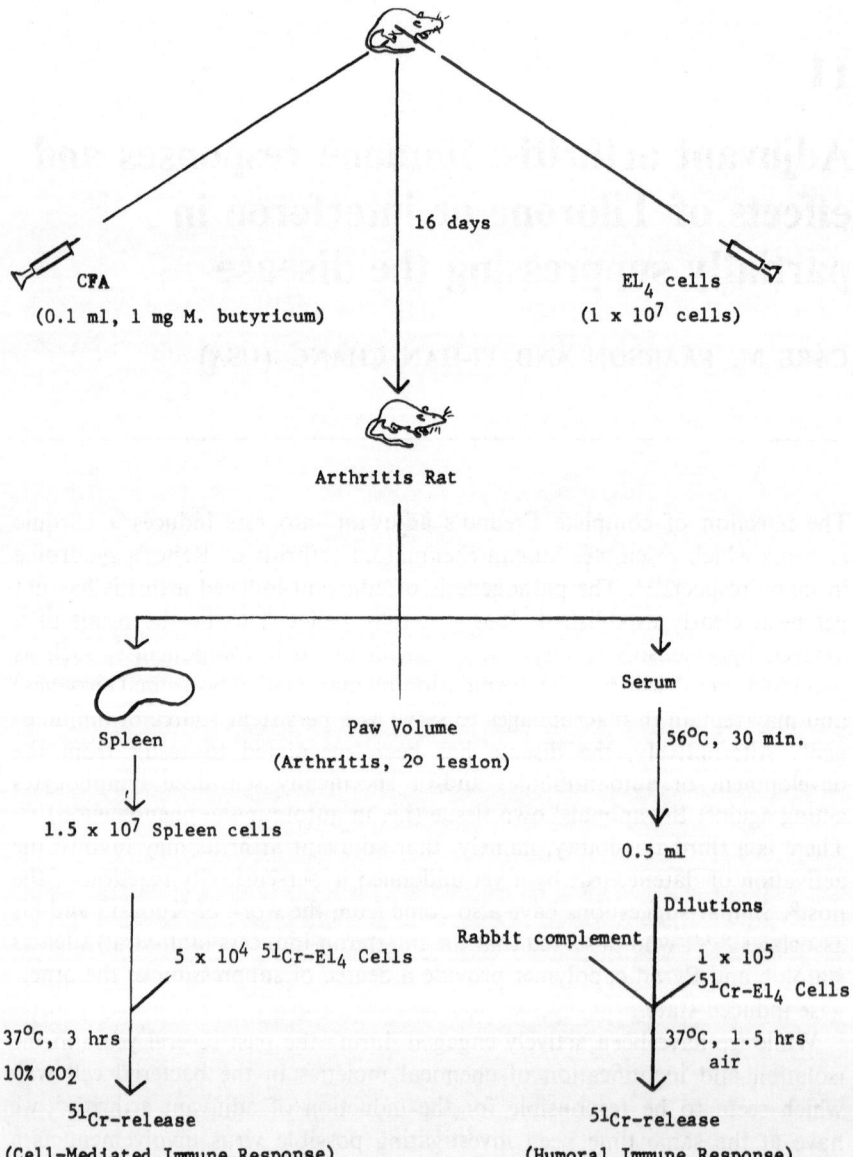

Figure 11.1 Diagrammatic scheme for simultaneous injection of complete Freund's adjuvant and ER_4 cells with techniques for testing cell-mediated immune responses as well as humoral immune responses

injected i.p. into the animals immediately following the subplantar injection of complete Freund's adjuvant (CFA).

On day 16 after paw injection of CFA and i.p. EL_4 cells, an increase in the size of the opposite or uninjected hindpaw was evaluated as a measure of secondary or induced systemic arthritis. Then, a sample of blood was collected and the spleen was removed. A suspension of spleen cells was incubated with ^{51}Cr labelled with EL_4 cells, and the percentage of ^{51}Cr released was determined. This *complement independent*, sensitized lymphocyte lysis of EL_4 cells served as a measure of cell-mediated immune response. The serum was decomplemented and serially diluted. The diluted serum was then added to a suspension of ^{51}Cr labelled EL_4 cells containing rabbit complement and this mixture was incubated for 1.5 h. The titre was taken as that dilution of serum which produced a 50% release of ^{51}Cr from the EL_4 cells. This *complement dependent* antibody lysis of the EL_4 cells served as a measure of the humoral immune response.

The EL_4 cell method of evaluation of responses in adjuvant arthritis was selected from a number of immunogens previously tested for three reasons: (1) unlike immunogens such as SRBC or BSA, sensitization to EL_4 cells had little or no effect on the development of adjuvant arthritis; (2) the cell-mediated immune response to EL_4 cells can be quantitatively measured by *complement independent* T-lymphocyte mediated lysis of EL_4 cells. The measurement of the cellular immune response was very reproducible; and (3) the humoral immune response can also be measured by complement (rabbit) lysis of prelabelled (^{51}Cr) EL_4 cells when placed in contact with rabbit serum.

The mean value (% ^{51}Cr release) for 22 experiments (7 animals per experiment) performed over a period of one year with spleen cells was 48.1%, with a standard error of 0.33%. The mean antibody titre for the same 22 experiments was 4252 with a standard error of 414. These results seemed to suggest that both delayed hypersensitivity and the humoral mechanisms are activated in the CFA injected rats. Whether one or both responses play a role in the development of adjuvant arthritis is still uncertain, since other antigens may be involved that we have no knowledge of yet. Nevertheless, this area will be explored further in the forthcoming experiments.

Tilorone

In order to investigate the possible role of an activated virus in adjuvant arthritis, perhaps as an additive or initiating factor, we examined the effects of Tilorone on this diseased model.

Tilorone hydrochloride, 2,7-bis (diethylaminoethoxy) fluoren-9-one hydrochloride (Figure 11.2) is a broad spectrum antiviral agent with activity associated with interferon induction[12,13]. It has also been reported that Tilorone may stimulate the humoral immune response[14], suppress the cell-mediated immune response[15], and to have anti-tumour[16] and anti-inflammatory properties[15].

Daily administration (p.o.) of Tilorone to groups of ten animals beginning on the day *before* the injection of complete Freund's adjuvant and ending on the day prior to measurement of arthritis suppressed the development of the disease in a dose-related manner as shown in Figure 11.3, where the dose

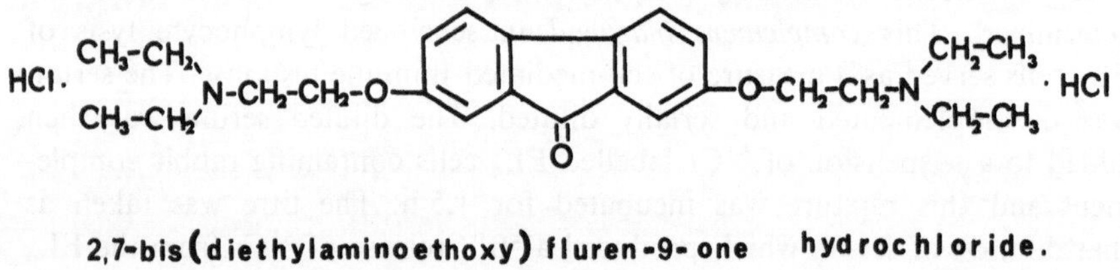

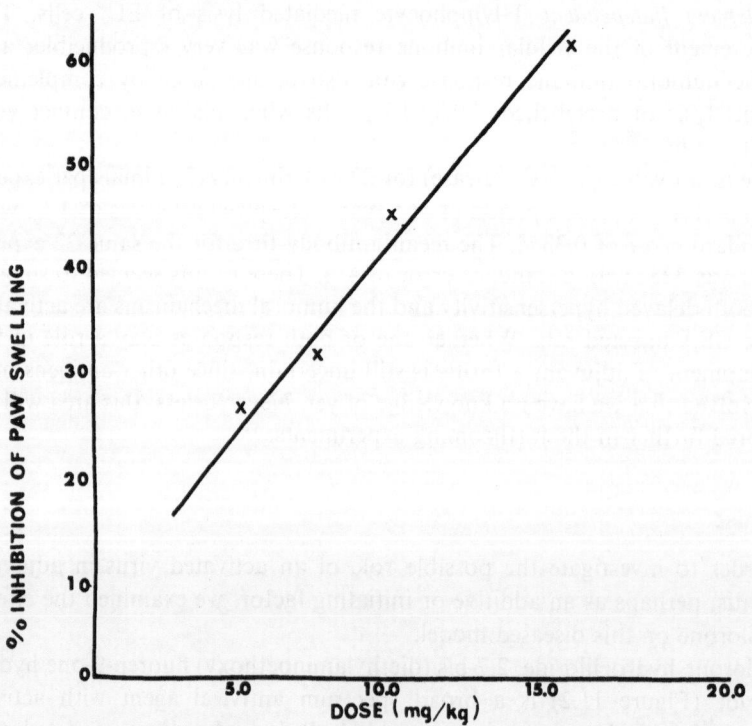

2,7-bis(diethylaminoethoxy) fluren-9-one   hydrochloride.

Figure 11.2   Tilorone Hydrochloride

Figure 11.3   Tilorone (p.o.) given on days −1 to +16 at daily intervals

response regression reaction is linear over quite a range when groups of ten Lewis rats were used at each dose level. The results are expressed as percentage inhibition compared with control animals dosed with saline.

The therapeutic effects of Tilorone showed a dependence on timing (respective to adjuvant injection) (Figure 11.4). A dose of 10 mg/kg administered (p.o.) daily for 5 consecutive days, beginning on the day before

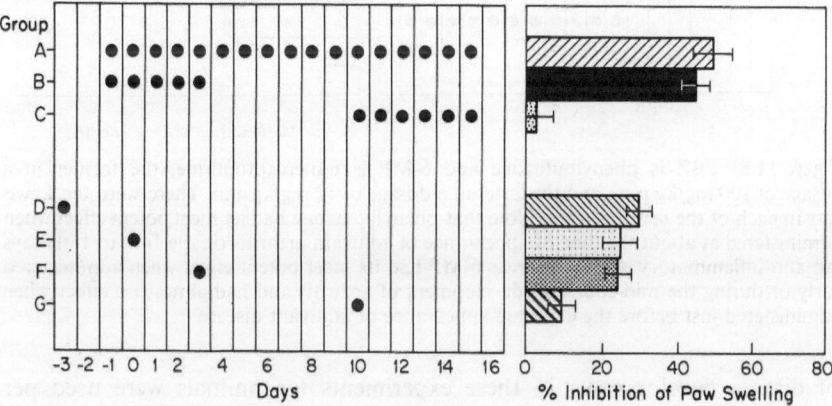

Figure 11.4 Tilorone (p.o.) 10 mg/kg. There were ten Lewis rats in each of groups A through G. Note that the greatest inhibition of paw swelling of the secondary (previously uninvolved) hind paw occurred when Tilorone was given before or soon after inoculation of adjuvant or when it was given continuously

the injection of adjuvant, resulted in a 50% suppression, whereas the same dose administered daily from day 10 to day 15 (respective to the day of adjuvant injection), had *no* suppressive effect. A single dose of Tilorone (10 mg/kg p.o.) was clearly effective when administered on day -3 (30.0 $\pm$ 3.1% suppression), day 0 (25.0 $\pm$4.5% suppression), or day 3 (24.3 $\pm$ 3.4% suppression), but not on day 10 (9.3 $\pm$ 3.4% suppression). These observations are very similar to those found with the use of immunosuppressive agents such as 6-mercaptopurine (Figure 11.5) and are in contrast to the results as seen in adjuvant arthritis with the use of anti-inflammatory drugs such as phenylbutazone (Figure 11.5)[17,18].

Both phenylbutazone (100 mg/kg p.o.) and 6-mercaptopurine (10 mg/kg p.o.) effectively suppressed the development of adjuvant arthritis when either of them were administered daily beginning on the day *before* adjuvant injection and ending on the day prior to the measurement of arthritis (day 16) (Figure 11.5). Oral administration of phenylbutazone (100 mg/kg/day) from day 13 to day 15 (respective to adjuvant injection) was much more effective than the same dose when given from day 0 to day 4. The opposite holds true for 6-mercaptopurine which was effective when administered early during the 'sensitization' period, but ineffective during the late stages

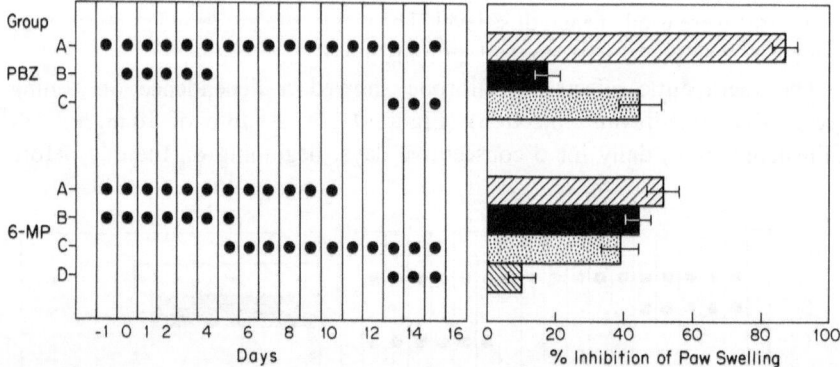

Figure 11.5 PBZ is phenylbutazone and 6-MP is 6-mercaptopurine, the former in a dosage of 100 mg/kg p.o., and the latter in a dosage of 10 mg/kg p.o. There were ten Lewis rats in each of the seven groups. Note that phenylbutazone had its most potent effect when administered at about the time of appearance of adjuvant arthritis on the 14th to 16th days (an anti-inflammatory effect), whereas 6-MP had its most potent effect when administered early or during the mid-course of development of arthritis and had almost no effect when administered just before the expected appearance of adjuvant disease

of disease development. In these experiments ten animals were used per group. Results were expressed as per cent inhibition compared with control animals treated with saline. Standard errors of the means are indicated in the figure.

As illustrated in Figure 11.6, adjuvant arthritis was clearly suppressed by Tilorone at dose levels (16.1, 10.9, and 7.4 mg/kg) that produced no suppression of the cell-mediated immune response. With the humoral immune response, the drug was stimulatory at lower doses (10.9 and 7.4 mg/kg), but suppressed at high doses (23.7 and 35.0 mg/kg). Also in this set of experiments 10 animals were used per group. The results were expressed as per cent inhibition compared with control animals treated with saline. Similarly, the standard errors of the means are indicated in the figure. Antibody titres shown are the means of two determinations with pooled serum.

From the above-mentioned results there is clearly *no correlation* between the effects of this drug on the immune response and the degree of suppression of adjuvant disease. The possibility that the lack of correlation between suppressions of cell-mediated immune response and anti-arthritic activity may be due to a difference in the sensitivity of the two measurements seems fairly unlikely, especially when one compares Tilorone with 6-mercaptopurine, the latter which appears to act in adjuvant arthritis primarily via immuno-suppression[19]. Equivalent suppressions of arthritis were achieved by Tilorone and by 6-mercaptopurine at 10 mg/kg/day. At this dose level, 6-mercapto-purine greatly suppressed (50%) the cell-mediated immune response to EL_4 cells in the arthritic rat[19], whereas Tilorone had *no* measurable effect.

At high dose levels Tilorone has been shown to be anti-inflammatory.

136

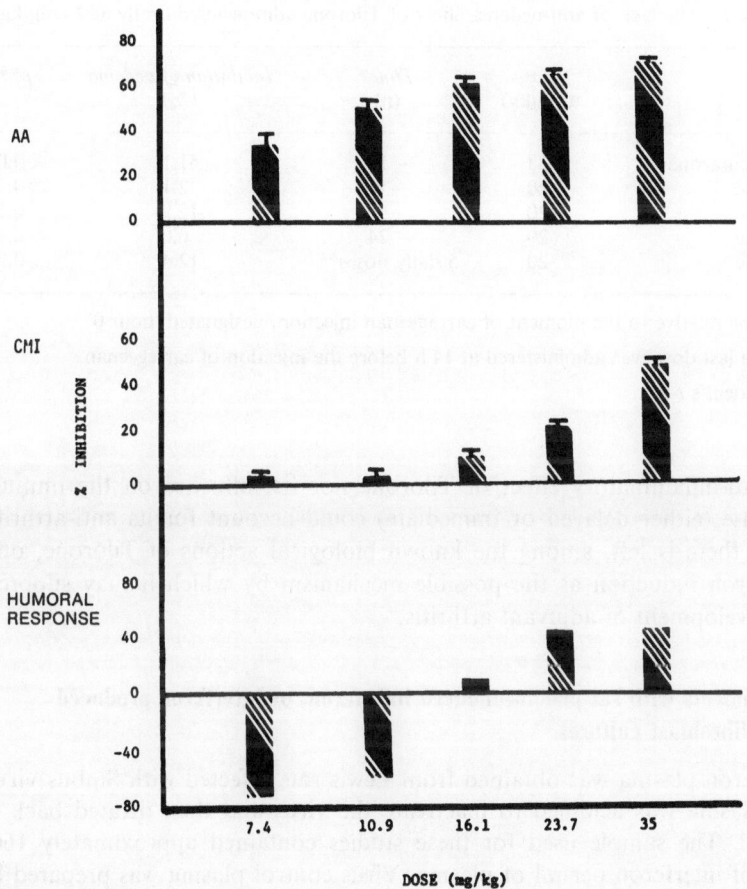

Figure 11.6 Effects of Tilorone on three different responses in EL_4 in adjuvant-injected Lewis rats

For example, two consecutive doses of Tilorone at 100 mg/kg administered at 24 h and 1 h prior to the injection of carrageenan had been shown to suppress the carrageenan-induced paw oedema in the rat[15]. In our own hands, single doses administered at 24 h before the injection of carrageenan were ineffective. No anti-inflammatory effect was detected at a dose level of 20 mg/kg even after five consecutive daily doses with the last dose being administered 14 h before the injection of carrageenan (Table 11.1), even though phenylbutazone, under similar circumstances, had a dramatic suppressive effect and demonstrated post anti-inflammatory activity. Since a single dose of Tilorone at 10 mg/kg administered as early as 16 days prior to the measurement of arthritis effectively suppressed the disease (Figure 11.5), it seems that the anti-arthritic effect of this drug clearly cannot be attributed to its anti-inflammatory action in these experiments. Since neither

137

Table 1 The lack of anti-oedema effect of Tilorone administered orally at 20 mg/kg

Drug	Dose (mg/kg)	Time* (h)	Inhibition of oedema (%)	p***
Phenylbutazone	33	−1	51.1	<0.001
Tilorone	20	−1	2.1	>0.5
Tilorone	20	−4	12.9	>0.2
Tilorone	20	−24	6.0	>0.2
Tilorone	20	5 daily doses**	12.4	>0.2

* Time relative to the moment of carrageenan injection, designated 'hour 0'.

** The last dose was administered at 14 h before the injection of carregeenan.

*** Student's t-test.

the anti-inflammatory effect of Tilorone nor its influence on the immune response (either delayed or immediate) could account for its anti-arthritic effect, there is left, among the known biological actions of Tilorone, only interferon induction as the possible mechanism by which it may suppress the development of adjuvant arthritis.

Experiments with rat plasma-induced interferon, or interferon produced in rat fibroblast cultures

Interferon plasma was obtained from Lewis rats infected with Sinbus virus. The plasma was acidified to inactivate the virus and then titrated back to neutral. The sample used for these studies contained approximately 1600 units of interferon per ml of plasma. Virus control plasma was prepared by adding Sinbus virus in an amount equivalent to that found in the interferon plasma and then inactivated in the same manner as described previously. A second control plasma was obtained by acidifying normal rat plasma followed by neutralization. A 0.2 ml dose of various plasma preparations was injected i.p. to rats daily from day −1 to day +15. These methods or production will now be described in considerable detail.

Viruses

Sinbus virus (SV)†, strain AR-339, and vesicular stomatitis virus (VSV), Indiana strain, were propagated in chick embryo fibroblast (CEF) cultures. A stock of SV containing $10^{11.2}$ median-tissue-culture-infective doses (TCID$_{50}$)/ml in CEF cells, was prepared in the yolk sac of 7-day old embryonated eggs by inoculation of 10^5 TCID$_{50}$ of CEF-grown virus and incubated for 72 h at 37 °C.

† These studies were conducted through the courtesy of Dr. William W. Hoffman.

Preparation of rat plasma interferon*

Interferon was induced in Lewis rats weighing approximately 250 g by intravenous injection of $2 \times 10^{11.2}$ $TCID_{50}$ of Sinbis virus (SV) in a volume of 2 ml. The rats were laparotomized under anaesthesia 8 h after injection and bled from the dorsal aorta. Samples were centrifuged at $1000 \times g'$ for 10 min; the plasma was removed and acidified to pH 2 with 1 N HCl and allowed to stand for 18 h at 4 °C to kill residual SV. Neutralization was performed by addition of 1 N NaOH. All samples were frozen and stored at −70 °C. Interferon levels on each rat were determined by CPE 50% viral cytopathology inhibition using mouse L-929 micro titre plates challenged with vesicular stomatitis virus (VSV).

Plasma levels of SV obtained at 8 h were determined by assaying untreated rat plasma on CEF monolayers. An equivalent number of killed viruses were added to acid-treated normal plasma to serve as control. A second control plasma was prepared by acid treatment and neutralization of normal plasma.

Preparation of rat fibroblast interferon*

Secondary rat fibroblast monolayers were prepared in 25 cm^2 culture flasks by seeding them with 5×10^6 primary cells in 5 ml of ENEM with 10% fetal calf serum (FCS), 200 U penicillin/ml and 200 μg streptomycin/ml. Subsequent procedures were done in maintenance medium. Interferon was superinduced in confluent cultures at 37 °C with poly I:C and the inhibitors, cycloheximide and actinomycin D, as described by Tan et al.[20] Briefly, cultures were exposed for 1 h to 20 μg cycloheximide/ml and 300 μg poly I:C/ml in 5 ml of maintenance medium. During the following 3 h they were exposed to cycloheximide alone and for an additional hour they were incubated with cycloheximide and 2 μg actinomycin D/ml. After each treatment the cultures were washed three times with Hanks' Balanced Salt Solution (HBSS). Following an additional 18 h incubation at 37 °C with 5 ml of maintenance medium, the culture fluids were pooled and assayed for interferon (Figure 11.7). Pooled fluids from cultures treated with inhibitors but not poly I:C served as controls. To detect the presence of any residual poly I:C, the interferon preparation was assayed against 10–20 $TCID_{50}$ of VSV on primary rabbit kidney cells; this system could detect 0.005 μg poly I:C/ml, but was not sensitive to rat interferon.

Rat interferon assay*

Interferon levels (mouse reference units) in plasma or culture fluids were determined as the reciprocal of the dilution inhibiting by 50% viral cytopathology (CPE) in mouse L929 microcultures challenged with 20–30

* These studies were conducted through the courtesy of Dr. William W. Hoffman.

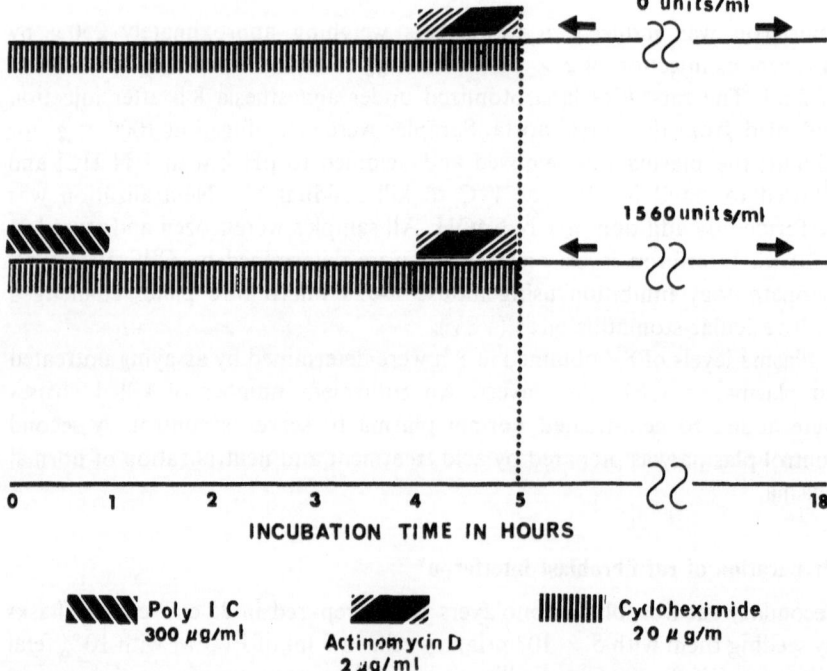

0 units/ml

1560 units/ml

0   1   2   3   4   5   18

INCUBATION TIME IN HOURS

Poly I C
300 μg/ml

Actinomycin D
2 μg/ml

Cycloheximide
20 μg/m

Figure 11.7   Preparation of interferon on rat fibroblast monolayer cultures and scheme of administration of various stimulants and inhibitors. Remainder of details of this methodology are explained in the text. (Courtesy of Dr. William W. Hoffman)

$TCID_{50}$ of VSV. Although most interferons are species specific, rat interferon cross reacts sufficiently on L929 cells to use them for this assay. The L929 cells used in this study were approximately as sensitive to rat interferon as rat embryo fibroblasts.

RESULTS

The interferon containing rat plasma *effectively suppressed* the development of adjuvant arthritis (Figure 11.8), whereas control plasma or plasma containing equivalent numbers of killed viruses had no significant effect. Since virus-infected animals are under stress, the possibility exists that the anti-arthritic effect of their plasma may be due to the presence of corticol steroids or other anti-phlogistic substances contained therein. To eliminate this possibility, interferon, prepared as described by tissue culture employing rat embryonic fibroblasts was also tested.

The fibroblast interferon method used in these studies has already been described and was prepared according to the method of Tan *et al.*[20]. It contained approximately 1600 units (actually 1560 units) of interferon per

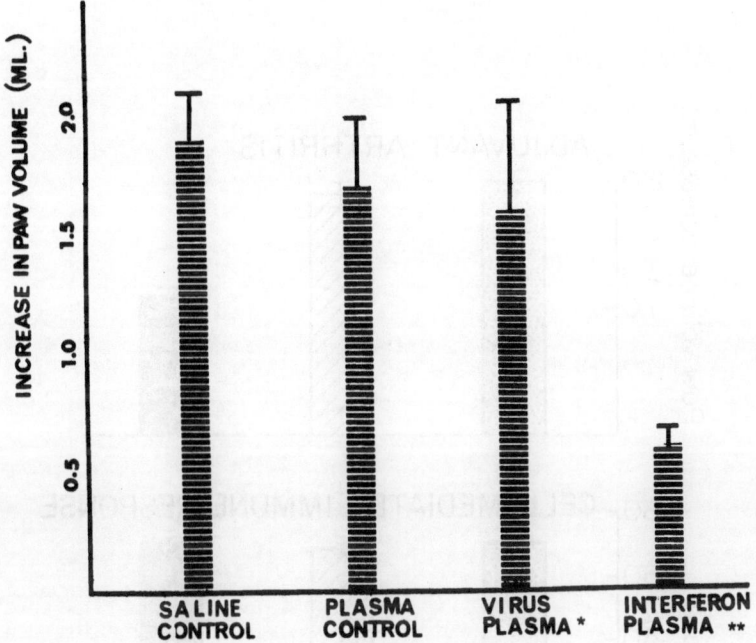

* Heat inactivated sinbus virus added to normal rat plasma.

** Approximately 1600 units of interferon/ml plasma.

Figure 11.8 Suppressive effect of interferon induced in normal rats at 8 h after injections of sinbus virus and then transferred parenterally to adjuvant injected rats as described in the text. The rat plasma contained approximately 1600 units of interferon per ml. Note suppressive effect of interferon on adjuvant disease and lack of any significant effect of serum control, plasma control, or rat plasma to which sinbus virus had been induced *in vitro* and then the virus inactivated

ml. Control cultures were not exposed to poly I:C, but otherwise were cultured in the same manner. No residual poly I:C was detected in the interferon preparation when assayed on rabbit kidney cells, with a sensitivity level of 0.005 μg/ml.

In this experiment, 0.4 ml of various preparations was administered i.p. daily from day -1 to day $+15$. Ten Lewis rats were used. All measurements were made on the day after the last injection. The interferon preparation obtained from rat fibroblast cultures *clearly suppressed* the development of adjuvant arthritis (Figure 11.9), but this interferon had no effect on cell-mediated immunity to EL_4 cells (Figure 11.9) or to humoral immune responses to EL_4 cells in Lewis rats in which the antibody titres shown in Figure 11.9 are the means of two determinations with pooled plasma.

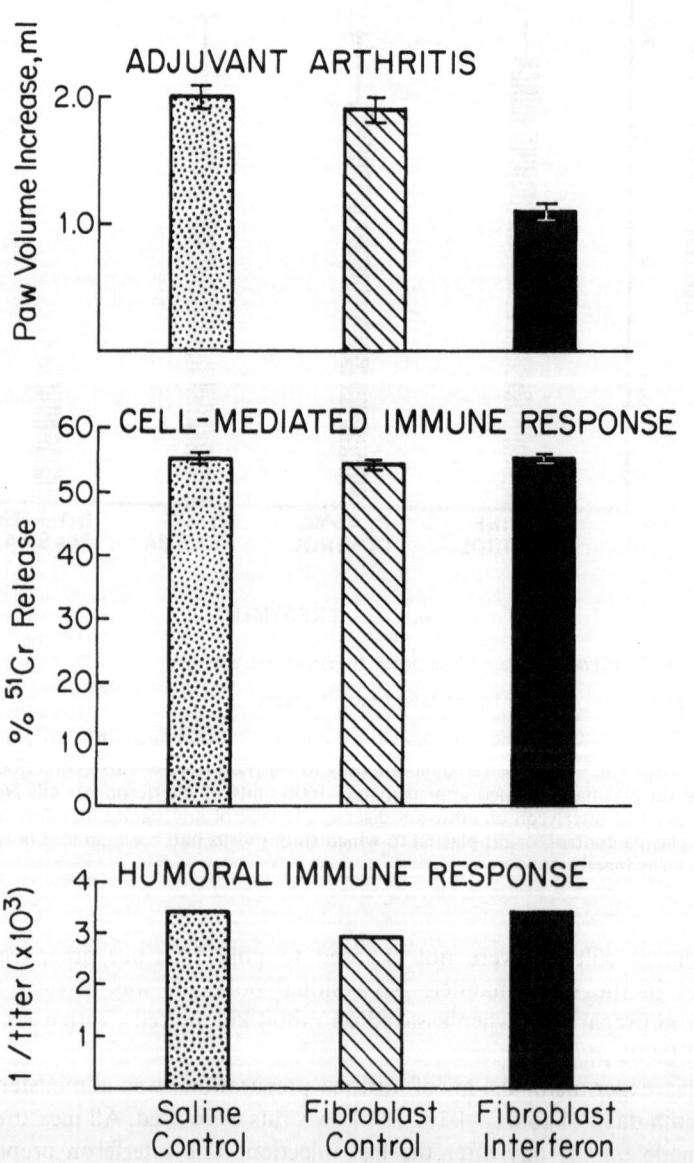

Figure 11.9 The suppressive effect of virus-induced interferon in embryonic fibroblast cultures demonstrating a significant inhibition by interferon on adjuvant arthritis (dosages are explained in the text) with total lack of response on cell-mediated immunity and the humoral immune response

Administration of interferon to mice in amounts (150 000–5 000 000 units/animal) that far exceed those presently employed have been reported to suppress the immune response[21]. In the present experiment, concurrent measurements of the humoral and cell-mediated immune responses to EL_4 cells in the arthritic animals showed no alteration in either branch of the immune system. These findings provide strong circumstantial evidence to the speculation that a virus or virus-like micro-organism plays a role in the pathogenesis of this experimental disease. The findings still leave open, however, the possibility that other types of cell-mediated responses or humoral responses could play secondary roles in the pathogenesis of adjuvant arthritis if such responses are directed at antigens (? viral) that have not as yet been delineated.

Acknowledgement

This work was supported in part by research funds from NIH Grant No. GM 15759.

References

1. Pearson, C. M. (1956). Development of arthritis, periarthritis, and periostitis in rats given adjuvants. *Proc. Soc. Exp. Biol. Med.*, **91**, 95
2. Pearson, C. M., Waxman, B. H. and Sharp, J. T. (1961). Studies of arthritis and other lesions induced in rats by injection of microbacterial adjuvant. V. *J. Exper. Med.*, **113**, 485
3. Pearson, C. M. and Wood, F. D. (1963). Studies of arthritis and other lesions induced in rats by the injection of mycobacterial adjuvant. VII. Pathologic details of the arthritis and spondylitis. *Am. J. Pathol.*, **42**, 73
4. Kohashi, O., Watanabe, Y., Beck, F. W. J. and Pearson, C. M. (1976). Studies on adjuvant arthritis in rats. III. Antigenic requirements for arthritogenicity of peptido-glycans from S. Aureus and L. Plantarium. *Int. Arch. Allergy Appl. Immunol.* (In press)
5. Adler, E., Heller, H., Weiner, E., *et al.* (1973). Degradation of ^{14}C-labelled group A streptococci and micrococci in muscular lesions in the mouse. *Israel J. Med. Sci.*, **9**, 483
6. Hadler, N. M. (1976). A pathogenetic model for erosive synovitis. *Arthritis Rheum.*, **19**, 256
7. Pearson, C. M. (1964). Experimental models in rheumatoid disease. *Arthritis Rheum.*, **7**, 80
8. Ryzewska, A. G. (1976). Influence of lymphatic tissue on the development of adjuvant-induced polyarthritis in rats. *Ann. Rheum. Dis.*, **26**, 506
9. Jones, R. S. and Ward, J. R. (1963). Studies on adjuvant induced polyarthritis in rats. II. Histogenesis of joint and visceral lesions. *Arthritis Rheum.*, **6**, 23
10. Kupusta, M. A. and Mendelson, J. (1967). Inhibition of adjuvant arthritis by Stantolon. *Proc. Soc. Exp. Biol. Med.*, **126**, 496
11. Kupusta, M. A. and Mendelson, J. (1969). The inhibition of adjuvant disease in rats by the interferon-inducing agent Pyran copolymer. *Arthritis Rheum.*, **12**, 463
12. Krueger, R. F. and Mayer, G. D. (1970). Tilorone hydrochloride: An orally active interferon inducer. *Science*, **169**, 1213
13. Mayer, G. D. and Krueger, R. F. (1970). Tilorone hydrochloride: mode of action. *Science*, **169**, 1214
14. Hoffman, P. F., Ritter, H. W. and Krueger, R. F. (1972). In: *Advances in Antimicrobial and Antineoplastic Chemotherapy* (M. Hejzlar, M. Semonsky, and S. Masak, eds.) p. 217. (Munich: Urban and Schwarzenberg)

15. Megel, H., Raychaudhwin, A., Shemano, I., Beaver, T. H. and Thomas, L. L. (1975). The anti-inflammatory actions of tilorone hydrochloride. *Proc. Soc. Exp. Biol. Med.*, **149**, 89

16. Adamson, R. H. (1971). Antitumor activity of tilorone hydrochloride against some rodent tumors. *J. Nat. Cancer Inst.*, **46**, 431

17. Waltz, D. T., DiMartino, M. J. and Misher, A. (1971). Adjuvant-induced arthritis in rats. II. Drug effects on physiologic, biochemical, and immunologic parameters. *J. Pharm. Exp. Ther.*, **178**, 223

18. Perper, R. S., Alvarez, B., Colombo, C. and Schroder, H. (1971). The use of a standard arthritis assay to differentiate between anti-inflammatory and immunosuppressive agents. *Proc. Soc. Exp. Biol. Med.*, **137**, 506

19. Chang, Y.-H. (1976). Mechanisms underlying the suppression of adjuvant-induced arthritis by 6-mercaptopurine. *Arthritis Rheum.* (submitted)

20. Tan, Y. H., Armstrong, J. A., Ke, Y. H. and Ho, M. (1970). Regulation of cellular interferon production: enhancement by antimetabolites. *Proc. Nat. Acad. Sci. U.S.A.*, **67**, 464

21. DeMaeyer-Guignard, J., Cachard, A. and DeMaeyer, E. (1975). Delayed-type hypersensitivity to sheep red blood cells: inhibition of sensitization by interferon. *Science*, **190**, 574

Discussion 11

Chairman:	I am sure Dr. Pearson is aware of the work which is being done on the immunosuppressive effects of Interferon itself and the fact that, for example, dosage and timing are extremely important. I mention the possibility that even if there is some immune response which is related to Mycobacterium, the timing of that would be different from the timing of antibody response against the EL for all cells, for example.
	I am suggesting that there may be other effects of Interferon than suppression of a virus, although that is obviously a very intriguing interpretation.
Pearson:	I would certainly agree. I believe that in most mouse systems 500 000 units, or 150 000 units, in contrast with 1600 units, are required in order to exhibit some of these effects. Obviously there is a great deal of work for us yet to do to measure Interferon levels in some of our animals by mouse unit assays and so forth, but these are only preliminary results and I am aware of those studies.
I. Ginsburg: (Israel)	How can Dr. Pearson explain some of his recent data to show that the mycobacterial cell wall is not needed, but that it is possible to settle very nicely with very small peptidoglycan pieces, which can be obtained from lactobacilli and from other Gram-positive bacteria? If this is just an activation of the virus why is the peptidoglycan part of the micro-organism needed?
Pearson:	I find myself in a dilemma because of some fairly recent publications by colleagues in my laboratory (Cogger, Kahachi et al.) which have speculated that the persistence of this non-degradable antigen over a long period of time, existing in macrophages etc., may well be a very important factor in the continuous stimulation of the immune response. I do not know which segment of the immune response to look at in order to initiate adjuvant disease.
	In this series of studies, which run counter—I will admit—to the persistence of some of those non-degradable agents in cells (that I assume are to be discussed later in the proceedings), one wonders if Interferon is so effective in this regard, whether an additive effect, an agent that we have all been looking for in rheumatoid arthritis and so forth, namely the activation of a latent virus and a continued activation by some of those factors, segments of cell walls, by the acid fast bacillus or the streptococcus or the staphylococcus, might be responsible for the continued propagation of adjuvant disease.
	I am presenting this paper as a rather provocative series of studies without any final conclusions.
J. L. Turk: (UK)	One of the points in Dr. Pearson's paper raises a problem—the use of carrageenan always in screening for non-specific inflammation. This probably acts by activating the alternate pathway of complement and I would think, in his system, it would be much nicer if there was a control for non-specific inflammation which was more like the lesion that the animal has. Probably one would prefer an activated macro-

phage giant cell control, a granuloma, rather than an acute inflammation by activation of the alternate pathway.

Has Dr. Pearson thought of another control for anti-non-specific inflammation?

Pearson: We plan to use other controls and that is an extremely valid point. We have not utilized those and this is the first one that came to mind. There is a great deal more study to be undertaken to try and rule out activation of the alternate pathway and so forth.

I would agree.

G. Macpherson: (UK) We are often told that stimulated macrophages and/or T-cells are themselves active releasers of Interferon. Is anything known of the Interferon levels in Dr. Pearson's arthritic rats on their own?

Pearson: No. That is part of the study that is to be forthcoming. I apologize for submitting this preliminary discussion, but it is one of the things that we have closely in mind to do when I get back home.

J. Niblack: (USA) I should like to remind Dr. Pearson, and to caution the audience, that the effects of Interferon inducers on lymphoid cells, particularly T-cells, and in a variety of cells in the lymphoid system is clearly documented—the effects of Interferon inducers and Interferon itself. There are obviously several effects taking place in the rat T-cell population that could explain things without having to invoke viruses at all.

Pearson: Yes. In part I would tend to agree, although it seems to me that the levels of Interferon are so relatively low in contrast with those that have shown effects on cell-mediated immunity etc., and we were able to show none at these rather low levels; although that does not rule out the possibility as I am first and ready to admit.

Nevertheless, the low levels and the lack of cell-mediated immunity responses *in our system only* seem to decrease the possibility that there was a major effect of Interferon on the lymphocytes at this rather low dosage, unless anyone would care to dispute that further.

A. Doble: (UK) Does Dr. Pearson consider that the secondary lesions in the soft tissue, such as the spleen capsule, are also due to virus activation? If so, why is it that the Interferon can stop—that there is no need to postulate Interferon production for the stopping of those lesions, whereas those in the joint tissues carry on for some time, and those are the lesions which appear to be effected by the Interferon?

Pearson: Some of the other lesions, the extra articular lesions, are also altered. We have looked at a few of those, namely the vasculitis in the ear, and so forth, which seems not to occur in the Interferon-treated animals. Some of the lesions in the spleen, in the liver, and occasionally in the lung and so forth, I believe to be granulomas associated with the inoculation of adjuvant itself, with a secondary immediate granulomatous reaction around some of those lesions in the spleen and likewise.

We have seen those lesions in some of our animals treated with Interferon, but not the arthritis, and not some of the secondary lesions and the vasculitis, or some lesions in and around the male genitalia, and so forth.

General Discussion

Chairman: A. C. Allison (UK)

Chairman:	We had interesting contrasts between the *in vivo* type of chemotaxis, discussed by Drs. Borel and Loewi, and the *in vitro* chemotaxis, mentioned very briefly by Drs. Wilkinson and others. One of the intriguing things is the difference between the two.
	Does anybody wish to ask any questions about chemotaxis, or to make any points?
E. W. Parish: **(UK)**	May I make a point on the difference between the Rebuck skin window test and the chamber. One of the features of activated macrophages is that they adhere to any surface, glass or collagen, very avidly, and it is possible that when the skin window test is used, the activated macrophages—quite sticky—get up to the window and take that one step on to another surface. When a chamber is put in they get up to the bottom of the chamber and they realize that there is no surface above them, so they go back and hold on to the tissues and are not released into the fluid.
D. A. Willoughby: **(UK)**	In skin window experiments, has anybody been able to keep the skin windows on for periods of longer than 48 hours without getting subsequent infection? Several of us who have attempted this have run into problems.
J. F. Borel: **(Switzerland)**	Yes, we have. We have kept them for up to 96 hours—provided that the rabbits did not scratch them off. We have used several agents, which were extremely active *in vitro* for the mononuclear cells, and we could never show any significant numbers of mononuclear cells.
	On the first remark, the histological sections do not show an aggregation of mononuclear cells up to the lesion so that they would not dare to release themselves into the serum, which is in the chamber, like the polymorphonuclear cells do.
G. Loewi: **(UK)**	I have had a chamber of my own on for three days and the culture was negative.
P. C. Wilkinson: **(UK)**	Confusion as to what we really mean by the term chemotaxis arises at every one of these meetings. Has chemotaxis anything at all to do with skin windows? We want to be very clear what we are discussing when we use the terms 'chemotaxis' and 'skin windows'.
	Chemotaxis is a reaction which cells show to chemical attractants by which the direction of their migration is determined. They migrate directionally in a gradient, and in order to show it convincingly the system has to be simplified considerably and a chemical attractant has to be put in a gradient with the cells shown moving in it. All kinds of other factors have to be excluded.
	In a skin window, one is really watching cell accumulation *in vivo* and there must be dozens of parameters which are studied. One of the important parameters, of which no one takes any notice, or which

147

	people find difficult to study experimentally, is the adhesion of cells, not only to the endothelial cells of the capillaries, but also in transit through the tissues. This is something which experimentally it is very difficult to measure.
Chairman:	But one is trying to find out why cells accumulate in an inflammatory lesion *in vivo*. Surely the skin window is closer in some respects?
Wilkinson:	It is closer to an inflammatory situation, but it does not measure chemotaxis. There are many reasons why cells can accumulate, one of which can be trapping. There may be sticky substances which trap cells. Cell biologists are familiar with such things. It may be that cell accumulation may be nothing whatsoever to do with chemotaxis.
M. Jayson: (UK)	I have a more general point, as a clinician, on Dr. Loewi's Paper. I was rather unhappy about making comparisons between the Crohn's Disease patients, and the sick controls, in that the sick controls consisted of a wide group of vastly different conditions varying from duodenal ulcer and peptic ulcerations to Behcet's and various other conditions, probably treated with a variety of different drugs. I wonder whether one can really make any meaningful comparisons.
Chairman:	There were fairly large numbers of rheumatoid arthritis patients?
Loewi:	Firstly that, and, secondly, we had about six ulcerative colitics, and several patients with tuberculous intestinal disease. I would have thought that they were quite comparable.
J.-P. Giroud: (France)	I entirely agree with Dr. Wilkinson about the problem of chemotaxis. When we speak about Boyden chambers and putting in some drugs, one of the problems lies in knowing whether the drugs perhaps act on the motility of the cells, and not only on their directionality. That is why I suggest that if we want to talk about chemotaxis, then we must first be sure that the drugs are only acting on directionality.
O. Voisin: (France)	There is a simple control—to put the same agent in the upper chamber. This should always be done. If it is done, and if there is an accumulation, then one can speak simply of chemotaxis.
K. Brune: (Switzerland)	I should like to put a question to the two speakers who presented papers about their technique to measure the influx of polymorphonuclear leukocytes, with former *in vivo* findings. We, but also Dr. Vinegar and many others, have found that if an inflammation is elicited, for example in the peritoneal cavity, in the pleural cavity, or in the joint cavity, then at least in the dose range of about 100 mg/kg of salicylate an increased influx of polymorphonuclear leukocytes will be found. I wonder whether a natural cavity differs considerably from the artificial cavity constructed by the new method presented.
Loewi:	It certainly would have to differ. In the peritoneal cavity there is an arrival, only early on, of polymorphs and that is followed by monocytes and some small lymphocytes, so there is quite a fundamental difference. We can leave the skin window on for 3 days, and nothing like this happens. Mr. Borel showed sections in which there was no accumulation at all of monocytic cells, but they were all polymorphs, so that there is a fundamental difference. I do not think that I can explain it any further. I do not know why it is.
Willoughby:	There is a fundamental difference, quite rightly, as Dr. Brune pointed out, but it is quite often a misleading one in that with delayed hypersensitivity reactions we are familiar with the initial disappearance phenomenon. Some of the work that has been carried out in our laboratory recently, and not published (Dr. Dunn), has shown a disappearance of the resting population of mononuclear cells, and if counts are expressed as a differential, this can lead one wildly astray.

148

GENERAL DISCUSSION

	Absolute counts of the cells have to be done; not only just differentials. This is one of the traps into which it is very easy to fall when looking at joint spaces and cavities.
Chairman:	The next subject presented this morning was the origin and kinetics of macrophages. It is a large subject to discuss in a short time, but are there any specific points, or any questions?
T. L. Vischer: (Switzerland)	Is there any situation where macrophages multiply, or can become less mature, in inflammatory sites or outside of the bone marrow?
R. van Furth: (The Netherlands)	In some situations—I think some types of granulomata—it can happen that immature macrophages may multiply when stimulated by T-cells, by lymphocytes. Some of these situations would have to be reinvestigated to have definite proof—but that experiment would be difficult— that one is not dealing with immature cells.

Secondly, all situations and all publications in which so-called mature cells multiply *in vitro* when conditioned medium is added— that is a stimulatory medium which has factors which stimulate proliferation of immature cells—have also to be reinvestigated. Although there are claims from American groups that peritoneal cells and macrophages do multiply, they usually stimulate the peritoneal cavity before, so that again there is recruitment of immature cells. If the peritoneal cavity is not stimulated and the cells taken out, there is no multiplication of cells.

It is therefore doubtful whether mature cells can multiply, but in some circumstances they may.

| G. Vaes: (Belgium) | Is anything known about the origin of the macrophages that are present in rheumatoid pannus or in the synovial membrane? From where do they come? |
| van Furth: | There have been claims that in the inflammatory situation they are from the circulation. However, what their origin is in the non-inflamed synovia has not been settled at all, as far as I know. |

Chairman's Summing-up and Future Trends—Cellular reactions in inflammation

A. C. ALLISON (UK)

At the first meeting of this series we reviewed the cellular events in acute and chronic inflammation[1]. I shall now summarize some advances made in this field of research during the past four years with reference to the discussions at this meeting. Inevitably the contributions from my own laboratory will be given undue prominence, because I am presenting a personal viewpoint and using familiar examples. Attention will then be drawn to major unsolved problems and some possible solutions. Predictions of future trends in the biomedical sciences are notoriously inaccurate, and my suggestions are offered not in any dogmatic spirit but in the hope that they will stimulate experiments to prove or disprove them.

CELLS INVOLVED IN INFLAMMATORY RESPONSES

Although many cell types participate in inflammatory responses (including lymphocytes, K-cells, platelets, endothelial cells and fibroblasts), the major cell types in acute and chronic inflammation are neutrophil granulocytes and cells of the mononuclear phagocytic lineage. This lineage includes immediate precursors in the bone marrow and elsewhere (monoblasts and promonocytes, only the latter being phagocytic) and circulating monocytes which are constantly replacing the Kupffer cells of the liver as well as macrophages in pulmonary alveoli, peritoneal and pleural cavities and other tissue spaces.

It was until recently thought that all the cells of this lineage in peripheral blood are phagocytic, but evidence is accumulating that some are not. We use non-specific esterase staining to distinguish three populations of mononuclear cells in human peripheral blood: mononuclear phagocytes, which show diffuse cytoplasmic staining; T-lymphocytes, which show granules of reaction product in the cytoplasm; and unstained cells, including B-lymphocytes. In freshly drawn blood only some cells with diffuse esterase staining engulf polystyrene latex particles, but if the mononuclear cells are cultured for one day all diffusely stained cells are phagocytic. Dr. Horwitz and I

150

interpret this finding as showing that quite a high proportion of monocyte precursor cells in human peripheral blood are not phagocytic but acquire phagocytic capacity in the course of a day. It would be interesting to determine the proportion of such cells in humans and experimental animals responding to inflammatory stimuli and in various diseases.

In some types of inflammation, notably allergic reactions and helminth infections, eosinophils are prominent. Evidence that certain T-lymphocyte responses to antigenic stimulation are associated with eosinophilia has been presented at this meeting by Dr. Parish. However, eosinophilia is not a characteristic feature of many classical delayed hypersensitivity reactions, including contact hypersensitivity. Perhaps stimulation of a subpopulation of T-lymphocytes leads to the formation of mediators which guide the differentiation of precursor cells along the eosinophil pathway and recruit these cells into lesions. Clearly it would be of interest to define such a sub-population of cells, which might be possible using specific surface markers (Ly antigens) or other procedures, and determine how they are activated. At least one function of eosinophils has recently been defined: capacity to kill antibody-coated schistosomula, the sensitive stage of schistosome worms shortly after they have penetrated the skin[2]. Selective depletion of eosinophils by antiserum increases the susceptibility of mice to schistosome infections, so these cells appear to play a protective role in schistosome and other helminth infections. A distinction is made on morphological grounds between 'active' and other eosinophils. Inflammatory infiltrates with many active eosinophils are associated with damage to heart muscle. The biochemical basis of such activation and tissue damage is an interesting problem, especially in tropical diseases. The constituents of neutrophil granules have been studied in considerable detail. Much less is known about the granules of eosinophils, although basic proteins are even more prominent than in neutrophils. They may well have proteinase and other activities. It would be of interest to know whether the lytic capacity of eosinophils for schistosomula, and heart muscle is due to a constituent of their granules (perhaps a basic protein inserted into the target cell plasma membrane), is present in the plasma membrane of the eosinophils (as appears to be the case for T-lymphocytes[3]), or is due to some other mechanism. This question could very easily be resolved by appropriate experiments with schistosomula and cultures of embryonic heart muscle cells, using fractions prepared from eosinophils.

PRODUCTION OF INFLAMMATORY CELLS

Neutrophils, eosinophils and mononuclear phagocytes all arise from a common precursor cell type which is most abundant in the bone marrow and present also in the spleen and circulating blood[4]. The agar culture technique allows cloning of the progenitor cells (colony-forming cells or CFU-c). Cell separation methods have identified the CFU-c as a transitional mononuclear cell distinct from multipotential stem cells. The CFU-c can differentiate into granulocytes (neutrophils or eosinophils) or mononuclear phagocytes. During inflammatory responses of various kinds the production of one or more of these cell types is considerably increased. This implies that the proliferation of CFU-c is stimulated, and that these differentiate predominantly into one of the mature cell types listed. It is therefore necessary to ask what factors stimulate the proliferation of CFU-c and induce them to differentiate into neutrophils, eosinophils or mononuclear phagocytes.

The requirement of a glycoprotein colony-stimulating factor (CSF) for *in vitro* granulocytic differentiation has led to suggestions that CSF is a granulopoietin. This interpretation is supported by reports of correlations between fluctuations in neutrophil production and levels of serum and urine CSF in several clinical and experimental situations[4]. In humans the main cell type producing CSF is the monocyte or tissue macrophage, suggesting that granulocyte–monocyte formation is controlled at least in part, by a system in which CSF produced by monocytes exposed to endotoxin or some other material stimulates proliferation of CFU-c; low levels of CSF direct the resulting cells into a monocytic pathway of differentiation whereas high levels favour differentiation into the granulocytic pathway, with a consequent decline in CSF production. Nevertheless, it is already clear that other factors are important: for example, properties of CSF samples vary, and granulopoiesis *in vitro* is inhibited by granulocytes themselves, by prostaglandin E, and by interferon. On the other hand mitogen-stimulated lymphocytes depleted of adherent cells can produce large quantities of CSF. The possible involvement of the complement system in stimulating CFU-c proliferation and/or differentiation into the granulocytic pathway and release comes from the observation that children deficient in C3, although subject to repeated pyogenic infections, do not show the usual leukocytic response to such infections[5].

In general, it is clear that factors stimulating the proliferation and differentiation of CFU-c along various pathways are of considerable interest. We can look forward to the chemical characterization of some at least of these factors and an analysis of the cellular regulatory mechanisms involved. This includes regulation of the production of mediators (for example, CSF liberation by macrophages and other cell types) and the mechanisms by which mediators control proliferation and differentiation. This takes us into a major area of research in cell biology, and there are bound to be interesting analogies with other systems. Two examples are control of the proliferation of erythroid cell precursors and their differentiation, with production of large amounts of haemoglobin, and proliferation of B-lymphocytes and their differentiation into cells producing large amounts of immunoglobulin. The role of cyclic nucleotides, nucleoprotein phosphorylation and other mechanisms of selective gene derepression will have to be analysed, and measurements made of specific products such as messenger

RNA's for lysozyme and basic proteins. Experimental pathologists have much to learn from developmental geneticists in this field.

RECRUITMENT OF CELLS INTO LESIONS

Two main groups of factors are involved in this process: those that facilitate entry of cells into sites of inflammation and those that immobilize cells, allowing them to accumulate in lesions. The former include factors facilitating attachment of cells to vascular endothelium and their emigration to the extravascular compartment. Most attention has been given to chemotaxis *in vitro*, usually using modified Boyden chambers. Four questions have to be asked about this system. Are the agents in question affecting overall motility of leukocytes or directional motility in a concentration gradient? Second, what is the chemical composition of the active agent? Third, to what extent are *in vitro* results applicable to recruitment of leukocytes *in vivo*? Fourth, what is the biological relevance of chemotaxis in different situations?

Only a few general remarks about chemotaxis are appropriate here. It is already clear that there are several classes of chemotactic agents, including:

(1) *Microbial products*[6]. The complexity and unknown structure of most of these have prevented analysis of their specificity and mode of action.

(2) *N-formyl methionyl peptides.* Recently several synthetic *N*-formyl methionyl peptides have been found to be chemotactic for neutrophils and macrophages[7,8]. *N*-formyl methionine is required for the initiation of protein synthesis in micro-organisms and it is possible that *N*-formyl methionyl peptides are released from the organisms and function as chemotactic agents in mammals. Some of the peptides are high active[9]: F-Met-Leu-Phe had an ED_{50} for induced migration of $7 \times 10^{-11}M$. There was a correlation between the capacity of various peptides to release lysosomal enzymes from rabbit neutrophils and their chemotactic activity. The relationship of structure to activity was highly specific. Binding of the peptides to a specific receptor on the plasma membrane of neutrophils may produce both chemotaxis and enzyme release, perhaps by altering calcium permeability. Obviously such specific structure-activity studies will provide a useful way of analysing the mechanism by which chemotaxis occurs.

(3) *Complement cleavage products.* Loewi has reported at this meeting that the relatively small polypeptide C3a is chemotactic for neutrophils and macrophages. An analogous polypeptide with anaphylatoxic activity is C5a, which is also a highly potent chemotactic agent for neutrophils and macrophages[8]. The chemotactic activity of the $C\overline{567}$ complex has long been known[6]. Activation of complement by the classical or alternative pathways is often associated with inflammatory responses (see contribution by Schorlemmer *et al.*, Chapter 14), and complement cleavage products may well play a major role in recruiting cells into lesions. It remains to define structure-activity relationships. In view of the chemotactic activity of *N*-formyl

methionyl peptides and peptides mediating eosinophil chemotaxis, small peptides derived from complement components may define the binding sites on the surfaces of neutrophils, eosinophils and macrophages which mediate chemotaxis and enzyme release. Again calcium permeability may be involved, as it is in mast cell degranulation induced by C3a and C5a. If the receptors on the three cell types are different, the possibility of selective chemotaxis arises, and has already been reported for eosinophils.

(4) *Peptides mediating eosinophil chemotaxis*[9]. The eosinophil chemotactic factor of anaphylaxis (ECF-A) was described as a mediator released during immediate-type hypersensitivity reactions in guinea pig and human lung slices. It was later found preformed in nasal polyps and shown to be associated with mast cell granules, released by IgE-mediated immunological reactions and to have a molecular weight of about 500 daltons. Two acidic peptides isolated from the preparations, with the sequences Ala-Gly-Ser-Glu and Val-Gly-Ser-Glu proved to be selectively chemotactic for eosinophils in Boyden chambers.

(5) *Other factors*. It makes biological sense also that where fibrin is being degraded the products should attract leukocytes which help to clear up the debris. There are several reports of chemotaxis of leukocytes by fibrin degradation products.

(6) *Lipid derivatives*. Prostaglandins have been extensively studied as mediators of inflammation and there are several reports that they modulate chemotaxis[10]. Another group of compounds that are currently attracting attention are other lipid endoperoxides. Transient intermediates of metabolism of these compounds may prove to be more important in inflammation than end products such as prostaglandins of the E and F series.

In general, many agents appear to be chemotactic for granulocytes and monocytes (e.g. microbial and complement cleavage products). Others are selective, for example products of activated T-lymphocytes which are chemotactic for monocytes and probably contribute to the recruitment of these cells into delayed hypersensitivity lesions[11]. However, the relative importance of selective cellular immigration and selective emigration in determining the composition of lesion is far from being established.

There is also uncertainty whether results obtained with Boyden chambers are always applicable *in vivo*. The skin window technique can be used with normal subjects and patients (being non-invasive) but it gives information only about neutrophils, since monocytes do not readily migrate into the windows. Nevertheless, the remarkable finding by Loewi and Segal of impaired migration of neutrophils into skin windows in patients with Crohn's disease illustrates the clinical potential of the system. Serum factors inhibiting chemotaxis (as in Crohn's disease) and enhancing chemotaxis should be characterized.

Simple experiments on the migration of cells into the peritoneal cavity or footpad of experimental animals after injection or slow release of putative chemotactic factors are also required. The use of leukocytes with a stable radioactive label would help to make observations quantitative. A recent advance has been the introduction of radioactive indium(^{111}In), as a label for cells. Carried through the plasma membrane as a chelate with oxine, ^{111}In is non-toxic, bound to cytoplasmic proteins and peptides and released only when the cells die (as shown by comparison of release of ^{125}I-iododeoxyuridine incorporated into DNA); ^{51}Cr leaks from cells that are still viable. A. Segal, who works in my laboratory, has used ^{111}In to label neutrophils from patients; the reinjected cells become concentrated in inflammatory sites and allow their localization by whole-body scanning.

The subcellular events producing chemotaxis of leukocytes are still unknown. As already mentioned, a current hypothesis is that the chemotactic agent binds to a specific receptor site on the leukocyte, thereby increasing calcium permeability through the plasma membrane. It is tempting to suggest that since microtubules are required for directional motility of leukocytes and calcium prevents assembly of tubulin subunits, these processes may be linked to chemotaxis[12]. If microtubules are selectively disassembled near the point of contact of the chemotactic agent, migration in that direction would be facilitated. This hypothesis can be tested by the use of calcium ionophores and drugs inhibiting microtubule assembly.

IMMOBILIZATION OF CELLS AT SITES OF INFLAMMATION

It seems clear that neutophils are less easily immobilized in lesions or by epithelial barriers than are monocytes. Examples are the migration of neutrophils through inflammatory periodontal lesions into the gingival sulcus and through inflamed synovia into synovial fluid. Inhibitors of cell movement are also more effective on monocytes than on neutrophils. The best known inhibitor is the macrophage migration inhibition factor (MIF) produced when lymphocytes respond to antigenic or mitogenic stimulation[11]. Since MIF production has been widely used as a criterion for responses by T-lymphocytes, it is worth reminding readers that human B-lymphocytes can also, when suitably stimulated, release MIF[13].

Neutrophils also release immobilizing factors[14], and the possibility that macrophages release similar factors, especially after stimulation, deserves further exploration. Experiments in our laboratory have shown that agents such as carrageenan elicit inflammatory responses as efficiently in nude as in conventional mice, without demonstrable antibody formation, which suggests that the marked accumulation of mononuclear phagocytes in these lesions occurs independently of mature T-lymphocytes. Polystyrene latex particles elicit only a mild inflammatory response, and many latex particles are removed from the site of injection quite rapidly, suggesting that cells after phagocytosis of latex leukocytes are able to emigrate, whereas after exposure to zymosan, asbestos or carrageenan mononuclear phagocytes are immobilized and therefore accumulate in lesions. The accompanying papers of Schorlemmer et al. (Chapter 14) and Davies et al. (Chapter 15) summarize evidence that cultured macrophages exposed to the latter group of agents secrete enzymes, complement cleavage products, prostaglandins and other factors.

A high priority task is to ascertain whether suitably stimulated macrophages liberate factors immobilizing other macrophages. If so, any agent inhibiting the formation of immobilizing factors or leukocytic responses to them might provide a means of resolving chronic inflammation.

ACTIVATION OF CELLS WITHIN INFLAMMATORY LESIONS

Neutrophils have three main effects. They ingest bacteria opsonized by antibody, especially in the presence of complement. They kill many ingested organisms. The details of this killing mechanism are beyond the scope of this review. We have been excited by demonstrating a major biochemical defect in chronic granulomatous disease, an inherited abnormality in the capacity of leukocytes to kill ingested organisms. In cells of the patients activity of plasma membrane NADH oxidase is markedly depleted[15]. We have found plasma membrane NADH oxidase also in macrophages, the activity of the enzyme being considerably increased in cells stimulated by BCG. Plasma membrane NADH oxidase appears to play a major part in the generation of superoxide anion and hydroxyl radicals which are important in killing organisms ingested by neutrophils or macrophages. Clearly much more work on this system, how it is activated and how it kills is required. The third effect of neutrophils is to release their hydrolases when exposed to immune complexes, especially in the presence of complement. This phenomenon has been studied experimentally by Henson[16] and others, and is thought to be important in Arthus reactions.

Since macrophages, unlike neutrophils, retain considerable capacity for protein and lipid synthesis, their activation in inflammatory lesions is much more spectacular. Three groups of agents activating macrophages are known. One is products of activated T-lymphocytes[11]. Another is immune complexes[17]. A third is the cleavage product of the third component of complement, C3b, as discussed by Schorlemmer et al. (Chapter 14). Consequences of macrophage activation include: (1) release of hydrolytic enzymes such as collagenase, elastase, plasminogen activator, proteinases that cleave complement components and glycosidases. The released enzymes can degrade connective tissue fibres and proteoglycan; (2) cleavage of complement components, including C3; (3) increased capacity to kill ingested micro-organisms, which appears to be due at least in part to increased plasma membrane NADH oxidase activity; (5) increased incorporation of labelled arachidonic acid into prostaglandins. The latter, especially the labile intermediates discussed by Kuehl et al. (Chapter 26) at this meeting, are likely to be important mediators of inflammation, others being complement cleavage products and kinins, formation of all of which would be promoted by macrophage activation. This process is therefore central to the pathogenesis of chronic inflammation. Detailed knowledge of the activators, how they regulate macrophage metabolism, the consequences of activation and its pharmacological control are all high priority needs.

THROMBOPLASTIN SYNTHESIS BY MACROPHAGES

Professor H. Prydz, a visitor in our laboratory from Norway this year, has found that mouse peritoneal macrophages and human monocytes stimulated by bacterial endotoxin release relatively large amounts of tissue thromboplastin. This is a phospholipoprotein of molecular weight 52,000 daltons which interacts with factor VII to bring about blood coagulation. When tissue thromboplastin is injected into experimental animals, disseminated intravascular coagulation is produced, and this can be prevented by intravenous administration of a highly purified bacterial enzyme, phospholipase C. Intravenous administration of endotoxins from Gram-negative bacteria produces a shock syndrome with disseminated intravascular coagulation (generalized Shwartzman reaction), and liberation of thromboplastin from macrophages may play a central role in this phenomenon, which has broad clinical relevance.

INTERACTIONS OF MACROPHAGES AND FIBROBLASTS IN COLLAGEN SYNTHESIS

Fibrogenesis is a common feature in chronic inflammatory reactions in the lungs, liver, joints and other sites. The fibrogenic effects of silica and asbestos particles are among the best known examples. We have presented biological evidence that silica fibrogenesis occurs in two stages: silica is taken up by macrophages which produce a diffusible product that stimulates fibrogenesis by fibroblasts[18]. It has also been shown that supernatants of macrophages cultured with silica stimulate proliferation of and collagen synthesis by fibroblasts. The next few years should bring characterization of such fibrogenic factors and how their production and effects could be pharmacologically controlled. The approaches mentioned previously might be applicable: purification of factors, measurement of binding to target cell membranes, search for effects on cyclic nucleotides and other regulators, activation of enzymes such as proline hydroxylase and formation of collagen messenger RNA. Techniques for each of these problems are available, and only time and ingenuity are required to solve them.

TRENDS

Certain general trends in research are clear. In the sixties much time and effort went into describing a range of products of activated lymphocytes, affecting many different cell types. Although this work continues, emphasis is shifting to the macrophage. This cell obviously produces a wide range of biologically important products: enzymes, CSF, pyrogens, thromboplastin, interferon, fibrogenic factor, lymphocyte-activating factors and others[1,17,18]. These are highly relevant to the pathogenesis of chronic inflammation and it is safe to predict that in the next few years much more information will be assembled about these factors, under what conditions they are produced and how they exert their effects.

Much has also been published about the biochemistry of neutrophils and further work on this subject (especially the mechanism of killing of ingested organisms) will certainly be undertaken. The eosinophil is emerging out of the area of descriptive pathology into that of contemporary immunology, and the biochemistry of these cells offers attractive opportunities for research. Mediators of inflammation are beyond the scope of this summary, but clearly their further characterization, and pharmacological control of their production and effects, will be the subject of major research in the years to come. No more than glimpses have been obtained of the effects of highly active intermediates in prostaglandin synthesis and other lipid endoperoxides. A new area of research is opening up. But the recognition of the importance of proteinases in the complement system, which is itself involved in macrophage activation, means that the detailed characterization of these enzymes and their selective inhibition are important. That is enough prediction of trends: they will reveal some interesting facts, but the surprises may well prove more interesting in the long run.

References

1. Allison, A. C. and Davies, P. (1974). Mechanisms underlying chronic inflammation. In: *Future Trends in Inflammation I* (G. P. Velo, D. A. Willoughy and J.-P. Giroud, eds.) p. 449. (Padua: Piccin Medical Books)
2. Butterworth, A. E., David, J. R., Franks, D., Mahmoud, A. A. F., David, P. H., Sturrock, R. F. and Houba, V. (1977). Antibody-dependent eosinophil-mediated damage to ^{51}Cr-labelled schistosomula of *Schistosoma mansoni*: damage by purified eosinophils. *J. Exp. Med.*, **145**, 136
3. Ferluga, J. and Allison, A. C. (1975). Cytotoxicity of isolated plasma membranes from lymph node cells. *Nature (London)*, **255**, 708
4. Moore, and Kurland, (1976)
5. Alper, C. A. (1974). The complement system. In: *Structure and function of plasma proteins* (A. C. Allison, ed.) pp. 107–158. (New York: Plenum Press)
6. Wilkinson, (1974)
7. Schiffman, E., Corcoran, B. E. and Wahl, S. M. (1965). N-formylonethionyl peptides as chelsaltractants for leukocytes (chemotaxis). *Proc. Natl. Acad. Sci. USA*, **72**, 1059
8. Showell, H. J., Freer, R. J., Zigmond, R. H., Schiffman, E., Aswanikumar, S., Corcoran, B. and Becker, E. L. (1976). *J. Exp. med.*, **143**, 1154
9. Goetzl, E. J. and Austen, K. F. (1977). Structural determinants of the eosinophil chemotactic activity of the acidic tetrapeptides of eosinophil chemotactic factor of anaphylaxis. *J. Exp. Med.*, **144**, 1424
10. Kaley, G. and Weiner, R. (1971). Effect of prostaglandin E on leukocyte migration. *Nature New Biol.*, **23**, 144

CELLULAR REACTIONS IN INFLAMMATION

11. David, J. R. and David, R. R. (1972). Cellular hypersensitivity and immunity. *Prog. Allergy.*, **16**, 300
12. Allison, A. C. (1974). Mechanism of movement and maintenance of an polarity in leukocytes. *Antibiot. Chemother.*, **19**, 197
13 Rocklin, R. E., MacDermott, R. P., Chess, L., Schlossman, S. F. and David, J. R. (1974). *J. Exp. med.*, **140**, 1303
14. Goetzl, E. J. and Austen, K. F. (1972). A neutrophil immobilizing factor derived from human leukocytes. 1. Generation and partial characterization. *J. Exp. Med.*, **136**, 1564
15. Segal, A. W., and Peeters, T. J. (1977). Analytical subcellular fractionation of human granulocytes with special reference to the localization of enzymes involved in microbioidal mechanisms. *Clin. Sci. Molec. med.*, **52**, 429
16. Henson, P. M. (1974). Mechanisms of activation and secretion by platelets and neutrophils. In: *Progress in Immunology* (L. Brent and J. Holborow, eds.) Vol. II, p. 95. (Amsterdam: North Holland Publishing Co.)
17. Cardella, C., Davies, P. and Allison, A. C. (1974). Immune complexes induce selective release of lysosomal hydrolases from macrophages. *Nature (London)*, **247**, 46
18. Allison, A. C., Clark, I. A. and Davies, P. (1977). Cellular interactions in fibrogenesis. *Ann. Rheum. Dis.*, **36**, suppl. 8

Section III
Chronic Inflammation: Mechanisms

CHAIRMAN: L. E. Glynn

CO-CHAIRMAN: I. Ginsburg

Co-Chairman's Introductory Remarks— The role played by leukocyte extracts and inflammatory exudates in the release of lipopolysaccharides from Gram negative bacteria: relation to tissue damage induced during infections

I. GINSBURG, Z. DUCHAN, S. BERGNER-RABINOWITZ, AND M. FERNE (Israel)

The role played by bacterial lipopolysaccharides (endotoxins) (LPS) in the initiation of tissue damage during bacterial infections, is well established[1]. It is accepted that LPS is released from the invading bacteria following autolysis, and the interaction of the solubilized LPS with tissues and body fluids lead to the initiation of the physiological, pharmacological and pathological sequelae seen after infections with Gram negative bacteria[1].

Previous studies from our laboratories have shown that the binding of LPS to membranes of RBC is markedly enhanced by heat-labile leukocyte factors[2], and that leukocyte factors are also capable of activating 'LPS' for binding to cell surfaces. Since the 'activation' of LPS caused by this factor was inhibited by protease inhibitors, it was postulated that proteases present in leukocytes and in inflammatory exudates may enhance tissue damage by increasing the passive sensitization of mammalian cells by LPS to subsequent lysis in the presence of antibodies and complement.

The present communication describes the role played by a heat-labile leukocyte factor (ENZ) in the 'extraction' of LPS from *Salmonella typhyi*. The role played by heat-stable cationic substances in the modulation of RBC sensitization by LPS and the possible role played by 'activated' LPS in the pathogenesis of tissue damage in inflammatory sites will be discussed. *Salmonella typhosa* 0–901 which had been cultivated in Todd Hewitt broth (Difco) were washed several times in phosphate buffered saline (PBS) pH 7.4

and adjusted to 1000 Klett Units/ml = 2.0 O.D at 540 nm. The bacterial
suspensions were treated for 30–180 min at 37 °C either with phenol[3] or with
freeze and thaw extracts of human peripheral blood leukocytes (containing
1–1000 μg/ml of protein). Following treatment the supernates were heated to
100 °C for 10 min, and used to sensitize red blood cells passively as described
in detail[2]. In some experiments LPS extracted from bacteria by phenol was
further treated with leukocyte extracts to 'activate' the LPS for binding to
RBC. To determine the degree of sensitization of RBC by LPS, we have
employed rabbit anti-salmonellae sera, which agglutinated the LPS-sensitized
RBC[2]. The addition of fresh rabbit serum to the sensitized cells led to the
lysis of the sensitized RBC. In some experiments we added nuclear histone
(10–100 μg/ml) to the reaction mixtures either before or after the binding of
LPS to RBC, and tested the percentage of inhibition of the haemagglutination
reaction. Samples of LPS released from bacteria either by phenol or by
leukocyte extracts were also subjected to gel filtration on Sephadex G-200
columns (5.9 × 40 cm) and the effluents were analysed for the presence of
LPS using the passive haemagglutination reaction.

Table 11.1 shows that while small amounts of LPS are spontaneously
released from washed salmonellae after incubation for 120 min at 37 °C in

Table 11.1 The release of LPS from salmonellae by leukocyte extracts (ENZ),
proteases and lysozyme

Concentration of extracting agent (Protein μg/ml)	ENZ	ENZ PMSF**	ENZ 100 °C***	TRYPSIN	PUS	LYSOZYME
0	240	240	240	240	240	240
1	240	240	240	240	240	240
5	3840	240	240	960	240	480
10	3840	240	240	3840	960	960
25	1920	240	240	3840	1920	1920
50	960	120	120	3840	1920	1920
100	960	120	120	3840	960	1920
250	—	—	—	1920	—	—
500	480	120	120	480	480	1920
1000	240	60	60	240	120	1920

Passive haemagglutination titres with LPS released by*

* 1000K.U/ml of salmonellae were treated for 120 min at 37 °C with increasing concentrations of the various agents. 500 μl of the supernates, which were obtained following
centrifugation at 2000g for 15 min, were incubated for 30 min at 37 °C with 1 ml of a 1%
human RBC suspension, which had been previously pretreated for 30 min with 25 μg/ml
of leukocyte extracts to activate LPS receptors. The titre of passive haemagglutination was
determined as the highest dilution of the rabbit anti-salmonellae serum, which agglutinated
the sensitized RBC. The potency of the LPS released from the bacteria by the leukocyte
extracts and proteases was compared with 10 μg/ml of a standard preparation of LPS
from *Salmonellae typhosa* 0–901 (Difco) which had been 'activated' by NaOH (3).

** PMSF - Phenyl-methyl sulphonyl fluoride–100 μg/ml.

*** ENZ boiled for 10 min.

PBS alone, substantial amounts of LPS were released into the supernates after the treatment of bacteria with leukocyte extracts, trypsin, lysozyme and by inflammatory exudates (pus.). The Table also shows that the release of LPS from the bacteria depended on the relative concentrations of the extracting agents. While small concentrations of leukocyte extracts (ENZ) (5–10 µg/ml) released relatively high amounts of LPS, ENZ concentrations which exceeded 50 µg/ml failed to release LPS, indicating the presence in ENZ of an inhibitory material. The capacity of ENZ to release LPS was completely abolished by heating to 100 °C or by pretreatment with phenyl-methyl sulphanyl fluoride (a known protease inhibitor). The Table shows that while trypsin and pus, at high concentrations, also failed to release substantial amounts of LPS, no inhibition of LPS release occurred with high concentrations of lysozyme. The data indicate, therefore, that leukocyte extracts and pus contain a heat-labile factor, probably a protease capable of detaching LPS from the bacterial surface. The nature of the inhibitory factor present in ENZ was further investigated. Since in a previous paper[2] it was shown that nuclear histone could block receptors in RBC and form inactive complexes with LPS released by phenol, it was postulated that leukocyte extracts may contain cationic proteins, which were responsible for the inhibition of the LPS reaction. To test this assumption, we have incubated RBC with high concentrations of ENZ or with pus. The RBC were then washed with PBS and then treated with crystalline trypsin. It was found that the trypsin-treated RBC could again bind a fresh batch of LPS, and became agglutinated by the addition of anti-LPS serum. The data suggest, therefore, that the inhibitory substance in ENZ (presumably cationic proteins) were digested by the trypsin and again unmasked the RBC receptors. These results are in accord with previous findings[2] that RBC pretreated with histone, which did not allow the binding of LPS, presumably due to the masking of LPS receptors, became 'reactivated' following treatment with trypsin.

To test whether the phenol and leukocyte extracts released the same LPS complex from the salmonellae, we have compared the patterns of gel filtration of LPS released by the two methods. It was found that both extracts yielded two distinct peaks of LPS actively following gel filtration. One peak emerged from the column with the void volume (high molecular weight), while the other had a molecular weight of approximately 15 000 daltons. The materials eluted in the two peaks were equally effective in sensitizing RBC to agglutination by anti-salmonellae serum. Although the nature of the low molecular weight material is still not known, it may be a depolymerized fraction of LPS.

The data presented indicate that the surface antigen of Gram negative bacteria (lipopolysaccharide-LPS) can be readily detached from the bacterial surface by very small amounts of human leukocyte extracts, lysozyme, inflammatory exudates as well as by crystalline trypsin.

The data are essentially similar to those which describe the capacity of leukocyte extracts and pus to release lipoteichoic acid (LTA) from strepto-cocci[2]. LTA has also been shown to sensitize mammalian cells to lysis by anti-streptococcal serum plus complement.

Although the nature of bonds which hold LPS on the bacterial surface are not fully known, the data presented suggest that proteolytic cleavage results in the release of 2 molecular species of LPS with different sizes but with the same cell-sensitizing properties. Since lysozyme was also capable of 'extracting' LPS from the bacteria, it may be postulated that a partial cleavage of the cell wall by lysozyme may also be involved in this reaction. It should, however, be also postulated that lysozyme, being a cationic poly-electrolyte, may bind the negatively-charged LPS and detach it from the bacterial surface (to be published).

The inhibition of LPS release from bacteria by high concentrations of ENZ and pus suggest that some cationic substances present in these fluids, probably bind the negatively charged LPS to form complexes which no longer can bind to RBC receptors.

The capacity of leukocyte factors to release LPS from Gram negative bacteria also points to the role which may be played by inflammatory exudates in the enhancing of tissue damage in inflammatory sites. It may be postulated that the interaction of proliferating Gram negative bacteria with leukocytes results in the release of a neutral protease, which detaches LPS from the surface of the bacteria. The LPS, which now becomes 'activated' by the same leukocyte factors, attaches itself to the surface of mammalian cells. Enhanced binding of LPS to cell surfaces occurs when leukocyte enzymes digest cell surfaces and unmask additional LPS receptors. The sensitized cells may then interact with antibodies and complement to cause cytolysis. Furthermore, LPS may trigger the transformation of lymphocytes and release lymphokines[4]. Pretreatment of lymphocyte surfaces by leukocyte extracts has been shown to cause enhanced transformation[5] and to enhance the transformation of cells induced by PHA[6] and perhaps by other mitogens. Since LPS has been implicated in numerous biological systems, including the triggering of Shwartzman phenomenon, and the activation of complement[7] it is postulated that the degranulation of PMN during the inflammation may further enhance tissue damage by amplifying the cell sensitizing properties of LPS. Further work along these lines is in progress.

Acknowledgement

This study was supported by grants from the Joint Research Fund of The Hebrew University-Hadassah School of Dental Medicine, founded by The Alpha Omega Fraternity and The Hadassah Medical Organization; by grants from the Chief Scientist, The Ministry of Health, Government of Israel; and Max Bogen Research Fund obtained through The Friends of The Hebrew University in The United States.

References

1. Kass, E. H. and Wolff, S. M. (1973). *Bacterial Lipopolysaccharides, Chemistry, Biology and Clinical Significance of Endotoxins*. (Chicago: The University of Chicago Press)
2. Ferne, M., Bergner-Rabinowitz, S. and Ginsburg, I. (1976). The effect of leukocyte hydrolases on bacteria. VI. The role played by leukocyte extracts in the sensitization of RBC by lipopolysaccharides and by the cell-sensitizing factor of group A streptococci. *Inflammation*, **1**, 247
3. Neter, E., Westphal, O., Luderitz, O., Gorzynski, E. A. and Eichenberger, E. (1956). Studies on enterobacter LPS: Effect of heat and chemicals on erythrocyte modifying antigenic, toxic and pyrogenic properties. *J. Immunol.*, **76**, 377
4. Peavy, D. L. Shands, J. W., Adler, W. A. and Smith, R. T. (1972). Selective effect of bacterial endotoxins on various subpopulations of lymphoreticular cells. *J. Infect. Dis.*, **128** (Supplement), 83
5. Vischer, T. L., Bretz, U. and Baggiolini, M. (1976). *In vitro* stimulation of lymphocytes by neutral proteinases from human polymorphonucleus leukocyte granules. *J. Exp. Med.*, **144**, 863
6. Garfunkel, A. A., Sela, M. N., Ovadia, H. and Ginsburg, I. (1977). Modulation of lymphocyte transformation by leukocyte hydrolases. *Israel J. Med. Sci.* (In press)
7. Mergenhagen, S. E. and Snyderman, R. (1972). Activation of complement by endotoxins. *J. Infect. Dis.*, **128** (Supplement), 78

12

The effect of local elevation of leukocyte cyclic AMP content on lysosomal enzyme release during acute inflammation *in vivo*

D. A. DEPORTER (Canada)

It is generally recognized that an insight into the control mechanisms involved in the release of lysosomal enzymes from inflammatory leukocytes could be of considerable benefit in the treatment of inflammatory diseases such as crystal-induced arthropathies, rheumatoid arthritis and periodontal disease. Recent studies from several laboratories have implicated the cyclic nucleotides, adenosine 3′,5′-cyclic monophosphate (cyclic AMP) and guanosine 3′,5′-cyclic monophosphate (cyclic GMP), in the control of lysosomal enzyme release from polymorphonuclear leukocytes (PMNs). It has been demonstrated that the discharge of these potentially destructive acid hydrolases from isolated PMNs that normally occurs in response to a variety of stimuli, including antigen–antibody complexes, zymosan particles and urate crystals, can be inhibited significantly by artificially elevating PMN cyclic AMP levels or enhanced by increasing their cyclic GMP levels[1–4]. However, these *in vitro* results have not as yet been supported by suitable animal experiments.

As part of a comprehensive study of the effect of local elevation of leukocyte cyclic AMP concentration on the release of various inflammatory mediators *in vivo*, we have investigated the effect of elevated cyclic AMP on leukocyte lysosomal enzyme discharge. Leukocyte cyclic AMP levels were elevated by administering dibutyryl cyclic AMP with or without the cyclic AMP phosphodiesterase inhibitor theophylline. Two rat models of acute inflammation were used; namely, a pyrophosphate crystal-induced pleurisy[5] and an immediate hypersensitivity-induced pleurisy[6]. Both these model systems have been shown to have relevance to human arthritis[7].

MATERIALS AND METHODS

The animals used were male Wistar rats weighing 250–300 g each.

Pyrophosphate pleurisy was induced by injecting 1 ml of a 1 % solution of a mixture of pyrogen-free monoclinic and triclinic crystals in saline[5]. Reverse passive Arthus reactions to BSA were produced in the pleural cavities of rats as described by Yamamoto et al.[6]. Briefly, 20–30 min following the intravenous injection of 0.2 ml of a solution of crystalline BSA in PBS, pH 7.4 (5 mg protein N_2/ml), 0.2 ml of a purified rabbit anti-BSA antiserum (1 mg protein N_2/ml PBS, pH 7.4) was injected intrapleurally.

To evaluate the effect of elevated leukocyte cyclic AMP content on the release of B-glucuronidase activity, 2.45 mg dibutyryl cyclic AMP (Sigma) with and without 0.99 mg theophylline (BDH) was injected into the pleural cavity with the respective irritant (i.e. either pyrophosphate crystals or anti-BSA). Three hours after the onset of each reaction the animals were anaesthetized with ether and exsanguinated via the carotid artery. Pleural exudates were withdrawn, blood-free, using siliconized Pasteur pipettes and separated into cells and supernatant by centrifugation at 200 g, 4 °C for 3 min.

Both the cellular and supernatant fractions were assayed for β-glucuronidase[8] and lactate dehydrogenase (LDH U-V system, Boehringer–Mannheim) activities. The cells were also assayed for their cyclic AMP content[9] to verify that the desired elevation had been produced by the two drug treatments.

In other animals the effect of the microtubular-disruptive drug colchicine on leukocyte cyclic AMP levels and lysosomal enzyme discharge during the reverse passive Arthus reaction was also assessed. Colchicine (BDH) was given intravenously at a dose of 0.2 mg/kg body weight 1 h before producing the intrapleural Arthus reactions.

RESULTS

Administration of dibutyryl cyclic AMP intrapleurally at the time of onset of the intrapleural Arthus reaction produced a 135% increase in leukocyte cyclic AMP concentration as compared with leukocytes from control Arthus reactions. When dibutyryl cyclic AMP was given in combination with theophylline, a 235% increase in leukocyte cyclic AMP content was observed (Figure 12.1).

Administration of dibutyryl cyclic AMP produced no reduction in the amount of β-glucuronidase released into the 3 h Arthus-induced pleural effusions. When dibutyryl cyclic AMP and theophylline were both injected intrapleurally at the time of onset of the Arthus reaction, there was a 30% increase in enzyme released (Figure 12.2). Injection of the drugs alone did not produce a significant increase in the release of β-glucuronidase activity as compared to saline injected controls (data not shown). The LDH results

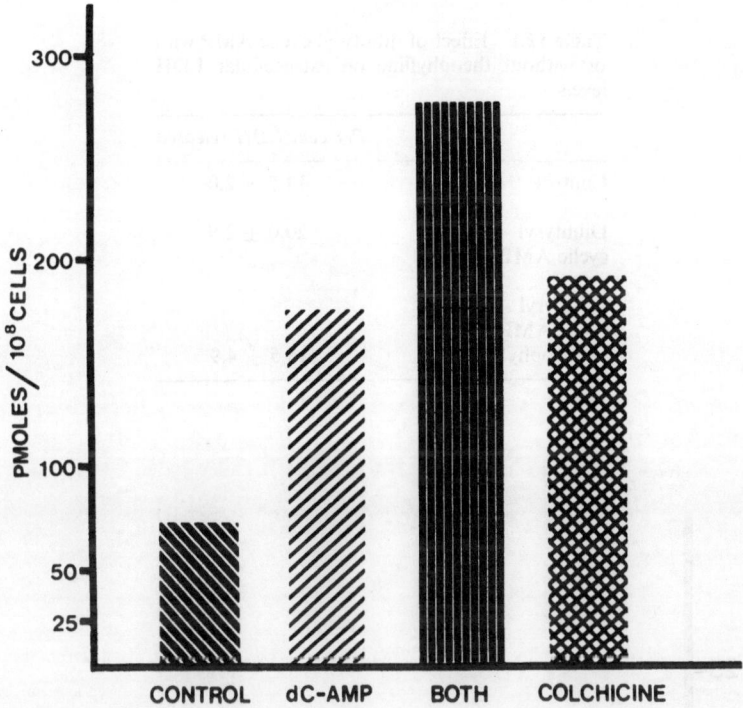

Figure 12.1 The effect of dibutyryl cyclic AMP, dibutyryl cyclic AMP with theophylline (both) and colchicine (0.2 mg/kg body wt.) on leukocyte cyclic AMP concentration at 3 h during the intrapleural Arthus reaction

are shown in Table 12.1. There was no significant difference between the three groups in the amount of LDH released.

Intrapleural administration of dibutyryl cyclic AMP and theophylline along with the pyrophosphate challenge produced a 400% increase in leukocyte cyclic AMP content (Figure 12.3). However, there was no significant effect on the per cent β-glucuronidase activity released into the inflammatory exudate (Figure 12.3). Furthermore, there was no difference in lactate dehydrogenase released or in cell viability as assessed by Trypan Blue exclusion tests (data not shown).

As can be seen in Figure 12.4, pretreatment of animals with intravenous colchicine at a dosage level of 0.2 mg/kg produced no decrease in the amount of β-glucuronidase activity released into the Arthus-induced pleural effusions. In contrast to this lack of effect of colchicine on enzyme release, the same pretreatment produced a 154% increase in leukocyte cyclic AMP concentration (Figure 12.1).

DISCUSSION

The present experiments using two different models of acute inflammation

Table 12.1 Effect of dibutyryl cyclic AMP with or without theophylline on extracellular LDH levels

	Per cent LDH released
Control	14.5 ± 2.0
Dibutyryl cyclic AMP	20.0 ± 2.9
Dibutyryl cyclic AMP + theophylline	18.5 ± 4.9

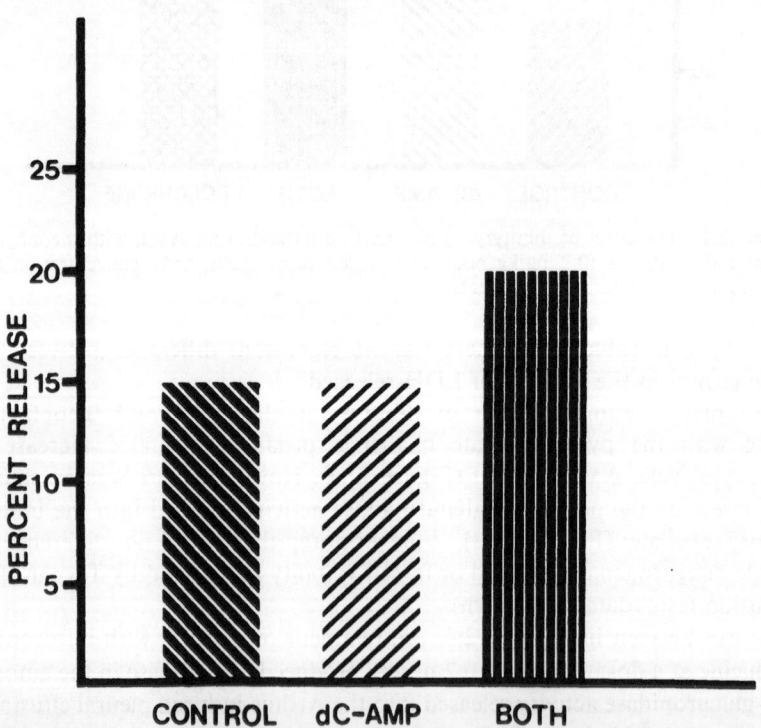

Figure 12.2 The effect of dibutyryl cyclic AMP alone and in combination with theophylline (both) on the per cent β-glucuronidase activity released into the Arthus-induced pleural effusions

$$\text{per cent released} = \frac{\text{extracellular enzyme}}{\text{cellular} + \text{extracellular enzyme}} \times 100$$

172

have demonstrated an apparent lack of inhibition of lysosomal enzyme discharge from leukocytes following local elevation of leukocyte cyclic AMP levels. These *in vivo* observations are in direct opposition to the *in vitro* work of others (see (10) for a review). Thus, it has been demonstrated using isolated human PMNs that the administration of exogenous dibutyryl cyclic AMP or theophylline or other cyclic AMP-elevating agents can markedly reduce the release of β-glucuronidase following stimulation with a variety of phagocytosable particles including antigen–antibody complexes. The reason for this lack of agreement is not readily apparent, but both the present animal models and the *in vitro* systems have inherent pitfalls. The *in vitro* studies did involve concentrations of dibutyryl cyclic AMP and theophylline approximating our own dose regimens. Furthermore, for the most part they utilized mixed populations of leukocytes rather than purified PMNs which again corresponds well to the population of cells present in a pleural effusion. One important point of difference, however, is that in the *in vitro* experiments the leukocytes were pre-incubated with agents chosen to increase cyclic AMP while in our own experiments the same drugs were not used as a predose but were given at the time of administration of the inflammatory irritant. Indeed, Zurier *et al.*[3] state that 'the time of preincubation was critical for reduction of enzyme release to be demonstrated' *in vitro*. Another technical point worth noting is that the inhibitory effect of cyclic AMP on enzyme release *in vitro*

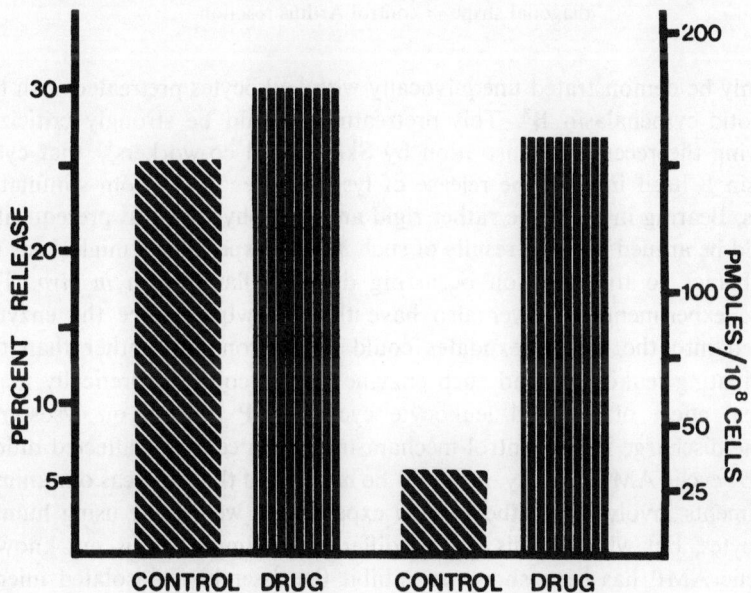

Figure 12.3 The effect of dibutyryl cyclic AMP with theophylline on leukocyte cyclic AMP concentration (right side) and on the per cent β-glucuronidase released by the cells (left side) at 3 h following intrapleural injection of pyrophosphate

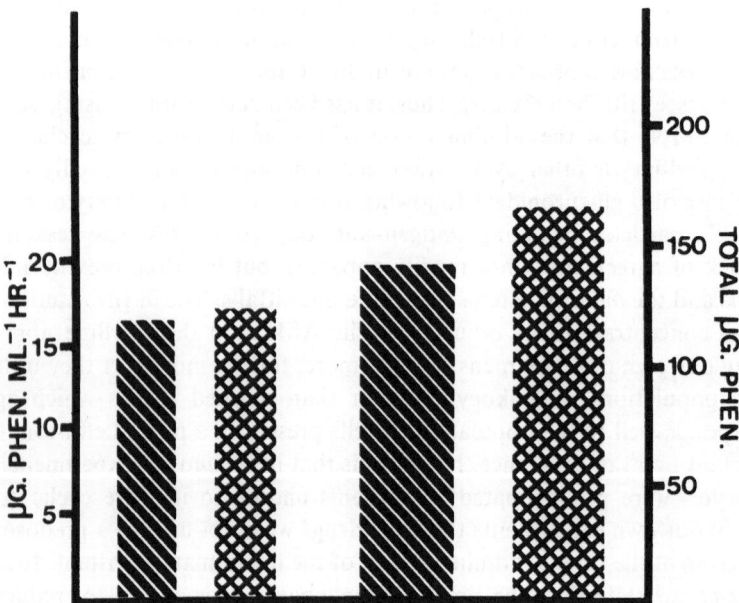

Figure 12.4 The effect of colchicine on the extracellular concentration of β-glucuronidase activity (left side) and the total extracellular β-glucuronidase activity (right side) at 3 h after the onset of the intrapleural Arthus reaction

cross-hatch = colchicine
diagonal stripe = control Arthus reaction

can only be demonstrated unequivocally with leukocytes pretreated with the antibiotic cytochalasin B[3]. This pretreatment could be strongly criticized following the recent demonstration by Skosey and co-workers[11] that cytochalasin B itself inhibits the release of lysosomal enzymes from stimulated PMNs. Bearing in mind the rather rigid and non-physiological prerequisites it could be argued that the results of such *in vitro* experiments might bear no resemblance to the situation occurring during inflammation *in vivo*. The *in vivo* experiments however also have their drawback since the enzyme released into the pleural exudates could come from cells other than the participating leukocytes and such enzyme release could theoretically mask the real effect of elevated leukocyte cyclic AMP content on lysosomal enzyme discharge if the control mechanism in such cells was affected differently by cyclic AMP. Finally, it should be mentioned that whereas our animal experiments involved rats the *in vitro* experiments were done using human leukocytes, but whether this species difference is important is not known.

Cyclic AMP has been shown to inhibit the assembly of isolated microtubular subunits from bovine brain[12], and intact microtubules are generally held to be a prerequisite for lysosomal enzyme discharge[13]. Therefore, it has been proposed following the *in vitro* experiments on PMN lysosomal enzyme release cited above that elevation of leukocyte cyclic AMP content produces an inhibition of lysosomal enzyme discharge by affecting leukocyte microtubular integrity, although direct evidence for this hypothesis is lacking. Since our results suggested that cyclic AMP does not produce a similar inhibition of leukocyte lysosomal enzyme release *in vivo*, we decided to investigate the effect of another microtubular disruptive agent, colchicine, on both leukocyte cyclic AMP content and lysosomal enzyme secretion in our immediate hypersensitivity-induced pleurisy model. The results were doubly weighted against a role for cyclic AMP and microtubules in the release of lysosomal enzymes from inflammatory leukocytes since colchicine not only did not reduce the amount of β-glucuronidase activity released but also produced a significant increase in leukocyte cyclic AMP content. Thus, whereas further work is needed to support the present results, the possibility exists that not only is cyclic AMP not involved in the release of lysosomal hydrolases from PMNs but that microtubules are also not involved. This latter suggestion is supported by recent results from other workers. For example, Moore et al.[14] have reported that it may be bundles of microfilaments of actin and myosin that are responsible for the movement of lysosomal granules in PMNs.

References

1. Weissmann, G., Zurier, R. B., Spieler, P. J. and Goldstein, I. M. (1971). Mechanisms of lysosomal enzyme release from leukocytes exposed to immune complexes and other particles. *J. Exp. Med.*, **134**, 149s
2. Ignarro, L. J. (1974). Regulation of lysosomal enzyme secretion: role of inflammation. *Agents Actions*, **4**, 241
3. Zurier, R. B., Weissmann, G., Hoffstein, S., Kammerman, S. and Tai, H. H. (1974). Mechanisms of lysosomal enzyme release from human leukocytes. II. Effects of c-AMP and c-GMP, autonomic agonists and agents which affect microtubule function. *J. Clin. Invest.*, **53**, 297
4. Hoffstein, S. and Weissmann, G. (1975). Mechanisms of lysosomal enzyme release from leukocytes. IV. Interaction of monosodium urate crystals with dogfish and human leukocytes. *Arthritis Rheum.*, **18**, 153
5. Deporter, D. A., Dieppe, P. and Willoughby, D. A. (1976). Pyrophosphate-induced inflammation: an *in vivo* study of the interrelationship of intracellular cyclic AMP and cyclic GMP. *Agents Actions*, **6**, 476
6. Yamamoto, S., Dunn, C. J., Deporter, D. A., Cappasso, F., Willoughby, D. A. and Huskisson, E. C. (1975). A model for the quantitative study of Arthus (immunologic) hypersensitivity in rats. *Agents Actions*, **5**, 374
7. Willoughby, D. A. (1976). Human arthritis applied to animal models. Towards a better therapy. *Ann. Rheum. Dis.*, **34**, 471
8. Fishman, W. H. (1965). In: *Methods of Enzymatic Analysis*. H. U. Bergmeyer, (ed.). New York and London: Academic Press
9. Brown, B. L., Albano, J. D. M., Ekins, R. P., Sgherzi, A. M., and Tampion, W. (1971). A simple and sensitive assay method for the measurement of adenosine 3′,5′-cyclic monophosphate. *Biochem. J.*, **121**, 561
10. Weissman, G., Goldstein, I., Hoffstein, S. and Tsung, P.-K. (1975). Reciprocal effects of c-AMP and c-GMP on microtubule-dependent release of lysosomal enzymes. *Ann. N.Y. Acad. Sci.*, **253**, 750
11. Skosey, J. L., Damgaard, E., Chow, D. and Sorensen, L. B. (1974). Modification of Zymosan-induced release of lysosomal enzymes from human polymorphonuclear leukocytes by cytochalasin B. *J. Cell. Biol.*, **62**, 625

12. Goodman, D. B., Rasmussen, H., DiBella, F., and Guthrow, C. D. (1970). Cyclic adenosine 3′,5′-monophosphate-stimulated phosphorylation of isolated microtubule subunits. *Proc. Nat. Acad. Sci. USA.*, **67**, 652

13. Malawista, S. E. (1975). Microtubules and the mobilization of lysosomes in phagocytosing human leukocytes. *Ann. N.Y. Acad. Sci.*, **253**, 738

14. Moore, P. L., Bank, H. L., Brissie, N. T. and Spicer, S. S. (1976). Association of microfilament bundles with lysosomes in polymorphonuclear leukocytes. *J. Cell. Biol.*, **71**, 659

Discussion 12

D. Roos: **(The Netherlands)**	Weissmann has unpublished evidence that the assembly of micro-tubules is not essential for lysosomal enzyme release *in vitro*. There may be concentrations of colchicine which disrupt microtubules but nevertheless do not inhibit lysosomal enzyme release. Has Dr. Deporter checked whether the β-glucuronidase is stable in the tissue which he examined? Would it be possible that there is a release of β-glucuronidase, but that it is degraded before it is measured? On the other hand, would it be possible that in the mixed leukocyte population that he examined, the lysosomal enzyme is being syn-thesized in the time of the experiment?
Deporter:	I have not checked that the β-glucuronidase is being destroyed during the time of the experiment. However, I have compared residual cellular levels in 'control versus experimental' and found them to be very similar. Synthesis is entirely possible. The only argument against it would be that these are acute inflammations and they are predominantly 70–80% polymorphonuclear leukocytes.
Roos:	I agree that in these cells it is highly improbable, but I do not know what other cells there are.
Deporter:	It is a possibility that cannot be ruled out. It is interesting that someone should bring up the effect of colchicine. It seems from experiments that have been reported that the concentration of the drug is highly critical, and that under some circumstances a particular concentration of colchicine can stimulate the release of lysosomal enzymes from PMNs *in vitro*. It also depends, interestingly enough, on the concentra-tion of the stimulus. Others have suggested that different concentrations of, for example, zymosan, in combination with a drug like colchicine, could produce opposite results.
Roos:	That may be possible.
G. Carter: **(USA)**	What is the evidence that lysosomal enzyme release is being seen, and not simply cell lysis?
Deporter:	We have evidence with the pyrophosphate model, where we studied the effect of dibutyryl cyclic AMP and theophylline on crystal uptake. We did studies of percentage of cells taking up crystals versus those that did not take up crystals, and which percentage of each group died and remained alive over a period of three hours after they had been removed from the pleural cavity. We found that there was no effect of dibutyryl cyclic AMP, or theophylline, on crystal uptake, and no effect on cell viability as assessed by trypan blue exclusion tests.
Carter:	We have tried to do some of these experiments and they seem to have an inherent problem in that there are basal levels of β-glucuronidase which makes it very difficult to determine whether it is being selectively released or whether it is a result of a basal level of cellular damage.
Deporter:	It is generally thought that the release of enzymes from cells that have

177

K. Brune: (Switzerland)	been exposed to calcium pyrophosphate dihydrate crystals is relatively selective. This was the hypothesis on which the experiment was based. The data are quite interesting but how can one be sure that the elevation of the cyclic nucleotide content did not happen to occur after the cells had been treated, had been removed from the cavity, had been centrifuged, and so on? Dr. Deporter pointed out quite eloquently that it can be dangerous to draw conclusions from *in vitro* studies for *in vivo* situations. I wonder whether his measurements justify concluding on a real *in vivo* situation.
Deporter:	The cells were centrifuged for less than 3 minutes. They were quickly fixed and theophylline was always added to the medium which was used to wash out the pleural cavity in an attempt not to alter the levels that were already there.
	This is a problem which is inherent with all experiments in the cyclic nucleotide and prostaglandin field.
E. Arrigoni-Martelli: (Denmark)	We have had results similar to those of Dr. Deporter using a different model of inflammation—Actinomyces-induced peritonitis. In this condition we have increased the level of cyclic AMP and at the same time increased the release of β-glucuronidase. This could suggest that we have to revise our opinion of the Yin-Yang hypothesis in the regulation of lysosomal enzyme release according to an increase of cyclic AMP and *vice versa*.
	There are probably people better qualified than I am to comment on this hypothesis.
Deporter:	It is fascinating that at first appearance, in our own experiments, there did seem to be a correlation between the cyclic GMP levels and β-glucuronidase release, because in the pyrophosphate model cyclic GMP is at its peak at 6 hours, cyclic AMP is at its lowest level, and β-glucuronidase is also at its highest level. So it would have seemed at first that cyclic GMP and β-glucuronidase were going together, and that probably would have suggested to us that the experiments would have come out exactly opposite to the results that we in fact achieved.
R. Turner: (USA)	It may not be bothering anybody else—and I think Dr. Deporter's work is beautiful—but I have one question. He did not show the standard errors on his graphs, and he did not show the numbers of repetitions.
	Could he tell us the levels of significance that he accepted and the number of times that the experiments were repeated?
Deporter:	I cannot remember how many times the experiments were repeated, but it was a considerable number. To be quite honest, I wanted the results to go the other way. But the level of significance was 95%.
J.-P. Giroud: (France)	When the dibutyryl cyclic AMP was injected, was any decrease in the number of cells noted?
Deporter:	This was very interesting. We have done it with several different models. It seems that a local elevation in leukocyte cyclic AMP content—at least in my own hands—will produce a reduction in cell migration only in the complement-dependent type of reaction, that is in the Arthus reaction. When pyrophosphate crystals or urate crystals were used, no effect by elevated leukocyte cyclic AMP was found on the number of cells migrating.
Giroud:	I would completely agree. Work done in my own department has been able to show that when dibutyryl cyclic AMP is injected, it is possible to block chemotaxis without blocking the motility of the cells. This is quite important in dealing with chemotaxis.

13

Recent studies on the secretory activity of mononuclear phagocytes with special reference to prostaglandins

P. DAVIES, R. J. BONNEY, M. E. DAHLGREN, L. PELUS, F. A. KUEHL, JR. AND J. L. HUMES (USA)

INTRODUCTION

The importance of phagocytosis and intracellular digestion by mononuclear phagocytes has been appreciated since the seminal observations of Metchnikoff over a century ago. In recent years it has become increasingly clear that mononuclear phagocytes also secrete a series of macromolecular mediators which play an essential role in homeostatic mechanisms and, under certain circumstances, contribute to the initiation and evolution of chronic inflammatory processes. We have reviewed in detail elsewhere[1-3] the secretory activities of macrophages under a variety of conditions. Table 13.1 summarizes the products of the secretory activity of macrophages with reference to inducing stimuli where appropriate. It is clear that in some, but not in all, instances products relevant to inflammatory processes are secreted in response to inflammatory stimuli.

We and others have discussed in detail elsewhere how stimuli of inflammation, either non-immune in origin or products of lymphocyte stimulation, cause the selective release of acid hydrolases from unstimulated macrophages. This information is summarized in Table 13.2. It is notable that in most instances the release of lysosomal enzymes occurs almost immediately after exposure of cells to inflammatory stimuli (the release of the lysosomal enzymes stimulated by carrageenan[4] and that caused by lymphokines[5] are notable exceptions). We have recently compared the inflammatory potencies of various stimuli with their ability to cause selective release of lysosomal enzymes from macrophages *in vitro*[6,7] and found a close correlation of activity for these two parameters. Thus, the chronic inflammatory capacity of three types of carrageenan as judged by morphological examination of

Table 13.1 Secretory products of mononuclear phagocytes

Product	Source	Stimulus for secretion	Reference No
Colony stimulating factor	Human peripheral blood monocytes	Endotoxin Polyinosinic: polycytidylic acid	18
Fibroblast growth factor	Rat peritoneal macrophages Rat peritoneal macrophages	Quartz dust Quartz dust None	19 20 21
	Mouse peritoneal macrophages	None	22
Interferon	Rabbit alveolar macrophage Mouse peritoneal macrophages	Newcastle disease virus	23 24
Listericidal factor	Guinea pig peritoneal macrophages	BCG *in vivo*	25
Stimulant of T-lymphocyte responses	Human peripheral blood monocyte	Endotoxin	26
	Mouse peritoneal macrophages	Certain phagocytic stimuli	27
Stimulant of B-lymphocyte responses	Human peripheral blood monocytes	Endotoxin	28
	Mouse peritoneal macrophages	Proteose peptone *in vivo*	29
Complement components: C1, C2, C3, C4, Factor B	Various	None	For review see 3 and 30
Pyrogen	Human peripheral blood monocytes	Endotoxin, Phagocytosis	31 32
Chemotactic substance for PMN	Human peripheral blood monocytes	Hydrocortisone	33
Prostaglandins	Guinea pig peritoneal macrophages	Lymphokines	14
	Human macrophages	None	13
	Mouse peritoneal macrophages	Antibody-coated erythrocytes	Glatt This volume
Cytotoxic factor(s) for syngeneic erythrocytes	Mouse peritoneal macrophages	None	34
Cytotoxic factor for tumour cells		Endotoxin	35
Hydrolytic enzymes: (a) Lysozyme	Human peripheral blood monocytes	None	36
	Mouse peritoneal macrophages		36
(b) Neutral proteinases: collagenase	Mouse peritoneal macrophages	*In vivo* inflammatory stimulus	For review see Ref. 2, 3 & 9
Plasminogen activator	Rabbit alveolar macrophages		
Elastase, azocaseinase	Human peripheral blood monocytes		
(c) Acid hydrolases	Mouse peritoneal macrophages	Various inflammatory stimuli	See Table 13.2
	Guinea pig alveolar macrophages		

Table 13.2   Selective release of acid hydrolases from macrophages by inflammatory stimuli

Stimulus	Source of Macrophages	Reference No.
Zymosan	Mouse peritoneal	7, 37, 38
Dental plaque	Guinea pig alveolar	39
	Mouse peritoneal	40
Group A streptococcal peptidoglycan-C-muco-	Mouse peritoneal	41
polysaccharide		42
Carrageenan	Mouse peritoneal	4, 6
Chrysotile asbestos	Mouse peritoneal	8
Antigen–antibody complexes	Mouse peritoneal	43
C3b	Mouse peritoneal	44
	Guinea pig peritoneal	45

7 day old lesion is related to their capacity to cause selective release of acid hydrolases from macrophages in culture over a 72 h time period[6]. In a more recent study[7], we have examined the intensity of chronic inflammatory lesions by both morphological and quantitative biochemical techniques. Chrysotile asbestos is highly inflammatory and a potent stimulator of the selective release of lysosomal enzymes from macrophages[8]. Treatment with 1N hydrochloric acid depletes the asbestos of a surface layer of brucite resulting in the loss of both the inflammatory capacity and ability to cause selective release of lysosomal enzymes. This illustrates further the correlation between these *in vivo* and *in vitro* phenomena, as well as showing that a relatively simple chemical modification removes the inflammatory potency of chrysotile asbestos.

The secretion of neutral proteinases by macrophages is usually of delayed onset but continues subsequently for prolonged periods of time[9]. Neutral proteinase secretion by macrophages is stimulated optimally by intraperitoneal injection of a sterile inflammatory stimulus to experimental animals several days before collection of peritoneal exudate cells for culture. Thioglycollate broth has been used extensively for this purpose. Intraperitoneal injection of endotoxin[10] and asbestos[11] has also been shown to stimulate plasminogen activator secretion by murine peritoneal macrophages. The addition of a nondigestible but inert phagocytic stimulus, such as latex particles, to macrophages obtained from experimental animals receiving endotoxin stimulates plasminogen activator secretion by these cells[10]. On the other hand, the *in vivo* administration of latex fails to stimulate plasminogen activator release[11] by macrophages collected from treated animals. Hamilton *et al.*[11] did not detect any secretion of acid hydrolases under the conditions where asbestos-stimulated macrophages secreted plasminogen activator. This emphasizes the possibility that secretory products of macrophages play different roles in chronic inflammatory responses, each making a specific contribution to the initiation, evolution or resolution of the process.

Synthesis and secretion of prostaglandins by macrophages

It is now clear that prostaglandins mediate certain aspects of inflammatory processes and modulate others (see paper by Kuehl *et al.*, chapter 25). Macrophage phospholipids contain high proportions (approximately 20% of total fatty acids) of arachidonic acid[12] and evidence that these cells synthesize prostaglandins has been presented[13,14]. The observations of Gordon *et al.*[14] are of particular relevance to inflammation since they showed that macrophages secreted prostaglandins in response to lymphokines.

The release of [³H]prostaglandins from macrophages prelabelled with [³H]arachidonic acid

Several investigators have shown that [³H]arachidonic acid is incorporated into phospholipids and neutral lipids of tissues and cells *in vitro*[15-17] and that its release and transformation into prostaglandins via the prostaglandin synthetase system can be quantitated.

Our initial investigations showed that unstimulated mouse peritoneal macrophages and macrophages obtained from mice injected intraperitoneally with thioglycollate broth four days previously incorporate [³H]arachidonic acid into cellular phospholipids. The incorporation of [³H]arachidonic acid into stimulated or unstimulated macrophages proceeds at approximately the same rate, 50–80% of total being located within cellular phospholipids 10 h after addition of label.

Inflammatory stimuli cause the synthesis and secretion of prostaglandins by macrophages

As seen in Table 13.2, a variety of inflammatory stimuli cause selective release of lysosomal acid hydrolases from macrophages. In marked contrast stimuli lacking chronic inflammatory activity fail to cause acid hydrolase release from macrophages (for details see Schorlemmer *et al.*[7]). We have taken two of these stimuli, zymosan, which is inflammatory, and latex particles, which are not inflammatory, and determined their effects on prostaglandin synthesis by macrophages.

MATERIALS AND METHODS

Macrophages were obtained by methods described previously[8] from unstimulated mice or animals which had received an intraperitoneal injection of 2 ml thioglycollate broth 4 days previously. Cultures were maintained for 24 h in M199 containing 10% heat-inactivated porcine serum (HIPS) before addition of 1 μC_i[³H]arachidonic acid in M199 containing 1% HIPS. After labelling for a 4 h period the medium containing [³H]arachidonic acid was removed and the cells washed to remove unincorporated label and then exposed to added stimuli in serum-free M199 for appropriate periods of time.

At the end of the incubation period, the culture medium was removed, acidified with citric acid and carrier PGE_2, $PGF_{2\alpha}$ and arachidonic acid added. A Folch extract was then prepared, evaporated to dryness, taken up in a small volume of ethyl acetate-methanol and spotted onto 2×20 cm strips of Whatman SG81 chromatographic paper. Components were separated by descending chromatography utilizing ethyl acetate/acetone/acetic acid [90/10/1] as the developing solvent.

On completion of chromatography, the carrier standards were visualized by iodine vapour and the appropriate areas of the paper cut out for scintillation counting of the separated tritiated products. These methods allow approximately 80% recovery of standard [3H]prostaglandins taken through the procedure outlined above. It must be emphasized that any reference made to [3H]prostaglandins measured in this system refers to products of mobility similar to that of authentic standards and does not take into account any other products of [3H]arachidonic acid with similar chromatographic mobilities.

RESULTS

Zymosan causes a dose- and time-dependent synthesis and secretion of [3H]PGE_2 and [3H]$PGE_{2\alpha}$ by both unstimulated and stimulated mouse macrophages. Figure 13.1 shows that exposure of 1×10^6 macrophages from thioglycollate-stimulated mice to 200 μg of zymosan for 4 h leads to a 6-fold increase in $PGF_{2\alpha}$ secretion. Synthesis and secretion begins as early as 15 min after addition of zymosan and continues for as long as 24 h. The release of [3H]prostaglandins from macrophages of thioglycollate-stimulated mice caused by zymosan is dose-dependent, increasing up to 10-fold for PGE_2 at a dose of 800 μg. It should be noted, however, that zymosan causes some cell death at doses of 400 μg and above as evidenced by release of cellular lactate dehydrogenase into the culture medium.

Unstimulated macrophages are more reactive to zymosan, lower doses causing greater increments of [3H]prostaglandin biosynthesis and secretion (Table 13.3). On the other hand, latex, which does not cause chronic

Table 13.3 Zymosan stimulates the synthesis and secretion of [3H]PGE_2 and [3H]$PGF_{2\alpha}$ by unstimulated macrophages

	PGE_2		$PGF_{2\alpha}$	
	c.p.m. released	Fold increase	c.p.m. release	Fold increase
Control	159 ± 8		115 ± 6	
Zymosan (25 μg/ml)	3084 ± 23	19	1550 ± 51	14

Approximately 4×10^6 unstimulated peritoneal macrophages prelabelled with [3H]-arachidonic acid were exposed to 25 μg zymosan in 2 ml culture medium for 4 h.

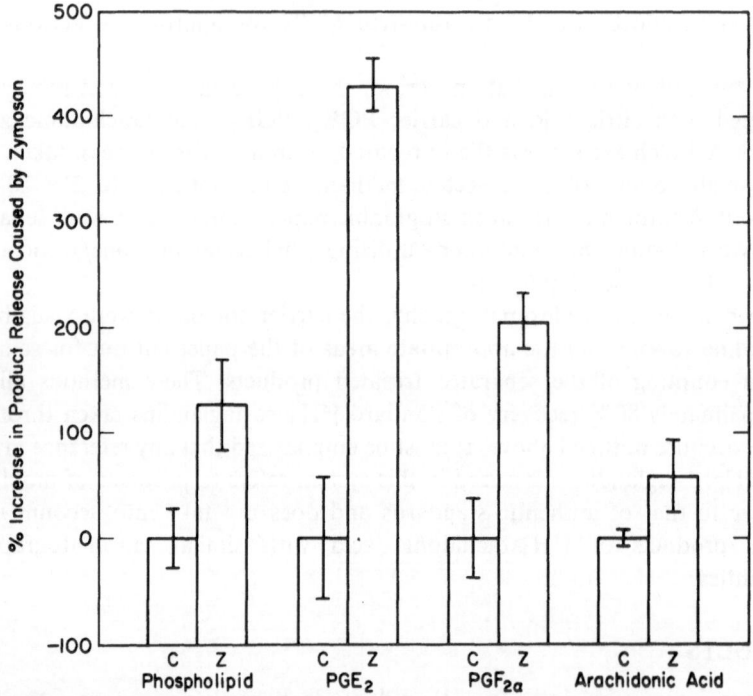

Figure 13.1 The synthesis and secretion of [³H]prostaglandins by peritoneal macrophages from thioglycollate-stimulated mice. 1×10^6 cells were exposed to 200 μg zymosan for 4 h at which time the culture medium was removed and [³H]prostaglandin content assayed

inflammation[7], fails to stimulate prostaglandin biosynthesis and secretion.

The zymosan-induced synthesis of [³H]prostaglandins by macrophages is inhibited by both non-steroidal and steroidal anti-inflammatory drugs. In contrast to the non-steroidal anti-inflammatory agents whose effects are seen immediately upon their addition, the effects of glucocorticoids such as dexamethasone and prednisolone are maximal only after a preincubation period of approximately 1 to 2 h before addition of zymosan. After this time, [³H]prostaglandin synthesis is inhibited by approximately 50% by 1×10^{-6}M concentrations of steroids. Significant inhibition of [³H]prostaglandin biosynthesis is seen with as little as 1×10^{-8}M steroid.

DISCUSSION

It is now clear from the studies of Myatt et al.[13] and Gordon et al.[14], those presented by Glatt in this volume and the results presented in this paper that macrophages synthesize and secrete prostaglandins in response to a series of inflammatory stimuli. In our study, we have utilized a different method than used by others[13,14] for measuring the synthesis of prostaglandins by prelabelling the cells with [³H]arachidonic acid. It remains to be determined whether the label is uniformly distributed in the cellular pool of phospholipids from which arachidonic acid utilized for prostaglandin biosynthesis is derived.

Macrophages which have been exposed to a sterile inflammatory stimulus *in vivo* do not show as great a sensitivity to zymosan as unstimulated macrophages despite the fact that they incorporate [^{3}H]arachidonic acid to approximately the same extent. It is not clear whether the observed differences in the synthesis and secretion of prostaglandins by stimulated and unstimulated macrophages is a reflection of a different cellular distribution of incorporated [^{3}H]arachidonic acid or is due to a more basic difference in synthetic capacity.

Further investigations are required to establish whether the differences between the capacity of inflammatory and non-inflammatory stimuli to cause selective release of lysosomal acid hydrolases is also true for prostaglandin biosynthesis and secretion. If this is so, similar investigations of the capacity of inflammatory stimuli to modulate the secretion of some of the other secretory products of macrophages listed in Table 13.1 should help to clarify further the secretory functions of macrophages which contribute to various aspects of chronic inflammatory processes.

Note: A chromatographic system allowing the separation of $PGF_{2\alpha}$ and 6-keto $PGF_{1\alpha}$ allows us to tentatively suggest that the product previously shown to have the same mobility as $PGF_{2\alpha}$ is 6-keto $PGF_{1\alpha}$, the stable metabolite of PGI_2.

References

1. Davies, P. and Allison, A. C. (1976). Secretion of macrophage enzymes in relation to the pathogenesis of chronic inflammation. In D. S. Nelson (ed). *Immunobiology of the Macrophage*, pp. 427–461. (New York: Academic Press)
2. Davies, P. and Allison, A. C. (1976). The secretion of lysosomal enzymes. In J. T. Dingle and R. T. Dean (eds.). *Lysosomes in Biology and Pathology*, Vol. 5, pp. 61–98. North Holland Research Monographs (Amsterdam: North Holland Publishing Company)
3. Page, R. C., Davies, P. and Allison, A. C. (1977). The macrophage as a secretory cell. *Int. Rev. Cytol.* (In press)
4. Allison, A. C. and Davies, P. (1975). Increased biochemical and biological activities of mononuclear phagocytes exposed to various stimuli, with special reference to secretion of lysosomal enzymes. In R. van Furth (ed.). *Mononuclear Phagocytes in Immunity, Infection and Pathology*, pp. 487–506. (Oxford: Blackwell Scientific Publications)
5. Pantalone, R. M. and Page, R. C. (1975). Lymphokine-induced production and release of lysosomal enzymes by macrophages. *Proc. Nat. Acad. Sci. USA*, **72**, 2091
6. Davies, P., Allison, A. C., Dym, M. and Cardella, C. (1975). The selective release of lysosomal enzymes from mononuclear phagocytes by immune complexes and other materials causing chronic inflammation. In D. C. Dumonde (ed.). *Infection and Immunology in the Rheumatic Diseases*, pp. 365–373. (Oxford: Blackwell Scientific Publications)
7. Schorlemmer, H.-U., Davies, P., Hylton, W., Gugig, M. and Allison, A. C. (1977). The selective release of lysosomal acid hydrolases from mouse peritoneal macrophages by stimuli of chronic inflammation. *Brit. J. Exp. Pathol.* (In press)
8. Davies, P., Allison, A. C., Ackerman, J., Butterfield, A. and Williams, S. (1974). Asbestos induces selective release of lysosomal enzymes from mononuclear phagocytes. *Nature (London)*, **251**, 423
9. Werb, Z. and Dingle, J. T. (1976). Lysosomes as modulators of cellular functions.

Influence on the synthesis and secretion of non-lysosomal materials. In J. T. Dingle and R. T. Dean (eds.). *Lysosomes in Biology and Pathology*, Vol. 5, pp. 127–156. North Holland Research Monographs. (Amsterdam: North Holland Publishing Company)

10. Gordon, S., Unkeless, J. C. and Cohn, Z. A. (1974). Induction of macrophage plasminogen activator by endotoxin stimulation and phagocytosis. Evidence for a two-stage process, *J. Exp. Med.*, **140**, 995

11. Hamilton, J., Vassalli, J.-D. and Reich, E. (1976). Macrophage plasminogen activator: Induction by asbestos is blocked by anti-inflammatory steroids. *J. Exp. Med.*, **144**, 1689

12. Stossel, T. P., Mason, R. J. and Smith, A. L. (1974). Lipid peroxidation by human blood phagocytes, *J. Clin. Invest.*, **54**, 638

13. Myatt, L., Bray, M. A., Gordon, D. A. and Morley, J. (1975). Macrophages on intra-uterine contraceptive devices produce prostaglandins. *Nature (London)*, **257**, 227

14. Gordon, D., Bray, M. A. and Morley, J. (1976). Control of lymphokine production by prostaglandins. *Nature (London)*, **262**, 401

15. Flower, R. J. and Blackwell, G. T. (1976). The importance of phospholipase A_2 in prostaglandin biosynthesis. *Biochem. Pharmacol.*, **25**, 285

16. Hong, S. L. and Levine, L. (1976). Stimulation of prostaglandin synthesis by bradykinin and thrombin and their mechanisms of action on MC5-5 fibroblasts. *J. Biol. Chem.*, **251**, 5814

17. Hong, S. L. and Levine, L. (1976). Inhibition of arachidonic acid release from cells as the biochemical action of anti-inflammatory corticosteroids. *Proc. Nat. Acad. Sci. USA*, **73**, 1730

18. Ruscetti, F. W. and Chervenik, P. A. (1974). Release of colony stimulating factor from monocytes by endotoxin and polyinosinic and polycytidylic acid. *J. Lab. Clin. Med.*, **83**, 64

19. Heppleston, A. G. and Styles, J. A. (1967). Activity of a macrophage factor in collagen formation by silica. *Nature (London)*, **214**, 521

20. Aalto, M., Potila, M. and Kulonen, E. (1976). The effect of silica-treated macrophages on the synthesis of collagen and other proteins *in vitro*. *Exp. Cell. Res.*, **97**, 193

21. Leibovich, S. J. and Ross, R. (1976). A macrophage-dependent factor that stimulates the proliferation of fibroblasts *in vitro*. *Am. J. Pathol.*, **84**, 501

22. Calderon, J. and Unanue, E. R. (1975). Two biological activities regulating cell proliferation found in cultures of peritoneal cells. *Nature (London)*, **253**, 359

23. Smith, T. J. and Wagner, R. R. (1967). Rabbit macrophage interferons. I. Conditions for biosynthesis by virus-infected and uninfected cells. *J. Exp. Med.*, **125**, 559

24. Hirsch, M. S., Zisman, B. and Allison, A. C. (1970). Macrophages and age-dependent resistance to herpes simplex virus in mice. *J. Immunol.*, **104**, 1160

25. Bast, Jr., R. C., Cleveland, R. P., Littman, B. H., Zbar, B. and Rapp, H. J. (1974). Acquired cellular immunity: Extracellular killing of listeria monocytogenes by a product of immunologically activated macrophages. *Cell. Immunol.*, **10**, 248

26. Gery, I. and Waksman, B. H. (1972). Potentiation of the T-lymphocyte response to mitogens. II. The cellular source of potentiating mediator(s). *J. Exp. Med.*, **136**, 143

27. Unanue, E. R., Kiely, J. M. and Calderon, J. (1976). The modulation of lymphocyte function by molecules secreted by macrophages. II. Conditions leading to increased secretion. *J. Exp. Med.*, **144**, 155

28. Wood, D. D., Cameron, P. M., Poe, M. T. and Morris, C. A. (1976). Resolution of a factor that enhances the antibody response of T-depleted murine splenocytes from several other monocyte products. *Cell. Immunol.*, **21**, 88

29. Schrader, J. W. (1973). Mechanism of activation of the bone marrow-derived lymphocyte. III. A distinction between macrophage-produced triggering signal and the amplifying effect on triggered B cells of allogeneic interactions. *J. Exp. Med.*, **138**, 1466

30. Colten, H. R. and Einstein, L. P. (1976). Complement metabolism: cellular and humoral regulation. *Transpl. Rev.*, **32**, 3

31. Bodell, P. (1974). Studies on the mechanism of endogenous pyrogen production. III. Human blood monocytes. *J. Exp. Med.*, **140**, 954

32. Dinarello, C. A., Goldin, N. P. and Wolff, S. M. (1974). Demonstration and characterization of two distinct human leukocytic pyrogens. *J. Exp. Med.*, **139**, 1369

33. Stevenson R. D. (1974). Polymorph migration stimulator. A new factor produced by hydrocortisone-treated monocytes. *Clin. Exp. Immunol.*, **17**, 601

34. Melsom, H. and Seljelid, R. (1973). The cytotoxic effect of mouse macrophages on syngeneic and allogeneic erythrocytes. *J. Exp. Med.*, **137**, 808

35. Currie, G. A. and Basham, C. (1975). Activated macrophages release a factor which lyses malignant cells but not normal cells. *J. Cell. Exp. Med.*, **142**, 1600

36. Gordon, S., Todd, J. and Cohn, Z. A. (1974). *In vitro* synthesis and secretion of lysozyme by mononuclear phagocytes. *J. Exp. Med.*, **139**, 1228

37. Weissmann, G., Dukor, P. and Zurier, R. B. (1971). Effect of cyclic AMP on release of lysosomal enzymes from phagocytes. *Nature (New Biol)*, **231**, 131

38. Ringrose, P. S., Parr, M. A. and McLaren, M. (1975). Effects of anti-inflammatory and other compounds on the release of lysosomal enzymes from macrophages. *Biochem. Pharmacol.*, **24**, 607

39. Ackerman, N. R. and Beebe, J. R. (1974). Release of lysosomal enzymes by alveolar mononuclear cells. *Nature (London)*, **247**, 475

40. Page, R. C., Davies, P. and Allison, A. C. (1973). Effects of dental plaque on the production and release of lysosomal hydrolases by macrophages in culture. *Arch. Oral Biol.*, **18**, 1481

41. Davies, P., Page, R. C. and Allison, A. C. (1974). Changes in cellular enzyme levels and extracellular release of lysosomal acid hydrolases in macrophages exposed to group A streptococcal cell wall substance. *J. Exp. Med.*, **139**, 1262

42. Page, R. C., Davies, P. and Allison, A. C. (1974). Pathogenesis of the chronic inflammatory lesion induced by group A streptococcal cell walls. *Lab. Invest.*, **30**, 568

43. Cardella, C. J., Davies, P. and Allison, A. C. (1974). Immune complexes induce selective release of lysosomal hydrolases from macrophages *in vitro*. *Nature (London)*, **247**, 46

44. Schorlemmer, H.-U., Davies, P. and Allison, A. C. (1976). Ability of activated complement components to induce lysosomal enzyme release from macrophages. *Nature (London)*, **261**, 48

45. Schorlemmer, H.-U. and Allison, A. C. (1976). Effects of activated complement components on enzyme secretion by macrophages. *Immunology*, **31**, 781

Discussion 13

K. Brune: (Switzerland)	We appreciate Dr. Davies mentioning our own work and we are pleased that we have results which seem complementary to his own.

However, we have a slightly different time course of prostaglandin release in our experiments, which also use macrophages, but we stimulate them with erythrocytes coated with antibody. Together with Dr. Davies's findings of the thioglycollate-stimulated leukocytes or macrophages, would it be possible that the method applied by him to measure prostaglandin release might not give the full amount of the prostaglandins released at the start of the experiment due to the fact that the labelled arachidonic acid may be in a different compartment not immediately available. |
| **Davies:** | I agree completely. I should make it clear that in contrast to our methodology, Drs. Brune and Glatt utilized a radio-immunoassay method to measure the levels of unlabelled PGE_2, whereas we used the pre-labelling method. We have no information at present as to the distribution of the labelled arachidonic acid within cell membrane phospholipids, although this is something that we are at present investigating. |
| **G. Macpherson:** (UK) | Would Dr. Davies comment on the differences between his own system and that of Simon Gordon. He has been looking at the release of another enzyme, plasminogen activator. There he finds that with stimulation of macrophages, the addition of an inert latex particle gives very long persistent release of this enzyme.

Does latex cause any lysosomal release from stimulated macrophages and would anyone comment on the significance of the difference between the two phenomena? |
| **Davies:** | If thioglycollate-stimulated macrophages are put into culture and the stimulation of lysosomal enzyme release by stimuli such as zymosan is looked for, there is little or no selective release. We have recently studied this quite extensively. Indeed, if non-stimulated cells are left in cultures over a period of days, their responsiveness to a stimulus such as zymosan—the particular instance that I have in mind that we studied was Group A streptococcal cell walls—they also lose their responsiveness to this kind of stimulus in terms of lysosomal enzyme release. We have to start thinking about the macrophage as an extremely versatile kind of cell that, under a certain set of circumstances, will release, or synthesize and release one set of mediators. If it has been previously stimulated, as with the thioglycollate cells, then it might go on and secrete another set of mediators. This is something that needs to be studied in great detail, and we are in the process of making some of these correlations at present.

I would add, however, that if latex is put in *in vivo* and the cells are then harvested several days later, the cells that are harvested do not secrete neutral proteinases. The neutral proteinase I have in mind is |

188

plasminogen activator. This has recently been studied (by John Hamilton).

H. Hahn:
(West Germany)
I presume that the studies with zymosan were done in a serum medium.

Davies:
No. The studies with the prostaglandins were run in a serum-free environment, and the studies with the zymosan were also studied in a serum-free environment.

Hahn:
So that there was no possibility of zymosan-bound C3b activating the macrophages via a C3 receptor.

Davies:
I hate to steal Dr. Schorlemmer's fire. He will be dealing with this in great detail.

I would add, however, that zymosan will also release lysosomal enzymes from macrophages in a serum-containing medium, and for that matter prostaglandins will also be synthesized in that kind of environment. But these particular experiments that I have described today were done both for lysosomal enzyme release and for prosta-glandin synthesis and secretion in serum-free environments.

Hahn:
But the possibility that C3 produced by macrophages, or carried by macrophages, was in turn bound to zymosan has not been completely ruled out?

Davies:
Absolutely. That is a possibility that we all wish to consider very seriously, especially in view of the data that Dr. Schorlemmer will present.

W. Brocklehurst:
(UK)
In most cases, with most tissues, when the formation of prostaglandins is blocked by indomethacin, this does not prevent the production of the hydroperoxy-eicosatrienoic acid (HETA). Does the same switch of synthesis of emphasis occur with the macrophage?

Davies:
It is a point that we have not investigated sufficiently for me to be able to make any definite comments about it now.

However, I can say that certainly in the presence of indomethacin, our cell cultures do make significant quantities of HETA.

14

Interactions of macrophages and complement components in the pathogenesis of chronic inflammation

H. U. SCHORLEMMER, J. FERLUGA AND A. C. ALLISON
(Germany and UK)

INTRODUCTION

Chronic inflammatory reactions make a substantial contribution to the pathogenesis of diseases all over the world. Among the diseases of temperate climates which have important chronic inflammatory components are rheumatoid arthritis, chronic hepatitis, regional ileitis (Crohn's disease), ulcerative colitis, periodontal disease and farmer's lung. In tropical countries schistosomiasis is produced by the chronic inflammatory reaction occurring around the eggs deposited by the causative helminth. In leishmaniasis and several other parasitic and fungal diseases chronic inflammatory reactions are prominent.

Chronic inflammation is accompanied by tissue degradation and repair. The degradation is especially important in the connective tissues of the joint, where loss of articular cartilage and bone results in the pain and deformity of rheumatoid arthritis. The fibrosis associated with repair is a major factor in the pathogenesis of cirrhosis, schistosomiasis, farmer's lung and other conditions.

It would therefore be of great clinical value if the mechanisms underlying chronic inflammation were understood and individual stages of the process could be controlled pharmacologically. Because the reactions *in vivo* are highly complex we have attempted to isolate components of the reactions for *in vitro* analysis. The predominant cells in chronic inflammatory responses are mononuclear phagocytes[1], so that the recruitment of these cells into lesions and their stimulation within the lesions is of central importance. In addition activation of the complement system has been associated with acute and chronic inflammatory reactions. Several activated complement components have the potential to mediate inflammatory tissue injury either directly or indirectly. Among the biologically active complement components the low-molecular-weight cleavage products of C3 and C5 play the most important role in the mediation of inflammation and tissue injury.

Chronic inflammatory reactions can be induced by agents that do not elicit strong immune responses. In this case pathogenesis appears to depend on interactions of macrophages and some components of the complement system. In the pathogenesis of other chronic inflammatory responses, for example that around the schistosome egg, thymus-derived T-lymphocytes play an important role. Experimental studies show that immune complexes can produce chronic inflammatory reactions, and this may also be a factor in the pathogenesis of naturally occurring lesions.

Macrophages are present at sites of chronic inflammation regardless of the inciting stimulus, be it of immunological or non-immunological origin. The properties of macrophages vary considerably depending upon their localization and the stimulus to which they have been exposed. Davies and Allison[1] have reviewed how macrophages participate in chronic inflammatory responses with particular reference to their function as secretory cells. Macrophages persist at sites of chronic inflammation for long periods of time. Many substances eliciting chronic inflammatory responses have been found also to induce selective release of acid hydrolases from macrophages in culture. On the other hand, a number of inert or readily digestible substances do not cause such release[2]. Recently macrophages have been shown to secrete neutral proteinases in response to a number of stimuli, including some of those causing release of acid hydrolases[3]. The timing and extent of acid hydrolase and neutral proteinase release differ markedly, the former being released in large amounts shortly after contact with an appropriate stimulus while the release of the latter commences usually after a latent period of at least 24 h and continues for a long time.

THE DIRECT INTERACTION WITH MACROPHAGES OF SUBSTANCES WHICH CAUSE SELECTIVE RELEASE OF ACID HYDROLASES

A consequence of mononuclear phagocyte stimulation by a variety of agents that can induce chronic inflammation is secretion of hydrolytic enzymes[1,4] which can degrade tissue constituents and interact with the complement system to generate mediators of inflammation[5].

An early event in such an activation of the complement system is the cleavage of the component C3 to a smaller fragment C3a and a larger fragment C3b. Highly purified C3b when incubated with mouse or guinea pig peritoneal macrophages in culture induces a selective dose- and time-dependent release of several glycosidases, but not of lactate dehydrogenase (Figures

192

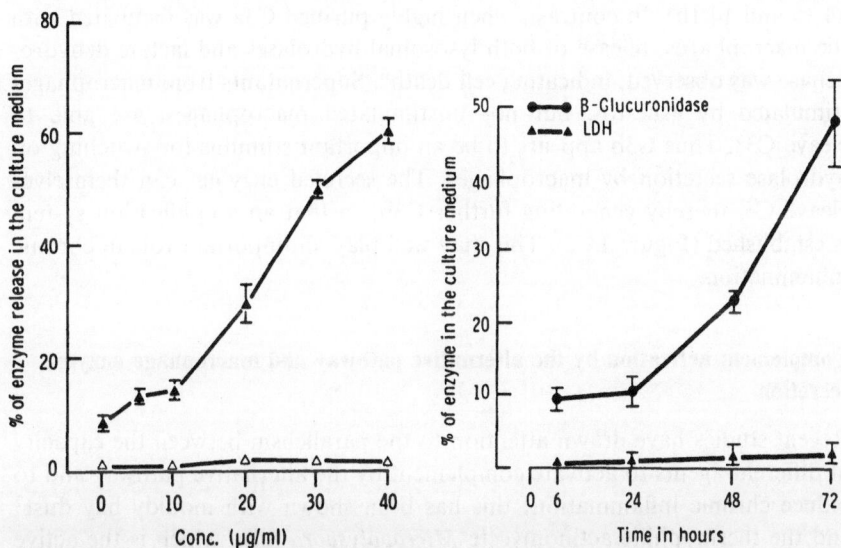

Figure 14.1a The release of β-galactosidase (▲) and lactate dehydrogenase (△) from macrophages exposed to increasing concentrations of C3b

Figure 14.1b The time-dependent release of β-glucuronidase (●) and lactate dehydrogenase (▲) from macrophages exposed to purified C3b (20 μg/ml)

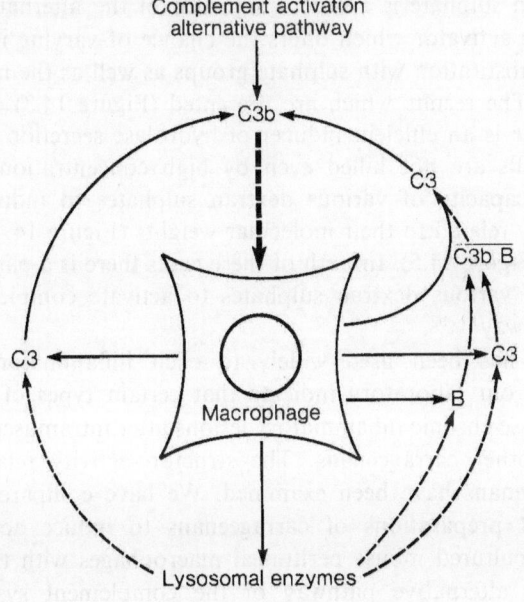

Macrophage activation

Figure 14.2 Possible amplification loops in the activation process of mononuclear phagocytes

14.1a and 14.1b). In contrast, when highly purified C3a was incubated with the macrophages, release of both lysosomal hydrolases and lactate dehydrogenase was observed, indicating cell death[6]. Supernatants from macrophages stimulated by asbestos, but not unstimulated macrophages, are able to cleave C3[5]. Thus C3b appears to be an important stimulus for switching on hydrolase secretion by macrophages. The secreted enzymes can themselves cleave C3, thereby generating further C3b, so that an amplification system is established (Figure 14.2). This may well play an important role in chronic inflammation.

Complement activation by the alternative pathway and macrophage enzyme secretion

Recent studies have drawn attention to the parallelism between the capacity of different agents to activate complement by the alternative pathway and to induce chronic inflammation: this has been shown with mouldy hay dust[7] and the thermophilic actinomycete *Micropolyspora faeni* which is the active agent in farmer's lung[8], with streptococcal cell walls[2,4], with dental plaque[9,10] and several other agents. We have investigated further the correlation between the capacity of various materials to activate the alternative pathway and to stimulate hydrolase secretion from mononuclear phagocytes in culture. Dextran sulphate is a potent activator of the alternative pathway. It is a synthetic activator which offers the chance of varying independently the degree of substitution with sulphate groups as well as the molecular size of the carrier. The results which are presented (Figure 14.3) establish that dextran sulphate is an efficient inducer of hydrolase secretion from macrophages. The cells are not killed even by high concentrations of dextran sulphate. The capacity of various dextran sulphates to induce hydrolase release is clearly related to their molecular weights (Figure 14.4) and degree of sulphation (Figure 14.5). In both of these cases there is a parallelism with the capacity of various dextran sulphates to activate complement by the alternative pathway[11,12].

Carrageenan has been used widely to elicit inflammatory responses. Experiments in our laboratory indicate that certain types of carrageenan elicit more intense chronic inflammatory lesions after intramuscular injection in mice than other carrageenans. The structure-activity relationships of various carrageenans have been examined. We have compared the ability of the different preparations of carrageenans to induce acid hydrolase secretion from cultured mouse peritoneal macrophages with their capacity to activate the alternative pathway of the complement system. Native undegraded carrageenan (Gelcarin HMR, manufactured by Marine Colloids Inc., Rocland, Maine, USA) induces the greatest increase in selective release of acid hydrolases. In contrast the calcium salt of carrageenan (obtained from Sigma Chemical Co., London) lacks the ability to induce selective release of

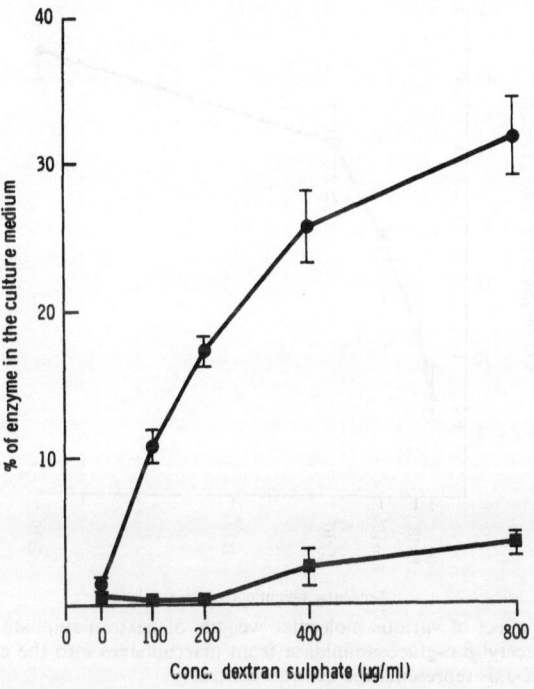

Figure 14.3 The release of N-acetyl-β-D-glucosaminidase (●) and lactate dehydrogenase (■) from macrophages exposed to increasing concentrations of dextran sulphate. The cultures of mouse peritoneal macrophages were assayed after incubation with dextran sulphate for 48 h

acid hydrolases, while the potassium salt of carrageenan (Sigma) shows intermediate activity[13]. Structure-activity relationships show that lambda-carrageenan, a linear polymer of D-galactose with α-1-3-linkages and sulphated on carbon-4 has the greatest activity (Figure 14.6). In macrophages cultured for 48 h in the presence of various concentrations of lambda-carrageenan there was a significant selective release of β-glucuronidase, a typical lysosomal hydrolase, which rises up to above 50% with 400 μg/ml of lambda-carrageenan. Káppa-carrageenan, containing alternate units of 4-sulphated D-galactose and 3,6-dehydro-D-galactose with α-1-3 and β-1-4 linkages, does not induce release of β-glucuronidase from cultured macrophages. Iota-carrageenan shows intermediate activity in inducing release of acid hydrolases from mononuclear phagocytes. Since the capacity of dextran sulphates to activate the alternative pathway of the complement system is dependent on the number of sulphate groups per molecule, we investigated the influence of the degree of sulphate substitution on the capacity of various carrageenans to activate the complement system. Varying amounts of lambda-carrageenan (9.6% sulphur), iota-carrageenan (8.9% sulphur) and kappa-carrageenan (7.1% sulphur) were incubated with constant amounts of C4-deficient guinea pig serum for 30 min at 37 °C. After the incubation remaining

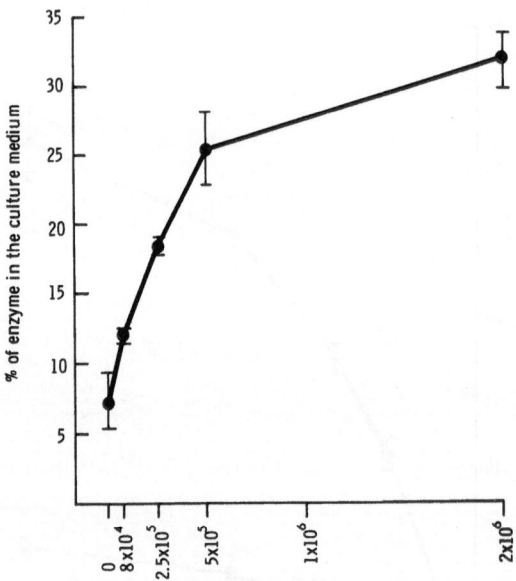

Figure 14.4 The effect of various molecular weights of dextran sulphate (400 μg/ml) on the release of *N*-acetyl-β-D-glucosaminidase from macrophages into the culture medium. The zero on the X-axis represents the dextran control

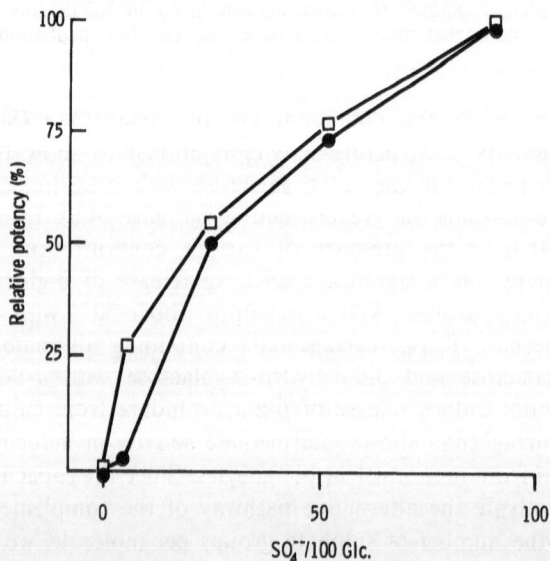

Figure 14.5 Influence of the degree of sulphation of different dextran sulphate preparations on the potency in activating C3 via the alternative pathway and releasing acid hydrolases from macrophages. The dextran sulphate sample of which the lowest concentration was required for activity was taken as 100% active. Other samples were compared with this, their relative activities being expressed as the reciprocal of the concentration required for comparable activity. The values for complement activation are calculated from data of Burger *et al.*[11]

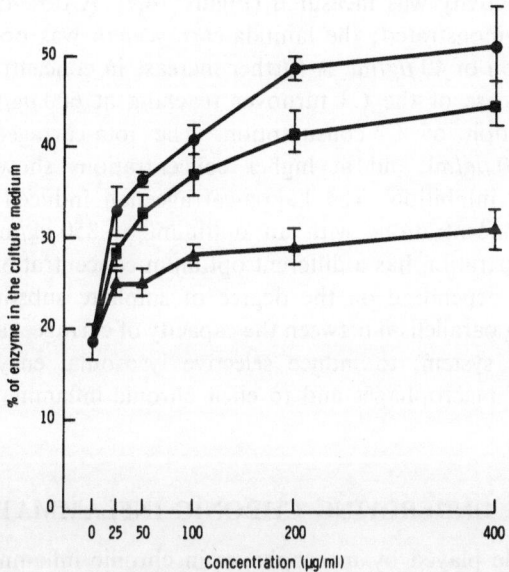

Figure 14.6 Effects of 48 h incubation with various concentrations of lambda-carrageenan (●), iota-carrageenan (■) and kappa-carrageenan (▲) on the release of β-glucuronidase from macrophages into the culture medium

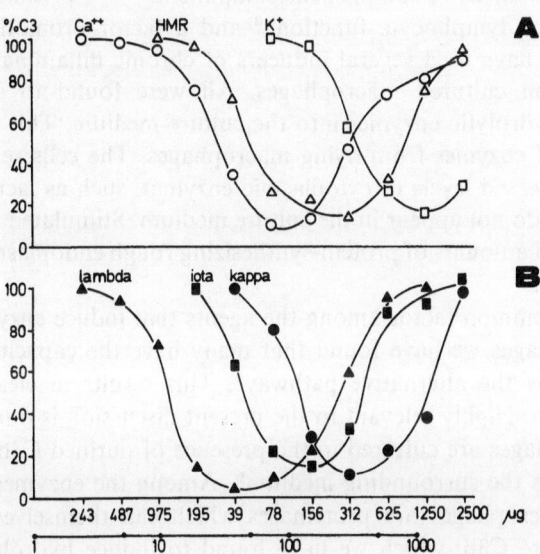

Figure 14.7 Dose-dependent C3 consumption of various purified preparations of carrageenan in C4-deficient guinea pig serum. Abscissa: final concentration of carrageenan in μg/ml incubation mixture (log scale). Ordinate: Per cent C3 remaining in the C4-deficient guinea pig serum after incubation with carrageenan. 100% refers to the H_2O treated control and equals 2.2×10^{11} SFU/ml C4-deficient guinea pig serum

haemolytic C3-activity was measured (Figure 14.7). A dose-dependent C3-turnover was demonstrated; the lambda-carrageenan was optimally active at a concentration of 40 μg/ml. A further increase in concentration led to a continuous decrease of the C3 turnover reaching at 600 μg/ml an almost complete inhibition of C3-consumption. The iota-carrageenan had its optimum at 150 μg/ml and at higher concentrations showed the same phenomenon of inhibition. The kappa-carrageenan induced C3 turnover only at high concentrations with an optimum at 350 μg/ml. Thus each carrageenan preparation has a different optimum concentration for complement activation depending on the degree of sulphate substitution. Again there is a striking parallelism between the capacity of carrageenans to activate the complement system, to induce selective lysosomal enzyme secretion from cultures of macrophages and to elicit chronic inflammatory response *in vivo*.

MECHANISMS UNDERLYING CHRONIC INFLAMMATION

The essential role played by macrophages in chronic inflammation is well recognized[1]. It has also become clear that macrophages secrete a number of products under various conditions *in vitro* and that several of these can interact with macrophages in the pathogenesis of chronic inflammatory responses. These include hydrolytic enzymes derived from lysosomes[1] and from other cellular sources[14], complement components[15-17], prostaglandins[18,19], factors effecting lymphocyte function[20] and a factor promoting fibroblast growth[21]. We have used several inducers of chronic inflammation to study their effects on cultured macrophages. All were found to stimulate the secretion of hydrolytic enzymes into the culture medium. This is not a nonspecific loss of enzymes from dying macrophages. The cells remain healthy and show increased levels of cytoplasmic enzymes, such as lactate dehydrogenase, which do not appear in the culture medium. Stimulated macrophages show increased amounts of protein-synthesizing rough endoplasmic reticulum and lysosomes.

Seeking a common factor among the agents that induce enzyme secretion from macrophages we have found that many have the capacity to activate complement by the alternative pathway[4]. This results in cleavage of C3, generating C3b. Highly relevant to the present discussion is our finding that when macrophages are cultured in the presence of purified C3b they secrete hydrolases into the surrounding medium[6]. Among the enzymes secreted by stimulated macrophages are proteinases which can themselves cleave C3[5] generating more C3b, which we have found to induce hydrolase secretion from macrophages. It is remarkable that factor B, C3 and hydrolytic enzymes are all synthesized by macrophages in abundance, and together comprise a self-activating system. The enzymes partially digest C3 producing C3b, which in the presence of factor B forms a cleavage complex acting on C3 to generate

198

more C3b; hence both cellular and humoral amplification loops exist. The system for activating macrophages by agents inducing chronic inflammation is produced by the macrophages themselves and does not require serum constituents. This could be highly relevant to the pathogenesis of chronic inflammation in lesions containing large numbers of macrophages. These could form a system generating chemotactic factors, which recruit more mononuclear phagocytes in the lesions and stimulate the secretion of enzymes which are themselves involved in the activating process. The secreted enzymes could also be important in the degradation of articular cartilage, proteoglycan, collagen, elastin and other connective tissue constituents.

CYTOLYTIC EFFECTS OF COMPLEMENT CLEAVAGE PRODUCTS RELEASED FROM STIMULATED MACROPHAGES

While unstimulated macrophages are not cytotoxic, macrophages stimulated *in vivo* or *in vitro* with various materials became cytotoxic, either killing tumour cells or inhibiting their multiplication. The mechanisms by which several agents exert their effects on macrophages and by which macrophages have cytotoxic effects on tumour cells are unknown. We have drawn attention to the fact that several stimulants of macrophages are able to activate complement by the alternative pathway[4]. The larger cleavage product of the third complement component, C3b, stimulates macrophages to secrete hydrolytic enzymes without loss of viability, whereas incubation of the smaller cleavage product, C3a, with macrophages results in death of the cells[5,6].

This observation prompted an investigation of the effects of C3a on murine and human lymphocytes and tumour cells and lymphoblastic cells in culture[22]. Purified C3a was incubated with various cell types of human and mouse origin. All the tumour cell types tested were lysed by low concentrations of C3a (Figure 14.8a), whereas normal human lymphocytes were relatively resistant (Figure 14.8b). These observations raised the possibility that a common factor in macrophage stimulation is C3b and that the stimulated macrophages are able to cleave the C3 which they themselves produce, liberating C3a which accounts for macrophage-mediated lysis.

To test this hypothesis we have investigated the effect of culturing macrophages with C3b and other stimuli, LPS and dextran sulphate (themselves activators of the complement system via the alternative pathway) on the capacity of macrophages to kill tumour cells. Macrophages were recovered from the peritoneal cavities of mice without prior stimulation and cultured in serum-free medium to which was added in some cultures highly purified C3b, LPS or dextran sulphate. After 24 h or 48 h ^{51}Cr-labelled lymphoma cells were added to the macrophages and both cell types were cultured together for a further 24 h. As shown in Table 14.1, unstimulated macrophages did not increase the release of ^{51}Cr into the medium above back-

Table 14.1 Lysis of P815 cells by culture media from mouse macrophages activated with C3b or with bacterial lipopolysaccharide (LPS)

	Stimulating agent	% specific release Mean	σ
24 h duration of incubation with stimulating agent	0	−3.7	2.1
	C3b*	102	2.0
	LPS†	85.4	4.4
48 h duration of incubation with stimulating agent	0	−5.4	1.7
	C3b*	102	1.0
	LPS†	86.5	5.0

* C3b = 20 μg/ml

† LPS 25 μg/ml

Ratio macrophages/P815 target cells = 5/1. Cytotoxicity test 24 h

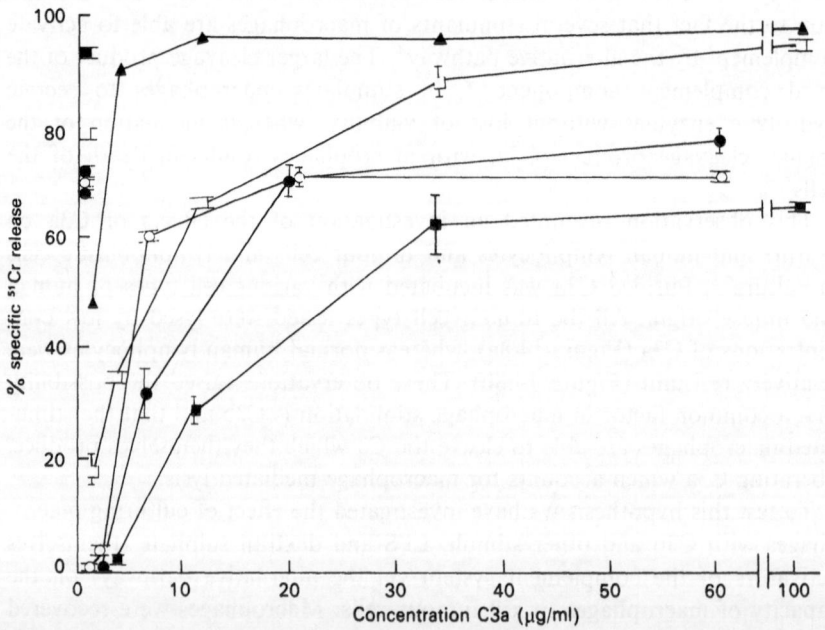

Figure 14.8a Lysis of various mouse cell types by C3a in 6 h. (▲) mastocytoma cells; (□) lymph node cells; (■) L-cells; (○) C234-cells; (●) D-55 cells. % label released by freezing and thawing the cells is indicated by the symbols on the ordinate

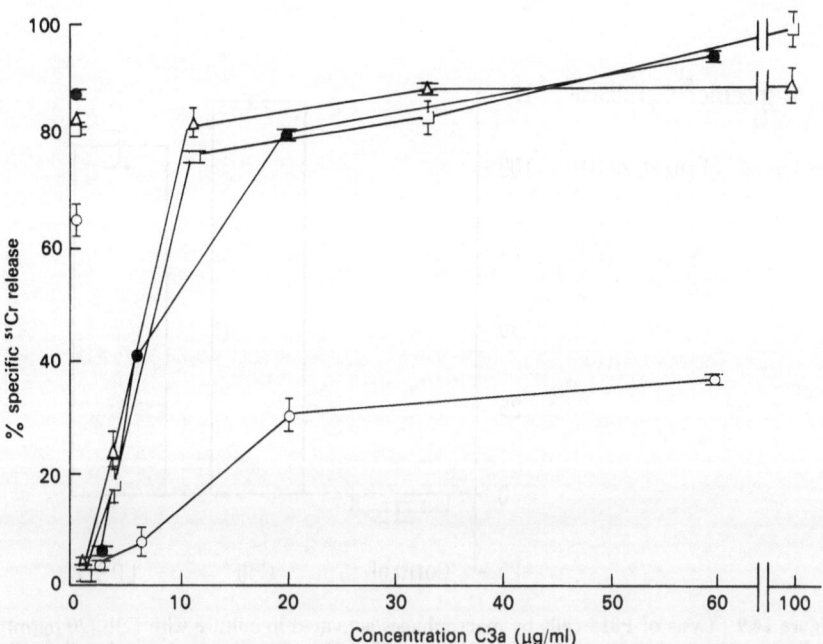

Figure 14.8b Lysis of human cells by C3a in 6 h. (○) unstimulated lymphocytes; (●) PHA-stimulated lymphocytes; (□) CLA-4 cells; (△) Chang cells. Symbols on the ordinate indicate the freezing and thawing controls

ground level, whereas C3b, LPS and dextran sulphate-treated macrophages lysed all or nearly all of the tumour cells. The macrophages also lysed another allogeneic mouse lymphoma (L5178 YE) and human lymphoblastic cell line cells (CLA-4). The lytic effect was considerably reduced in the presence of serum. Stimulated macrophages could kill tumour cells by direct contact or by the release of a lytic factor (or factors) (Figure 14.9). The presence of a lytic factor in the culture media of stimulated macrophages has been found in our experiments and in other laboratories[23,24]. Lytic activity has been consistently found in the culture media; the appearance of the lytic activity is dose- and time-dependent (Figure 14.10 and 14.11). As previously reported[22], C3b even in concentrations much higher than those used in these experiments is not lytic for the tumour cells used. As mentioned above, the other product of C3 cleavage, C3a, is highly lytic for tumour cells. Since macrophages synthesize C3 and enzymes acting on C3, the latter could be cleaved in stimulated macrophages, with the release of C3a into the culture medium. The media of macrophages cultured with dextran sulphate, LPS or C3b (but not in the absence of these agents) were found to contain material with anaphylatoxic activity, inducing contraction of guinea-pig terminal ileum (Figure 14.12a and b). The tachyphylaxis and cross desensitization observed with reference samples of C3a identify the active agent in the

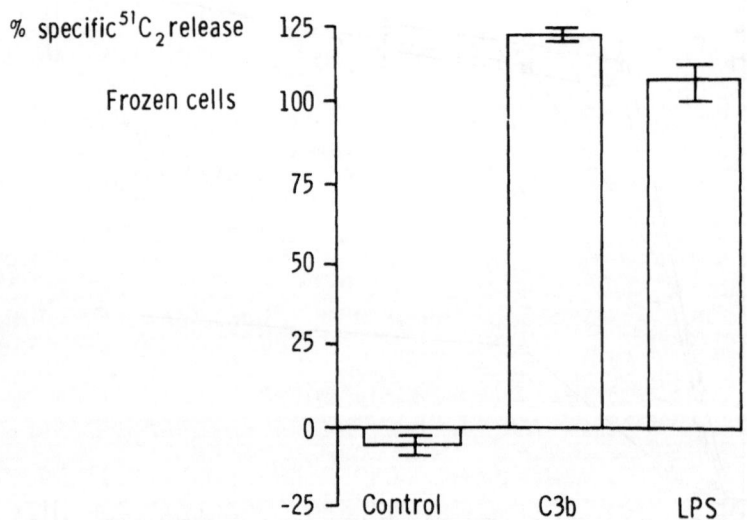

Figure 14.9 Lysis of P815 cells by macrophages activated in culture with C3b (20 μg/ml) or lipopolysaccharide *E. coli* 055 B5 (25 μg/ml) for 24 h. Freezing and thawing the cells released 70–80% of total incorporated label (^{51}Cr)

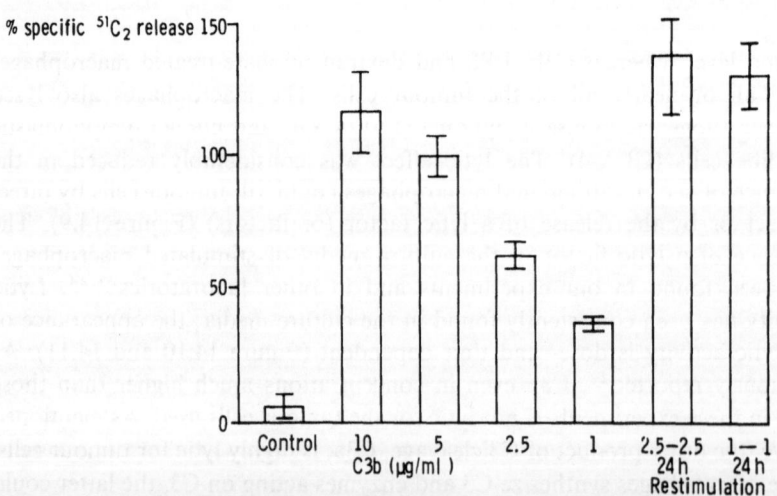

Figure 14.10 Dose dependence of C3b-stimulation on macrophage cytotoxicity. Macrophage cultures grown in the presence of various concentrations of C3b for 48 h have shown a tumorolytic effect on labelled tumour cells used

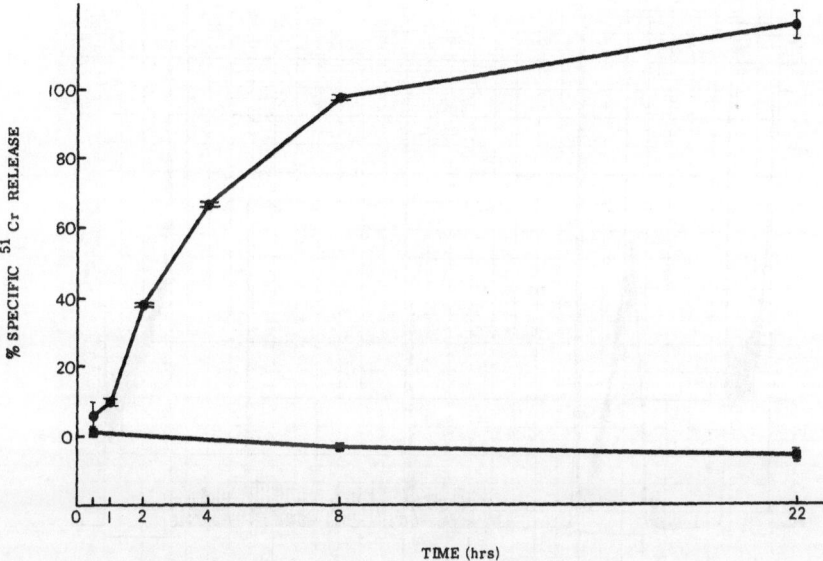

Figure 14.11 The time course of ^{51}Cr release from mastocytoma cells incubated with normal and C3b-stimulated macrophages

media of stimulated macrophages as C3a. Further evidence that the lytic activity is due to C3a comes from experiments using specific antiserum against C3a. As shown in Figure 14.13, the lytic activity of culture media was virtually abolished by anti C3a but not by normal serum. The main conclusion from these experiments is that macrophages stimulated by various agents (LPS, C3b, dextran sulphate) secrete a factor indistinguishable pharmacologically and immunologically from C3a.

These results establish that the complement cleavage product C3b stimulates macrophages to secrete hydrolytic enzymes[5] and to become cytolytic[25]. Generation of C3b by activation of the classical or alternative pathway of complement could be a common factor in many anti-tumour systems. We have also found that the smaller cleavage product, C3a, is lytic for macrophages, lymphocytes, fibroblasts and tumour cells[6,22].

In general, the observations now presented focus attention on C3b as a potent naturally-occurring stimulator of macrophage activities, including capacity to lyse cells. In media of stimulated macrophages C3a has been found[26] and could account for the cytolytic effects observed. Experiments with specific antibodies suggest that C3a is the main lytic agent. C3b is a potent macrophage stimulator, amongst other things inducing the release from these cells of further C3b, so that serial stimulation can occur. This may well be a potent factor in the pathogenesis of chronic inflammation, inducing the associated cytolytic effects.

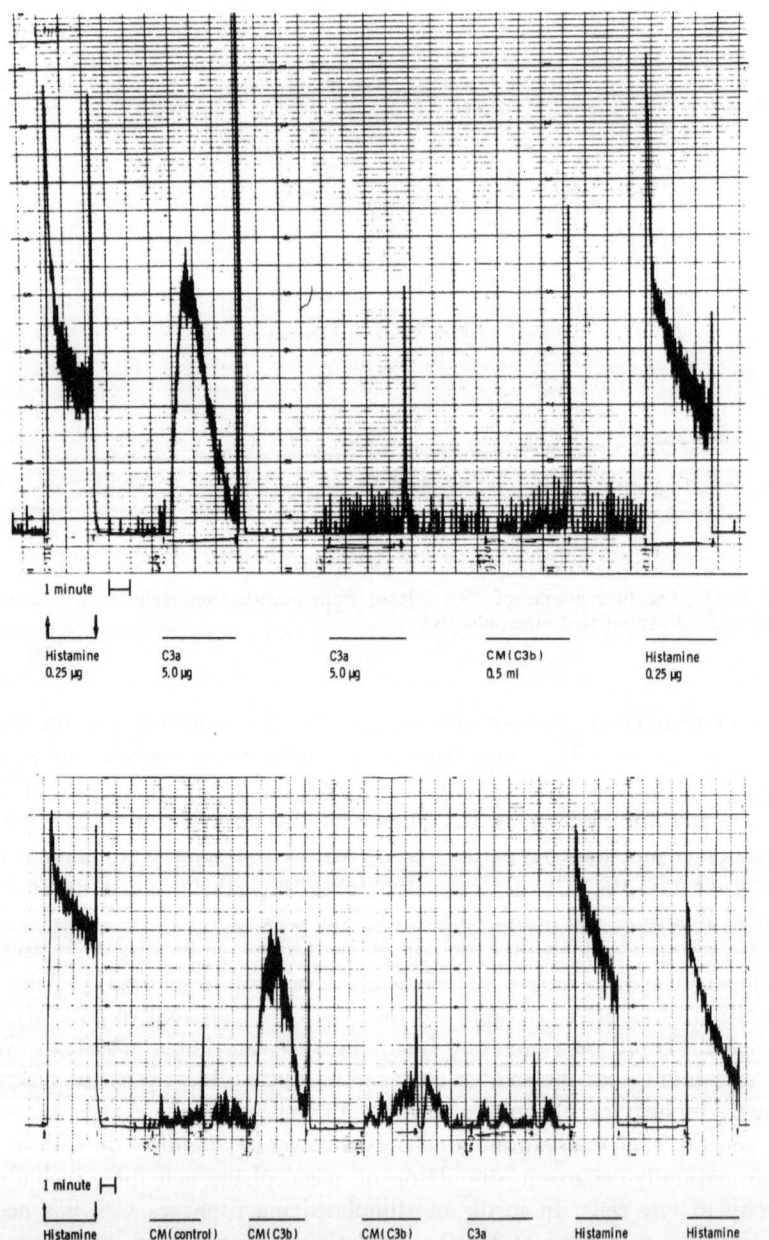

Figure 14.12 a and b C3a-like contraction of isolated guinea pig ileum induced by a culture medium from macrophages incubated with C3b (CM-C3b). The tachyphylaxis and cross-desensitization observed with reference samples of C3a identify the active agent in the medium of stimulated macrophages as C3a

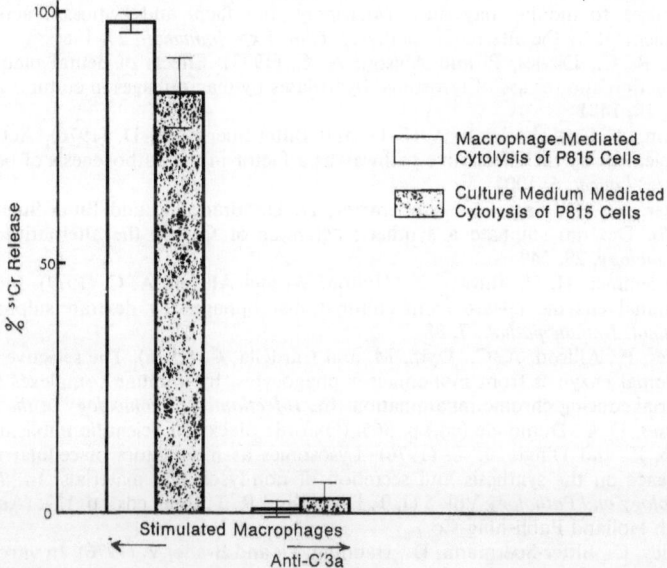

Figure 14.13 Evidence that the lytic activity is due to C3a is shown by using specific antisera against C3a. The lytic activity of culture media of activated macrophages was virtually abolished by anti-C3a but not by normal serum

ACKNOWLEDGEMENT

We are indebted to Dr D. Bitter-Suermann for provision of purified complement components. This research was undertaken while H. U. Schorlemmer was supported by a grant (Scho 215/1) of the Deutsche Forschungsgemeinschaft, Bad-Godesberg, Germany.

References

1. Davies, P. and Allison, A. C. (1976). Secretion of macrophage enzymes in relation to the pathogenesis of chronic inflammation. In: *Immunobiology of the Macrophages* D. S. Nelson (ed.) pp. 427. (New York: Academic Press)
2. Davies, P., Page, R. C. and Allison, A. C. (1974). Changes in cellular enzyme levels and extracellular release of lysosomal acid hydrolases in macrophages exposed to group A streptococcal cell wall substance. *J. Exp. Med.*, **139**, 1262
3. Unkeless, J. C., Gordon, S. and Reich, E. (1974). Secretion of plasminogen activator by stimulated macrophages. *J. Exp. Med.*, **139**, 834
4. Schorlemmer, H. U., Bitter-Suermann, D. and Allison, A. C. (1977). Complement activation by the alternative pathway and macrophage enzyme secretion in the pathogenesis of chronic inflammation. *Immunology*, **32**, (in press)
5. Schorlemmer, H. U. and Allison, A. C. (1976). Effects of activated complement components on enzyme secretion by macrophages. *Immunology*, **31**, 781
6. Schorlemmer, H. U., Davies, P. and Allison, A. C. (1976). Ability of activated complement components to induce lysosomal enzyme release from macrophages. *Nature (London)*, **261**, 48
7. Edwards, H. J. (1976). A quantitative study on the activation of the alternative pathway of complement by mouldy hay dust and thermophilic actinomycetes. *Clin. Allergy* **6**, 19

8. Schorlemmer, H. U., Edwards, J. H., Davies, P. and Allison, A. C. (1977). Macrophage responses to mouldy hay dust, Micropolyspora faeni and zymosan, activators of complement by the alternative pathway. *Clin. Exp. Immunol.*, **27**, 198

9. Page, R. C., Davies, P. and Allison, A. C. (1973). Effects of dental plaque on the production and release of lysosomal hydrolases by macrophages in culture. *Arch. Oral Biol.*, **18**, 1481

10. Allison, A. C., Schorlemmer, H. U. and Bitter-Suermann, D. (1976). Activation of complement by the alternative pathway as a factor in the pathogenesis of periodontal disease. *Lancet*, **6**, 1001

11. Burger, R., Hadding, U., Schorlemmer, H. U., Brade, V. and Bitter-Suermann. D. (1975). Dextran sulphate a synthetic activator of C3 via the alternative pathway. *Immunology*, **29**, 549

12. Schorlemmer, H. U., Burger, R., Hylton, W. and Allison, A. C. (1977). Induction of lysosomal enzyme release from cultured macrophages by dextran sulphate. *Clin. Immunol. Immunopathol.*, **7**, 88

13. Davies, P., Allison, A. C., Dym, M. and Cardella, C. (1976). The selective release of lysosomal enzymes from mononuclear phagocytes, by immune complexes and other material causing chronic inflammation. In: *Infection and immunology in the rheumatic diseases*. D. C. Dumonde (ed.) p. 365. (Oxford: Blackwell Scientific Publications)

14. Werb, Z. and Dingle, J. T. (1976). Lysosomes as modulators of cellular functions. Influence on the synthesis and secretion of non-lysosomal materials. In: *Lysosomes in Biology and Pathology* Vol. 5 (J. T. Dingle and R. T. Dean eds.) p. 127. (Amsterdam: North Holland Publishing Co.)

15. Bentley, C., Bitter-Suermann, D., Hadding, U. and Brade, V. (1976). In vitro synthesis of factor B of the alternative pathway of complement activation by mouse peritoneal macrophages. *Eur. J. Immunol.*, **6**, 393

16. McClelland, D. B. L. and van Furth, R. (1976). In vitro synthesis of B_1C/B_1A globulin (the C3 component of complement) by tissues and leukocytes of mice. *Immunology*, **31**, 855

17. Einstein, L. P., Schneeberger, E. E. and Colten, M. R. (1976). Synthesis of the second component of complement by long term primary cultures of human monocytes. *J. Exp. Med.*, **143**, 114

18. Gordon, D., Bray, M. A. and Morley, J. (1976). Control of lymphokine production by prostaglandins. *Nature (London)*, **262**, 401

19. Bonney, R. J., Davies, P., Dahlgren, M. E., Pelus, L., Keuell, F. A. and Humes, J. L. (1977). Zymosan-induced prostaglandin secretion from peritoneal macrophages. *Fed. Proc.*, **36**, 673

20. Waksman, B. H. and Namba, Y. (1976). On soluble mediators of immunological regulation. *Cell Immunol.*, **21**, 161

21. Leibovich, S. J. and Ross, R. (1976). A macrophage dependent factor that stimulates proliferation of fibroblasts in vitro. *Am. J. Pathol.*, **84**, 501

22. Ferluga, J., Schorlemmer, H. U., Baptista, L. C. and Allison, A. C. (1976). Cytolytic effects of the complement cleavage product C3a. *Br. J. Cancer*, **34**, 626

23. Currie, G. A. and Basham (1975). Activated macrophages release a factor which lyses malignant cells but not normal cells. *J. Exp. Med.*, **142**, 1600

24. Sethi, K. K. and Brandis, H. (1975). Cytotoxicity mediated by soluble macrophage products. *J. Nat. Cancer Inst.*, **55**, 393

25. Schorlemmer, H. U., Ferluga, J., Baptista, L. C., Bitter-Suermann, D. and Allison, A. C. (1977). Role of complement cleavage products in killing of tumour cells by macrophages. *Immunology* (Submitted)

26. Ferluga, J., Schorlemmer, H. U., Baptista, L. C. and Allison, A. C. (1977). Production of the complement cleavage product C3a by stimulated macrophages and its tumorolytic effects. *Clin. exp. Immunol* (Submitted)

Discussion 14

R. L. Souhami: (UK)	With two colleagues (Drs. Bradfield and Addison) I have looked at the effect of a variety of dextran sulphates to inhibit the phagocytic activity of the liver *in vivo*, and the ability of the sulphated dextrans corresponded almost exactly with the graph shown by Dr. Schorlemmer on C3b activation as far as molecular size was concerned. It seemed that below a molecular weight of 80 000 there was very little activity, and certainly the prevention of hepatic uptake of red cells is prevented by dextran sulphates of molecular weights higher than 70 000 which would suggest that a similar mechanism to that seen in the experiments is involved in the uptake of dextrans *in vivo*.
	Secondly, neutral dextrans were without effect, but phosphated dextrans had a similar effect, although they were much more toxic. But, they had to be highly negatively charged dextrans.
	Thirdly, Dr. Schorlemmer mentioned that he thought that the dextran sulphates were not toxic to the cells. That highlights a possible danger and difficulty of extrapolating from *in vitro* data to the *in vivo* situation, because there is no doubt that these substances *in vivo* are followed by Kupffer cell death and their replacement by newly-formed cells, and the same thing goes for other so-called inert compounds, e.g. carbon.
Schorlemmer:	I would agree with the last point. We have cultured macrophages, and this is only one cell type. Professor Hahn has done *in vivo* experiments and he also has observed a more or less cytotoxic effect of these dextran sulphates. He always uses a very high molecular weight dextran sulphate.
G. Vaes: (Belgium)	Have Dr. Schorlemmer and his colleagues done any experiments with dextran instead of dextran sulphate. If so, have they looked at what happens to the secretion of β-glucuronidase?
Schorlemmer:	·Yes. We have. In all these cases we have used the dextrans—the same size, same molecular weight dextrans—as a control, and we have had no release of lysosomal enzymes. These experiments were always in parallel with the dextran sulphates.
Vaes:	Did these dextrans, or dextran sulphates, accumulate inside the cells by phagocytosis, or not?
Schorlemmer:	The dextran sulphates and the dextrans are more or less soluble. I am sure that they accumulate in the cells. I have not tested that.
Vaes:	Have any other polysulphated molecules, such as chondroitin sulphate or heparin, been tried in this particular system?
Schorlemmer:	Yes. I have tried several others—what we call polyanions. All of those which activate the alternative pathway also induce a secretion of lysosomal enzymes from these macrophages.
Vaes:	But do any of the polyanions that do not activate the pathway do the same thing?
Schorlemmer:	I believe that heparin does not activate the alternative pathway and it also does not activate, or induce, enzyme secretion from macrophages.

207

Vaes:	At least lysosomal enzymes.
Schorlemmer:	That is right. That is all that we have tested.
P. C. Wilkinson: (UK)	I wanted to ask about C3a. Dr. Schorlemmer's findings of lytic activity for this substance are most interesting. Some people think that it is a chemotactic factor, but it is difficult to see how a product of a cell could be chemotactic for that cell.
	Can Dr. Schorlemmer say something about the mechanism of lysis, and whether close cell-to-cell contact is needed? Is a very high concentration of C3a needed to lyse a target cell by a macrophage?
Schorlemmer:	We have done two types of experiment. We have stimulated the macrophages with C3b or with lipopolysaccharides, and we have added to the cells, to the macrophages, to these activated cells, the target cells. In this case it was a close contact and we got the lysis of these target cells.
	In other experiments we added supernatants of the activated macrophages to target cells and we also got a lysis.
	At the moment I cannot give the exact amount that we had in these activated macrophage supernatants of C3a. It must vary from comparison experiments with a representative C3a sample. It must be in a range of about 5 µg/ml.
G. Loewi: (UK)	Dr. Wilkinson has just put a question about chemotaxis. I was kindly provided with C3a and C3 by Dr. Schorlemmer and we got the following results.
	With C3a for polymorphs we got a curve, with 50 µg/ml as the maximal stimulant.
	With macrophages we got the same curve, again with 50 µg/ml maximally, but a lower peak.
	With C3 we got some stimulation but only about 1/10th or less of that obtained with C3a.
Wilkinson:	My point was about the actual macrophage producing the C3 and then chemotaxing. This would be impossible. Do they chemotax towards really pure C3a? I do not know. They can chemotax towards factors at a distance, but I find it difficult to visualize a cell, which produces something which is then the centre of a gradient, moving anywhere else.
Loewi:	But it is not producing C3a. It is producing C3. Surely something else then splits it into C3a.
Wilkinson:	But the highest C3a concentration will be at the cell—in the vicinity of the cell itself.
Schorlemmer:	Can I comment? Several groups working in West Germany and in the Netherlands have shown that macrophages can produce C3. It is produced by the macrophages as a native molecule. It is our hypothesis that when there is a secretion of C3, of the native molecule, and when there is a secretion of several enzymes, they can interact and there will be a cleavage of the native molecules to the C3b, which on the one hand can activate the macrophages, and the C3a, which could be—as in Dr. Loewi's case—the chemotactic factor, or, as in our case, a tumorolytic factor.
A. C. Allison: (UK)	We think this is relevant in the pathogenesis of granulomas. There are some macrophages there. They then release C3a and other chemotactic factors of the complement system, and others, and they can then bring in more macrophages. This is how there is a progressive increase in the size of a granulomatous response, which we know can go on for very long periods of time.
	Does that meet with Dr. Wilkinson's approval, or with his disapproval?
Wilkinson:	As long as these cells are moving to something at a distance from them. A cell attracting another cell is O.K.
Allison:	The point is that this provides a mechanism for the recruitment of cells into inflammatory sites.

Wilkinson:	If a cell is stimulated to release its stuff and then stimulates a cell at a distance to come in, no problem.
I. Ginsburg: **(Israel)**	Would Dr. Schorlemmer please make further comment about the mechanism of lysis of cells. Has he tried to inhibit the lysis by cholesterol, lecithin, or analogues of membranes? Secondly, has he added any inhibitor to proteases?

I ask because many years ago we showed that if cells were injured with very small amounts of complement and antibodies to the extent that they did not really lyse, but were damaged to a small extent, but then if any non-specific protease was added, the cell would be completely disintegrated.

Is it possible that this is the synergistic effect between haemolysin, a phospholipase, a lysolecithin-like substance, or who knows what, together with an additional protease which will enhance the activity of the primary injury? |
| **Schorlemmer:** | We have done no experiments with lysolecithin or anything like that. |
| **M. Glatt:** **(Switzerland)** | My question is technical. In one of his slides, Dr. Schorlemmer showed that the release reaction is biphasic. He gets an early increase and a plateau at about 6 hours and then the release of enzymes continues for a further 72 hours. Could he say something about the uptake or degradation of C3 *in vitro*? Could it be that some of this material is degraded by the early release of proteinases? |
| **Schorlemmer:** | The C3b stimulation?

I showed a slide where we used the C3a, the C3b and the native C3. We looked for enzyme secretion over a period of 72 hours. We only found a secretion with the selective release of enzymes with C3b, and this release starts at about 24 hours and then it increases. With the native C3 we found no release of enzymes, which would be an indication that it is not degraded, at least not in the active component which will induce the release of enzymes. |
| **R. L. Souhami:** **(UK)** | All these sulphated dextrans over a certain molecular weight can be demonstrated inside macrophages histochemically and not below the molecular weight which Dr. Schorlemmer showed to be ineffective. The same thing applies with low molecular weight in dextrans and heparins, which he says are ineffective in his system.

Is it possible that C3b is producing macrophage activation merely by combining with the dextran, or whatever particle it is, to enable it to be phagocytosed in the first place, and that is the reason why the macrophage is activated—because C3b has a permissive role in allowing phagocytosis? |
| **Schorlemmer:** | I cannot say at the moment. We are doing some studies with the endogenous and exogenous C3b in the stimulatory phase. My hypothesis is that there will be activation of the alternate pathway outside of the cell, and there will then be a generation of the C3b, and the C3b will then activate the macrophages. It is an hypothesis, and we shall have to test and prove it. |

15

Matrix vesicles and apatite nodules in arthritic cartilage

S. YOUSUF ALI (UK)

Early ultrastructural observations of rabbit articular cartilage had shown a pericellular distribution of electron-dense lipidic debris in the matrix surrounding the chondrocytes[1]. The debris was found to contain rounded membranous bodies (up to 200 nm in diameter) which sometimes had a granular appearance and their accumulation in articular cartilage was age-related. Both fibrillated and non-fibrillated specimens of human articular cartilage showed similar electron-dense particles surrounding healthy cells and it was suggested that these were derived from cytoplasmic processes extending from the chondrocyte into the surrounding matrix[2,3]. Meachim[4] found them in human osteoarthrotic articular cartilage, and their distribution appeared similar to that found for phospholipid and neutral lipid by light microscopic histochemistry[5]. Similar vesicular bodies were seen in other studies of articular cartilage and they have been variously described as cellular debris[6], Corona vesicles[7], matrix granules[8], membranous debris[9] and lipid material[10], and extracellular lipid[11]. The function of these pericellular bodies has not been satisfactorily explained. Initially Ghadially et al.[2] considered these osmiophilic bodies to consist of physiologically extruded lipid from the cells. Chrisman, Semonsky and Beusch[12], using electron histochemical methods, showed the presence of esterase and cathepsin-type of activity in the extracellular particles in articular cartilage and thought of them as lysosomes. Bonner and Owen[13] in an abstract mentioned that these bodies stained with lipid stains and at electron microscopic level reacted with substrates for acid phosphatase, β-glucuronidase and N-acetyl-β-glucosaminidase. They too postulated them as extracellular lysosomes but none of the pictures or evidence has been published in detail. Thyberg and Friberg[14] using epiphyseal cartilage showed some acid phosphatase and aryl sulphatase activity to be associated with extracellular vesicles.

Recent evidence derived from detailed studies of growth cartilage and re-examination of human articular cartilage, however, suggests an alternative role for these extracellular, membranous, matrix vesicles, specially in arthritis[15-18]. This new concept implies that the pericellular matrix vesicles in human articular cartilage are similar to those in epiphyseal cartilage and that under certain circumstances, they may induce abnormal calcification which either by altering the ionic composition or formation of mineral nodules could lead to a rapid destruction of cartilage in some forms of degenerative joint disease. Firstly the role and function of these matrix vesicles in growth cartilage will be summarized and then their presence and pathological role in human articular cartilage will be critically evaluated.

It is only recently that the sequence of biochemical events responsible for the mineralization of growth cartilage and its subsequent transformation into cancellous bone have been partially elucidated. Bonucci[19] and Anderson[20] demonstrated that the longitudinal septa of epiphyseal cartilage contain extracellular membranous matrix vesicles (100 nm in diameter) which display the first microcrystals of hydroxyapatite. Similar matrix vesicles or dense bodies have been found in a variety of mineralizing tissues, such as medullary bone, dentin, calcifying aorta, and antler horns (see review by Anderson[21]). Electron histochemistry demonstrated the presence of alkaline phosphatase in these vesicles but no acid phosphatase[22]. Biochemical isolation and characterization has shown that matrix vesicles contain most of the alkaline phosphatase, pyrophosphatase and ATPase activity of growth cartilage and that they are derived from the cell processes of chondrocytes and are not lysosomes[23,24]. The mechanism by which matrix vesicles concentrate calcium to induce apatite formation has been studied by using ^{45}Ca and it is clear that calcium can bind to the membranes of the vesicles or diffuse passively into the lumen under physiological conditions and that in the presence of low calcium concentration and an energy supply (ATP) they can actively take in calcium against a concentration gradient[24-26]. Systematic electron probe analysis of a single longitudinal septum of epiphyseal cartilage has established how matrix vesicles take in first calcium and then phosphorus to form crystals of apatite which then grow to form mineral nodules which subsequently coalesce to form calcified septa[24,26]. The role of matrix vesicles in various disorders of calcification and growth is under investigation.

With our knowledge of matrix vesicles in growth cartilage we have re-examined human articular cartilage to see if they play a role in mineralization of the joint tissue, specially in pathological conditions. Some of this information and most of the technical methods used in this study have been published elsewhere[15,16,17,24]. The questions that needed an answer were: are the matrix vesicles in human articular cartilage similar to those in epiphyseal cartilage, morphologically (that is in size, appearance and distribution), chemically (enzyme content, whether alkaline phosphatase is cellular

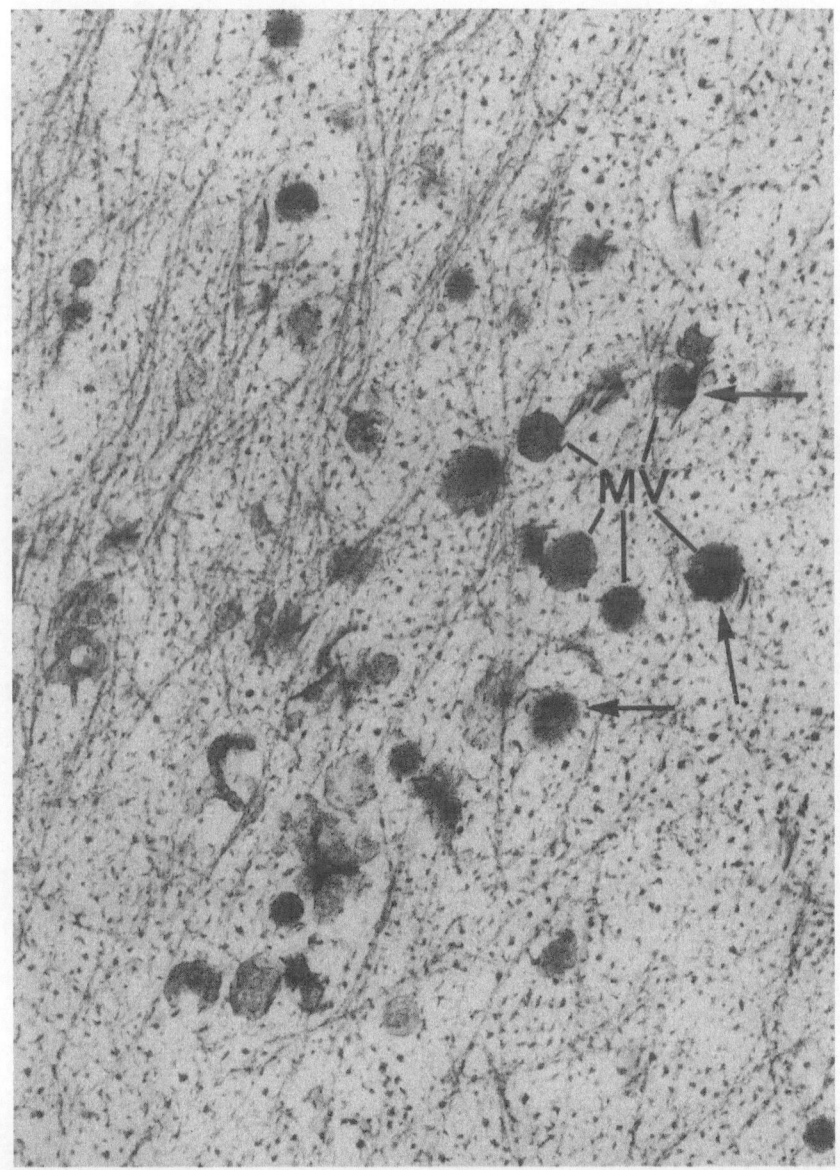

Figure 15.1 Electron microscope picture of matrix vesicles (MV); some with crystal needles inside them (arrows) are shown in the longitudinal septa matrix in the hypertrophic region of rabbit proximal tibial growth plate. All the electron micrographs are stained with uranyl acetate and lead citrate. Compare these vesicles with those in human articular cartilage in Figures 15.3, 15.4, 15.5 shown at the same magnification. × 51 300

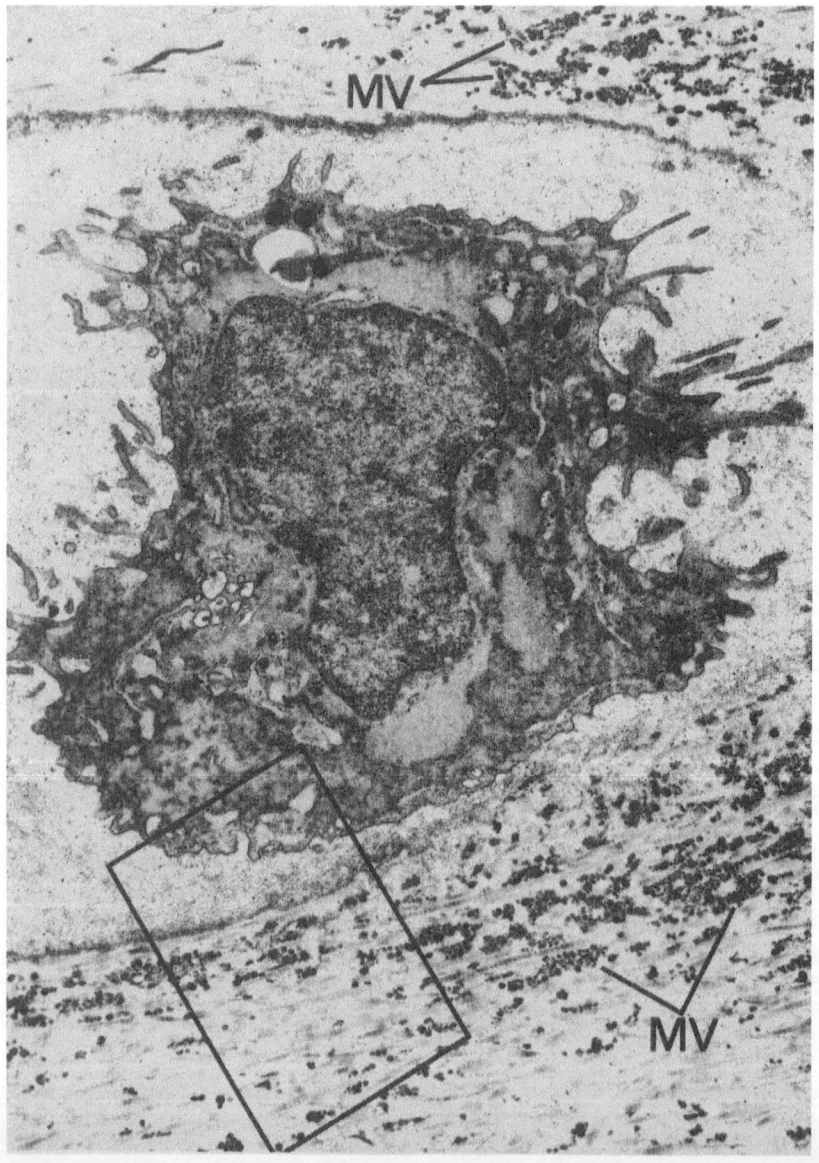

Figure 15.2 Chondrocyte from the middle zone of adult human articular cartilage, showing the pericellular distribution of matrix vesicles (MV) scattered amongst the collagen fibrils. The inset area is shown at a higher magnification in Figure 15.3. × 13 750

or extracellular and associated with these vesicles) and functionally (are microcrystals and apatite nodules associated with them)? It was also important to evaluate any changes in these parameters in arthritic cartilage. Ultrastructural examination of articular cartilage confirmed that the dense bodies surrounding the pericellular area were very similar to matrix vesicles in growth cartilage (compare Figures 15.1, 15.3, 15.4, 15.5 and 15.6). Their appearance showed the same osmiophilic characteristics and their size, which varied from 50 nm to 250 nm in diameter, was very similar to the matrix vesicles, although they appeared more heterogeneous (Figures 15.2, 15.3, 15.4 and 15.5). A double membrane could be seen (Figures 15.4 and 15.5; see also References 16 and 17), and the vesicles were present at all levels of the articular cartilage, but were more frequent in the IV zone in the tidemark region adjoining the subchondral bone. In this region microcrystals were present inside the vesicles and mineral nodules could be seen either forming from vesicles or lying next to them (Figures 15.4 and 15.6) and this was again very similar to growth cartilage. Obviously it was not possible to put any number to their frequency and occurrence, and we had to turn to biochemistry for quantitation.

Digestion of human articular cartilage with collagenase and separation of cells from the extracellular fractions has revealed that the major portion of the alkaline phosphatase activity of this tissue is not present in chondrocytes but in the matrix vesicles[24]. Indeed the pattern of distribution of this enzyme in the various fractions is indistinguishable from growth cartilage but is quite different to that obtained with elastic ear cartilage or other tissues[24]. This indicates that articular cartilage is similar to growth cartilage in this respect. An analysis of the alkaline phosphatase activity levels in normal articular cartilage from humans of different ages is shown in Figure 15.7. There is high enzyme activity in juvenile and adolescent articular cartilage, but this settles down to a low level in adult life. In osteoarthritic cartilage the enzyme level is sometimes 30 times that of the normal in the same age group. This may be an indication that there is an increase in the number of matrix vesicles in osteoarthritic cartilage, although a specific enzyme increase could not be ruled out. Ultrastructurally, matrix vesicles were more frequently encountered in the mid-zone of osteoarthritic cartilage than in the normal (see also References 16 and 17). They also appeared to be more granular and frequently contained needle-like crystals inside them which were more common in IV zone (Figure 15.6). In osteoarthritic cartilage some mid-zone vesicles also displayed granular or microcrystalline appearance and nodules of apatite-like mineral in the deeper zones. Osteophytic cartilage, which had high alkaline phosphatase activity, also had many granular matrix vesicles (Figure 15.5).

This combined biochemical and electron microscopic analysis indicated that the calcification mechanism was abnormal in osteoarthrotic cartilage and could therefore have serious consequences. Abnormal calcification

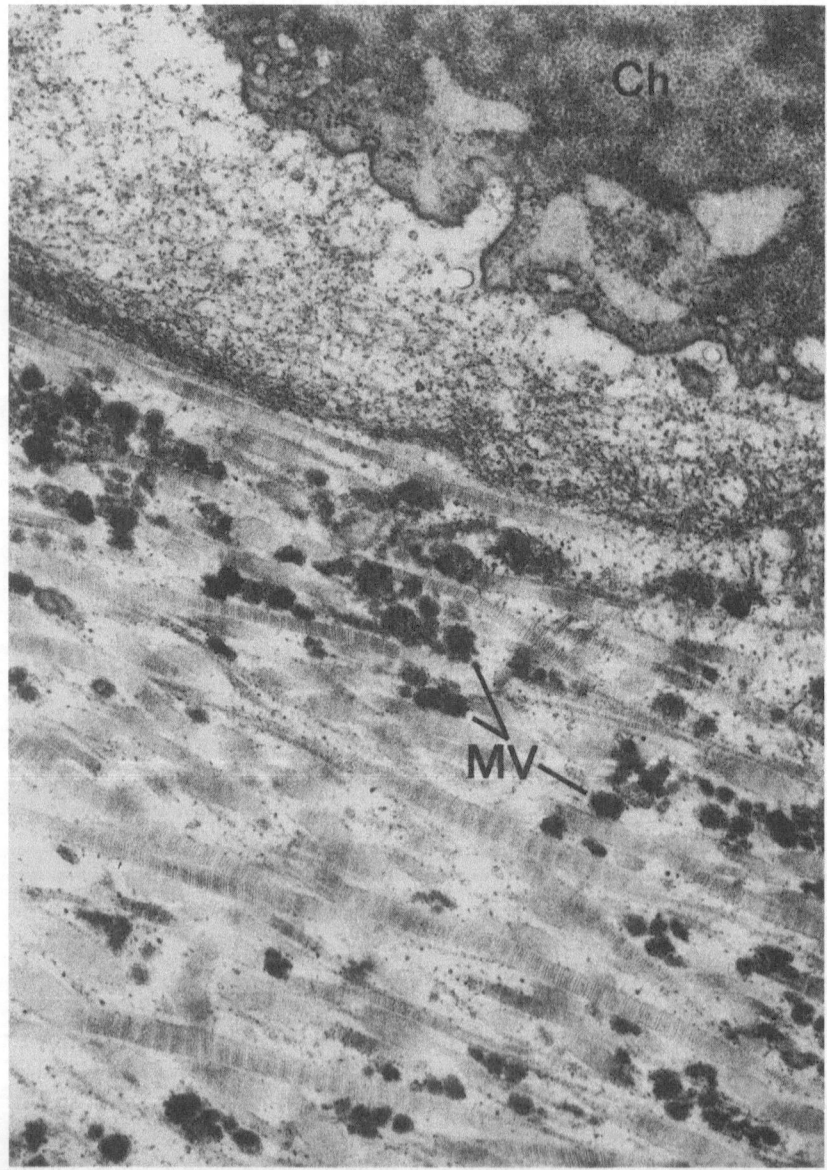

Figure 15.3 Higher magnification picture of the inset area in Figure 15.2 showing the matrix vesicles scattered amongst the collagen fibrils in the pericellular region outside the chondrocyte (Ch) lacuna, in human articular cartilage. The collagen fibrils are thicker than in growth cartilage. × 51 300

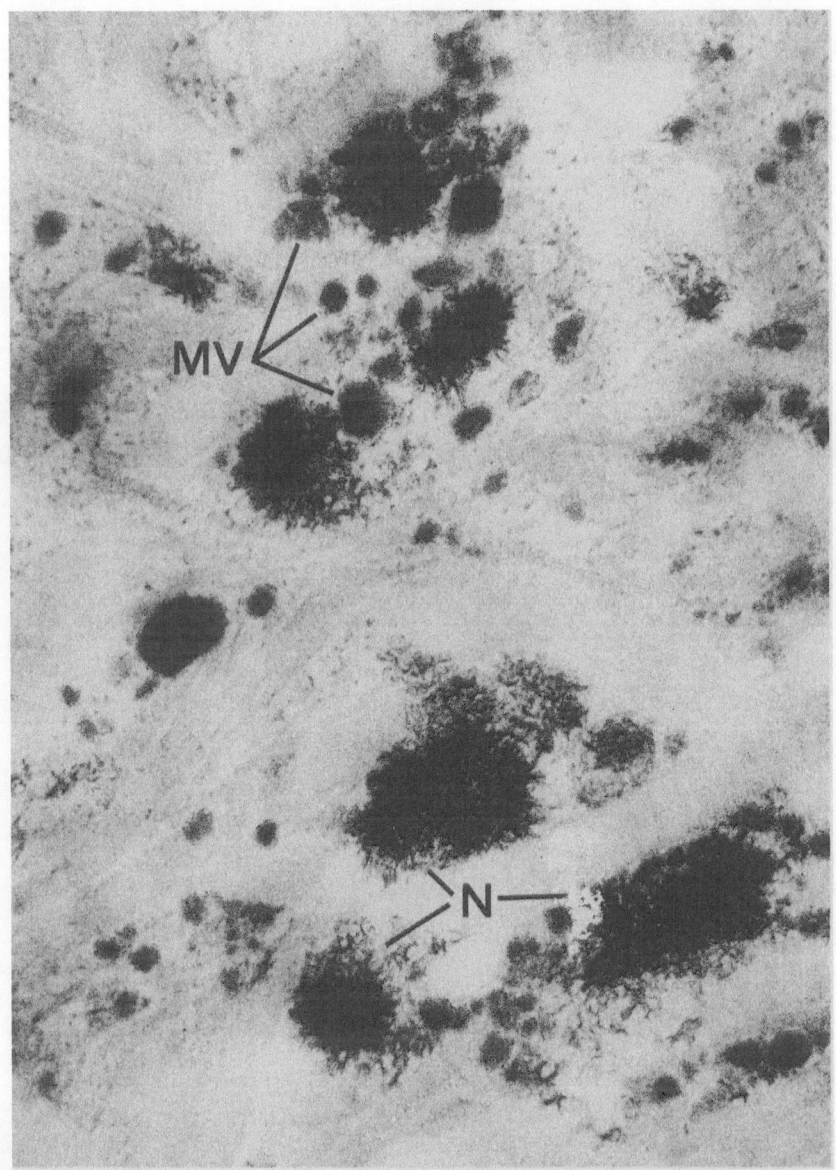

Figure 15.4 Matrix vesicles (MV) and mineral nodules (N) in the deeper zone of human articular cartilage. The vesicles have a double membrane and the collagen fibres are thicker than in the middle zone of articular cartilage and of the growth plate. (Compare with Figure 15.1.) × 51 300

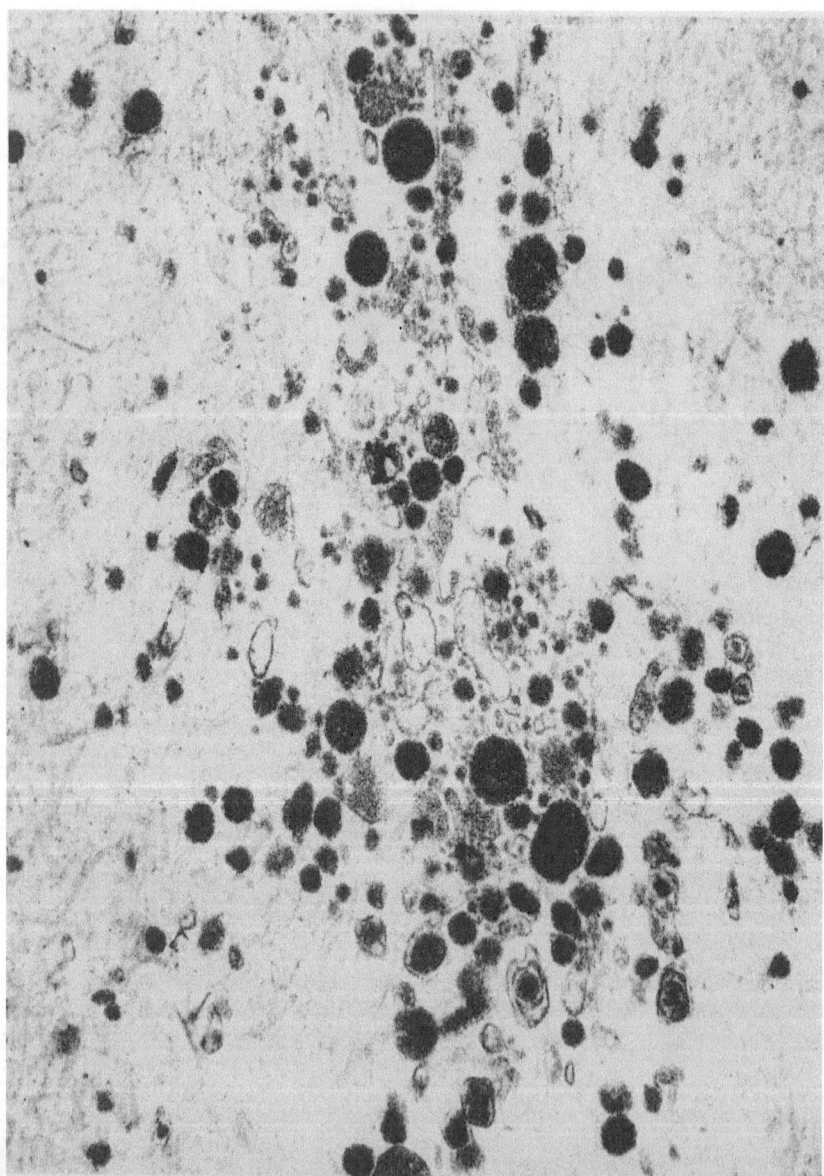

Figure 15.5 Matrix vesicles (MV) some with granular or crystalline appearance from the middle zone of human periarticular osteophyte. The collagen fibrils appear different to those in articular cartilage and the growth plate but the matrix vesicles are very similar. (Compare with Figures 15.1, 15.3 and 15.4). × 51 300

mechanism can produce cartilage degeneration in a number of ways. For example, if there is an increase in matrix vesicles and mineral nodules in the deeper zones of cartilage, this may lead to focal conversion of the basal portions of the tissue into calcified cartilage and eventually bone. This may alter the 'tidemark' region to reduplication and permit an advance of the mineral front, implying that articular cartilage which can be considered a latent growth plate, has reverted to a growth phase again. This remodelling near the subchondral bone will put greater pressure on the remaining layer of cartilage which may then become more susceptible to degradation by normal wear process. This concept fits in very well with that put forward originally by L. C. Johnson[27] and others. Moreover, any change in local concentration of calcium in articular cartilage could alter the various physicochemical properties of the tissue, such as the water-binding capacity, the colloidal charge density, the swelling pressure and thus the elasticity of the tissue[28,29]. These changes will make the articular cartilage more prone to wear under pressure. In addition, the presence of mineral crystallites and nodules in the middle and upper layers of cartilage will lead to physical, abrasive wear of the whole tissue.

Finally, some of our findings with regards to matrix vesicles and the findings of apatite-like crystals and nodules in cartilage can be correlated with some of the implication of crystal-induced inflammation in joints. McCarty[30] introduced the concept of 'crystal-deposition disease' and found that apart from urate and pyrophosphate deposits, two other crystal types could be found in human articular cartilage and adjoining tissues and fluids, namely hydroxyapatite and dicalcium phosphate dihydrate. Recurrent acute inflammation associated with focal apatite crystal deposition has been found in some patients[31]. Dieppe, Huskisson, Crocker and Willoughby[32] not only analysed and demonstrated hydroxyapatite nodules in symovial fluid, but also showed the inflammatory reaction which the mineral particles could produce. Their work has permitted them to postulate an 'apatite deposition disease' as one form of osteoarthrosis. The particle size described by Dieppe et al. varied from 0.15 μm to 0.8 μm and the matrix vesicles found by us in human articular cartilage were from 0.05 to 0.25 μm, and when nodules were formed from them, the diameter increased to 0.6 μm. Thus the mineral nodules shown in Figures 15.4 and 15.6 are very near in size and description to those shown by Dieppe et al. It would have to be stressed that in normal articular cartilage these mineral nodules associated with the matrix vesicles are commonly found in the deeper layers. It is possible that in osteoarthrotic cartilage they occur in the middle zones and if there were deep fibrillation or vertical clefts in the cartilage, then it is easy to visualize these nodules being shed into the joint cavity and setting up an inflammatory cycle. It should also be stressed that in chondrocalcinosis there appears to be a slight decrease in alkaline phosphatase activity[33] of articular cartilage, whereas we have found an elevation in osteoarthrotic cartilage and our findings are therefore quite

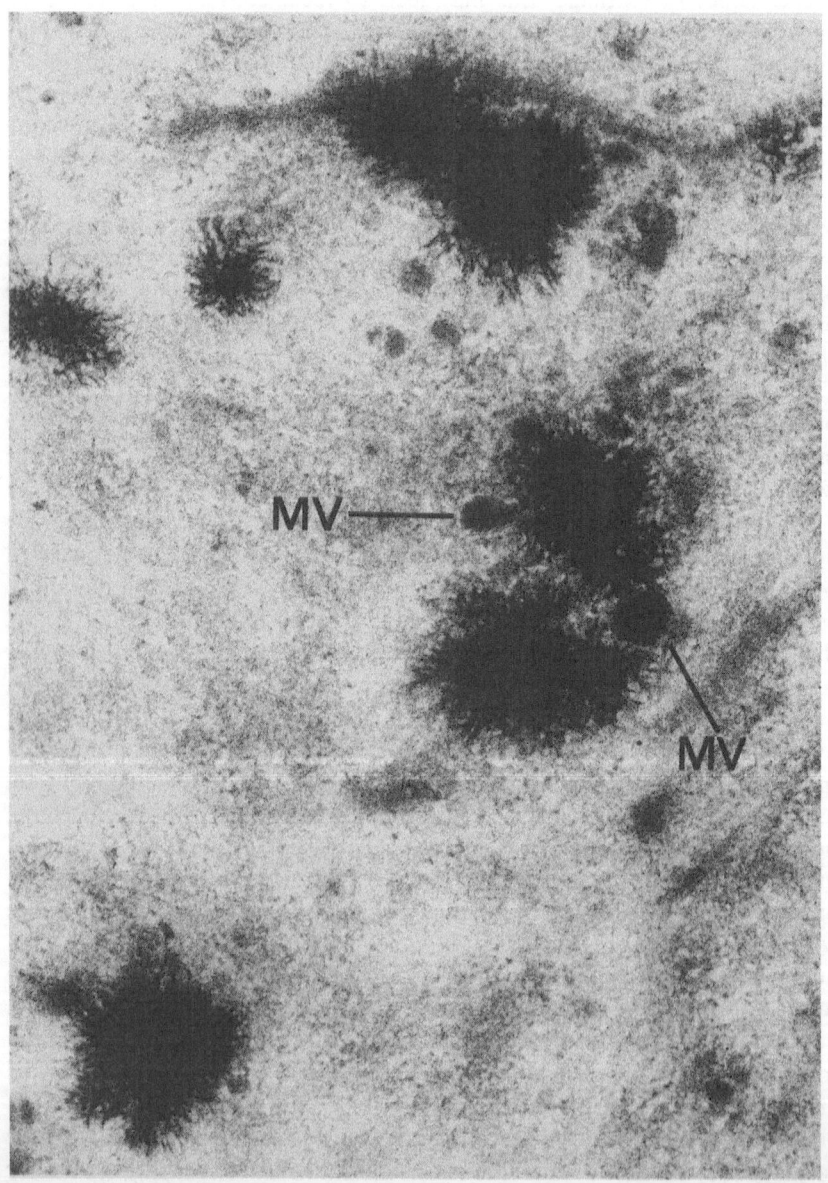

Figure 15.6 Matrix vesicles (MV) and mineral nodules from the pericellular region of the deep zone of osteoarthrotic human articular cartilage. The matrix vesicles have a double membrane and are closely associated with the apatite-like crystal clusters and nodules. × 112 500

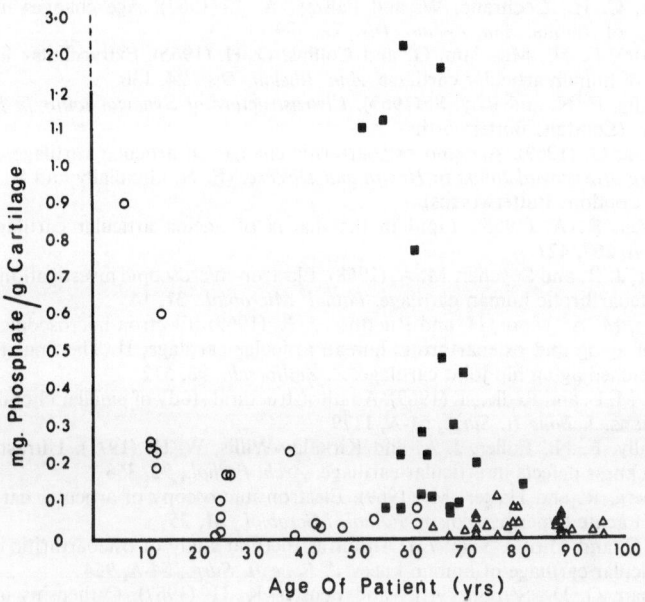

Figure 15.7 The amount of alkaline phosphatase activity in fresh human articular carti-lage is plotted against the age of the patient. O, Normal cartilage obtained from femoral heads at amputation (Type I). △, Normal cartilage obtained from femoral heads after sub-capital fractures of the neck of femur (Type II). ■, Osteoarthrotic cartilage (Type IV) obtained from femoral head after total hip replacement

different to pseudogout. It is easy to see that lack of alkaline phosphatase (pyrophosphatase) will lead to an accumulation of pyrophosphate, whereas increase in alkaline phosphatase will permit the hydrolysis of phosphate-containing substrates (e.g. ATP, PPi, G-6-P, G-1-P, etc.) and lead to the formation of apatite[24]. Howell et al.[34] have found that articular cartilage is capable of extruding pyrophosphate, specially in some forms of osteoarthrosis. We therefore agree with Dieppe et al. (1976) and feel that apatite deposition disease should be added to the crystal deposition diseases defined by McCarty (1970) and suggest that the formation of apatite nodules in cartilage and in synovial fluid is dependent to a large extent on the distribution and function of matrix vesicles.

Acknowledgements

I am grateful to the Nuffield Foundation and the P.F. Charitable Trust for financial support, and to Mrs. Angela Wisby for technical help.

References

1. Barnett, C. H., Cochrane, W. and Palfrey, A. J. (1963). Age changes in articular cartilage of rabbits. *Ann. Rheum. Dis.*, **22**, 389

2. Ghadially, F. N., Meachim, G. and Collins, D. H. (1965). Extracellular lipid in the matrix of human articular cartilage. *Ann. Rheum. Dis.*, **24**, 136

3. Ghadially, F. N. and Roy, S. (1969). *Ulstrastructure of Synovial Joints in Health and Disease.* (London: Butterworths)

4. Meachim, G. (1969). Age and osteoarthritic changes in articular cartilage. In: *Ultrastructure of Synovial Joints in Health and Disease.* (F. N. Ghadially and S. Roy, eds.) p. 61. (London: Butterworths)

5. Stockwell, R. A. (1965). Lipid in the matrix of ageing articular cartilage. *Nature (London)*, **207**, 427

6. Rüttner, J. R. and Spycher, M. A. (1968). Electron microscopic investigations on aging and osteoarthrotic human cartilage. *Pathol. Microbiol.*, **31**, 14

7. Spycher, M. A., Moor, H. and Ruettner, J. R. (1969). Electron microscopic investigations of aging and osteoarthrotic human articular cartilage, II. The fine structure of freeze-etched aging hip joint cartilage. *Z. Zellforsch.*, **98**, 512

8. Zimny, M. L. and Redler, I. (1969). An ultrastructural study of patellar chondromalacia in humans. *J. Bone Jt. Surg.*, **51-A**, 1179

9. Ghadially, F. N., Fuller, J. A. and Kirkaldy-Willis, W. H. (1971). Ultrastructure of full-thickness defects in articular cartilage. *Arch. Pathol.*, **92**, 356

10. Silberberg, R. and Hasler, M. (1969). Electron microscopy of articular cartilage: the effect of acute hyperthyroidism. *Pathol. Microbiol.*, **31**, 25

11. Weiss, C. and Mirow, S. (1972). An ultrastructural study of osteoarthritic changes in the articular cartilage of human knees. *J. Bone Jt. Surg.*, **54-A**, 954

12. Chrisman, O. D., Semonsky, C. and Beusch, K. G. (1967). Cathepsins in articular cartilage. In: *The Healing of Osseous Tissue.* (R. A. Robinson, ed.). p. 169. (Washington D.C.: National Academy of Science and National Research Council Publications)

13. Bonner, Jr., W. M. and Owen, C. (1968). Hydrolytic enzymes in extracellular granules of aging articular cartilage. *Arthritis Rheum.*, **11**, 816

14. Thyberg, J. and Friberg, U. (1972). Electron microscopic enzyme histochemical studies on the cellular genesis of matrix vesicles in the epiphyseal plate. *J. Ultrastruct. Res.*, **41**, 43

15. Ali, S. Y. and Evans, L. (1973). Enzymic degradation of cartilage in osteoarthritis, *Fed. Proc.*, **32**, 1494

16. Ali, S. Y. and Bayliss, M. T. (1974). Enzymic changes in human osteoarthrotic cartilage, In S. Y. Ali, D. W. Elves and D. H. Leabech (eds.) *Normal and Osteoarthrotic Articular Cartilage*, p. 189. (London: Institute of Orthopaedics Publication)

17. Ali, S. Y. and Wisby, A. (1975). Ulstrastructural aspects of normal and osteoarthrotic cartilage, *Ann. Rheum. Dis.*, **34**, Suppl. 2, 21

18. Ali, S. Y. and Wisby, A. (1976). The role of matrix vesicles in human osteoarthrotic cartilage. *Proc. Roy. Mic. Soc.*, **11**, Pt. 5, 62

19. Bonucci, E. (1967). Fine structure of early cartilage calcification. *J. Ultrastruct. Res.*, **20**, 33

20. Anderson, H. C. (1969). Vesicles associated with calcification in the matrix of epiphyseal cartilage. *J. Cell. Biol.*, **41**, 59

21. Anderson, H. C. (1976). Matrix vesicles of cartilage and bone. In: *The Biochemistry and Physiology of Bone*, (G. H. Bourne, ed.) Vol. IV, p. 135. (New York: Academic Press)

22. Matsuzawa, I. and Anderson, H. C. (1971). Phosphatases of epiphyseal cartilage studied by electron microscopic cytochemical methods. *J. Histochem. Cyotchem.*, **19**, 801

23. Ali, S. Y., Sajdera, S. W. and Anderson, H. C. (1970). Isolation and characterization of calcifying matrix vesicles from epiphyseal cartilage. *Proc. Nat. Acad. Sci. U.S.*, **67**, 1513

24. Ali, S. Y. (1976). Analysis of matrix vesicles and their role in the calcification of epiphyseal cartilage. *Fed. Proc.*, **35**, 135

25. Ali, S. Y. and Evans, L. (1973). The uptake of (^{45}Ca) calcium ions by matrix vesicles isolated from calcifying cartilage, *Biochem. J.*, **134**, 647
26. Ali, S. Y., Wisby, A., Evans, L. and Craig-Gray, J. (1977). The sequence of calcium and phosphorus accumulation by matrix vesicles. *Calc. Tiss. Res.*, (In press)
27. Johnson, L. C. (1962). Joint remodelling as the basis for osteoarthritis. *J. Am. Vet. Med. Assoc.*, **141**, 1237
28. Gersh, I. and Catchpole, H. R. (1960). The nature of ground substance of connective tissue. *Perspec. Biol. Med.*, **3**, 282
29. Sokoloff, L. (1963). Elasticity of articular cartilage: effect of ions and viscous solutions. *Science*, **141**, 1055
30. McCarty, D. J. (1970). Crystal deposition diseases. In: *Disease-a-Month*. (H. F. Dowling, ed.) p. 5. (Chicago: Year Book Medical Publishers Inc.)
31. McCarty, D. J. and Gatter, R. A. (1966). Recurrent acute inflammation associated with focal apatite crystal deposition. *Arthritis Rheum.*, **9**, 804
32. Dieppe, P. A., Huskisson, E. C., Crocker, P. and Willoughby, D. A. (1976). Apatite deposition disease, a new arthropathy. *Lancet*, **i**, 266
33. Reginato, A. J., Schumacher, H. R. and Martinez, V. A. (1974). The articular cartilage in familial chondrocalcinosis, light and electron microscopic study. *Arthritis Rheum.*, **17**, 977
34. Howell, D. S., Muniz, O. and Pita, J. C. (1974). Extrusion of pyrophosphate into extracellular media by cartilage incubates. In: *Normal and Osteoarthrotic Articular Cartilage*. (S. Y. Ali, M. W. Elves and D. H. Leaback, eds.) p. 177 (London: Institute of Orthopaedics Publication)

16

Crystal induced inflammation and osteoarthritis

P. A. DIEPPE (UK)

INTRODUCTION

Examination of synovial fluids by light microscopy led to the discovery of urate crystals in patients with gout[1], and of pyrophosphate crystals in 'pseudogout'[2]. This work was followed by experiments to show that the crystals can cause inflammation, and it is now generally accepted that the presence of these particles in the joint cavity initiates the inflammatory response in these two diseases. In gout, the sodium biurate crystals form within the synovial fluid itself, whereas in 'pseudogout', calcium pyrophosphate dihydrate is precipitated first in articular cartilage, and only escapes into the synovial fluid if dislodged from its former site. However, the presence of pyrophosphate crystals in articular cartilage (chondrocalcinosis), is more often associated with a chronic 'degenerative' type of arthritis than with acute pseudogout[3]. An examination of cartilage and synovial fluid from patients with the universal chronic form of joint disease, osteoarthritis, therefore seemed worthwhile.

THE IDENTIFICATION OF CRYSTALS IN OSTEOARTHRITIC SYNOVIAL FLUIDS

A large number of patients attending a rheumatology clinic with a clinical diagnosis of osteoarthritis, including the typical X-ray features, have been examined. Those in whom exacerbations were common and synovial fluid easy to obtain were studied further, and synovial fluid aspirated from affected joints, usually the knees. The group is therefore a selected one and not necessarily representative of osteoarthritis in general.

Synovial fluids were examined as soon as possible after collection, first by polarized light microscopy, and then by analytical electron microscopy, according to the method of Crocker et al.[4] Positively birifringent monoclinic or triclinic crystals were observed in five cases, and elemental analysis of the crystals showed the presence of calcium and phosphorus in the ratio $P/Ca = 0.8$. Using identical conditions for analysis, pure calcium pyrophosphate dihydrate crystals[5] have a similar P/Ca ratio. In 20 cases a different mineral has been identified; nodules, varying in size from 0.1 to 1 micron in diameter were identified using electron microscopy, and found to consist of calcium and phosphorus in the ratio $P/Ca = 0.44$. In many cases high resolution microscopy showed the presence of micro-crystals in the nodules, and their morphology was similar to the apatite nodules found in osteoarthritic cartilage by Ali[6]; occasional intracellular nodules were observed, contained in membrane bound vesicles. Pure hydroxyapatite (kindly supplied by Prof. Fleisch) has a similar morphology, and identical P/Ca ratio.

In the selected group of osteoarthritic patients so far studied, crystal deposition has been common; nodules or aggregates of hydroxyapatite crystals have been found more often than pyrophosphate crystals, and the cells in the synovial fluids have been similar in the two groups (Table 16.1).

Table 16.1 A comparison of the total and differential cell counts in osteoarthritic patients with apatite nodules or pyrophosphate crystals in the synovial fluid

---

1. 20 patients with typical osteoarthritis and effusions in the knees in which apatite nodules have been found
   Cell count: range $0.3 - 12.3 \times 10^9$ cells/l
   Mean 2.64
   Mean differential: 83% mononuclear, 17% polymorphs

2. 6 patients with chondrocalcinosis and osteoarthritis, in whose effusions pyrophosphate crystals were seen
   Cell count: range $0.5 - 2.1 \times 10^9$ cells/l
   Mean 1.60
   Mean differential: 90% mononuclear, 10% polymorphs

THE INFLAMMATORY PROPERTIES OF HYDROXYAPATITE

Having identified hydroxyapatite crystals in osteoarthritic synovial fluids, it is important to establish whether or not they have any tissue damaging potential. Pyrogen-free hydroxyapatite has therefore been used as the irritant in a number of models of inflammation. Injection of 1 ml of a 1% suspension of hydroxyapatite into the pleural space of the rat causes a brisk inflammatory response (Figure 16.1); this is accompanied by release of lysosomal enzymes,

226

and phagocytosis of the hydroxyapatite[7]. Intradermal injection in mice causes an acute inflammation followed by formation of granulomas lasting for up to six weeks. Intradermal injection of 10 mg of hydroxyapatite in 0.2 ml of sterile saline in human volunteers also causes an inflammatory response. This is biphasic (Figure 16.2); a transient, variable initial erythema, probably related to histamine release, is followed by a more prolonged phase accompanied by swelling and hyperalgesia. The second phase of the response is reduced by anti-inflammatory drugs such as indomethacin. Small persistent granulomas, lasting several weeks, sometimes form.

The inflammatory potential of hydroxyapatite, which can cause both acute and chronic responses, has therefore been established.

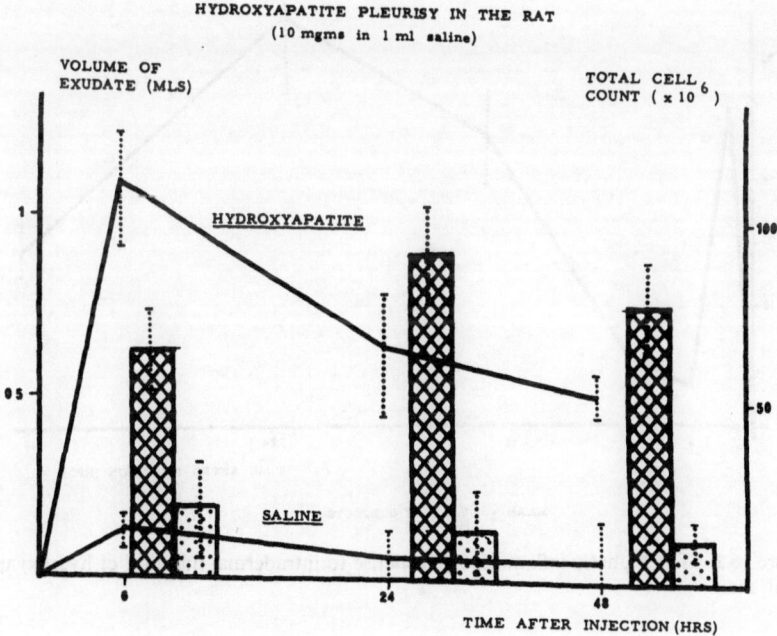

Figure 16.1 The intrapleural inflammatory response to hydroxyapatite in the rat. The lines show the volume of exudate produced, and the hatched blocks the total cell count in the exudates. (Mean ± 1 SD, groups of 12)

MINERAL DEPOSITION AND OSTEOARTHRITIS

The formation of nodules of hydroxyapatite in osteoarthritic articular cartilage has been demonstrated by Ali[6]. Similar nodules of apatite have been identified in the synovial fluid of patients with osteoarthritis[8], and the present study suggests that this may be a common finding. The work described also suggests that hydroxyapatite can cause tissue damage.

Osteoarthritis is primarily a disease of cartilage, but it can no longer be regarded as simply a phenomenon of ageing, or due to wear and tear. A metabolic abnormality seems more plausible, and the present work suggest that the articular cartilage in osteoarthritis may have changed its metabolic

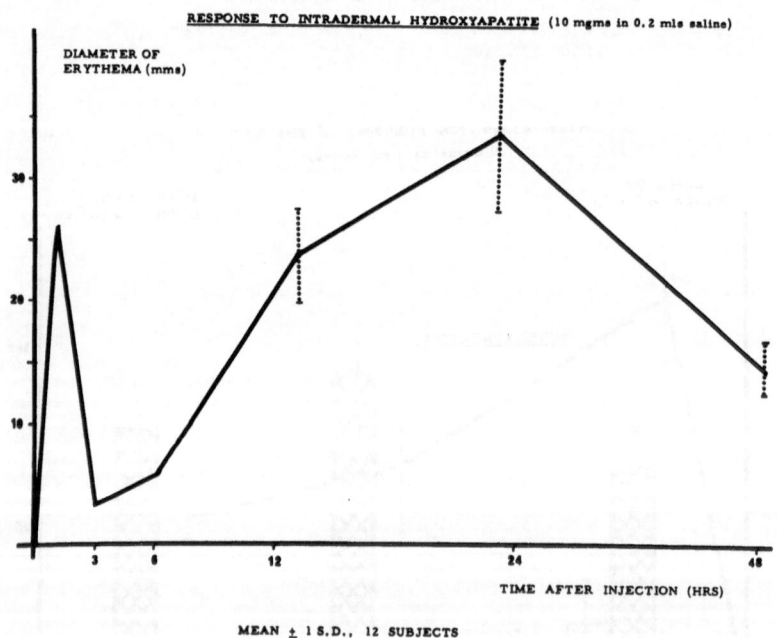

RESPONSE TO INTRADERMAL HYDROXYAPATITE (10 mgms in 0.2 mls saline)

DIAMETER OF ERYTHEMA (mms)

TIME AFTER INJECTION (HRS)

MEAN ± 1 S.D., 12 SUBJECTS

Figure 16.2 The biphasic inflammatory response to intradermal injection of hydroxyapatite in man

status to that of growth cartilage or calcifying cartilage. The formation of mineral deposits may cause direct damage to the cartilage; in addition escape of apatite nodules into the synovial fluid may initiate inflammatory events causing soft-tissue changes and thus further damage to the cartilage.

Many of the clinical features of osteoarthritis suggest an inflammatory component: the disease is episodic in nature, and responds to anti-inflammatory agents; morning stiffness and inactivity stiffness occur; synovial effusions are common; and 'hot' joints are sometimes seen, for example 'hot'

PATHWAYS IN THE PATHOGENESIS OF OSTEOARTHRITIS

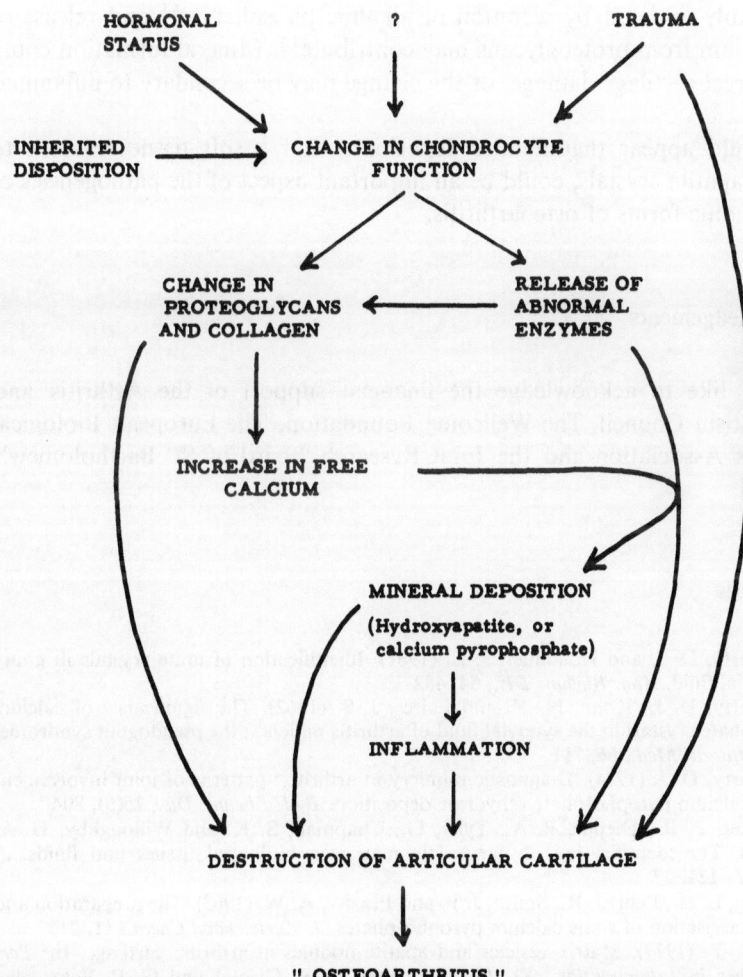

Figure 16.3 An hypothesis as to some of the pathways in the pathogenesis of osteoarthritis. (See text)

Heberden's nodes. In addition specific inflammatory sub-types of the disease have been described[9,10]. Many of these inflammatory features could be explained by a reaction to release of apatite crystals.

A hypothetical scheme of the pathogenesis of osteoarthritis is shown in Figure 16.3. A number of factors, including genetic disposition and hormonal influences, may be responsible for a change in chondrocyte function, and change of the cartilage to a growth-type state. The formation of mineral is probably initiated by secretion of alkaline phosphatase[11] and release of free calcium from proteoglycans may contribute[12]. Mineral formation could cause direct cartilage damage, or the change may be secondary to inflammation.

It would appear that apatite deposition, and a soft tissue reaction to hydroxyapatite crystals, could be an important aspect of the pathogenesis of at least some forms of osteoarthritis.

Acknowledgements

I would like to acknowledge the financial support of the Arthritis and Rheumatism Council, The Wellcome Foundation, The European Biological Research Association and the Joint Research Board of St. Bartholomew's Hospital.

References

1. McCarty, D. J. and Hollander, J. L. (1961). Identification of urate crystals in gouty synovial fluid. *Ann. Rheum. Dis.*, **54**, 452
2. McCarty, D. J., Kohn, N. N. and Faires, J. S. (1962). The significance of calcium phosphate crystals in the synovial fluid of arthritis patients: the pseudogout syndrome. *Ann. Intern. Med.*, **56**, 711
3. McCarty, D. J. (1974). Diagnostic mimicry in arthritis: patterns of joint involvement with calcium pyrophosphate dihydrate deposition. *Bull. Rheum. Dis.*, **25(5)**, 804
4. Crocker, P. R., Dieppe, P. A., Tyler, G., Chapman, S. K. and Willoughby, D. A. (1977). The identification of particulate matter in biological tissues and fluids. *J. Pathol.*, **121**, 37
5. Brown, E. H., Lehr, J. R., Smith, J. P. and Frazier, A. W. (1963). The preparation and characterisation of some calcium pyrophosphates. *J. Agric. Food Chem.*, **11**, 215
6. Ali, S. Y. (1977). Matrix vesicles and apatite nodules in arthritic cartilage. In: *Perspectives in Inflammation*. (D. A. Willoughby, J. P. Giroud and G. P. Velo, eds.) p. 211. (Lancaster: MTP Press Limited)
7. Dieppe, P. A., Willoughby, D. A., Glatt, M. and Huskisson, E. C. (1977). The inflammatory properties of hydroxyapatite crystals (Abstract). *Ann. Rheum. Dis.* (In press)
8. Dieppe, P. A., Huskisson, E. C., Crocker, P. R. and Willoughby, D. A. (1976). Apatite deposition disease: a new arthropathy. *Lancet*, **i**, 266
9. Peter, J. B., Pearson, C. M. and Marmor, L. (1966). Erosive osteoarthritis of the hands. *Arthritis Rheum.*, **9**, 365
10. Ehrlich, G. E. (1975). Osteoarthritis beginning with inflammation: definitions and correlations. *J. Am. Med. Assoc.*, **232**, 157

11. Ali, S. Y. and Wisby, A. (1975). Ultrastructural aspects of normal and osteoarthrotic cartilage. *Ann. Rheum. Dis.*, **34**, Suppl. 2, 21
12. Benderly, H. and Maroudas, A. (1975). *Ann. Rheum. Dis.*, **34**, Suppl. 2, 46

17

Microanalysis of particulate material involved in inflammation

P. A. DIEPPE, P. R. CROCKER AND D. A. WILLOUGHBY (UK)

Inflammation is often associated with the presence of minute inert particles. These particles may be the primary cause of the inflammation, as in some joint and lung diseases, or arise as a result of the reaction, as in the case of some renal calculi. Precise analysis of such particles is desirable, and has been aided by the application of recent technological advances.

Crystalline material can be analysed by X-ray diffraction, which gives precise details of the space lattice. However, this method is only applicable to fairly large crystals, isolated from other material, and it is difficult and time consuming. A simpler, quicker, and more flexible means of analysis of pure material is offered by infra-red spectrophotometry, which can also be used to isolate certain chemical constituents in biological samples. For the identification of individual particles within biological matter, analytical electron microscopy has been used. Correlation of results from the two pieces of apparatus has aided analysis of a wide variety of clinical and experimental specimens.

1. INFRA-RED SPECTROPHOTOMETRY

Dry samples are ground up to achieve a small particle size, mixed with potassium bromide, and compressed to form small transparent discs which can be mounted in the spectrophotometer. The absorption spectrum is then plotted on graduated, log paper. As little as $10 \, \mu g$ of any given substance is enough for its spectrum to be recorded, and analysis of the results can be aided by computerized comparison with spectra from known standard chemicals. The method depends on changes in the vibration of inter-atomic bonds, and therefore identifies individual chemical groups. Individual substances can only be found if the spectrum of the pure compound is known, and by cross-checking the spectra with other methods of analysis. However, once a chemical has been 'finger-printed', it can be quickly and reliably identified from samples of differing type and purity; the whole process only taking about 15 min.

2. ANALYTICAL ELECTRON MICROSCOPY

This technique is particularly suited to analysis of individual particles found in biological samples. Such particles are often small, few in number, and difficult to identify by any other method. Specimens are prepared in the usual way for electron microscopy, although thicker sections than usual may be necessary to preserve the particles in the tissue, and precautions need to be taken with the chemical processing to avoid invalidation of elemental analysis data. There are many advantages in the use of a system that combines transmission microscopy with scanning microscopy and X-ray energy spectroscopy. This allows high resolution images to help morphological identification, analysis of very small areas, and diffraction data can be obtained from the same sample. This technique has been used to cross-check data from infra-red spectrophotometry, and to identify particles in biological tissue that are sometimes too small to be seen at all by light microscopy.

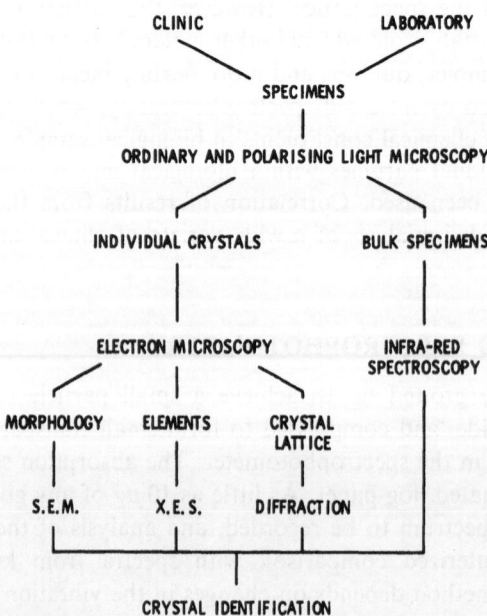

Figure 17.1 The microanalytical system. XES = X-ray energy spectroscopy. SEM = scanning electron microscopy

These two pieces of apparatus are being used to complement each other and form a complete analytical system (Figure 17.1). Bulk samples are analysed by infrà-red spectrophotometry; cross-checks are made with standard chemicals, and if unknown spectra are obtained the substance is analysed further, including electron diffraction, in the analytical electron microscope. The microscope is the only way of identifying small individual particles in tissues, and is also useful where a mixture of different materials is present. Quantitative analysis of the tissue matrix is difficult, but for analysis of relatively inert, discrete particles there are less pitfalls, and elemental ratios, rather than precise quantification, are used. The techniques are not yet perfected, and many hazards exist in biological work, but the combination of data obtained from the two pieces of apparatus, as well as from more conventional techniques, has proved invaluable.

At present the analytical system is being used to identify material in calculi, synovial fluids, urine, tissue specimens, and foreign bodies from patients. It is also being used for analysis of irritants and their products in use in a programme of work on experimental inflammation. In addition, further advancement of the techniques should allow much wider applications in biological research in general.

Acknowledgements

We would like to thank Perkin-Elmer Ltd, Jeol (UK) Ltd, Link Systems Ltd., and numerous individual workers in a variety of disciplines, for their help in the development of this system. Financial support has come from The Wellcome Foundation, The European Biological Research Association, The Arthritis and Rheumatism Council and the Joint Research Board of St. Bartholomew's Hospital.

Discussion 17

T. L. Vischer: (Switzerland)	Dr. Ali demonstrated that there are vesicles and granules of apatite in cartilage in the growth zone. Has he looked at regenerating cartilage, perhaps after traumatism, or very early, to see if these vesicles are a sign of growth or regeneration, which might also be the explanation in osteoarthrosis, where there is often regeneration too.
Ali:	I think this is the postulate, that where cartilage is being altered, especially in the subchondral region, it is a form of regeneration. A more specific answer can be found in fracture calluses, where there is cartilage formation in the callus and matrix vesicles and apatite crystals are found in them.
Vischer:	Dr. Dieppe's experiments are very stimulating. In osteoarthrosis we got stuck with pyrophosphate, and it is something new. How much apatite did Dr. Dieppe use in the induction of his experimental lesions, and has that any relation to what can be found on the electron-micrographs.
	Secondly, he showed one cell, from a patient, with apatite inside. Where is it localized, more precisely? I did not notice it on the slide.
Dieppe:	The first point is important. We have used quantities in the order of 5 or 10 mg of the crystalline substance to produce the lesion. I do not know how much occurs in a synovial fluid, or in cartilage of osteo-arthritis. We have the same problem as Dr. Ali. We cannot really quantify how much occurs, and this is obviously important in knowing how much damage is produced by its presence.
	Intra-cellular localization of the apatite, when it is taken up by cells, seems to be mainly in mononuclear cells. Mononuclear cells, rather than polymorphs, seem to occur chiefly in these fusions in osteo-arthritis.
Vischer:	I meant in a membrane, or in a lysosome, or in a phagosome, or just free in the cytoplasm.
Dieppe:	No. It seems to be membrane bound. We have one or two pictures where we think that we have seen lysosomal discharge into that area, but they are few and far between that we have been able to recognize.
G. Haberland: (West Germany)	Is Dr. Dieppe familiar with some work done about nine years ago (Eisen of London and Spirouack of St. Louis) in which synovial inflammation was induced by inducing either urate or other crystals; by adding a proteinase inhibitor it was possible to prevent the reaction. This would mean that there is no direct action between the crystals and the macrophages, but that something happens before the macro-phages are interacted. At that time it was not known that the crystals—as has been shown by the studies with sulphated dextrans—were acting as potentiators which together with high molecular weight kininogen and kallikrein are the activators of the Hageman factor and, thus, activators of the activator system at large which in turn, via the activation of kallikrein, leads to an activation of the complement system too.

Dieppe: I am aware of that work. The surface property of the particles is critical to exactly what is happening. There has been some interesting work recently from the USA on urate and pyrophosphate crystals which produce differing effects dependent on whether they are coated with various proteins.

We have not yet investigated this, nor have we investigated the mechanism of the inflammation in much detail. All we have observed is that we get an inflammatory response with this very simple *in vivo* technique.

C. M. Pearson: I agree with the comments that these are very interesting papers.
(USA)

I have a question on chondrocalcinosis. It is clearly evident that this is an hereditary disease, in a number of instances, in various parts of the world. Has anybody looked at, for instance, enzymatic defects, increase in alkaline phosphatase, or whatever else might be going wrong in some of the individuals with these disorders?

Ali: A group in Miami has looked at pyrophosphate crystal deposition and has found that there is a depression of alkaline phosphatase activity in that type of tissue. It is important to remember that where there is a depression in alkaline phosphatase pyrophosphate crystals will form, whereas with an elevation of alkaline phosphatase the crystals will be apatite.

E. Munthe: How would Dr. Dieppe explain the often severe cases of chondro-
(Norway) calcinosis that have no sign of osteoarthritis? They can have quite heavy calcification in the cartilage, but without signs of osteoarthrosis.

Dieppe: I agree that this sometimes occurs. It has been shown from family studies that very often the precipitation of the salt comes a long time before there is any evidence of arthritis.

Obviously there are two sides to the postulate as to how these things may produce an arthritis. One is a direct effect on the cartilage, which the evidence that has been put forward would suggest may not be too important. The other is that if they escape into the synovial fluid, then there may be a reaction. Some very nice work (McCarty) has been done on this which suggests that some local influence may increase the solubility of the crystals and therefore allow them to be released out into the fluid and cause the secondary reaction. In the absence of any such factor it may be that there is not much reaction to them because they are stuck where they are formed.

18

The influence of chemical composition of plasma membranes on the functional activities of macrophages

M. DIANZANI, F. FEO, R. A. CANUTO, R. GARCEA,
L. GABRIEL AND M. V. TORRIELLI (Italy)

Cellular membranes play an important role in the inflammatory processes. Deformation, stretching, fusion, synthesis of membrane occur during endocytosis, exocytosis, interaction of cells with crystals, cell migration, etc. Previous work in this laboratory[1] has shown that liver mitochondria whose outer membrane had been enriched *in vivo* with cholesterol are less resistant to the lysis by monosodium urate (MSU) crystals. Furthermore the *in vivo* enrichment of macrophage plasma membrane with cholesterol markedly inhibits the phagocytosis of latex particles or lipid droplets[2,3].

Weissmann[4] has proposed that the pathogenesis of acute gout is initiated by the phagocytosis of MSU crystals from serum. Hydrogen binding between crystals and phagolysosome membrane is thought to induce rupture of the latter, discharge of lysosomal enzymes and cytolysis. Cholesterol-rich membranes, such as erythrocyte membranes[5], cholesterol-containing phosphatidyl choline liposomes[6] and outer mitochondrial membrane from liver of hypercholesterolaemic rats[1] are sensitive to the lytic effect of MSU crystals. It seems that the presence of cholesterol is a prerequisite for hydrogen binding between MSU crystals and liposomes to occur[6].

The above data seem to envisage the existence of close relationships between the phagocytic activity, cholesterol content of membranes and effect of MSU crystals on cellular membranes. In this paper we investigate whether *in vitro* induced modifications in cholesterol content of macrophage plasma membranes alter their phagocytic activity and the resistance to lysis by MSU crystals.

MATERIALS AND METHODS

The isolation of peritoneal macrophages from rats, phagocytosis measurements, plasma membrane isolation and purification, isolation, purification and determination of various lipid· fractions were described in previous papers[2,7,8].

Lipid dispersions

Egg phosphatidyl choline was extracted and purified according to Singleton et al.[9] and stored in chloroform at −20 °C under nitrogen. 45 mg of phospholipid (plus 25 mg of cholesterol where required) were transferred into 50 ml round-bottomed tubes. The samples were evaporated under nitrogen and least traces of solvent were removed in vacuo. 10 ml aliquots of Ringer solution (120 mM NaCl, 4.9 mM KCl, 1.7 mM $CaCl_2$, 1.2 mM $MgSO_4$, 2.7 mM KH_2PO_4, 13.3 mM Na_2HPO_4) were added to the dry films. The lipids were dispersed by vortexing the stoppered tubes for 15 min above the temperature of phase transition of the lipids. Then they were transferred into plastic tubes and subjected to ultrasonic oscillation for 10–40 min (Biosonik III sonifier, Bronwill Scientific, Inc., Rochester, at maximal output) while cooled at 0 °C and bubbled with nitrogen. The lipid dispersions were centrifuged 6 min at 134 000 × g; clear supernatants were used as source of lipid vesicles.

Removal and addition of cholesterol

A method patterned on that used by Bruckdorfer et al.[10] was followed. This method was based on the incubation of ghosts with phosphatidyl choline dispersions in order to remove the erythrocyte cholesterol. When dispersions of phosphatidyl choline plus cholesterol were used, exchange of cholesterol between lipid vesicles and cell membranes took place. Preliminary experiments with macrophages showed that incubation of these cells with phosphatidyl choline vesicles, containing equimolar amounts of cholesterol, resulted in a partial equilibration of the cholesterol content between the vesicles and macrophages. Consequently, an increase in cholesterol content of macrophage plasma membranes was observed. Freshly isolated macrophages (3 × 10^8 cells) were suspended in 20 ml of Ringer solution containing 10 mM glucose, and incubated 3 h at 37 °C with 0.375 ml of lipid dispersions per ml of suspension. At the end of incubation the cells were sedimented by centrifuging 10 min at 300 × g, washed twice and suspended in glucose-containing Ringer solution. The viability of macrophages was evaluated by determining the exclusion of the diffusion into the cytoplasm of trypan blue. It was, at this stage, 90% (viability of freshly isolated cells, 95–98%).

Incubation with monosodium urate crystals

Crystals of monosodium urate were prepared according to McCarty and Faires[11] and ground in a mortar to yield particles of 2–15 μm. In order to measure the release of enzymes, macrophages (10^8 cells) were suspended in 9.5 ml of Ringer solution. The reaction was started by addition of MSU crystals (106 mg). The incubation was carried out at 37 °C while shaking (100 strokes per min). At the times indicated, 1 ml aliquots were taken and cells and crystals were sedimented by centrifugation. Maximal enzyme release was obtained by addition of 1 mg of Triton X-100 per ml of reaction mixture.

Enzyme assays

Lactic dehydrogenase activity was determined according to Kornberg[12], beta-galactosidase according to Sellinger et al.[13].

Analytical procedures

Cyclic adenosine-3′,5′-monophosphate was determined according to 'Biochemica Test Combination' (Boehringer, Mannheim, Germany). The data were corrected for values obtained with phosphodiesterase-treated samples. A biuret method was used to determine the protein[14].

RESULTS

Lipid composition

The data in Table 18.1 show that incubation of macrophages with egg phosphatidyl choline vesicles induces a free cholesterol decrease of 1.5 times in intact macrophages and 1.4 times in macrophage plasma membranes. The incubation in the presence of cholesterol-containing vesicles results in about 1.8 and 1.6 times increases of free cholesterol in macrophages and in isolated plasma membranes, respectively. The phospholipid contents do not change in cholesterol-enriched and in cholesterol-depleted macrophages. Consequently, the cholesterol to phospholipid ratios vary directly with the cholesterol.

No variations in the relative percentages of different phospholipid classes were observed in macrophage plasma membranes after incubation with phosphatidyl choline vesicles, either in the presence or absence of cholesterol (data not reported). Some modifications of phospholipid fatty acid composition in macrophage plasma membranes were observed. As illustrated in Figure 18.1 the incubation of macrophages with lipid vesicles induces 71% and 70% decreases of myristic acid, as well as 86% and 50% decreases of

Table 18.1 Variations in the cholesterol content of macrophages and isolated plasma membranes after incubation with vesicles of phosphatidyl choline, or phosphatidyl choline *plus* cholesterol

Samples	Treatment	No. of expts.	Cholesterol (µg/mg of protein)	Phospholipid (mg/mg of protein)	Cholesterol (µg/mg of phospholipid)
Macrophages	None	3	10.72 ± 2.04	0.083 ± 0.019	129.1 ± 38.4
	PC	4	$\dagger 6.98 \pm 1.63$	0.083 ± 0.021	108.2 ± 37.5
	PC + Chol.	4	$*19.21 \pm 3.90$	0.082 ± 0.022	234.9 ± 78.9
Plasma membranes	None	6	26.52 ± 4.90	0.076 ± 0.007	348.9 ± 72.0
	PC	3	$\dagger\dagger 19.00 \pm 3.20$	0.081 ± 0.009	252.2 ± 50.9
	PC + Chol.	4	$**41.51 \pm 5.91$	0.086 ± 0.013	482.8 ± 88.7

Data are mean values $\pm$ SD. The SD of the ratio cholesterol to phospholipid (µg/mg) was calculated according to Worthing and Jeffner[27].
Differ significantly from control: $\dagger p < 0.01$
$\qquad\qquad\qquad\qquad *p < 0.001$
$\qquad\qquad\qquad\qquad \dagger\dagger p = 0.05$
$\qquad\qquad\qquad\qquad **p < 0.001$

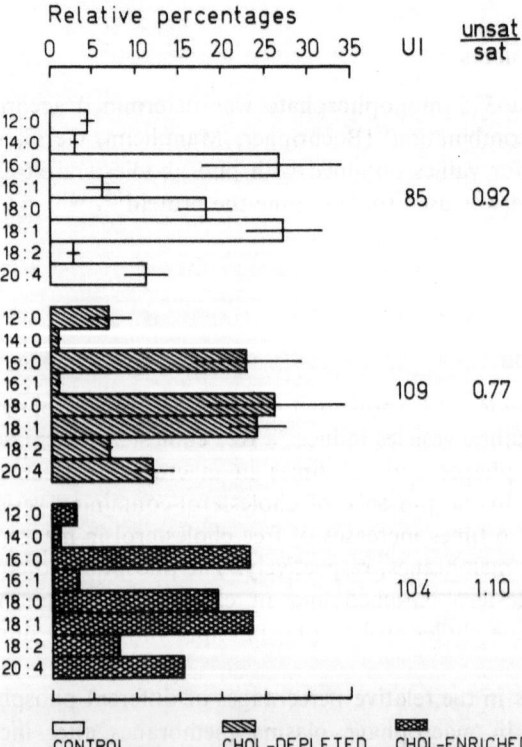

Figure 18.1 Fatty acid composition of plasma membranes isolated from normal, cholesterol-depleted and cholesterol-enriched macrophages.
The results are mean values $\pm$ SD. Number of experiments: 6 for control macrophages, 4 for cholesterol-depleted macrophages and 2 for cholesterol-enriched macrophages

palmitoleic acid, in cholesterol-depleted and cholesterol-enriched cells, respectively. This is compensated by 150% and 196% increases of linoleic acid. As a consequence, the unsaturation indexes increase 22% and 18%, respectively.

Effect of monosodium urate crystals

The data in Figure 18.2 show the time course of the discharge of lysosomal β-galactosidase (beta-GA) and cytoplasmic lactic dehydrogenase (LDH) from macrophages during incubation with MSU crystals. Control macrophages incubated with crystals release at the end of 4 h, 40% of beta-GA vs. 30% from macrophages without crystals. The released LDH is 60% vs. 40%. After 6 h the release of both enzymes increases to about 80% vs. approx. 30% and 40% for beta-GA and LDH, respectively, in macrophages without crystals. This indicates the existence of extensive cell lysis induced by MSU crystals, as it was also shown by a 40% loss in cell viability after 6 h incubation with MSU. As for cholesterol-depleted macrophages, beta-GA and

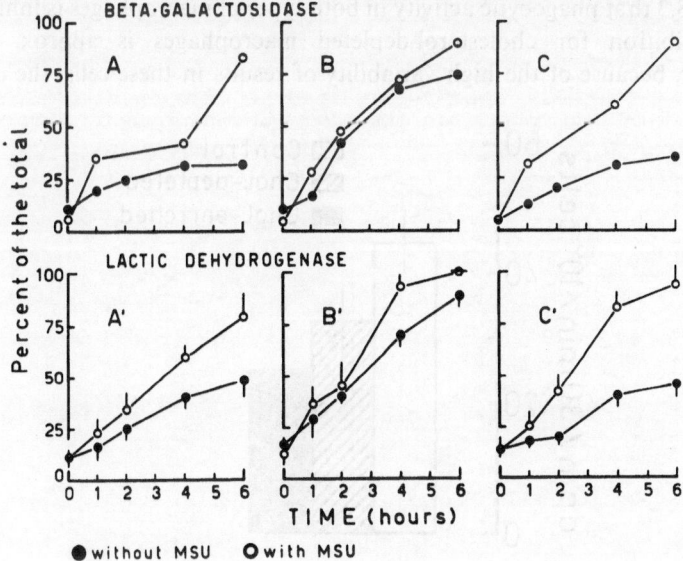

Figure 18.2 Effect of monosodium urate crystals on the time-course of the enzyme release from normal, cholesterol-depleted and cholesterol-enriched macrophages. Macrophages were submitted to 3 h incubation at 37 °C with dispersions of phosphatidyl choline or phosphatidyl choline *plus* cholesterol to obtain depletion or enrichment in cholesterol, respectively (see Materials and Methods). The addition of lipid dispersions was omitted in control macrophages. At the end of incubation, macrophages were washed several times, suspended in glucose-containing Ringer solution (10^8 cells/ml) and submitted to additional 6 h incubation in the presence of MSU crystals (11.1 mg/ml). At the times indicated, aliquots of suspensions were sedimented by centrifugation and the beta-GA and LDH activities were determined in the supernatants. The data are means of 2 and 5-11 experiments for beta-GA and LDH release, respectively. The maximal release was obtained by adding to some samples 1 mg/ml of Triton X-100. Vertical bars = SD AA' = Control; BB' = Cholesterol-depleted; CC' = cholesterol-enriched

LDH discharge is faster than in control macrophages both in the presence and absence of MSU crystals. This indicates a poor resistance of cholesterol-depleted macrophages to simple incubation even in the absence of crystals. The loss of viability in these cells was 60% after 6 h incubation with MSU. By contrast, cholesterol-enriched macrophages appear to be as resistant to incubation as control macrophages. However, the time-course of the enzyme release in the presence of MSU crystals, shows a 42% release of LDH after only 2 h incubation. After 4 h the release is 83% and is almost complete after 6 h. The discharge of beta-GA is also faster, even though to lesser extent, than that of LDH, in cholesterol-enriched macrophages compared to control macrophages.

Phagocytosis

The phagocytosis of latex particles was studied in cholesterol-depleted and in cholesterol-enriched macrophages. It appears from data reported in Figure 18.3 that phagocytic activity in both types of macrophages is inhibited. The inhibition for cholesterol-depleted macrophages is approx. 22%. However, because of the high variability of results in these cells, the degree

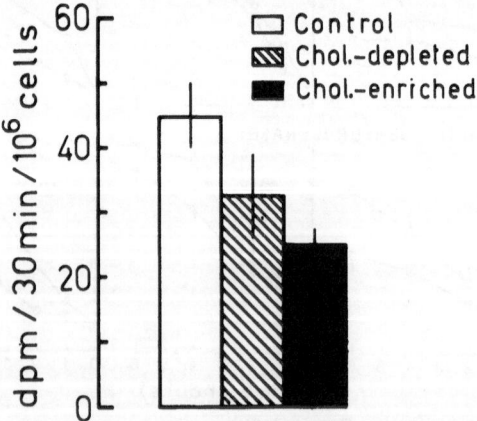

Figure 18.3 Uptake of [^{125}I]albumin during phagocytosis of polystyrene latex particles by control, cholesterol-depleted and cholesterol-enriched macrophages.

Macrophages were submitted to preliminary treatment for depletion or enrichment in membrane cholesterol (see Materials and Methods). Washed macrophages (10^8 cells) were suspended in the following reaction medium: 1.5 ml of Ringer solution, 1.5 ml of rat serum, 10 mM glucose, 45 μCi of [^{125}I]human serum albumin (Sorin Saluggia) and about 3×10^9 latex particles. Final volume, 3.2 ml. After 30 min at 37 °C, 2 ml aliquots were added to 20 ml of a medium containing 154 mM NaCl, 15 mM EDTA, 40 mM Na-fluoride and 2 mM K-cyanide. The suspensions were centrifuged and washed several times. Radio-activity was determined in the final pellets by a beta-counter. The results were corrected for radioactivity in samples to which 40 mM Na-fluoride and 2 mM K-cyanide were added. Data are means ± SD of nine experiments for control and cholesterol-depleted macrophages, and six experiments for cholesterol-enriched macrophages

of significance is low ($P = 0.1$). By contrast, for cholesterol-enriched macrophages a 45 % decrease of phagocytic activity was detected. The difference between cholesterol-enriched and control macrophages was highly significant ($P < 0.001$).

Cyclic AMP content

cAMP was shown to inhibit phagocytosis and lysosomal enzyme release from polymorphonuclear phagocytes[15]. It alters intracellular distribution of microtubules[16]. These structures are essential for phagolysosome formation in mononuclear phagocytes[17]. On the other hand, the lipid composition of membranes was observed to modulate the activity of adenyl cyclase of turkey erythrocytes[18]. These observations prompted us to investigate whether variation in cAMP content occurs in macrophages with altered membrane cholesterol content. It was observed that the cAMP produced by resting or phagocytizing macrophages was the same in the control as in cholesterol-depleted or cholesterol-enriched cells.

CONCLUSIONS

The results in this paper indicate that modification in the cholesterol to phospholipid ratio of macrophage plasma membranes induces changes in their resistance to the lytic action of MSU crystals. Moreover, it has been possible to inhibit phagocytosis by increasing the cholesterol content of the membranes. This agrees with our previous observation that phagocytic activity is largely inhibited in macrophages enriched *in vivo* with cholesterol[2,3]. However, a slight inhibition of particle endocytosis is probably present in cholesterol-depleted macrophages. An inhibition of endocytosis has also been described by Heiniger *et al.*[19] in mouse fibroblasts cultured *in vitro* in the presence of cholesterol synthesis inhibitors.

Our preparations of cholesterol-enriched and cholesterol-depleted macrophages show modifications of only phospholipid fatty acids which are present in low relative percentages in macrophage plasma membranes. This results in a rise of the unsaturation index. These modifications probably depend on some exchange between the phosphatidyl choline of plasma membrane and the highly unsaturated phosphatidyl choline from egg. The cholesterol content influences the physical state of artificial[20] and natural[21-23] membranes. The incorporation of cholesterol among phospholipid molecules containing unsaturated paraffin chains causes lipid to be less fluid[24] and increases total hydrophobic interactions, thus giving greater cohesion to membranes. As a consequence, the membranes of cholesterol-enriched macrophages should be more resistant to the deformation and stretching which occur in plasma membranes during phagocytosis. According to recent evidence mitochondrial membranes with increased cholesterol content, but without changes in the phospholipid fatty acids, lose their elasticity and are less prone to deformation[23,25]. The cholesterol effect on phagocytosis could also be due to a reduction of membrane fusion secondary to the enrichment of membranes with cholesterol. The fusion of artificial membranes with a high cholesterol content, was found to be diminished[26].

If the above interpretations are correct, we should expect increased membrane fluidity in cholesterol-depleted macrophages. Therefore, the decrease of the phagocytic activity in these cells cannot be explained through the existence of high membrane rigidity. Under these circumstances, the hypothesis could be advanced that normal cholesterol content of membranes, by providing the optimal physical state, is an important prerequisite for endocytic processes to occur (see also Reference 19).

Weissmann[4] suggested a model for the lysis of polymorphonuclear phagocytes by MSU crystals. MSU crystals covered by films of plasma proteins cannot adhere to the outer surface of circulating phagocytes. Once the phagolysosomes are formed, the dehydration and digestion of plasma protein by lysosomal enzymes enables the crystal to become directly apposed to the inner surface of the phagolysosomal membranes. Hydrogen binding between crystal and polar moieties of phospholipid molecules is thus possible. This is followed by rupture of the membrane and cytolysis due to liberation of lysosomal enzymes (Figure 18.4A). In our experimental system MSU crystals are not covered by serum proteins; direct apposition to the outer surface of the plasma membrane is possible. The apposition should be enhanced with cholesterol-enriched cells whose membranes are more rigid. This should be followed by the rupture of membrane and discharge of cytoplasmic enzymes (Figure 18.4B). However, the release of certain amounts of lysosomal enzymes could occur through the mechanism of Figure 18.4C. According to this model, the fusion of lysosome to phagocytic vacuole could

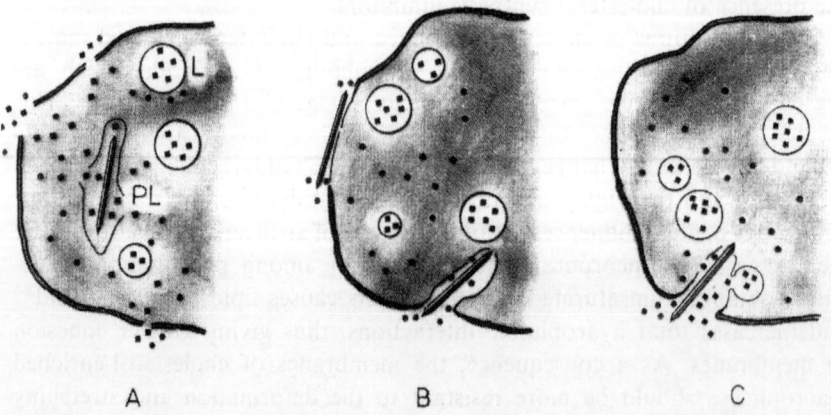

Figure 18.4 Postulated mechanism of enzyme release from macrophages in the presence of MSU crystals (explanation in the text)

preceed, in some instances, the fusion of plasma membrane. Consequently, lysosomal enzyme discharge occurs. It could be associated with the release of cytoplasmic enzymes if MSU crystals induce the rupture of phagolysosome membrane. The incubation of cholesterol-enriched macrophages with MSU crystals induced faster release of both beta-GA and LDH than in control macrophages. However, when the time-course of beta-GA discharge was compared to that of LDH, it appeared that the former enzyme was released slower than the latter. This behaviour could indicate plasma membrane rupture, in cholesterol-enriched macrophages, precedes the cytolysis induced by the discharge of lysosomal enzymes, probably due to partial inhibition of phagocytosis. A few MSU crystals, taken up by membrane areas of cholesterol-enriched macrophages having low cholesterol to phospholipid ratio (see Reference 8), could be responsible for cytolysis by the mechanism outlined by Weissmann[4], as well as by the mechanism reported in Figure 18.4C.

Whatever the mechanism of MSU-induced enzyme release, our data stress the importance of the cholesterol content of membranes and support the Weissmann hypothesis[4] on the mechanism of action of MSU crystals on artificial and natural membranes.

SUMMARY

Incubation of rat peritoneal macrophages with phosphatidyl choline vesicles induced a 1.4 times decrease in the cholesterol to phospholipid ratio of plasma membranes. If macrophages were incubated with cholesterol-containing vesicles of phosphatidyl choline (molar ratio 1:1) cholesterol content was almost doubled. These changes were associated with minor modifications in the phospholipid fatty acids percentages, without changes in the relative amounts of different phospholipids. Cholesterol-depleted macrophages became highly fragile and underwent lysis during incubation, irrespective of the presence or absence of MSU crystals. Cholesterol-enriched macrophages were as resistant as control macrophages to the incubation but showed higher sensitivity to the lysis by MSU crystals than the control. Cholesterol-enriched macrophages showed a 45% inhibition of latex particles phagocytosis. A less marked inhibition of phagocytosis was found in cholesterol-depleted macrophages. No variations in the cAMP content occurred in macrophages as a consequence of altered plasma membrane cholesterol content.

Acknowledgement

This work was supported by a grant from 'Consiglio Nazionale delle Ricerche' of Italy.

References

1. Dianzani, M. U., Feo, F., Rita, G. A. and Zuretti, F. M. (1974). The role of cholesterol in biological membranes. In *Future Trends in Inflammation* (G. P. Velo, D. A. Willoughby and J. P. Giroud, eds.) pp. 385–404. (Brescia: Piccin Medical Books)
2. Feo, F., Canuto, R. A., Torrielli, M. V., Garcea, R. and Dianzani, M. U. (1975). Effect of a cholesterol rich diet on cholesterol content and phagocytic activity of rat macrophages. In: *Future Trends in Inflammation*, II (J. P. Giroud, D. A. Willoughby and G. P. Velo, eds.) pp. 135–142. (Basel: Birkhauser Verlag)
3. Dianzani, M. U., Torrielli, M. V., Canuto, R. A., Garcea, R. and Feo, F. (1976). The influence of enrichment with cholesterol on the phagocytic activity of rat macrophages. *J. Pathol.*, **118**, 193
4. Weissmann, G. (1975). The molecular basis of acute gout. In *Cell Membranes, Biochemistry, Cell Biology and Pathology* (G. Weissmann and R. Claiborne eds.) pp. 257–266. (New York: HP Publishing Co., Inc.)
5. Wallingford, W. R. and McCarty, D. J. (1966). Differential membranolytic effects of microcrystalline sodium urate and calcium pyrophosphate dihydrate. *J. Exp. Med.*, **133**, 100
6. Weissmann, G. and Rita, G. E. (1972). Molecular basis of gouty inflammation: interaction of monosodium urate crystals with lysosomes and lyposomes. *Nature New Biol.*, **240**, 167
7. Feo, F., Canuto, R. A., Bertone, G., Garcea, R. and Pani, P. (1973). Cholesterol and phospholipid composition of mitochondria and microsomes isolated from Donis Hepatoma 5123 and rat liver. *FEBS Letters*, **33**, 229
8. Gravela, E., Feo, F., Canuto, R. A., Garcea, R. and Gabriel, L. (1975). Functional and structural alterations of liver ergastoplasmic membranes during DL-ethionina hepatocarcinogenesis. *Cancer Res.*, **35**, 3041
9. Singleton, W. S., Gray, M. S., Brown, M. L. and White, J. L. (1965). Chromatographically homogeneous lecithin from egg phospholipids. *J. Amer. Oil Chem. Soc.*, **42**, 53
10. Bruckdorfer, K. R., Edwards, P. A. and Green, C. (1968). Properties of aqueous dispersions of phospholipid and cholesterol. *Eur. J. Biochem.*, **4**, 506
11. McCarty, D. J. and Faires, J. S. (1963). A comparison of the duration of local antiinflammatory effect of several adrenocorticosteroid esters—a biossay technique. *Curr. Ther. Res.*, **5**, 284
12. Kornberg, A. (1955). Lactic dehydrogenase of muscle. *Methods in Enzymology*. **1**, 441
13. Sellinger, Z., Beaufay, H., Jaques, P., Doyen, A. and De Duve, C. D. (1960). Tissue fractionation studies. Intracellular distribution and properties of beta-N-acetylglucosaminidase in rat liver. *Biochem. J.*, **74**, 450
14. Gornall, A. G., Bardawill, C. J. and David, M. (1949). Determination of serum proteins by means of biuret reaction. *J. Biol. Chem.*, **177**, 751
15. Ignarro, L. J. and Cech, S. Y. (1976). Bidirectional regulation of lysosomal enzyme secretion and phagocytosis in human neutrophils by guanosine 3′5′-monophosphate and adenosine 3′5′Monophosphate[1] (39232). *Proc. Soc. Exp. Biol. Med.*, **151**, 448
16. Willingham, M. C. and Pastan, I. (1975). Cyclic AMP and cell morphology in cultured fibroblasts. *J. Cell. Biol.*, **67**, 146
17. Pesanti, E. L. and Axline, S. G. (1975). Phagolysosome formation in normal and colchicine-treated macrophages. *J. Exp. Med.*, **142**, 903
18. Orly, J. and Schramm, M. (1975). Fatty acids as modulators of membrane functions: Catecholamine-activated ademplate cyclase of the turkey erythrocyte. *Proc. Nat. Acad. Sci. USA*, **72**, 3433
19. Heiniger, H. S., Kandutsch, A. A. and Chen, H. W. L. (1976). Depletion of L-cell sterol depresses endocytosis. Nature, **263**, 515
20. Chapman, D. (1973). Some recent studies of lipid, lipid-Cholesterol and membrane system. In: *Biological Membranes* (D. Chapman and D. H. F. Wallach eds.) vol. 2, pp. 91–144 (New York: Academic Press)
21. Kroes, J. and Ostwald, R. (1971). Erythrocyte membranes—effect of increased cholesterol content on permeability. *Biochim. Biophys. Acta*, **249**, 647

22. Poznansky, M., Kikwood, D. and Solomon, A. K. (1973). Modulation of red cell K$^+$ transport by membrane lipids. *Biochim. Biophys. Acta*, **330,** 351

23. Feo, F., Canuto, R. A., Garcea, R. and Gabriel, L. (1975). Effect of cholesterol content on some physical and functional properties of mitochondria isolated from adult rat liver, fetal liver, cholesterol-enriched liver and hepatomas AH-130 3924 A and 5123. *Biochem. Biophys. Acta.*, **413,** 116

24. Phillips, M. C. (1972). The physical state of phospholipids and cholesterol in monolayers, bilayers and membranes. In: *Progress in Surface and Membranes Sciences* (J. F. Danielli, M. D. Rosemberg and D. A. Cadenhead, eds.) pp. 139–221. (New York: Academic Press)

25. Feo, F., Canuto, R. A., Garcea, R., and Gabriel, L. (1976). The influence of lipid composition on some physical and functional properties of cellular membranes in rat liver and hepatomas. In: *Recent Advances in Biochemical Pathology. Toxic Liver Injury.* (M. U. Dianzani, G. Ugazio and L. M. Sena, eds.) pp. 171–188. Minerva Medica.

26. Papahadjopoulos, D., Poste, G., Schaeffer, B. E. and Vail, W. J. (1974). Membrane fusion and molecular segregation in phospholipid vesicles. *Biochim. Biophys. Acta*, **352,** 10

27. Worthing, A. C. and Jeffner, J. (1943). *Treatment of Experimental Data* pp. 207–230. (New York: Wiley)

Discussion 18

I. Ginsburg: (Israel)	Professor Dianzani described an interesting experiment in which the content of certain lipids was artificially elevated. Has he looked at animals with different ratios of lipids in the membranes. Rumen, for example, seem to have very little cholesterol but very high sphingo-myelin. Mouse cells seem to have a lot of cholesterol. They say that camels have a lot of different lipids in the membrane. It would be interesting to compare leukocytes from various animal species with naturally occurring odd lipids in the membranes and their responses to the crystals.
Dianzani:	It is a good idea. We have not studied mice. It might be a good idea to do comparative studies of various animals.
P. C. Wilkinson: (UK)	May I add a corollary. The blood neutrophil in the human is said to have a higher cholesterol:phospholipid ratio than the monocyte or macrophage. Nevertheless, the neutrophil is a pretty good phagocyte, and I am not sure that the simple ratios are quite the answer to the efficiency of phagocytes. I am sure that there are many mysteries in the micro-organization of the cell membrane of which we have no know-ledge.
Dianzani:	There is not a complete inhibition. Of course it is only an hypothesis. The content of cholesterol in the membranes cannot be increased above a certain level nor can more than a certain amount of cholesterol be added to artificial membranes, since too high an amount will produce labilization of the membranes. I do not know what would happen if the cholesterol content of membranes could be increased in some way. I do not think that the phagocytosis could be stopped completely. There would be an increase in rigidity and a decrease in the fluidity of the membranes.
Wilkinson:	There is a really interesting phenomenon here. The surface chemists tell us that the interaction of proteins with pure lecithin mono-layers is very different from the interaction of a protein with a mixed cholesterol/lecithin monolayer. The business of ratios of lipids in cell membranes and phagocytosis and other phenomena is both important and interesting.

Opening to Discussion—

Mechanisms in chronic inflammation

A. CATS (Netherlands)

About a decade ago we were only able to distinguish between the various rheumatic syndromes on the basis of their clinical signs and symptoms and a few laboratory parameters. Since then, new laboratory tests have been developed by which the presence of urate crystals, IgM anti-IgG anti-globulins, and anti-nuclear factors can be demonstrated more easily. These developments marked the beginning of a new era, in which we learned more about the pathogenetic mechanisms to which the various signs and symptoms of these diseases can be attributed.

In this afternoon session a number of new data were presented. Dr. Deporter presented a very interesting paper, in which he discussed the role of cyclic nucleotides in the control of leukocyte lysosomal enzyme release, but because chronic inflammatory mechanisms are the subject of this afternoon one may ask whether in chronic inflammation the same mechanisms are involved. I will focus on rheumatic disorders, because they have been studied in detail with respect to chronic inflammation.

Immune and non-immune irritants seem to be important for the development of a chronic inflammation. These irritating agents might originate either from the host himself or from his environment. In auto-immune processes host antigens cause an altered reaction, because they are not recognized as 'self'. Otherwise chronic inflammation might be due to the persistence of foreign antigens either as a result of insufficient catabolism of these antigens or of an abundant supply. Non-immunogenic agents might be derived from a metabolic product, such as urates, or be acquired from the environment, as is the case, for instance, for silica crystals. Many years ago it was already recognized that of all the patients infected with group A streptococci, only a small number developed rheumatic fever or scarlet fever or nephritis.

These observations draw the attention to the importance of host factors in addition to environmental irritating agents. From experimental studies we know how the induction of a chronic inflammation can differ in various strains and from animal to animal[1,2].

Recent data on the histocompatibility antigens until now not mentioned in this symposium throw some new light on the significance of host factors[3]. Histocompatibility antigens are now associated with a number of rheumatic inflammatory diseases (Table 1).

Table 1 Disease associated with histocompatibility antigens

Ankylosing spondylitis ⎫ Morbus reiter ⎬ B27 Yersinia arthritis ⎭	
Rheumatoid arthritis	Dw4
SLE	A1; A8
Psoriasis	B13; B17

Even in ankylosing spondylitis there is not a complete association between the disease and a histocompatibility antigen. This might indicate that HLA-B27 is not involved directly in the pathogenesis, but that this gene is possibly only a marker for an immune response gene, that is localized in the close vicinity of the locus coding for HLA-B27. There is increasing evidence from HLA studies that the development of a chronic inflammation is influenced by genetically determined factors. This means that besides persisting irritants, genetical factors are probably also involved in chronic inflammation.

Serum sickness is one of the best-studied models in animals[4] as well as in man[5], in both of which an immunogen might induce tissue lesions.

The migratory polyarthritis found in rheumatic fever has been compared with the same phenomenon observed in the serum-sickness model. Recently, Whittle and co-workers[6] investigated the presence of meningococcal antigen in the serum, cerebrospinal, and synovial fluid of patients with group A meningococcal infections. The amount of serum antigen was found to decrease as haemagglutinating antibodies increased in the serum. When arthritis and vasculitis developed in their patients, they were able to demonstrate the presence of the meningococcal antigen, immunoglobulins and complement at the site of the lesions by using immunofluorescent techniques.

It is generally accepted that in systemic lupus erythematosus a pathogenetical mechanism similar to that of serum sickness is involved. In SLE, activity of the disease has been reported to be related to the presence of high levels of anti-ds DNA antibodies and low complement levels in the serum, but the reverse has also been shown. Swaak[7] found that exacerbations of the clinical symptoms in SLE occurred when the anti-ds DNA antibody level in the patient's serum dropped. It was suggested by Hughes[8] that release of DNA is a relatively common phenomenon in man. The release of this antigen in SLE patients with circulating anti-ds DNA antibodies may provide an opportunity for immune complex formation.

Immune complexes have been identified by several techniques in patients suffering from various chronic inflammatory diseases. It is not yet certain, however, whether these techniques really measure antigen–antibody complexes, or only demonstrate the presence of protein aggregates. Nevertheless there is enough evidence from experimental work to make it certain that immune complexes are active in clinical manifestations of these diseases. The question arises, however, what features the complexes must possess to become pathogenic for the individual. It seems that at least the size, ratio-antigen–antibody, avidity (binding energy) and solubility of these complexes are important factors for their becoming pathogenic. Precipitating antibodies that combine with antigens to form large insoluble complexes are rapidly cleared from the circulation by the reticuloendothelial system. Non-precipitating antibodies exhibit slower clearance of antigen; they form soluble complexes which are deposited in blood vessels and the kidneys. The question also arises why, in contrast to such diseases as serum sickness, neisseria vasculitis, and arthritis, the inflammatory process shows a chronic course in a great many other diseases. It is obvious that a chronic inflammation needs a persisting stimulus. There seem to be two main sources for such a continuous stimulation. Firstly it might be that there is a continuous supply of new antigen. We can only speculate on how virus probably acts, but it seems that, for example in SLE, drugs might be able to render cell-constituents immunogenic. *Secondly*, Cooke, and co-workers[9] have postulated on the basis of experimental work that trapping of immune complexes in avascular collagenous joint structures, including cartilage and menisci, may be of pathogenetic importance. If altered IgG is retained in these avascular structures, it may act as a continuous stimulus for a local immune response in the synovium.

The immune complex deposits or a continuous production of immune complexes could be the most important stimulus for the maintenance of a chronic inflammation. *Furthermore*, chronic inflammation is histologically characterized by signs of delayed hypersensitivity. Since delayed hypersensitivity is mainly mediated by T-cells, it has been suggested that a functional defect of T-cells or a defect localized in a sub-population of these lymphocytes might be present, although the precise function of T-cells in chronic inflammation is unclear.

In a recent study we were able to demonstrate that T-cells—probably reactive ones, as judged from their morphology—are present between plasma-cell-rich areas and lymphocytic aggregates in the rheumatoid synovium[10]. This suggests that T-cells interact locally with the B-cell system and probably modulate the antibody response. A possible role for T-cells in the rheumatoid joint inflammation has also been suggested by recent clinical studies on the effect of thoracic-duct drainage in rheumatoid patients[11].

Thoracic-duct lymphocytes are predominantly T-lymphocytes, and Edgren and Wegelius[12] have shown that clinical improvement is associated with reduction of the number of peripheral-blood T-lymphocytes. These findings, and the fact that B-lymphocyte parameters do not change essentially in these patients during this treatment, suggest that T-lymphocyte depletion may be responsible for the beneficial clinical effect of this procedure.

Finally, as has been nicely shown by Dr. Davies, Schorlemmer and Dianzani this afternoon, various types of cells, such as macrophages, lymphocytes, and granulocytes, can generate and activate different mediators, which in their turn produce the features of a chronic inflammation.

As you can see from this summary, many questions still need to be answered before we can understand the mechanisms which are responsible for chronic inflammation.

References

1. Kaplan, M. H. and Svec, K. H. (1964). Immunologic relation of streptococcal and tissue antigens. Presence in human sera of streptococcal antibody cross reaction with heart tissue. *J. Exp. Med.*, **119**, 651
2. Beachey, E. H., Alberti, H. and Stollerman, G. H. (1969). Delayed hypersensitivity in purified streptococcal M protein in guinea pigs and in man. *J. Immunol.*, **102**, 42
3. Dausset, J., Degos, J. and Horst, J. (1974). The association of the HL-A antigens with diseases. *Clin. Immunol. Immunopathol.*, **3**, 127
4. Dixon, F. M. (1971). The immunopathology of glomerulonephritis. In: *Immunological Diseases* (M. Samter, ed.) Vol. 2, 2nd edn. (Boston: Little Brown and Co.)
5. Seegal, B. (1952). Antigen-antibody reaction. Combined Staff Clinic. ed. G. H. Mudge, *Am. J. Med.*, **13**, 352
6. Whittle, H. C., Greenwood, B. M., Davidson, N., Tomkins, A. *et al.* (1975). Meningococcal antigen in diagnosis and treatment of group A meningococcal infections. *Am. J. Med.*, **58**, 823
7. Swaak, A. J. G., Arden, L. A., Lakmaker, F., de Groot, E. R. and Feltkamp, T. E. (1976). Significance of anti-ds DNA profiles. Annual Meeting of the Heberden Society, London, November 1976.
8. Hughes, Graham, R. V., Cohen, S. A., Lightfoot Jr., R. W., Meltzer, J. S. and Christian, Ch. L. (1971). The release of DNA into serum and synovial fluid. *Arthritis and Rheum.*, **14**, 259
9. Cooke, T. D. V., Richer, S., Hurd, E. and Jasin, H. E. (1975). Localization of antigen-antibody complexes in intra-articular collagenous tissues. *Ann. N.Y. Acad. Sci.*, **256**, 10
10. de Vries, E., van Leeuwen, A. W. F. M., van de Putte, L. B. A., Lafeber, G. J. M. and Meijer, C. J. L. M. (1977). Atypical T cells in rheumatoid synovial membranes. Accepted for publication in *Virchow's Arch., Abt. B, Cell Pathol.*, **24**, 19
11. Pearson, C. M., Paulus, M. E. and Machleder, H. I. (1975). The role of the lymphocyte and its products in the propagation of joint disease. *Ann. N.Y. Acad. Sci.*, **256**, 150
12. Edgren, J., Klockars, M., Weber, T., Wangel, A., Lindstrom B., Stenstrang, K., Peterson, T., Riska, H., Kajander, A. and Wegelius, O. (1976). Extracorporal irradiation of the thoracic duct lymph as immunosuppressive treatment of rheumatoid arthritis. *Scan. J. Rheumatol.*, **5**, 108
13. Goldberg, M. A., Arnett, F. C., Bias, W. B. and Schulman, E. (1976). Histocompatibility antigens in systemic lupus erythematosus. *Arthritis and Rheum.*, **19**, 129

General Discussion

Chairman: L. E. Glynn

Chairman:	This afternoon's papers seemed to fall into two groups: those dealing with activation of macrophages and the others dealing with crystals and their significance, and they are also indirectly associated with release of enzymes from macrophages.
I. Ginsburg: (Israel)	My question is addressed to Dr. Davies. When one screens the literature on the factors which bring about activation of macrophages they can probably be divided into two groups: those which act from within and those which work from without. We know that we can stimulate membranes by antigen–antibody complexes and get release of enzymes. We can get release of enzymes because of phagocytosis of various particles, inert particles, streptococcal walls, carrageenan, and other materials which are taken up by macrophages.

Is there competition between two agents? Suppose that a macrophage is engaged with two stimuli, one from within and one from without. Would it prefer the inside or the outside? Are there synergistic effects? Is there inhibition because the macrophage is not angry, but frustrated?

Secondly, has Dr. Davies looked at the possibility that macrophages that have eaten up any kind of noxious material will either enhance their migration towards the chemotactic factor, ignore it, or be inhibited. I am very much intrigued by the question of whether macrophages, which took up microbial cell wall components, can still really move towards the stimulus of the chemotactic factor and whether the translocation experiments, which were described many years ago, were true, or merely an accidental laboratory curiosity. |
| **P. Davies:** (USA) | To answer the second question first, as to whether a macrophage which has encountered one of these noxious stimuli, which triggers the synthesis and secretion of one or more of these mediators. From the work that we did at the Clinical Research Centre, we have some evidence that if a macrophage engulfs a particle (the particle studied was the Group A streptococcal walls, and this work was done with J. Ferluga and has not been published), we found that cells either fed the particle, or, on the other hand, macrophages to which the supernatants from other cells which had been fed the Group A streptococcal cell wall, had their movement slowed down.

The reason for this was unclear to us at this time, but one could speculate that the enzymes that were being released, especially the proteinases, might be doing something to the membrane and slowing the rate of migration of the macrophage. Professor Vischer has some rather interesting data relevant to this point.

As to the question of competition from within—what something from within does to further encounters of the cell with another |

255

stimulus from the outside—I have very little information on this in relation to acid hydrolases or to the prostaglandins, although there is some interesting information in this area in relation to neutral proteinases. This came up in an earlier discussion. If macrophages are taken from mice which have been stimulated *in vivo* with endotoxin, and they are then given *in vitro* a non-digestible particle in the form of a latex particle, which we showed today not to be inflammatory, then in this way the storage of this inert particle within the lysosomal system will enhance the secretion of the neutral proteinases, which almost certainly are generated from another cellular compartment. Their transport from the endoplasmic reticulum, where they are synthesized, to the outside of the cell almost certainly is not via a lysosomal route, but simply the fact that something is stored within the lysosomes is sufficient to enhance the secretion of these neutral proteinases.

That is about as much as I can say.

T. L. Vischer:
(Switzerland)

I want to confirm that exposure of macrophages to proteases of any kind inhibits their migration, at least *in vitro*.

Do activated macrophages, i.e. macrophages that do something—either secrete proteinases or release lysosomal hydrolases—do they get turned off? Do they have to die to be turned off, or can they stop these processes? I have seen beautiful slides of streptococcal products inside the cells and Dr. Ginsburg has implied that these macrophages were still secreting something. Had he any evidence for that, and is there any mechanism for turning off macrophages? That would be useful.

Davies:

That is an extremely relevant question and one that we have thought about.

What Professor Vischer suggests should be so, simply for the reason that macrophages are present at sites of chronic inflammation not only during initiation of this process but also during its evolution and during its revolution. In my summary slide I showed that they secrete acid hydrolases and that they secrete prostaglandins, but this seems to occur on rather an acute basis in terms of the macrophage's lifespan. It is something that occurs quickly. For example, with most of the acid hydrolase phenomena, most of the release seems to occur within 24–48 h of the addition of the stimulus, and in certain instances the sensitivity of the macrophage to release acid hydrolases from lysosomes, or prostaglandins seems to diminish with the state of the stimulation of the cell. In other words, when the cell has seen the inflammatory stimulus for an extended period of time, its capacity to secrete these two types of mediator diminishes.

On the other hand, it is very clear from the studies both *in vivo* and *in vitro* that the secretion of neutral proteinases is a much more long-term affair. This makes a lot of sense. Some of the degradation that one sees in a process of chronic inflammation must surely be to the benefit of the host. As well as gross destruction there has to be remodelling, so it makes a lot of sense that a macrophage should secrete things like plasminogen-activator to get rid of fibrin, for example; to secrete collagenase, which we know is laid down and then removed during the exquisite process of tissue remodelling that takes place.

Finally, we know now (from the work of Leibovitch and Ross, and also Richards) that macrophages make factors which turn on fibroblasts not only to divide, but also to secrete collagen. It would seem to me that it would be very worthwhile to study the phase of activation—in other words, how does a non-stimulated macrophage, or how does a stimulated macrophage behave in terms of making these factors which affect fibroblast behaviour. Obviously the fibroblast will have the last word in terms of laying down new connective tissue components which help to resolve any inflammatory process.

I think that Professor Vischer's idea is an excellent one.

Ginsburg: I believe that it is very difficult to measure secretion of the lysosomal enzymes by macrophages *in vivo* because the burden of proof will lie in determining whether it came from the macrophage or from the polymorph. If materials could be found which are selectively secreted by one and not by the other, then maybe the answer would be in the affirmative. I might pinpoint one material: cationic proteins. We know that cationic proteins are probably exclusively present in granulocytes —exclusively may be too firm a word—but cationic proteins cannot be found in macrophages so that it is possible that by taking this measure, the release of cationic proteins, we shall be able to say whether the something which came off the cell is from the macrophage or from the polymorph.

I am not one hundred per cent sure that the macrophages which are obtained from the joints or from the muscle, or from livers with granulomas, really continue to secrete. Morphologically they have projections and they look quite well. Under electron microscopy it is very difficult to see other changes (i.e. metabolic changes), unless some immuno-chemical techniques to localize enzymes are used.

This brings me to another important factor that has probably been touched upon only marginally. In most experiments in the lab it is much easier to use a buffer because it is easy to obtain, it is cheap, it does not increase the protein content, and where whole serum or whole synovial fluids are used as the medium, the medium gets contaminated with so many enzymes that any marginal release of enzyme from cells would not be picked up.

I should like to raise a general question. I raised the same question two years ago in Paris and I did not get any good answers. It may be that I should have produced the answer before coming here!

Is it true that all the systems on which we are working—chemotaxis, release of lysosomal enzymes—are effective in 100% serum or 100% exudate? Exudate contains so many inhibitors of proteases, so many cationic materials that can hook on, recept, or negatively charge receptors, that it may be that some of the activities may not be generated when 100% serum or 100% synovial fluids are used.

I believe that the problem pertains to prostaglandins too. What is the half-life of prostaglandin in a tissue? Can prostaglandins be incriminated as being mediators of chronic inflammation, or only in the acute phases of inflammation? Do prostaglandins function in the presence of a thick soup of a pus or an exudate?

I raise these questions because we have recently done some experiments similar to Professor Vischer's on lymphocytes and on pus. If peripheral blood lymphocytes are stimulated with PHA, or with a variety of other mitogens, uptake of thymidine will result to a certain extent. However, when lymphocytes are pre-treated with pus obtained from a dental abscess, a staphylococcal abscess, and the cells are washed, then the results are entirely different. If histones are put on to lymphocytes which have been acted upon by what seem to be neutral proteases of leukocytes, then the response to PHA can be completely modified. Things are very complicated in tissues, which is why I believe that some of our models should be transferred to 100% exudates of various sorts. And even that is not sufficient.

P. C. Wilkinson: I do not know what Dr. Ginsburg means by '100% exudate'. This
(UK) seems to be a very non-quantitative thing to estimate in terms of percentages.

The other thing about serum is, that, generally speaking, I do not know about all the assays but in assays of cell locomotion 100%

serum is usually rather inhibitory to locomotion; certainly to stimulated locomotion. The cells move better in dilutions like 10 or 20%. On the other hand, if one considers where they are moving *in vivo*, they are not actually moving in the bloodstream. They are moving out in the tissues around the bloodstream, which presumably are not 100% serum anyway.

One thing which is very important for cell locomotion and which has not been emphasized is the importance of serum albumin itself as a protein. One can get quite nice dose responses showing that serum albumin will increase the rate of locomotion of phagocytic cells and lymphocytes in a dose-dependent manner at doses of around 500 μg, 1 or 2 mg/ml. So the serum albumin in the medium is very important, I think, for reasons that we do not understand, for locomotion of cells.

I do not wish to comment on any other functions because I do not really know about them.

T. L. Vischer:
(Switzerland)

I think it is possible to get protease activity. We have about 20% in highly inflammatory synovial fluids; free protease activity digesting caseine, and not just some artificial substrate.

It is the wrong question. In tissues the cells interact very closely, not as they do in tissue culture and in artificial systems, but there is the structure of the vessels, the collagen, the connective tissue and everything, and cells sitting there. We might get very short-range interactions which might imitate a little, or approach in some way, *in vitro* situations.

Davies:

I would agree with that. We have to consider situations where there are cell-to-cell interactions. Quite clearly we now know that induction of certain phases of immune responses, for example, involves the intimate contact of one cell with another. Under those circumstances serum probably does not play a very important role.

On the other hand, in other situations I would agree with Dr. Ginsburg.

There is one pathological fluid which is readily available to most of us—rheumatoid synovial fluid. It is a nice distillate of the secretory products of a chronic inflammatory response, and there are many interesting questions that can be asked with this kind of fluid in many of the systems being studied *in vitro*.

Chairman's Summing-up and Future Trends

L. E. GLYNN (UK)

The questions posed by this afternoon's session may be summed up in a single question. Why does an inflammatory reaction sometimes fail to subside? The same question can also be put in reverse. Why do inflammatory reactions ever subside?

The commonest or at least the most easily understood cause of a persistent inflammation is the persistence of a living causative agent. Such persistence can be either local, e.g. tubercle bacilli in any local form of tuberculosis, or at a distance from which organisms are continually fed into the lesion in question. This latter was the basis of the hypothesis of focal infection, now largely discarded, but partly resurrected by the observations of Ginsburg on the transportation of organisms from the rabbit tonsil to sites of experiment injury in the heart.

The continuing survival of organisms in an inflammatory focus implies failure of those defensive mechanisms normally responsible for their elimination. Such failure can be either genetically determined as for example in the DiGeorge or Wiskott–Aldrich syndromes or acquired as in the adult form of primary agammaglobulinaemia. Alternatively a living agent can survive despite the unimpaired efficacy of the host's defences, because it has entered a protected environment, i.e. one into which the defensive agents of the host have difficulty in penetrating. Typical examples are gummata tuberculomata and chronic abscesses in general, and moreover the longer the lesion persists the more resistant it becomes, in part at least by virtue of the thickening fibrous wall by which it is encircled. With virus infections the problem of inaccessibility reaches its zenith with the incorporation of viral DNA within the actual genome of host cells.

Chronicity of inflammation owing to the persistence of the aetiological agent is by no means confined to living agents. The cell walls of dead micro-organisms, especially β haemolytic streptococci can be remarkably resistant to the enzymes made available for their destruction. Their retention within

259

macrophages leads to release of lysosomal enzymes, as shown by Allison and his associates, and these enzymes then account for the continuing local tissue injury. It is not only the enzyme resistant residues of micro-organisms that can act in this way. The chronic inflammations of gout, pseudo gout and silicosis are undoubtedly similarly mediated but characterized by even greater chronicity by virtue of the almost absolute resistance of the foreign materials to enzymatic destruction and their consequent recycling through phagocytic cells.

An extremely important cause of non resolution of an inflammatory lesion, more familiar to surgeons than to immunopathologists, is inadequate drainage. This results in the local accumulation of necrotic and exuded material which must be removed before the mechanisms of repair can be adequately involved. Such accumulations of necrotic and exuded material encourage the maintenance of the inflammatory state in two ways: firstly the materials themselves or peptides derived from them are irritants in their own right, and secondly they form ideal media for the growth of micro-organisms for which they may well constitute a protected environment. Chronic osteomyelitis is a perfect example of the importance of drainage, and the resistance of established cases to antibiotics of proven activity against the causative organisms emphasizes the significance of the concept here advanced.

Inflammation is generally regarded as induced by release of mediators such as histamine, bradykinin, etc. In order to localize their action to the site of irritation a number of inhibitors are available both in the general circulation and by local production, thus constituting a negative feedback system. Unwanted prolongation of inflammation may therefore, in theory at least, result from a failure in the switch-off of the mediators and/or a deficiency in the provision of inhibitors.

A typical example of such a mechanism is that suggested by John Morley. It has been shown that lymphokines released from activated lymphocytes stimulate macrophages to synthesize and release prostaglandins, and prostaglandins in their turn inhibit the release of lymphokines by activated lymphocytes, i.e. a typical example of negative feedback. What would be the result, asked Dr. Morley, of a loss of sensitivity by lymphocytes to the inhibitory effect of prostaglandins? A self perpetuating inflammation or at least one persisting as long as sensitized lymphocytes and antigen are still present.

Immunological research over the last 70 years has clearly established that many inflammatory lesions are mediated by immunological reactions and these reactions have been conveniently classified by Coombs and Gell into four types. Without going into the details of the mechanisms of these reactions it is sufficient to say that they all require the presence of antigenic material both to sensitize the host and to elicit the reaction once sensitization has become established. Where sensitization is to an exogenous antigen a resulting state of chronic inflammation implies constant or repeated exposure to the offending agent, e.g. an industrial dermatitis. Prevention of such exposure terminates the inflammation. With the introduction of the concept of autoimmunity a much less amenable situation can be readily envisaged. An autoimmune thyroiditis or adrenalitis are self perpetuating lesions, at least until the antigen has been completely destroyed by the inflammatory process. Such autoimmunity may well underlie much chronic inflammation and it is conceivable that the autoantigen might itself be a product of the inflammatory process as suggested for rheumatoid arthritis.

The actual mechanism, however, by which the immunologically mediated inflammatory process is activated need not necessarily involve an antigen, exogenous or endogenous. Many biological mechanisms achieve rapidity of response by making use of the cascade principle by which the product of an initiating reaction activates a precursor enzyme next along the line. This activated enzyme in turn activates the next precursor and so on until the final product is obtained. In essence this is similar to the principle of the photo-multiplier tube. The longer the chain, however, the more opportunity for inappropriate activation of one of the intermediate steps. Such activation could then account for an ongoing inflammation of obscure or unknown causation. A well established example of such a chain of events is given by the complement system with its classical and its alternative modes of activation. It may well be asked 'How many other alternative pathways remain to be discovered'.

An interesting suggestion recently put forward by Dudley Dumonde is essentially an example of such inappropriate activation of a usually antigenically mediated response. He asks, in effect, whether the activation of lymphocytes to release lymphokines is invariably due to antigenic stimulation or can other stimuli lead to lymphokine release. The passage of lymphocytes for example through the complex structure of a post capillary venule must be associated with considerable physical deformation of all membranes which might well lead to activation, and if at all common some homeostatic mechanism presumably exists to control it. 'What' Dr. Dumonde asks, would be the result of failure of such a control mechanism?

What of the future? It is becoming increasingly evident that a maximally efficient inflammatory reaction, i.e. one which most rapidly restores the *status quo ante* requires a highly ordered and controlled sequence of events, both humoral and cellular. This in turn must require a highly developed, but at present almost unknown system of intercellular communication, based presumably on the ability of cells to release specific messenger molecules into their environment and the presence on cell surfaces of so called receptors. What is a receptor? Presumably a molecular configuration on a cell surface such that an interaction with an appropriate configuration in the environment will undergo a sufficient energy change to activate a chain of enzymes whose effect will ultimately result in some detectable change in the functional activity of the recipient cell. The paper by Allison on the effect of complement components on macrophages is a good example of this basic phenomenon. Our knowledge of receptors is still in its infancy, and at present is largely confined to those capable of reacting to specific parts of immunoglobulin molecules or to components of the complement system. I would suggest that as a means of controlling undesired inflammation by pharmacological agents an extension of our knowledge of intercellular communication and the specific determinants involved could prove most highly rewarding.

Section IV
General Aspects   I

CHAIRMAN: J. P. Giroud

CO-CHAIRMAN: K. Brune

19

Dual function of E-type prostaglandins in models of chronic inflammation

I. L. BONTA, M. J. PARNHAM, M. J. P. ADOLFS AND
L. VAN VLIET (The Netherlands)

INTRODUCTION

The debate over the dual function of prostaglandins (PGs) in inflammatory conditions is continuing with unremitting vehemence[1]. Recent data[2] indicate that a pivotal pro-inflammatory mediator role may be exerted by the cyclic endoperoxide PGG_2, although PG itself is also pro-inflammatory, since it potentiates the acute inflammatory effect of other mediators[3]. The suggestions concerning the anti-inflammatory function of PGE were born out of *in vitro* studies, which have shown that PGE-mediated elevation of intracellular cyclic-AMP (cAMP) prevents the release of lysosomal enzymes from PMN leukocytes and the discharge of lymphokines from T-lymphocytes[4-6]. The inhibitory effect of PGE on the synthesis of collagen is another *in vitro* observation[7] which supports a possible anti-inflammatory function. Further- more, pharmacological doses of PGE were shown, *in vivo*, to inhibit granu- loma formation, when applied locally into an implanted foreign body[8] and to suppress the adjuvant-induced arthritis of rats[9,10].

Provided that endogenous PGE has indeed a dual function, its lack *in vivo* should result in suppression of some components of inflammation and rein- forcement of others. The discovery that aspirin inhibits the generation of PGs[11] resulted in this drug and related inhibitors of cyclo-oxygenase being used as pharmacological tools of paramount importance in proving the pro-inflammatory role of PGs. Implicit in the use of cyclo-oxygenase in- hibitors as tools in studying the pro- and anti-inflammatory role of endo- genous PGs is the assumption that the entire anti-inflammatory effect of aspirin-like drugs can be explained on the basis of their suppression of PG output[12]. More recently some doubt has been cast on this assumption[13-15].

Therefore, we have chosen dietary withdrawal of precursors of PGs as a more suitable tool in achieving permanent shortage of endogenous PGs and in examining some models of chronic inflammation under this condition in rats. In addition to a discussion of these studies, an account will be given of the mutual effects of PGE_1 and a phosphodiesterase inhibitor on adjuvant arthritis in rats, in an attempt to test the hypothesis that elevation of cAMP is involved in the anti-inflammatory effect of E-type PGs *in vivo*.

CHRONIC INFLAMMATION DURING DEPRIVATION OF PG-PRECURSORS

The precursors of endogenous prostaglandins are essential fatty acids and in rats kept on an essential fatty acid deficient (EFAD) diet the arachidonic acid content of membrane phospholipids is replaced by 5,8,11-eicosatrienoic acid, which is not a substrate for the cyclo-oxygenase step in the biosynthesis of PGs[16]. During collagen-induced aggregation of platelets from EFAD rats, the output of thromboxane A_2 and cyclic endoperoxides is very markedly reduced[17]. We have now compared the amounts of PGE in exudates obtained from kaolin-induced pouch-granulomata and from carrageenan-impregnated poly-ether sponge implants of normal and EFAD rats (Table 19.1). The exudates from normal rats contained large amounts of PGE, but the PGE content of exudates from EFAD rats was exceedingly low and in several cases no PGE-like activity was detectable in the EFAD exudates. During these experiments two other observations were made, which are shown in Table 19.2.

First, the exudate production was markedly reduced in animals deprived of endogenous PGs. This finding is in agreement with other works which have

Table 19.1 Prostaglandin-like activity of inflammatory exudates

Source of exudate	PGE_2 equivalent (ng/ml) Normal	EFAD
Pouch-granuloma 4 days	129 ± 49 (4)	6.2{1.35–10.7} (2)
Sponge implant 8 days	32.8 ± 5.1 (5)	4.0 ± 4.0 (4)

Mean values are given ± SEM, except for pouch-granulomata of EFAD rats where the range of values is shown { }. Numbers of observations are given in brackets. The pouch-granuloma exudates were passed through an Amberlite XAD-2 column to which indomethacin was added. The lipids absorbed to the column were recovered by washing with methanol, evaporated and resuspended in chloroform before bioassay. The sponge implant exudates were obtained from the capsules of the granulomata, centrifuged and the supernatant used for bioassay. The rat stomach strip served as assay organ (superfusion technique with appropriate antagonists), using PGE_2 as a standard. With EFAD rats, only two out of four pouch-granulomata contained sufficient amounts of fluid for bioassay. With sponge implants, PG-like material was only present in detectable amounts in 1 out of 4 EFAD exudates. The detection limit of this assay was 200 pg PGE_2. The EFAD condition was achieved by a dietary method described earlier[18].

Table 19.2 Exudate volume and leukocyte count

Source of material		Parameter	Normal	EFAD
Pouch-granuloma	day 4	Exudate ml	1.38 ± 0.17 (8)	0.25 ± 0.02 (8)
	day 8		4.59 ± 0.88 (8)	1.94 ± 0.54 (8)
Sponge implant	day 8	Leukocytes 10^6/ml	12.0 ± 3.1 (5)	5.5 ± 0.6 (5)

Mean values are given $\pm$ SEM. Numbers of observations are shown in brackets. To measure the exudate volume the rats were killed with chloroform, the skin over the pouch was cut and the exudate was withdrawn from the pouch with a syringe. To estimate the number of leukocytes, fluid was squeezed out of both sponges from each rat, the fluids were pooled and after lysing the erythrocytes with zaponin, the total leukocytes were counted from 40 μl aliquots in a Coulter counter.

shown that, in EFAD rats, a variety of rat paw oedemas, in which fluid leakage through microvessels obviously occurs, are partially suppressed[18-20] All these observations support the view that increase of microvessel permeability is a pro-inflammatory mechanism exerted by PGE in the rat. Second, the leukocyte count in exudates squeezed from sponge implants of EFAD rats was reduced, but leukocytes were still present in large numbers. EFAD rats are, in any case, somewhat leukopenic[21], thus in these experiments the ratio of infiltrating leukocytes/total circulating leukocytes in EFAD rats was probably not much different from controls. Since the relatively moderate fall in leukocyte migration was not proportional to the marked reduction in PG production in EFAD rats, the findings do not support the suggestion of a major role for endogenous PGs in leukocyte infiltration into the inflamed area in rats.

Carrageenan-impregnated sponge implants were used to examine the granulomatous tissue proliferation over an 8-day period in EFAD rats. In this type of study it is a common practice to relate granuloma weight to body weight[8]. From earlier studies we were aware of the stunted growth in EFAD rats. Therefore, we related the weight increase (i.e. granuloma formation) in sponge implants to the increase in body weight over the same period and thus calculated a 'proliferation index'. The results in Table 19.3 show that during a permanent shortage of endogenous PGE (EFAD rats) the proliferation index was significantly increased. Collagen synthesis is known to be involved in the proliferation component of inflammation and in this context, PGE_2 has been shown to inhibit bone collagen synthesis *in vitro*[7]. PGE_2 has also been shown to inhibit granuloma formation in rats[8] and low doses of indomethacin, the prototype inhibitor of PG biosynthesis, stimulated collagen synthesis in sponge granulomata[22]. It is possible that the increased proliferation index in the EFAD rats reflected a larger amount of collagen in the granulomata. This in turn suggests that one component of the anti-inflammatory function of endogenous PGE might be exerted through inhibition of collagen production at the inflamed site. However, reduced

Table 19.3 Granuloma proliferation in carrageenan impregnated sponge implants

| | 1st experiment | | 2nd experiment | |
	Normal	EFAD	Normal	EFAD
Growth, 8 days				
Δbody weight (g)	19.1 ± 1.6	18.4 ± 1.6	20.2 ± 2.3	6.2 ± 1.8
Granuloma, 8 days				
Δdry weight (mg)	101 ± 23	184 ± 39	379 ± 33	240 ± 25
Proliferation index				
(Δdry wt./Δbody wt.)	5.2 ± 1.2	10.1 ± 2.1	19.8 ± 2.9	53.5 ± 11

Mean values are given ± SEM. In the 1st expt. each group contained 6 rats, in the 2nd expt. 5 rats. In each rat two sponges were implanted and recorded separately. On day 8 the rats were killed, the sponges were removed with the surrounding connective tissue and after drying for 24 h at 80 °C they were weighed. The preimplantation sponge weights were subtracted from the dry weight values recorded after removal. The resulting Δdry weight values were used to calculate the proliferation index. In the 1st expt. the rats were caged in Makrolons containing sawdust. The animals were chewing the sawdust and the EFAD rats suddenly displayed a higher growth rate than usually observed with such animals. In the 2nd expt. the sawdust bedding was replaced with sol 'Speedi-Dry', an undigestible grit. The nature of the body weight growth promoting factor in the sawdust is not known. It is unlikely to have been a precursor of endogenous PGs, because EFAD rats which were kept on sawdust, still exhibited very markedly reduced amounts of PGs in the pouch-granuloma exudates (see Table 19.1).

incorporation of labelled proline into non-inflamed tissues has been reported in EFAD rats[23]. This is not necessarily in contradiction to our present proposal, because collagen synthesis in inflamed-tissue (the granulomata) may differ in its sensitivity to PGs from that in normal tissue.

To examine the influence of shortage of endogenous PG-precursors in an immunological model of chronic inflammation, adjuvant-induced arthritis in rats was used. The complete adjuvant was injected into the left hind paw of male rats from an inbred Wistar strain. The increase in volume of the contralateral paw was used to evaluate the chronic arthritis 20 days after the induction of the disease. EFAD rats displayed a markedly stunted growth during the development of the syndrome (Figure 19.1). Therefore, it appeared reasonable to relate the paw volume increase to the increase in body weight over the same period. The results (Figure 19.2) show that in normal rats there was very little chronic inflammation, which is in agreement with the recognized insensitivity of the Wistar strain to the arthritis component of the adjuvant syndrome. Chronic arthritis was more pronounced in the EFAD rats, although in these animals the acute (6 h) inflammation in the injected paw was slightly smaller than that in normal animals. Denko[24] observed suppression of adjuvant arthritis in EFAD rats. However, in his study the injected paw was used to evaluate both the acute and chronic components of the syndrome. This probably accounts for the discrepancy between the data obtained in the two different studies. Apart from the differential influence of PG-precursor shortage on the acute and chronic inflammatory components

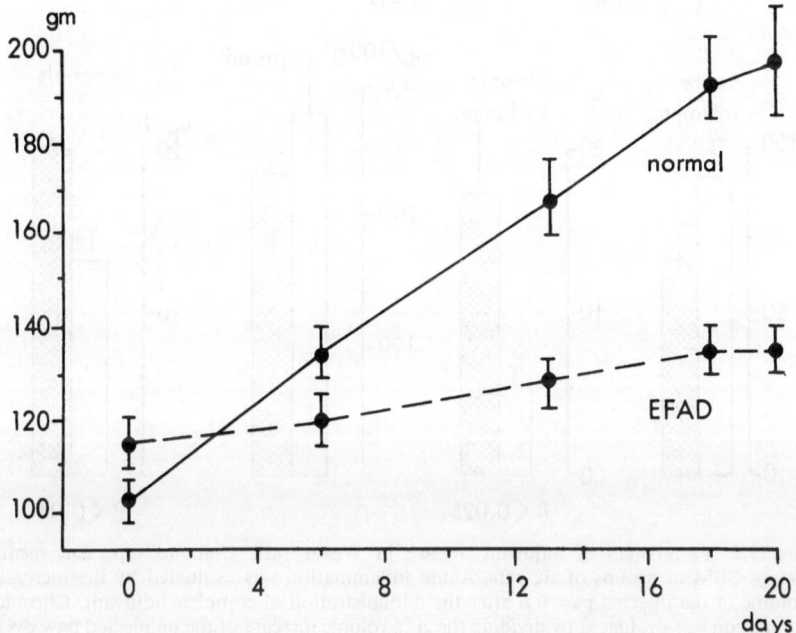

Figure 19.1 Body weight changes during development of adjuvant arthritis in Wistar rats. Each point represents the mean value ± SEM. There were in each group six rats. Complete Freunds adjuvant (0.1 ml of 6 mg/ml *M. butyricum* in liquid paraffin) was administered in the left hind paw on day 0

of the adjuvant disease, the adrenal weights of the EFAD rats were higher than in the corresponding control animals (Figure 19.2). The adjuvant disease might have caused greater stress in the EFAD rats, thus accounting for the larger adrenals. The adrenal hyperplasia may, however, have been due to reduced corticosteroid production, resulting from disturbed lipid metabolism in EFAD rats[25], thus leading to overproduction of ACTH. The role of endogenous corticosteroids in modulating chronic inflammatory models is still unclear[26]. Thus, the present results are open to several interpretations, a shortage of endogenous PGs being only one of them. A more rigorous study of adjuvant arthritis in EFAD rats appears to be warranted.

The present findings show that shortage of endogenous PGs, achieved by dietary withdrawal of PG-precursors, is associated with enhancement of the proliferative granulomatous and immune arthritic components of inflammation. In turn this suggests that endogenous PGs may inhibit these components of chronic inflammation. For the study of this problem EFAD rats seem to constitute an effective model. Such animals are probably more useful, in this context, than animals treated with agents which interfere with PG production, since some of the latter drugs may affect inflammation

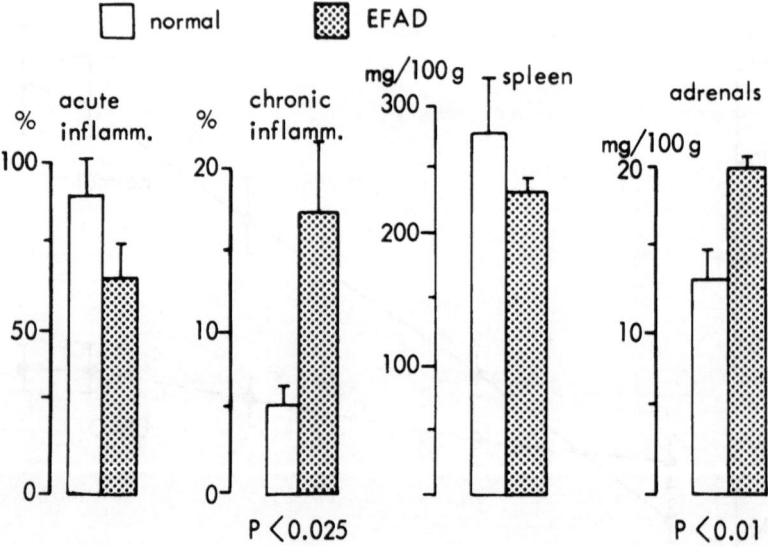

Figure 19.2 Parameters of adjuvant disease in Wistar rats. Columns represent mean values ± SEM of groups of six rats. Acute inflammation was evaluated by the increase in volume of the injected paw 6 h after the administration of complete adjuvant. Chronic inflammation was evaluated by dividing the $\Delta\%$ volume increase of the uninjected paw over a 20 day period, by $\Delta\%$ body weight over the same period. On day 20 the animals were killed to remove and weigh the spleens and adrenals

through mechanisms which are independent of their interaction with the discharge of PGs[15].

SUPPRESSION OF ADJUVANT-ARTHRITIS

The earlier proposal that the anti-inflammatory effect of pharmacological doses of PGE_1 is mediated through elevation of c-AMP[10] prompted us to examine whether a phosphodiesterase inhibitor would enhance the suppressing influence of PGE_1 on the adjuvant disease of rats. A Lewis rat strain, known for its high sensitivity to the development of adjuvant arthritis, was used for these experiments. PGE_1 (0.75 mg/kg), theophylline (75 mg/kg) or both agents together were administered s.c. daily from the day of complete Freund's adjuvant injection into one hind paw. Chronic arthritis in the uninjected paw was evaluated by volume measurement and X-ray photographs of the tibiotarsal joint. Detailed figures of this study were presented elsewhere[27], but the main results are outlined in Table 19.4. The chronic arthritis was inhibited by each drug alone and when given together there was a mutual enhancement of their effects. The suppression of the arthritis was not only evident in the joint swelling, but also in the prevention of bone destruction (Figure 19.3). The results in Table 19.4 also show that the effects

Table 19.4 Suppressing effects of PGE_1 and theophylline on several parameters of adjuvant disease in Lewis rats

| Drug daily s.c. (mg/kg) | Percent suppression | | |
	Chronic arthritis	Spleen weight	Tibiotarsal joint destruction
Prostaglandin E_1 (0.75)	36*	24**	79*
Theophylline (75)	33*	23**	19
PGE_1 + theo. (0.75 + 75)	52**	37***	100***

Percent suppression is related to a control group of rats which received complete Freunds adjuvant in one hind paw, but received neither PGE_1 nor theophylline. The original data, from which the above percent values are derived, are presented elsewhere[27]. Chronic arthritis in the uninjected paw was evaluated by volume measurement on day 28. Tibiotarsal joint destruction in the uninjected paw was examined from X-ray photographs taken on day 35. This was also the day the rats were killed to remove and weigh the spleens. Significance versus control-group refers to the original data.
* $P < 0.05$; ** $P < 0.01$; *** $P < 0.001$

day 35 untreated paw

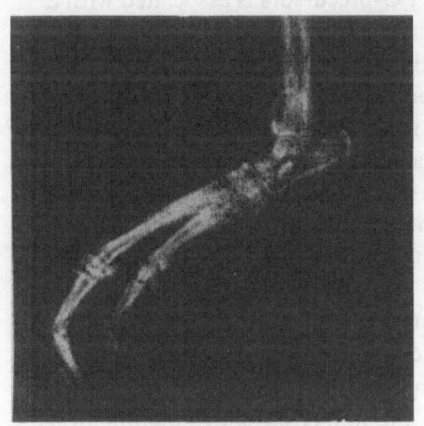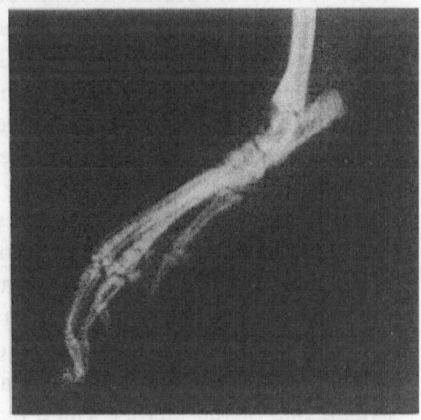

vehicle   theophylline + PgE 1

Figure 19.3 X-ray photographs of adjuvant arthritic paws of Lewis rats. The picture on the left shows the non-adjuvant injected paw of a rat which received the saline vehicle only. Note the bone resorption at the tibiotarsal and metatarsal joints. The picture on the right is the uninjected paw of a rat which received PGE_1 and theophylline in doses as presented in Table 19.4. Bone resorption is absent

of PGE_1 and theophylline on spleen weight paralleled their suppression of the chronic arthritis. The earlier *in vitro* findings, showing that PGE effects which are related to anti-inflammatory function are mediated through elevation of c-AMP[4,5,6], gain support from the present *in vivo* observations. However, gross changes in c-AMP levels in paw perfusates were not correlated with the severity of the arthritis[28]. It is more likely that, provided the combined treatment with PGE_1 and theophylline was indeed mediated through an effect on c-AMP, such changes might have occurred at a site remote from the inflicted paw. The fact that suppression of splenomegaly paralleled the inhibition of the chronic inflammation in the paws, suggests that immunological activation and subsequent synovial infiltration by splenic lymphocytes might have been the process which was affected by the concomitant administration of PGE_1 and theophylline. The above is an exceedingly oversimplified explanation, but a more realistic working hypothesis has been currently developed[29].

CONCLUDING REMARKS

Dietary deprivation of PG-precursors in rat appears to suppress the exudative component of inflammation, while the proliferative component seems to be promoted. Permanent deprivation of PG-precursors is associated with a markedly reduced output of PG-endoperoxides from aggregating platelets[17] and a pronounced reduction of PGE levels in exudates from inflamed sites (present results). These observations underline the concept (Figure 19.4) of the dual role of endogenous E-type PGs in models of inflammation in the rat. However, caution should be exercised in the interpretation of results derived from EFAD rats, because the EFAD condition is a complicated metabolic situation[30] in which other factors, besides shortage of endogenous PGs, undoubtedly play a role. Some of the changes associated with EFAD diet (stunted growth, increased adrenal weight) present problems with immediate consequences in the appropriate evaluation of changes in parameters of inflammation. Bearing these precautions in mind, the experiments with EFAD rats seem to show that when PG-output is limited to a great extent, one of the factors which maintain the homeostasis of inflammation is missing. Thus the differential consequences of EFAD, namely suppression of the exudative component of inflammation together with enhancement of non-immune (granuloma) and immune (adjuvant arthritis) components probably represent the pro- and anti-inflammatory effects of endogenous PGEs. The anti-inflammatory function of exogenously administered PGE_1 was enhanced in the present experiments by the concomitant administration of an inhibitor of phosphodiesterase. This observation indicates the *in vivo* validity of the concept that PGE might exert its anti-inflammatory role through shifting the balance of the intracellular cyclic nucleotides in favour

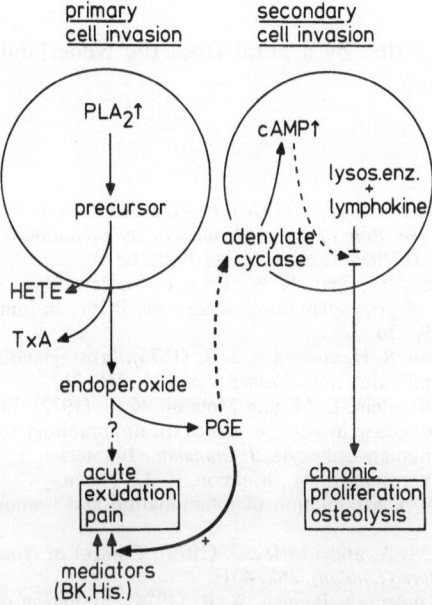

Figure 19.4 Conceivable dual function of PGE in inflammation. During primary cell invasion the PGE thus released potentiates other mediators and amplifies the acute components of inflammation. The released PGE may stimulate the adenylate cyclase of other invading cells in which the increased c-AMP would prevent the discharge of materials which contribute to the chronicity of inflammation. This oversimplified model, in common with most models, is a poor replica of the reality

of c-AMP. Whether this attractive concept can also be extended to the inflammatory role of endogenous PGE is conceivable, but needs to be proven.

Finally, the apparent dual function of endogenous PGs invites the following speculation. Anti-inflammatory drugs currently in use, which primarily inhibit the cyclo-oxygenase or interfere, by another mechanism, with the discharge of endogenous PGs, while relieving symptoms of acute inflammation, may also disturb the homeostatic balancing function of PGs in the chronic phase of inflammatory conditions. Some of these drugs seem to suppress acute inflammation in animals which are deprived of PG-precursors[15,18]. Thus, even potent inhibitors of the cyclo-oxygenase may exert anti-inflammatory effects through other mechanisms, in addition to preventing the increase in PG levels. The warning has been expressed that anti-inflammatory drug design based simply on PG-biosynthesis inhibition is a practice which disregards the complicated network between different cell populations and mediators involved in the chronicity of inflammation[31]. The dual function of endogenous PGs in regulating inflammation is a concept which, when more firmly established, may help in finding new ways to pharmacologically control chronic inflammatory conditions.

273

Acknowledgement

This study was supported by a grant from the Nederlandse Vereniging tot Rheumatiekbestrijding.

References

1. Willoughby, D. A. and Dieppe, P. (1976). Prostaglandins in the inflammatory response —pro or anti? In: *The Role of Prostaglandins in Inflammation* (G. P. Lewis, ed.) pp. 14–25. (Bern-Stuttgart-Vienna: Hans Haber Publishers)
2. Kuehl, F. A., Humes, J. L., Egan, R. W., Ham, E. A., Beveridge, G. C. and van Arman, C. G. (1977). Role of prostaglandin endoperoxide PGG_2 in inflammatory processes, *Nature (London)* **265**, 170
3. Moncada, S., Ferreira, S. H. and Vane, J. R. (1973). Prostaglandins, aspirin-like drugs and the oedema of inflammation. *Nature (London)*, **246**, 217
4. Bourne, H. R., Lichtenstein, L. M. and Melmon, K. L. (1972). Pharmacologic control of allergic histamine release in vitro: evidence for an inhibitory role of 3′,5′-adenosine monophosphate in human leukocyte. *J. Immunol.*, **108**, 695
5. Bourne, H. R., Lichtenstein, L. M., Melmon, K. L., Henney, C. S., Weinstein, Y. and Shearer, G. M. (1974). Modulation of inflammation and immunity by cyclic AMP. *Science*, **184**, 19
6. Gordon, D., Bray, M. A. and Morley, J. (1976). Control of lymphokine secretion by prostaglandins, *Nature (London)*, **262**, 401
7. Raisz, L. G. and Koolemans-Beijnen, A. R. (1974). Inhibition of bone collagen synthesis by prostaglandin E_2 in organ culture. *Prostaglandins*, **8**, 377
8. DiPasquale, G., Rassaert, C., Richter, R., Welaj, P. and Tripp, L. (1973). Influence of prostaglandins (PG) E_2 and F_{2a} on the inflammatory process. *Prostaglandins*, **3**, 741
9. Aspinall, R. L. and Cammarata, P. S. (1969). Effect of prostaglandin E_2 on adjuvant arthritis. *Nature (London)*, **224**, 1320
10. Zurier, R. B., Hoffstein, S. and Weissmann, G. (1973). Suppression of acute and chronic inflammation in adrenalectomized rats by pharmacologic amounts of prostaglandins. *Arthritis. Rheum.*, **16**, 609
11. Vane, J. R. (1971). Inhibition of prostaglandin synthesis as a mechanism of action for aspirin-like drugs. *Nature New Biol.*, **231**, 232
12. Vane, J. R. (1973). Inhibition of prostaglandin biosynthesis as the mechanism of action of aspirin-like drugs. In: *Advances in the Biosciences* (S. Bergström and S. Bernhard, eds.) Vol. 9, pp. 395–411. (Oxford: Pergamon Press)
13. Brocklehurst, W. E. and Dawson, W. (1974). New data concerning the inhibition of prostaglandin formation by anti-inflammatory drugs. In: *Future Trends in Inflammation* II (G. P. Velo, D. A. Willoughby and J.-P. Giroud, eds.) pp. 37–43. (Padua: Piccin Medical Books)
14. Smith, M. J. H. (1975). Prostaglandins and aspirin: An alternative view. *Agents Actions*, **5**, 315
15. Bonta, I. L., Bult, H., Vincent, J. E. and Zijlstra, F. J. (1977). Acute anti-inflammatory effects of aspirin and dexamethasone in rats deprived of endogenous prostaglandin precursors. *J. Pharm. Pharmacol.*, **29**, 1
16. Ziboh, V. A., Vanderhoek, J. Y. and Lands, W. E. M. (1974). Inhibition of sheep vesicular gland oxygenase by unsaturated fatty acids from skin of essential fatty acid deficient rats. *Prostaglandins*, **5**, 233
17. Bult, H. and Bonta, I. L. (1976). Rat platelets aggregate in the absence of endogenous precursors of prostaglandin endoperoxides, *Nature (London)*, **264**, 449
18. Bonta, I. L., Chrispijn, H., Noordhoek, J. and Vincent, J. E. (1974). Reduction of prostaglandin phase in hind-paw inflammation and partial failure of indomethacin to exert anti-inflammatory effect in rats on essential fatty acid deficient diet. *Prostaglandins*, **5**, 495
19. Denko, C. W. (1974). Effect of prostaglandins in urate crystal inflammation. *Pharmacology*, **12**, 331

DUAL ROLE OF PROSTAGLANDINS

20. Bonta, I. L., Bult, H., van der Ven, L. L. M. and Noordhoek, J. (1976). Essential Fatty Acid Deficiency: A condition to discriminate prostaglandin and non-prostaglandin mediated components of inflammation. *Agents Actions*, **6**, 154
21. Vincent, J. E., Zijlstra, F. J. and Bonta, I. L. (1975). The effect of non-steroid antiinflammatory drugs, dibutyryl cyclid 3′,5′-adenosine monophosphate and phosphodiesterase inhibitors on platelet aggregation and the platelet release reaction in normal and essential fatty acid deficient rats. *Prostaglandins*, **10**, 899
22. Kulonen, E. and Potila, M. (1975). Effect of the administration of antirheumatic drugs on experimental granuloma in rat. *Biochem. Pharmacol.*, **24**, 219
23. Denko, C. W. (1976). ^{35}S and ^{3}H-proline incorporation in rats deficient in essential fatty acids. *J. Rheumatol.*, **3**, 205
24. Denko, C. W. (1976). Modification of adjuvant inflammation in rats deficient in essential fatty acids. *Agents Actions*, **6**, 636
25. Hayashida, T. and Portman, O. W. (1959). Effects of essential fatty acid deficiency on rat adrenal composition and secretory activity. *Am. J. Physiol.*, **197**, 893
26. Parnham, M. J. (1977). Metyrapone: A possible tool in investigating the role of endogenous corticosteroids in inflammation. *Agents Actions*. Suppl. issue (In press)
27. Bonta, I. L., Parnham, M. J., van Vliet, L. and Vincent, J. E. (1977). Mutual enhancement of the effects of prostaglandin E_1 and theophylline on the Freund adjuvant-induced arthritis syndrome of rats. *Br. J. Pharmacol.*, **59**, 438P
28. Adolfs, M. J. P., Bonta, I. L. and Parnham, M. J. (1977). Cyclic AMP production during adjuvant-induced arthritis in rats. *Br. J. Pharmacol.*, **59**, 439P
29. Parnham, M. J., Bonta, I. L. and Adolfs, M. J. P. (1977). Interactions between prostaglandin E and cyclic nucleotides in chronic inflammatory disease. In: *Perspectives in Inflammation* (D. A. Willoughby, J.-P. Giroud and G. P. Velo) pp. 279–287. (London: MTP Press Limited)
30. Holman, R. T. (1971). In: *Progress in the Chemistry of Fats and Other Lipids* (R. T. Holman, ed.) p. 275. (Oxford: Pergamon Press)
31. Morley, J. (1977). Interaction between lymphocytes and macrophages. *Agents Actions*. Suppl. issue (In press)

Discussion 19

G. P. Velo: (Italy)	How long does it take to get a complete reduction of fatty acids? It is a critical point. The amount of the reduction, and the length of time taken, should be specified.
Bonta:	Our method of depleting these animals has been published repeatedly in our papers. We take the animals from others that are five days before their delivery, and are already on the deficient-diet. We take the litters; they are kept on this diet, and we do our experiments three months after delivery. This time we investigated the erythrocytes. We investigated the ratio of the different fatty acids, and our animals are highly deficient. So it takes approximately three months.
P. Davies:	Professor Bonta's very interesting presentation raises several questions. First, in relation to his sponge granuloma experiment. I should like to know whether the cellular populations within that granuloma are also affected. Has he, for example, done DNA measurements in these sponge granulomas?
Bonta:	We have done some experiments and they will be reported in a paper. We are submitting a paper covering prostaglandins too. There are more details about this. We counted the leukocytes—the total leukocyte count was established in the granulomata. We squeezed out the fluid and counted the leukocytes. There was some reduction in the leukocyte count in our prostaglandin-deficient animals. However, the reduction in the leukocyte count was not proportional with the very marked reduction in the prostaglandin content of the fluid. Furthermore—and this is published work—these deficient animals are a little bit leukopenic, not very much, but, in relation to the already existing leukopenia it appears that the lack of the prostaglandins did not much affect the leukocyte migration to the sponges. However, we shall have to do more detailed experiments to differentiate the cell count.
M. Dianzani: (Italy)	In Turin we have used the cell-model of essential fatty acid deficiency in order to study whether there is a different susceptibility to carbon tetrachloride lipid-induced peroxidation in the liver. Carbon tetrachloride induces lipid peroxidation and we hoped by deprivation of arachidonic acid to get different results. However, in our case there was no difference. Eicosatrienoic acid is the only good substrate for lipid peroxidation. Can Professor Bonta be sure that all his results are explained by depletion of prostaglandins? In this model there are in the liver, and in the kidney, and in several other tissues, a lot of other changes. For instance, a lot of mitochondrial damage, sharp decrease in ATP, and probably all protein biosynthesis, may be affected too.
Bonta:	We are aware that in these animals more is happening than simply depletion of the prostaglandins, and we are certainly investigating this.

There is also an effect on the adrenals. I am not claiming that the only reason for the modification in the inflammatory response is entirely due to the lack of prostaglandins, but this is certainly one way to investigate the role of the endogenous prostaglandins, because when the endogenous prostaglandins are depleted, for example by treating the animals with a prostaglandin biosynthesis inhibitor, one is faced with a very similar problem, because some of the prostaglandin biosynthesis inhibitors—something else that we have shown with this approach which has also been published—some of these drugs might have other effects besides the inhibition of prostaglandin biosynthesis in the patient.

D. A. Willoughby:
(UK)

I loved Professor Bonta's model—essential fatty acid depletion—but I too would like to follow up Dr. Davies's question. How fit are these cells once they have been squeezed out? Are they viable when they have been squeezed out from the sponge?

Secondly, it seems to me that during the course of this meeting ever-increasingly we seem to be coming up against the problem of relevance of all of the models to anti-rheumatic drugs, as opposed to anti-inflammatory drugs. Could Professor Bonta comment?

Bonta:

We have not yet investigated whether the cells that we obtain from the granulomata are vital, viable, and so forth. We are now in the process of doing it. We had first to establish that there was something happening here. We are now investigating these cells more closely and I hope that sometime in the future we shall say some more about this.

On the second point, this kind of approach might be successful both in investigating the classic anti-rheumatic drugs and in providing some alternative approach to treatment via the whole adrenal-cyclic AMP system.

20

Interactions between prostaglandin E and cyclic nucleotides in chronic inflammatory disease

M. J. PARNHAM, I. L. BONTA AND M. J. P. ADOLFS
(The Netherlands)

INTRODUCTION

Despite the mass of available data, the debate over the pro- and/or anti-inflammatory role of prostaglandins (PGs) continues unabated[1] (see Chapter 19). However, it is becoming increasingly clear, that the actions of PGs in inflammation appear to involve alterations in cyclic AMP (cAMP) levels at various sites. Our interest has been directed towards the relationship between PGs and cAMP in adjuvant arthritis in rats.

PGs of the E series have been shown to markedly inhibit the development of adjuvant arthritis in pharmacological doses[2,3]. Recently Bonta et al.[4] showed that this action of PGE_1 is significantly enhanced by concomitant treatment of arthritic rats with theophylline. This finding apparently supports the earlier suggestion[5] that the PGs act by increasing cAMP levels in lymphocytes. However, although the inhibitory effects of PGE on several parameters of lymphocyte activation in vitro have been correlated with increased intra-cellular levels of cAMP[6], such a correlation has been observed with several other inflammatory phenomena. These include lysosomal enzyme release[7] and histamine release[8] from human leukocytes in vitro. Furthermore, increases in cAMP levels have also been observed following addition of PGE to rat bone cells[9] and human synoviocytes[10] in vitro. Thus, it is not clear whether the effects of PGE on adjuvant arthritis are due to a selective effect on lymphocyte cAMP or whether they also involve an effect on cAMP levels in cells of the inflamed joint.

In man, rheumatoid synovia have been shown to produce relatively large

279

amounts of PGE[11,12]. However, although increased PG production has been correlated with increased cAMP levels in rheumatoid synovial cultures[13], little is known about changes in endogenous cAMP during the development of inflammatory responses.

We have studied both the changes in cAMP levels in the joints of rats during the development of adjuvant arthritis and the effect of PGE_1 on these levels. The implications of these findings, in the light of current knowledge, will be incorporated into a working hypothesis for the relationship between PGs and cAMP in chronic inflammatory joint disease.

RESULTS AND DISCUSSION

Arthritis was induced in male Lewis rats (150–200 g) by the injection of 0.1 ml complete Freund's adjuvant into the left hind paw and a control group received 0.1 ml incomplete adjuvant. Subsequently, the arthritic animals were anaesthetized with 25% urethane 10, 14, 18 or 22 days after the adjuvant injection and the control group were anaesthetized after 22 days. These time periods were chosen because the development of the chronic phase of the arthritis begins on day 10 and reaches a peak around day 22. A stainless steel coaxial catheter was inserted through an incision in the right (uninjected) thigh and pushed, sub-cutaneously, until the tip covered the tibiotarsal joint (Figure 20.1). The catheter was tied in place and the joint

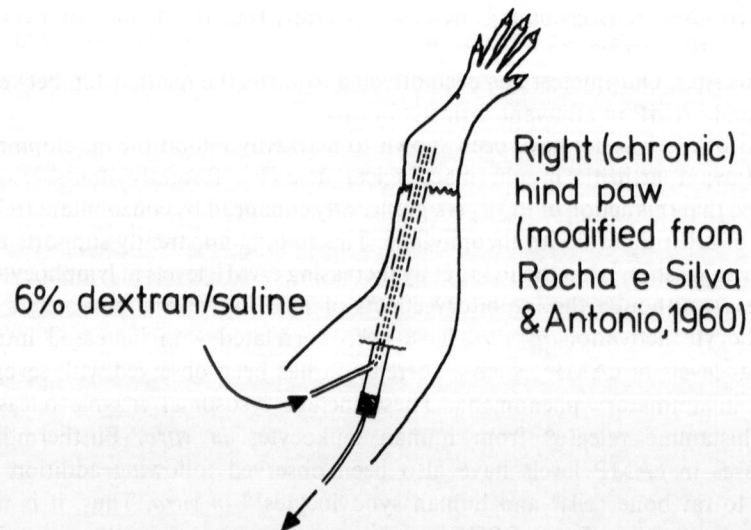

6% dextran/saline

Right (chronic) hind paw (modified from Rocha e Silva & Antonio, 1960)

Figure 20.1 Perfusion of the right (chronic) hind paw of the rat. 6% dextran-saline was pumped down the inner tube (inner diameter = 1 mm) at 0.2 ml/min and collected over ice via the outer tube (inner diameter = 4 mm). Perfusion, in one experiment, with Evans Blue revealed that only a discreet area around the (inflamed) tibio–tarsal joint was perfused

perfused for 2 h with sterile 6% dextran/saline. The perfusate was collected over ice. Following extraction of total lipids with chloroform:methanol (2:1), emulsion of the dextran with ethanol and centrifugation at 2500 r.p.m. for 5 min, the cAMP content of the dried supernatant was assayed in duplicate by the method of Gilman[35], using a commercial kit (Boehringer-Mannheim). Since gross changes in cAMP levels were being measured, the levels were expressed as pmol/h/100 g body wt. These values, thus, represent both intracellular cAMP in cells removed in the perfusate and cAMP released into extracellular fluid from a variety of cells. In this context, it is worth noting that PGE has been shown to stimulate the release of cAMP from cultured fibroblasts[14], macrophages[15] and bone cells[9]. This effect is not specific for PGE and the physiological significance of the phenomenon is unknown[16].

The values for cAMP levels during the development of adjuvant arthritis are shown in Figure 20.2. Gross cAMP levels in the inflamed joint decreased till day 18, during the early development of the inflammation. However, by day 22, when the paw swelling was at a peak, cAMP levels had returned towards control values. This suggests that the early development of the chronic inflammatory lesion in adjuvant arthritis is associated with a generalized decline in cAMP levels in the joint. Using ^{51}Cr labelled cells, Perper et al.[36] have shown that, during this early stage of the chronic phase of adjuvant

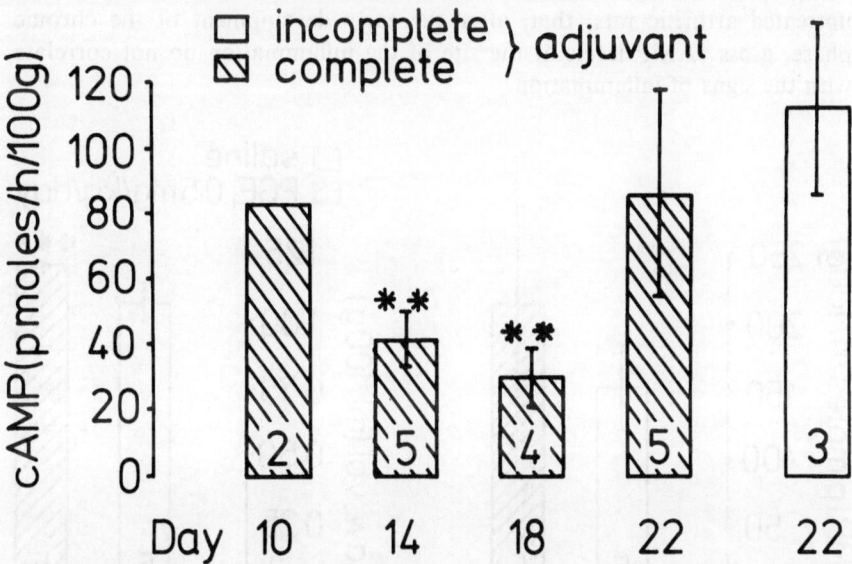

Figure 20.2 Levels of cAMP in perfusates of rat hind paws after injection of Freunds adjuvant into the contralateral paw. Each column indicates mean levels of cAMP ($\pm$ SEM) on the given day after adjuvant injection. On day 10 the range of individual values was 80.0−85.9 pmol/h/100 g. Numbers at the base of the columns indicate numbers of observations. Significance of differences from day 22 incomplete adjuvant controls was determined by Students' t-test: ** $p < 0.01$

arthritis, lymphocyte accumulation in the uninjected paw is much greater than monocyte accumulation. Lysosomal enzyme activity in the uninjected paw also begins to increase during this initial period[17]. Since both lymphocyte activation and lysosomal enzyme release are associated with decreased intracellular cAMP levels[6], it is likely that the decreased cAMP levels we observed may reflect changes in infiltrating lymphocyte and granulocyte populations. The increase in cAMP levels towards day 22 is probably due to complex changes initiated by the inflammatory process in various cell populations in and around the inflamed joint.

In order to investigate the effect of exogenous PGE on gross cAMP levels in the uninjected paw, arthritic rats were treated with either PGE_1 (0.5 mg/kg/day, s.c.) or saline (1 ml/kg/day, s.c.) on days 16–22 and the uninjected paws were perfused on day 22. Paw volume was also determined by mercury displacement. As shown in Figure 20.3, paw volume in PGE_1-treated animals was significantly increased when compared with controls, which contrasts with earlier work showing an inhibitory effect of PGE_1[3-5]. It is possible that this may reflect increased local lysosomal enzyme release, since there is some indication that low doses of PGE_1 *increase* lysosomal enzyme release from granulocytes[18]. Certainly, the dose of PGE_1 used in our present study was much lower than that used by other investigators. However, there was no significant change in cAMP levels in paws of PGE_1-treated animals when compared with controls. This confirms the initial finding, in untreated arthritic rats, that, after the early development of the chronic phase, gross cAMP levels at the site of the inflammation do not correlate with the signs of inflammation.

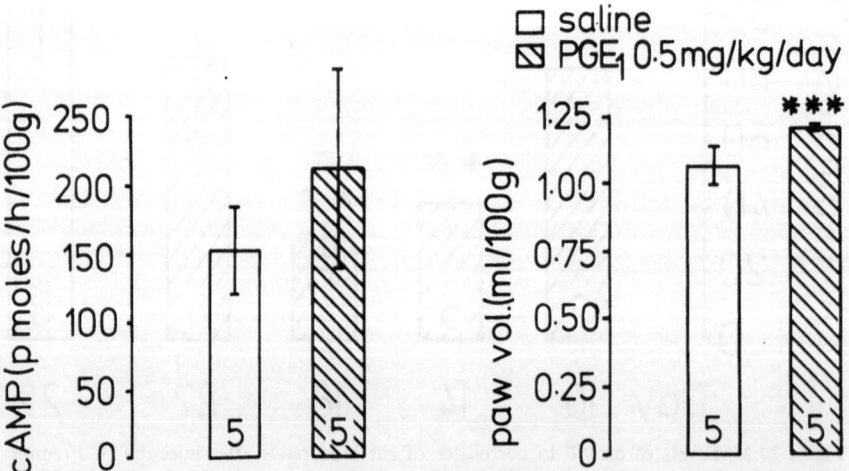

Figure 20.3 Effect of PGE_1 pretreatment on gross cAMP levels and paw volume in day 22 arthritic (uninjected) paws. Each column represents mean values ($\pm$ SEM). Numbers at the base of the columns indicate numbers of observations. Significance of differences between saline and PGE_1-treated animals was determined by Students' *t*-test: *** $p < 0.001$

POSSIBLE INTERACTIONS BETWEEN PROSTAGLANDINS AND CYCLIC NUCLEOTIDES IN CHRONIC JOINT INFLAMMATION

To account for our results and the data from other investigations into the role of PGs and cyclic nucleotides in chronic inflammation, we have developed a working hypothesis on the possible interactions between these two groups of substances. This involves consideration of the systemic interactions, in spleen and lymph nodes, in distinction to those changes which probably occur in the inflamed joint.

Spleen and lymph nodes

Gordon et al.[20] have shown that guinea pig macrophages produce much greater amounts of PGE in vitro than PMN leukocytes, monocytes or lymphocytes. These macrophage PGs inhibit lymphokine secretion by cultured lymphocytes and it has been suggested that this effect indicates a possible feedback mechanism on lymphocyte activation in vivo during the development of chronic inflammatory diseases[19]. It is probable that, in vivo, macrophage PG production would be stimulated by phagocytosis of antigen since antigen stimulation markedly increases PG production in vitro[20]. Although they appear to produce less PG than macrophages, activated

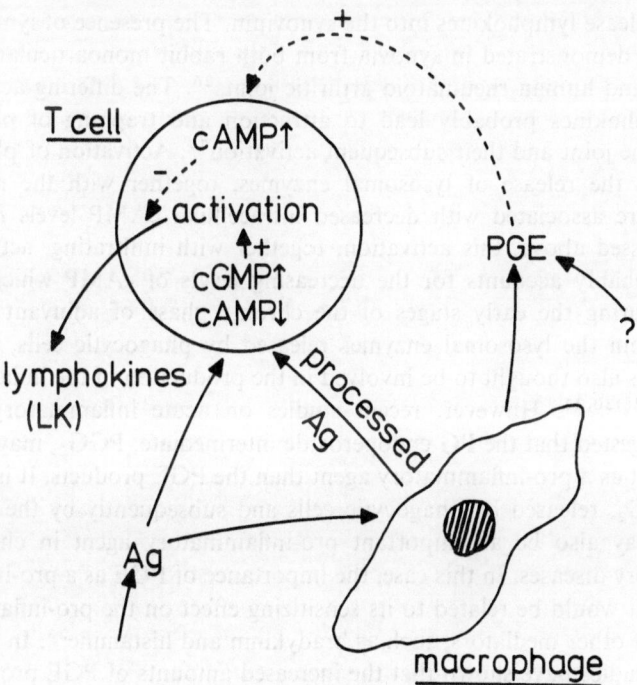

Figure 20.4 Probable interactions between PGE and cyclic nucleotides in spleen and lymph node cells during the development of chronic inflammatory joint disease

T-lymphocytes may also make a contribution to the release of PGs[21]. The relationship between inhibition of T-cell activation by PGE and increased lymphocyte cAMP levels is now well documented[6]. This action probably accounts for a major part of the *in vivo* inhibitory effect of PGE$_1$ on adjuvant arthritis, since spleen weight was also reduced by PGE$_1$ treatment[4]. Both these effects of PGE$_1$ were enhanced by concomitant treatment of the rats with theophylline. However, it is possible that PGE may act by preventing movement of T-cells to the joint, since cAMP and drugs which increase cAMP levels immobilize both T and B cells in a static configuration *in vitro*[22]. Cyclic 3'5'-guanosine monophosphate (cGMP) and agents which increase cGMP have the opposite effect. A growing body of evidence indicates that increased cGMP levels are associated with T-lymphocyte activation *in vitro*[23]. It is probable that this also occurs *in vivo*. Thus T-cell activation by antigen and the associated release of lymphokines would involve an increase in intracellular cGMP. PGE released by macrophages would then stimulate T-cell cAMP, suppressing lymphocyte activation according to the Yin-Yang hypothesis[24]. These interactions are summarized in Figure 20.4.

Inflamed joint

On arrival at the joint, under some chemotactic influence, the activated T-cells release lymphokines into the synovium. The presence of lymphokines has been demonstrated in synovia from both rabbit monoarticular arthritic joints[25] and human rheumatoid arthritic joints[26]. The differing activities of the lymphokines probably lead to attraction and trapping of phagocytic cells in the joint and their subsequent activation[27]. Activation of phagocytic cells and the release of lysosomal enzymes, together with the release of PGs[28], are associated with decreased intracellular cAMP levels *in vitro*[29]. As discussed above, this activation, together with infiltrating, activated T-cells, probably accounts for the decreasing levels of cAMP which we observed during the early stages of the chronic phase of adjuvant arthritis. Apart from the lysosomal enzymes released by phagocytic cells, the PGE released is also thought to be involved in the production of the inflammatory response[28,30,31]. However, recent studies on acute inflammatory models have suggested that the PG endoperoxide intermediate, PGG$_2$, may be more important as a pro-inflammatory agent than the PGE products. It is possible that PGG$_2$, released by phagocytic cells and subsequently by the inflamed tissue, may also be an important pro-inflammatory agent in chronic inflammatory diseases. In this case, the importance of PGE as a pro-inflammatory agent would be related to its sensitizing effect on the pro-inflammatory actions of other mediators, such as bradykinin and histamine[33]. In addition, *in vitro* studies have shown that the increased amounts of PGE produced by rheumatoid synovia cause bone resorption and an increase in intracellular cAMP levels[13]. However, although bone resorption may represent an additional pro-inflammatory action of PGE in chronic inflammation, it has been suggested that the increase in bone cell cAMP is related to inhibition of bone formation rather than bone resorption[9]. Nevertheless, inhibition of bone and/or synovial cell growth would exacerbate the necrosis of the joint. (It is worth noting that treatment of adjuvant arthritic rats with PGE_1 and/or theophylline inhibited bone destruction[4], indicating that this was probably not a direct action of the PG on the inflammatory process, but rather an indirect effect mediated by an action on activated lymphocytes).

Apart from these pro-inflammatory actions of PGE, it is likely that locally released PGE also exerts a negative-feedback inhibition on activated T-cells entering the inflamed joint. This would probably involve an increase in intracellular cAMP levels as discussed for the spleen and lymph nodes. The probable relationships between PGs and cyclic nucleotides in an arthritic joint are summarized in Figure 20.5. It is clear from this diagram that once the inflammatory response has developed and tissue damage has occurred, changes in intracellular cyclic nucleotide levels will vary from cell to cell. Thus phagocytic cells would exhibit low cAMP levels, synovial and bone

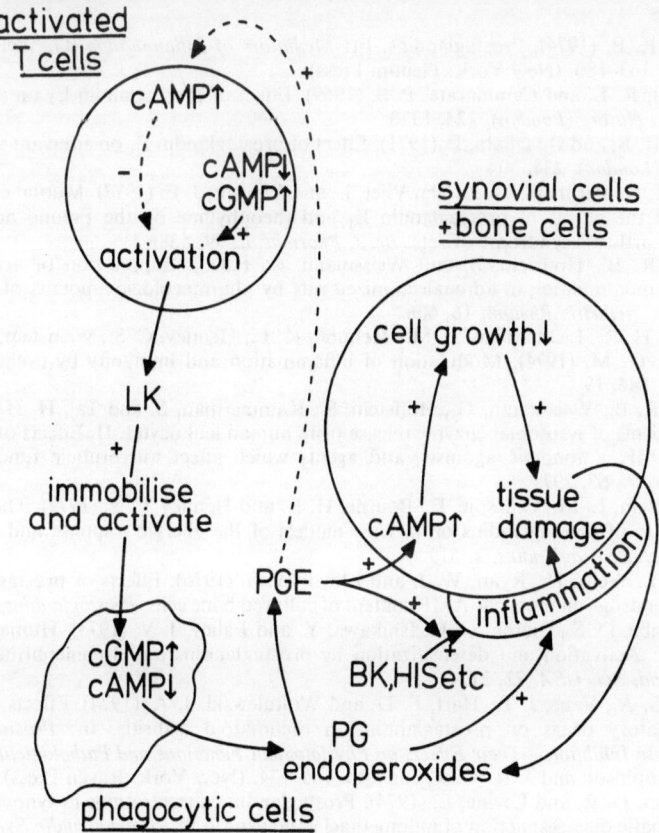

Figure 20.5 Probable interactions between PGs and cyclic nucleotides in chronic inflamed joints

cells might have high cAMP levels and lymphocyte cAMP levels might vary, depending on the extent of inhibition by PGE. This would explain why during the later development of adjuvant arthritis, around day 22, gross cAMP levels in the paws of rats could not be correlated with inflammatory symptoms. It is possible that cyclic nucleotide levels in either the spleen, lymph nodes or circulating lymphocytes would give an accurate reflection of the development of the disease. In this context, Ryzewski & Roszkowski-Sliz[34] found that adenylate cyclase activity in lymph node lymphocytes from day 15 arthritic rats was higher than in normal animals. To what extent endogenous PGs are involved in modulating lymphocyte cyclic nucleotide levels remains to be determined.

Acknowledgements

We thank Dr. D. H. Nugteren of Unilever Research Laboratories, Vlaardingen for a gift of PGE_1. This work was supported by a grant from the Nederlandse Vereniging tot Rheumatiekbestrijding.

References

1. Zurier, R. B. (1974). Prostaglandins. In: *Mediators of Inflammation* (G. Weissmann, ed.) pp. 163–180. (New York: Plenum Press)
2. Aspinall, R. L. and Cammarata, P. S. (1969). Effect of prostaglandin E_2 on adjuvant arthritis. *Nature (London)*, **224,** 1320
3. Zurier, R. B. and Quagliata, F. (1971). Effect of prostaglandin E_1 on adjuvant arthritis. *Nature (London)*, **234,** 304
4. Bonta, I. L., Parnham, M. J., Van Vliet, L. and Vincent, J. E. (1977). Mutual enhancement of the effects of prostaglandin E_1 and theophylline on the Freund adjuvant-induced arthritis syndrome of rats. *Br. J. Pharmacol.*, **59,** 438P
5. Zurier, R. B., Hoffstein, S. and Weissmann, G. (1973). Suppression of acute and chronic inflammation in adrenalectomized rats by pharmacologic amounts of prostaglandins. *Arthritis Rheum.*, **16,** 606
6. Bourne, H. R., Lichtenstein, L. M., Melmon, K. L., Henney, C. S., Weinstein, Y. and Shearer, G. M. (1974). Modulation of inflammation and immunity by cyclic AMP. *Science*, **184,** 19
7. Zurier, R. B., Weissmann, G., Hoffstein, S., Kammerman, S. and Tai, H. H. (1974). Mechanisms of lysosomal enzyme release from human leukocytes. II. Effects of cAMP and cGMP, autonomic agonists, and agents which affect microtubule function. *J. Clin. Invest.*, **53,** 297
8. Lichtenstein, L. M., Gillespie, E., Bourne, H. R. and Henney, C. S. (1972). The effects of a series of prostaglandins on *in vitro* models of the allergic response and cellular immunity. *Prostaglandins*, **2,** 519
9. Yu, J. H., Wells, H., Ryan, W. J. and Lloyd, W. S. (1976). Effects of prostaglandins and other drugs on the cyclic AMP content of cultured bone cells. *Prostaglandins*, **12,** 501
10. Newcombe, D. S., Ciosek, C. P., Ishikawa, Y. and Fahey, J. V. (1975). Human synoviocytes: Activation and desensitization by prostaglandins and 1-epinephrine. *Proc. Nat. Acad. Sci. USA*, **72,** 3124
11. Higgs, G. A., Vane, J. T., Hart, F. D. and Wojtulewski, J. A. (1974). Effects of anti-inflammatory drugs on prostaglandins in rheumatoid arthritis. In: *Prostaglandin Synthetase Inhibitors—Their Effects on Physiological Functions and Pathological States.* (H. J. Robinson and J. R. Vane, eds.) pp. 165–174. (New York: Raven Press)
12. Robinson, D. R. and Levine, L. (1974). Prostaglandin concentrations in synovial fluid in rheumatic diseases: action of indomethacin and aspirin. In: *Prostaglandin Synthetase Inhibitors—Their Effects on Physiological Functions and Pathological States.* (H. J. Robinson and J. R. Vane, eds.) pp. 223–228. (New York: Raven Press)

13. Robinson, D. R., McGuire, M. B. and Levine, L. (1975). Prostaglandins in the rheumatic diseases. *Ann. N.Y. Acad. Sci. USA*, **256**, 318
14. Franklin, T. J. and Foster, S. J. (1973). Leakage of cyclic AMP from human diploid fibroblasts in tissue culture. *Nature New Biol.*, **246**, 119
15. Gemsa, D., Steggemann, L., Meuzel, J. and Till, G. (1975). Release of cyclic AMP from macrophages by stimulation with prostaglandins. *J. Immunol.*, **114**, 1422
16. Chlapowski, F. J., Kelly, L. A. and Butcher, R. W. (1975). Cyclic nucleotides in cultured cells. *Adv. Cyclic Nucl. Res.*, **6**, 245
17. Ignarro, J. L. and Slywka, J. (1972). Changes in liver lysosomal fragility, erythrocyte membrane stability, and local and systemic lysosomal enzyme levels in adjuvant-induced polyarthritis. *Biochem. Pharmacol.*, **21**, 875
18. Weissmann, G. (1972). Discussion. In: *Prostaglandins in Cellular Biology* (P. W. Ramwell and B. B. Pharriss, eds.) p. 172. (New York: Plenum Press)
19. Morley, J. (1974). Prostaglandins and lymphokines in arthritis. *Prostaglandins*, **8**, 315
20. Gordon, D., Bray, M. A. and Morley, J. (1976). Control of lymphokine secretion by prostaglandins. *Nature (London)*, **262**. 401
21. Ferraris, V. A. and De Rubertis, F. R. (1974). *J. Clin. Invest.*, **54**, 378
22. Schreiner, G. F. and Unanue, E. R. (1975). The modulation of spontaneous and anti-Ig-stimulated motility of lymphocytes by cyclic nucleotides and adrenergic and cholinergic agents. *J. Immunol.*, **114**, 802
23. Hadden, J. W., Hadden, E. M., Johnson, L. D. and Johnson, E. M. (1975). Cyclic nucleotides in lymphocyte function and metabolism. In: *Lymphocytes and their Interactions* (R. C. Williams, ed.) pp. 27–55. (New York: Raven Press)
24. Goldberg, N. D., Haddox, M. K., Dunham, E., Lopez, C. and Hadden, J. W. (1974). The Yin-Yang hypothesis of biological control: Opposing influences of cyclic GMP and cyclic AMP in the regulation of cell proliferation and other biological processes. In: *Control of Proliferation in Animals Cells* (B. Clarkson and R. Baserga, eds.) (New York: Cold Spring Harbor Press)
25. Stastny, P., Cooke, T. D. and Ziff, M. (1973). Production of a macrophage migration inhibitory factor in rabbits with experimental arthritis. *Clin. Exp. Immunol.*, **14**, 141
26. Stastny, P., Rosenthal, M., Andreis, M. and Ziff, M. (1975). Lymphokines in the rheumatoid joint. *Arthritis Rheum.*, **18**, 237
27. Pick, E. and Turk, J. L. (1972). *Clin. Exp. Immunol.*, **10**, 1
28. Higgs, G. A., McCall, E. and Youlten, L. J. F. (1975). A chemotactic role for prostaglandins released from polymorphonuclear leucocytes during phagocytosis. *Br. J. Pharmacol.*, **53**, 539
29. Weissmann, G., Goldstein, I. and Hoffstein, S. (1976). Prostaglandins and the modulation by cyclic nucleotides of lysosomal enzyme release. In: *Advances in Prostaglandin and Thromboxane Research* (B. Samuelsson and R. Paoletti, eds.) Vol. 2, pp. 803–814. (New York: Raven Press)
30. Kaley, G. and Weiner, R. (1971). Prostaglandin E: A potential mediator of the inflammatory response. *Ann. N.Y. Acad. Sci.*, **180**, 338
31. Velo, G. P., Dunn, C. J., Giroud, J. P., Timsit, J. and Willoughby, D. A. (1973). Distribution of prostaglandins in inflammatory exudate. *J. Pathol.*, **111**, 149
32. Kuehl, F. A., Humes, J. L., Egan, R. W., Ham, E. A., Beveridge, G. C. and van Arman, C. G. (1977). Role of prostaglandin endoperoxide PGG_2 in inflammatory processes. *Nature (London)*, **265**, 170
33. Ferreira, S. H. and Vane, J. R. (1974). New aspects of the mode of action of non-steroid anti-inflammatory drugs. *Ann. Rev. Pharmacol.* **14**, 57
34. Ryzewski, J. and Roszkowski-Sliz, W. (1974). The influence of cysteine on adenyl cyclase activity in rat lymphocytes. *Arch. Immunol. Ther. Exp.*, **22**, 619
35. Gilman, A. G. (1970). A protein binding assay for adenosine 3′; 5′-cyclic monophosphate. *Proc. Nat. Acad. Sci., USA*, **67**, 305
36. Perper, R. J., Sanda, M., Stecher, V. J. and Oronsky, A. L. (1975). Physiologic and pharmacologic alterations of rat leukocyte chemotaxis (Cx) *in vivo. Ann. N.Y. Acad. Acad. Sci.*, **256**, 190
37. Rocha e Silva, M. and Antonio, A. (1960). Release of bradykinin and the mechanism of production of thermic edema in the rat's paw. *Med. Exp.*, **3**, 371

Discussion 20

J. Westwick: (UK)	In the first slide did Dr. Parnham show a significant difference between cyclic AMP levels at Day 15 to the earlier days? Was there a significant difference?
Parnham:	The changes during the chronic spate? There was a significant difference on Day 14 and Day 18, compared to the Day 22 controls. Unfortunately we were not able to get sufficient animals from the suppliers in one group, other than to do the controls on Day 22, so we decided to do them on Day 22, which was the maximum response. Because there is no inflammation in these controls we assumed that it would be the same throughout the period. There is no indication why that should not be. Certainly on Day 14 and Day 18 there was a very significant decrease in cyclic AMP, when compared with these controls.
Westwick:	Am I right in thinking that the controls were only two animals?
Parnham:	I did not put any significance on that because there were only two animals on Day 10. These were preliminary results. We have to get some more results on Day 10 before I can say whether there is a significant effect there. It looks as though there is no significant difference on Day 10, compared with the controls.
D. Roos: (The Netherlands)	I presume that the cyclic AMP was measured in the fluid phase of the filtrate. Was there any indication of an equilibrium between the cyclic AMP level in the cells in the joint and the fluid that was measured?
Parnham:	Since these experiments have been done we have looked at cells in perfusates (another series of experiments that we are doing). There are cells in the perfusates. Presumably when we extracted the cyclic AMP we were actually measuring extra-cellular and intra-cellular cyclic AMP levels. That was the point of the experiment. It was supposed to be a blunderbuss. We actually looked at the gross cyclic AMP levels and not at any one particular cellular population.
Roos:	And is anything known about the stability of the cyclic AMP in the fluid?
Parnham:	No. We certainly did recovery experiments, and extraction, and the recovery of cyclic AMP added to the fluid was something like 70%.
Z. M. Bacq: (Belgium)	Only PGE_1 has been used. What about PGE_2, which seems to be quantitatively more important in the organism and has very different actions in certain respects?
Parnham:	That is quite an important question. When the anti-inflammatory effects of PGE were first shown PGE_2 was used. In work published in 1972 (*Proceedings of the National Academy of Science*) it was shown that both PGE_1 and PGE_2 have anti-inflammatory effects on adjuvant arthritis. It so happens that PGE_1, used as a drug, is more effective than PGE_2, but certainly when looking at endogenous prostaglandins then PGE_2 is likely to be most important.

21

The time course of the vascular events associated with inflammation due to ultraviolet irradiation of guinea pig ears

D. F. WOODWARD AND D. A. A. OWEN (UK)

INTRODUCTION

A variety of inflammatory stimuli of moderate intensity elicit biphasic permeability and erythema responses[1-3]. The time course of the biphasic permeability and erythema responses produced by ultraviolet (UV) injury were described by Logan and Wilhelm[4]. Permeability was measured by assessing the colour-intensity of the exuded Evans Blue dye in the inflammatory lesion and the erythema was assessed visually. Gupta and Levy[5] measured the permeability changes more precisely by injecting ^{131}I-radiolabelled human serum albumin intravenously at various intervals after exposure to UV radiation and expressed permeability in units of c.p.m./g of dry wt. However, erythema was again assessed visually. In an attempt to quantify the erythema response, it was decided to measure skin temperature. Differences in temperature between irradiated and non-irradiated skin on the flank are very small[6] which makes it difficult to quantify the erythema response. However, marked differences in cutaneous temperature were observed between irradiated and non-irradiated ears and consequently, the whole ear was chosen as the site to be irradiated. Furthermore, using the ears eliminates the need to depilate the skin.

The present studies were undertaken to follow the time course of the development of (a) the biphasic permeability response, (b) the biphasic erythema response, and (c) the oedema produced by mild UV injury. In addition, the primary and secondary phases of the erythema and permeability responses and the oedema have been quantified.

METHODS

Conscious, male, albino guinea pigs housed in individual cages with free access to food and water were used. The environmental temperature was maintained at 22 ± 1 °C.

A Kromayer model 10 lamp, emitting mainly radiation of wavelength 365 nm, was used as the source of UV rays. Infra-red radiation was filtered out by circulating water. The back of one ear of each animal was irradiated by placing it in light contact with the UV lamp for 30 s; the other ear served as a control.

The cutaneous temperature of the ears was measured by means of a Light Laboratories electric thermometer utilizing a 'surface touch on' probe. The probe was applied to the ears at sufficient pressure to just physically move each ear and was left there until the recorded temperature remained constant. The time course of the erythema response was obtained by measuring cutaneous temperature at various intervals after UV radiation.

The time course of the permeability response was evaluated by injecting ^{51}Cr labelled erythrocytes and ^{125}I labelled human serum albumin intravenously at appropriate times 30 min before the animals were sacrificed. Both ears were then removed, weighed and counted in a gamma counter

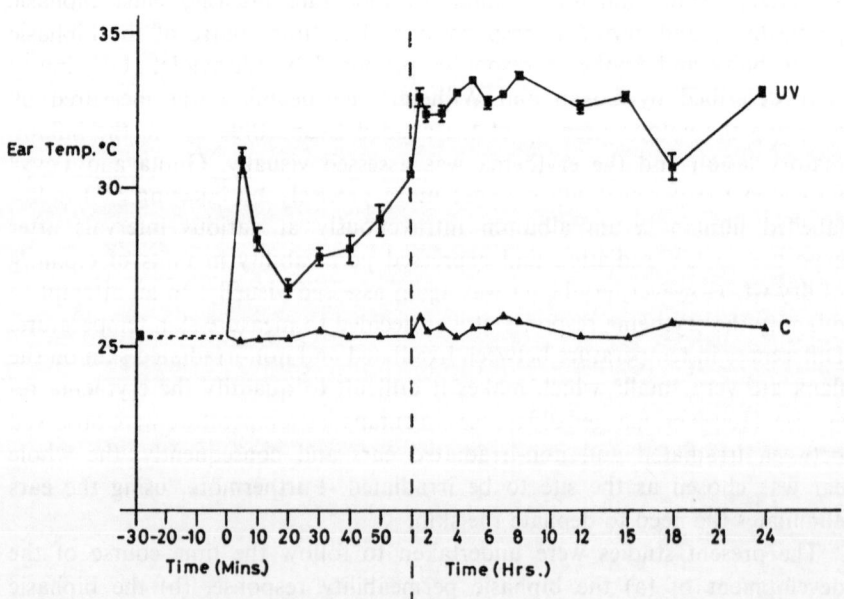

Figure 21.1   Time course of ear temperature changes. The temperature of the irradiated ears (■———■) increased in a biphasic manner after UV injury. The temperature of the non-irradiated ears (▲———▲) remained unchanged

together with 1 ml of venous blood. The ears were then dried to constant weight in a vacuum oven. Drying and using 1 ml of venous blood as a reference enabled blood content, total albumin content and consequently, extravascular albumin content to be expressed in units of ml/g dry weight of tissue.

The time course of the oedema response was obtained by calculating the total water content (g water/g dry wt. tissue) at the time of sacrifice.

RESULTS AND DISCUSSION

The erythema response

Figure 21.1 shows the time course of the ear temperature changes. There was an initial rapid increase in ear temperature, which declined but then gradually increased to reach a maximum at 90 min after irradiation.

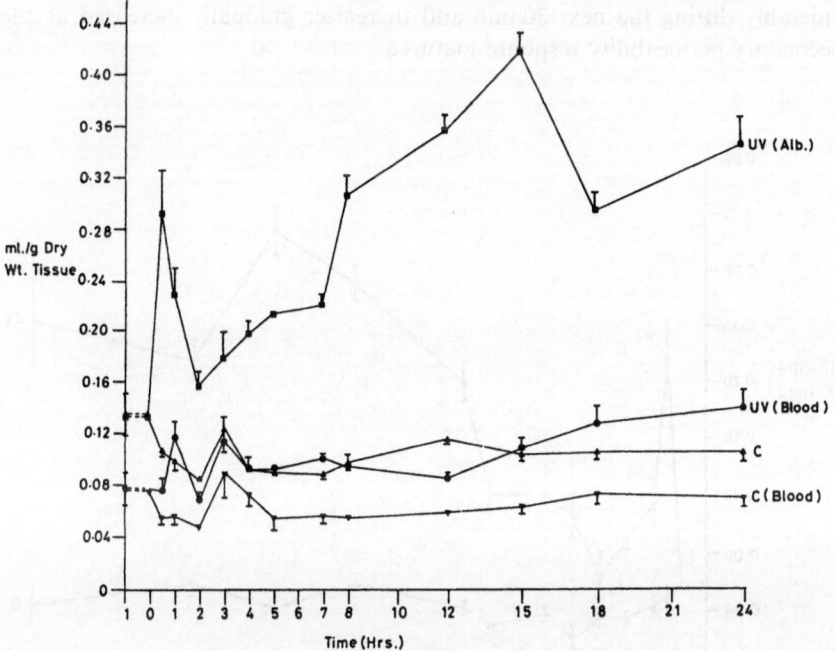

Figure 21.2 Time course of blood content and permeability changes. Total albumin content in the irradiated ears (■————■) exhibited a considerable biphasic increase whereas total albumin content in the non-irradiated ears (▲————▲) and blood content in the irradiated ears (●————●) and non-irradiated ears (▼————▼) showed no marked change

The permeability response

Figure 21.2 shows the time course of the blood content and permeability changes. Total albumin content in the irradiated ears increased considerably in a biphasic manner whereas changes in total albumin content in the non-irradiated ears and blood content in both ears were comparatively small. By subtraction of the blood content in the irradiated ears from the total albumin content in the irradiated ears, the extravascular albumin content in the irradiated ears was obtained. Likewise, the extravascular albumin content in the control ears was calculated.

Figure 21.3 shows the time course of the permeability changes measured as the extravascular albumin which accumulates in the 30 min period prior to each of the points. The permeability response was biphasic, the secondary permeability response being later in onset and more gradual than the secondary increase in ear temperature.

Figure 21.4 shows the time course of the development of the oedema response. There was no obvious biphasic response. Water content did not increase during the first 30 min of the inflammatory response although permeability at this stage was high. However, water content increased considerably during the next 30 min and thereafter gradually increased as the secondary permeability response matured.

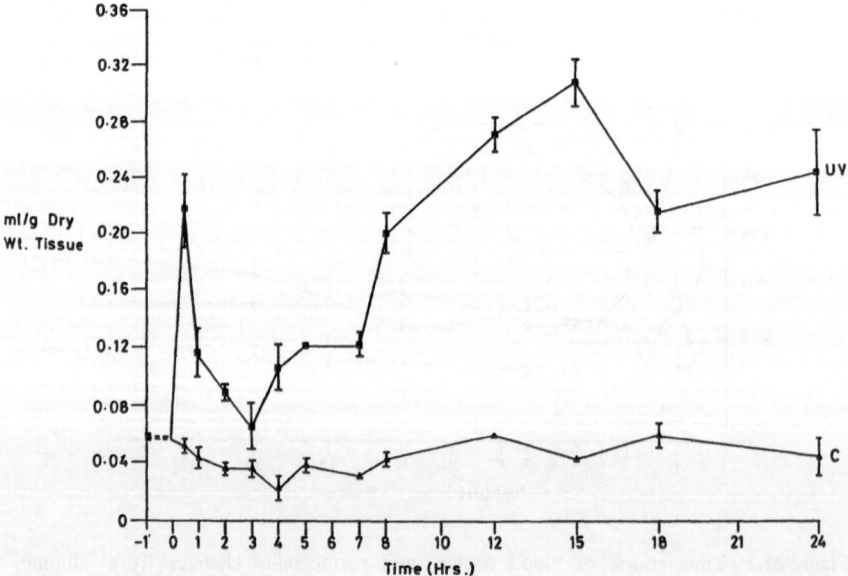

Figure 21.3 Time course of permeability changes. Extravascular albumin in the irradiated ears (■————■) accumulated in a biphasic manner. There was no change in extravascular albumin content in the non-irradiated ears (▲————▲)

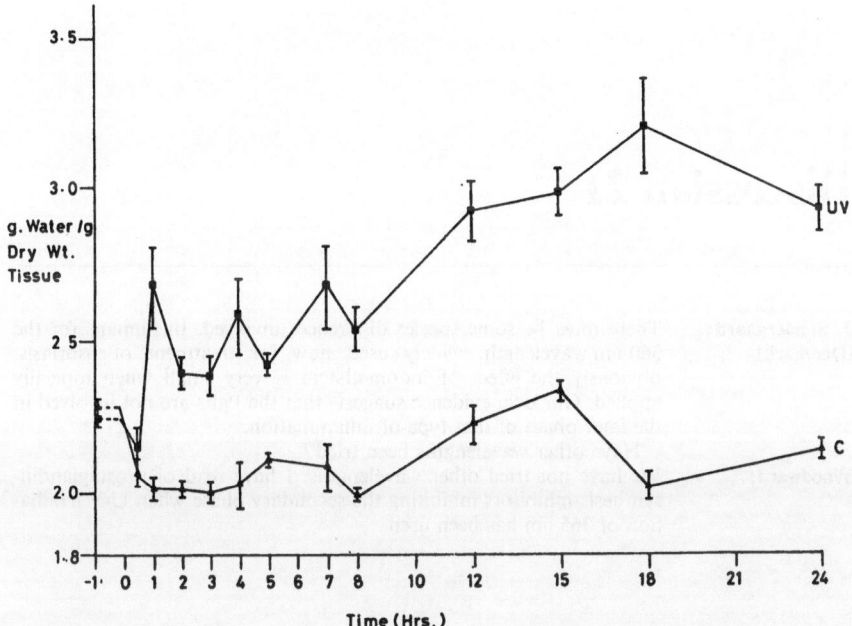

Figure 21.4 Time course of water content changes. Water content does not increase until 1 h after injury (irradiated ears (■————■) and subsequently gradually increases as the permeability response matures. The water content of the non-irradiated ears does (▲————▲) not change significantly

These experiments confirm that mild UV injury of guinea pig ears produces a biphasic erythema response, a biphasic permeability response and oedema; Logan and Wilhelm[7] obtained qualitatively similar results, although they did not accurately quantify the changes in these parameters.

References

1. Wilhelm, D. L. and Mason, B. (1960). Vascular permeability changes in inflammation. *Br. J. Exp. Pathol.*, **41**, 487
2. Steele, R. H. and Wilhelm, D. L. (1966). The inflammatory reaction in chemical injury. *Br. J. Exp. Pathol.*, **47**, 612
3. Vinegar, R., Schreiber, W. and Hugo, R. (1969). Biphasic development of carrageenan oedema in rats. *J. Pharmacol. Exp. Ther.*, **166**, 96
4. Logan, G. and Wilhelm, D. L. (1966). The inflammatory reaction in ultraviolet injury. *Br. J. Exp. Pathol.*, **47**, 286
5. Gupta, N. and Levy, L. (1973). Delayed manifestation of ultraviolet reaction in the guinea pig caused by anti-inflammatory drugs. *Br. J. Pharmacol.*, **47**, 240
6. Lambelin, G., Vassart-Thys, D. and Roba, J. (1971). Cutaneous thermometry for topical therapy evaluation of U.V. erythema in the guinea pig. *Arzneim. Forsch.*, **21**, 44
7. Logan, G. and Wilhelm, D. L. (1966). Vascular permeability changes in inflammation. *Br. J. Exp. Pathol.*, **47**, 300

Discussion 21

J. Sondergaard:
(Denmark)

There must be some species differences involved. In humans for the 360 nm wavelength, widely used now for treatment of psoriasis, obviously the effect of indomethacin is very small when topically applied. Our own evidence suggests that the PgEs are not involved in the later phase of that type of inflammation.

Have other wavelengths been tried?

Woodward:

We have not tried other wavelengths. I have read of prostaglandin-synthesis-inhibitors inhibiting the secondary phase when U-V irradiation of 365 nm has been used.

22

Role of macrophages in D-penicillamine-induced stimulation of DNA synthesis in lymph node cells

E. ARRIGONI-MARTELLI, L. BINDERUP, E. BRAMM (Denmark)

Abbreviations used: LNC: lymph node cells
Con A: Concanavalin A
PHA: phytohaemagglutinin P
LPS: lipopolysaccharide
^{3}H-TdR: [^{3}H]thymidine

In a previous paper[1] we have shown that rat lymph node cells (LNC) were stimulated to mitosis and their response to Con A potentiated by preincubation with such drugs as D-penicillamine and levamisole, reported to stimulate the cellular immune response[2,5].

In this paper we extend these observations and present data showing that the presence of macrophages is required for the D-penicillamine induced enhancement of DNA synthesis in lymphocytes.

METHODS

Lymphocytes were obtained from Lewis rat lymph nodes and cultured as already described[1]. Briefly, lymphocyte suspensions of 10^6 cells/ml were cultured in RPMI 1640, supplemented with 10% FCS, 2 mM glutamine, 100 units/ml penicillin and 100 μg/ml streptomycin. D-penicillamine or levamisole was added with or without mitogens for the whole period of culture (48 h, direct assay) or during a preincubation period of 24 h, after which the cells were washed and reincubated for 48 h with or without mitogens.

The mitogens used were Con A (1 μg/ml, Sigma, Grade IV), PHA (50 μg/ml, Difco) and LPS (10 μg/ml, *E. coli* 005:B5, Difco). DNA-synthesis

295

was measured by the uptake of [^{3}H]thymidine, 1 μCi/ml added 4 h before the end of incubation.

Lymph node cells depleted of adherent cells were obtained from lympho-cyte suspensions of 3×10^6 cells/ml, incubated for 24 h on glass Petri dishes at 37 °C. Non-adherent cells were collected from the Petri dishes, washed twice in culture medium and resuspended at a concentration of 10^6 cells/ml (more than 95 % viable cells).

Syngeneic macrophages were obtained by injection of 10 ml of sterile saline into the peritoneal cavity. The abdomen was gently massaged and the cells collected from the cavity were washed and resuspended in culture medium at a concentration of 0.6×10^6 cells/ml. After incubation for 24 h in glass culture tubes (1 ml/tube, 37 °C), in the presence of D-penicillamine when indicated, the non-adherent cells were removed by two washes. 10^6 depleted lymphocytes were added to the remaining adherent cells (0.2×10^6). The cultures were then incubated for 48 h with or without addition of differ-ent mitogens.

RESULTS AND DISCUSSION

The culture of rat LNC for 48 h in presence of D-penicillamine resulted in a significant increase of the basal ^{3}H-TdR incorporation and in a significant decrease of the LPS-stimulated ^{3}H-TdR uptake. The responsiveness of the LNC to Con A and PHA was not significantly modified. In similar experi-mental conditions levamisole increased ($p < 0.05$) the basal ^{3}H-TdR uptake and the responsiveness to Con A and PHA, leaving unaffected the LPS-induced stimulation. The LNC preincubated for 24 h with D-penicillamine

Table 22.1 Basal and mitogen stimulated ^{3}H-TdR incorporation in rat LNC: effects of D-penicillamine and levamisole

(A) Direct assay
(B) Preincubation assay

	Basal	Con A (1 μg/ml)	PHA (50 μg/ml)	LPS (10 μg/ml)
(A)				
D-penicillamine				
500 μg/ml	1.46*	0.87	0.98	0.64*
Levamisole				
25 μg/ml	1.69*	1.81*	1.34*	1.29
(B)				
D-penicillamine				
500 μg/ml	1.87*	1.85*	1.69*	4.47*
Levamisole				
25 μg/ml	1.51*	1.69*	1.76*	1.19

The results are expressed as the ratio of ^{3}H-TdR incorporated (d.p.m./10^6 cells) by treated/ control cultures. Triplicate cultures of 3–5 experiments.
* $p < 0.05$.

showed a significantly increased basal and mitogen stimulated ^{3}H-TdR incorporation. Preincubation with levamisole had no effect on LPS-stimulated cultures whereas it had an effect qualitatively similar to that observed in the direct assay on basal, Con A- and PHA-stimulated DNA synthesis (Table 22.1).

An important qualitative difference between D-penicillamine and levamisole is apparent from these results. The response of LNC to LPS—which besides directly stimulating B-lymphocytes[6] has also some biological effects on T-cells[7,8]—is unmodified by levamisole whereas it is markedly affected, particularly in the preincubation assay, by D-penicillamine.

We have already described[1] that the effects of D-penicillamine on Con A-stimulated LNC are concentration dependent only in the preincubation assay, but not in the direct assay. As shown in Figure 22.1 the same was true for PHA and LPS stimulated cultures. As we[1] and others[9] have demonstrated the inhibitory effect of D-penicillamine on ^{3}H-TdR uptake only takes place when it is added before or simultaneously with the stimulant. Addition of D-penicillamine after the stimulation is ineffective. It seems therefore that more or less pronounced inhibition of mitogen stimulation observed in the direct assay might depend on a nonspecific interference of D-penicillamine with the binding of mitogen to lymphocyte membrane. If this hypothesis is correct the enhancement of DNA synthesis induced by D-penicillamine in conditions where any non-specific interference can be excluded—as in preincubation assay—might be dependent on a stimulatory influence on a

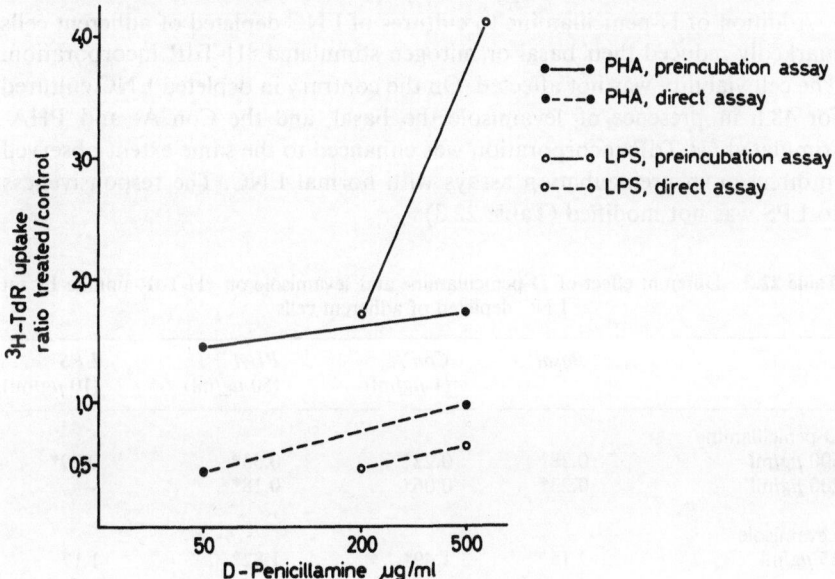

Figure 22.1 Effect of different concentrations of D-penicillamine on LPS- and PHA-induced DNA synthesis in direct or in preincubation assay

discrete cell population present in LNC. Candidates for the role as target cells might be the macrophages ('adherent cells') representing approximately 20% of the total LNC. Several evidences suggest that the adherent cells, or factors released by them, either in basal or stimulated conditions interfere with the mitotic response of lymphocytes[10-15].

To test this hypothesis the effects of D-penicillamine and levamisole have been evaluated in LNC depleted of macrophages ('adherent cells'). Preliminary experiments (Table 22.2) showed that the depletion did not

Table 22.2 Influence of depletion of adherent cells on basal and mitogen-stimulated ^{3}H-TdR incorporation in rat LNC

Basal	Con A (1 μg/ml)	PHA (50 μg/ml)	LPS (10 μg/ml)
1.14	0.98	1.83*	3.31*

See footnotes Table 22.1.

* $p < 0.05$.

modify the basal and Con A-stimulated ^{3}H-TdR incorporation but resulted in a substantial increase of PHA- and LPS-stimulated DNA synthesis. In slightly different experimental conditions the removal of adherent cells has been found to reduce the responsiveness of LNC to PHA[13] but to enhance, in agreement with our findings, the responsiveness to LPS[14].

Addition of D-penicillamine to cultures of LNC depleted of adherent cells markedly reduced their basal or mitogen stimulated ^{3}H-TdR incorporation. The cell viability was not affected. On the contrary in depleted LNC cultured for 48 h in presence of levamisole the basal, and the Con A- and PHA-stimulated ^{3}H-TdR incorporation was enhanced to the same extent observed in direct or in preincubation assays with normal LNC. The responsiveness to LPS was not modified (Table 22.3).

Table 22.3 Different effect of D-penicillamine and levamisole on ^{3}H-TdR uptake by rat LNC depleted of adherent cells

	Basal	Con A (1 μg/ml)	PHA (50 μg/ml)	LPS (10 μg/ml)
D-penicillamine				
500 μg/ml	0.38*	0.22*	0.53*	0.29*
200 μg/ml	0.23*	0.06*	0.18*	—
Levamisole				
25 μg/ml	2.15*	1.49*	1.82*	1.17

See footnotes Table 22.1.

* $p < 0.05$.

The removal of adherent cells thus reversed the stimulatory effect of D-penicillamine observed in preincubation assay and greatly potentiated the inhibitory effect observed in direct assay. This finding suggest as a likely possibility that D-penicillamine activates adherent cells, probably macrophages, present in normal LNC. The activated macrophages are in turn able to stimulate the DNA synthesis in lymphocytes, a phenomenon repeatedly described in several different experimental situations[11,12,14,15]. The consequence of this activation is the enhancement of ^{3}H-TdR uptake in the preincubation assay and the suppression of the non-specific inhibitory influence on lymphocytes in direct assay.

Further support to this hypothesis is provided by experiments where the responsiveness to Con A was assessed in depleted LNC reconstituted in ratio 5:1 with syngeneic purified peritoneal macrophages preincubated for 24 h with D-penicillamine (Figure 22.2). In these experimental conditions the response to Con A is potentiated approximately to the same extent observed in preincubation assay with unfractionated LNC.

A number of experiments have suggested that macrophages play a significant role in the specific and non-specific responses of B- and T-lymphocytes[10-15] and that the majority, if not all, of the non-specific immune

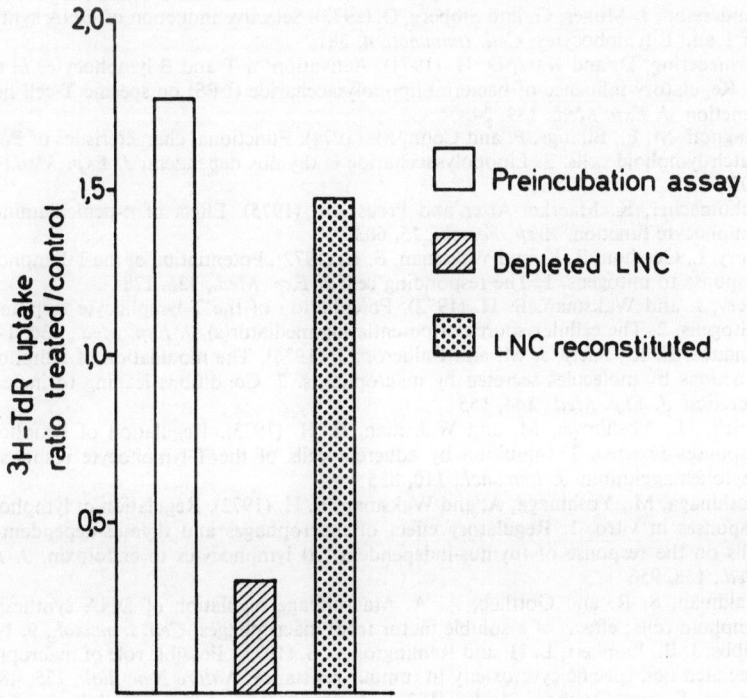

Figure 22.2 Effect of reconstitution of depleted LNC with peritoneal macrophages preincubated with 500 μg/ml of D-penicillamine on Con A-stimulated DNA synthesis

stimulants function as macrophage activators, among other activities[16-20]. The present experiments suggest that macrophages are instrumental in the influence of D-penicillamine on the basal and mitogen-stimulated lymphocyte DNA-synthesis, whereas they are inert bystanders of similar activity of levamisole.

Acknowledgements

The authors wish to thank Ms. E. Greve Pedersen and Ms. U. L. Christiansen for their valuable technical assistance.

References

1. Binderup, L., Bramm, E. and Arrigoni-Martelli, E. (1977). Effects of antirheumatics on lymphocyte culture—tissue reactions. (In press)
2. Arrigoni-Martelli, E., Bramm, E., Huskisson, E. C., Willoughby D. A. and Dieppe, P. A. (1976). Pertussis vaccine edema: an experimental model for the action of Penicillamine-like drugs. *Agents Actions*, **6**, 613
3. Dieppe, P. A., Willoughby, D. A., Huskisson, E. C. and Arrigoni-Martelli, E. (1976). Pertussis vaccine pleurisy: a model of delayed hypersensitivity. *Agents Actions*, **6**, 618
4. Arrigoni-Martelli, E. and Bramm, E. (1976). Development of models for penicillamine-like drugs. *Rheumatol. Rehabil.*, **15**, 207
5. Renoux, G. and Renoux, M. (1974). Modulation of immune reactivity by phenylimidothiazole salts in mice immunized by sheep red blood cells. *J. Immunol.*, **113**, 779
6. Andersson, J. Möller, G. and Sjöberg, O. (1972). Selective induction of DNA synthesis in T and B lymphocytes. *Cell. Immunol.*, **4**, 381
7. Armedering, D. and Katz, D. H. (1974). Activation of T and B lymphocytes *in vitro*. 1. Regulatory influence of bacterial lipopolysaccharide (LPS) on specific T-cell helper function. *J. Exp. Med.*, **139**, 24
8. Kagnoff, M. F., Billings, P. and Cohn, M. (1974). Functional characteristics of Peyer's patch lymphoid cells. 2. Lipopolysaccharide is thymus dependent. *J. Exp. Med.*, **139**, 407
9. Schumacher, K. Maerker-Alzer and Preuss, R. (1975). Effect of D-penicillamine on lymphocyte function. *Arzn. Forsch.*, **25**, 603
10. Gery, I., Gershon, R. K. and Waksman, B. H. (1972). Potentiation of the T-lymphocyte response to mitogens. 1. The responding cell. *J. Exp. Med.*, **136**, 128
11. Gery, I. and Waksman, B. H. (1972). Potentiation of the T-lymphocyte response to mitogens. 2. The cellular source of potentiating mediator(s). *J. Exp. Med.*, **136**, 143
12. Unanue, E. R., Kiely, J. M. and Calderon, J. (1976). The modulation of lymphocyte functions by molecules secreted by macrophages. 2. Conditions leading to increased secretion. *J. Exp. Med.*, **144**, 155
13. Folch, H., Yoshinaga, M. and Waksman, B. H. (1973). Regulation of lymphocyte responses *in vitro*. 3. Inhibition by adherent cells of the T-lymphocyte response to phytohemagglutinin. *J. Immunol.*, **110**, 835
14. Yoshinaga, M., Yoshinaga, A. and Waksman, B. H. (1972). Regulation of lymphocyte responses in vitro. 1. Regulatory effect of macrophages and thymus-dependent (T) cells on the response of thymus-independent (B) lymphocytes to endotoxin. *J. Exp. Med.*, **136**, 956
15. Waldman, S. R. and Gottlieb, A. A. Macrophage regulation of DNA synthesis in lymphoid cells: effects of a soluble factor from macrophages. *Cell. Immunol.*, **9**, 142
16. Hibbs, J. B., Lambert, L. H. and Remington, J. S. (1973). Possible role of macrophage mediated non specific cytotoxicity in tumour resistance. *Nature New Biol.*, **235**, 48
17. Ariyan, S. and Gershon, R. K. (1973). Augmentation of the adoptive transfer of specific tumour immunity by non-specifically immunized macrophages. *J. Nat. Cancer Inst.*, **51**, 1145

18. Basic, J., Milas, C., Grdna, D. J. and Withers, H. R. (1975). *In vitro* destruction of tumour cells from mice treated with Corynebacterium granulosum. *J. Nat. Cancer Inst.*, **55**, 589
19. Mansell, P. W. A., Diluzio, N. R., MacNawee, R., Rowden, G. and Proctor J. W. (1976). Recognition factors and non-specific macrophage activation in the treatment of neoplastic disease. *Ann. N.Y. Ac. Sci.*, **277**, 20
20. Juy, D. and Chedid, L. (1975). Comparison between macrophage activation and enhancement of non-specific resistance to tumours by mycobacterial immunoadjuvants. *Proc. Nat. Acad. Sci. USA*, **72**, 4105

Discussion 22

G. P. Velo: (Italy)	Dr. Arrigoni-Martelli showed results with only one dosage of penicillamine. Dosages are important in this kind of experiment. Were there any experiments with lower dosages?
Arrigoni-Martelli:	Yes. In the reconstitution experiments we explored a range of dose from 100 to 500 μg/ml D-penicillamine and we found that at 100 μg/ml there was still a significant effect in this context.
T. L. Vischer: (Switzerland)	I am wondering about the culture system. There was a stimulation index of 2, 1½, and so on, which is unusually low in lymphocyte cultures. Could Dr. Arrigoni-Martelli comment. I am referring to stimulation with PHA and Con A. Most people get much more.
	Is it possible, from such experiments, to draw conclusions about the drugs that are added?
Arrigoni-Martelli:	The result reported here is a ratio between control and treated, and it is quite difficult to get the actual value from that. I do not remember the actual values of stimulation, but they were compatible with those reported in the literature.
	Secondly, the results are reported here as the mean of several experiments, and they were statistically evaluated. They are reported as a significant increase in the order of 0.05 level of significance.
P. Davies: (USA)	The dosage of penicillamine is a very high one, but I wondered whether, if the incubation time is prolonged before adding the mitogen, then the penicillamine might become more effective.
	Has that possibility been looked at?
Arrigoni-Martelli:	We selected doses ranging from 100 to 500 μg/ml and the viability of the cells was assessed and was in order. We have done other things, such as incubating lymphocytes for 48 h rather than for 24 h, and measuring the incorporation of thymidine 24 h later. In every instance the lymphocytes were incubated with penicillamine and then the culture medium was washed out. After 24-, 48- or 72-h cultures there is a substantial increase of thymidine incorporation.
	The essential point is that the lymphocytes have to be stimulated in some way with penicillamine, and then the penicillamine has to be removed in order to show such stimulation.
Davies:	I was trying to get at whether the penicillamine effect was at all time-dependent.
Arrigoni-Martelli:	I do not know. In some conditions. If prolonged incubation is meant, then I would say not.

23

Anti-inflammatory effects of tumour bearing

S. NORMANN AND E. SORKIN (USA)

INTRODUCTION

Macrophages are increasingly recognized as important effector cells against neoplastic growth[1]. *In vivo* macrophages comprise anywhere from 4 to 55% of the cells harvested from various tumours[2,3] and the histologic prominence of macrophages as a component of monocytic infiltrates is consonant with a better prognosis[1]. *In vitro* macrophages inhibit the incorporation of tritiated thymidine into the DNA of nearly all rapidly replicating cell lines (cytostatic reaction) and kill selectively those cells exhibiting abnormal growth characteristics (cytocidal reaction)[4-7]. For both cytostasis and cytotoxicity, appropriately activated macrophages are more effective than lymphocytes based on aggressor to target cell ratios and they are generally immunologically non-specific.

From *in vitro* studies, three parameters have emerged as essential for growth control by macrophages:

(1) an appropriate ratio of macrophages to tumour cells,

(2) contact between the target cell and the macrophage and

(3) the state of macrophage activation.

If these same parameters are important *in vivo*, the outcome of tumour growth would depend in large part on the host's ability to mobilize, activate, and distribute macrophages throughout the tumour. The purpose of the present report is to present evidence that the process of tumour bearing leads to a cell selective inhibition in monocyte inflammation. Because such a defect could alter the ratio and distribution of macrophage relative to tumour cells, it affords a mechanism by which neoplasms might escape growth regulation by the host.

1. GROWTH OF SUBCUTANEOUS TUMOURS IMPAIRS MONOCYTE INFLAMMATION

In 1972, Bernstein and co-workers[8] observed that guinea pigs with large intramuscular tumours have impaired delayed cutaneous hypersensitivity and decreased numbers of inflammatory cells in induced peritoneal exudates. These findings were confirmed by Eccles and Alexander[9] with two chemically induced tumours transplanted to syngeneic rats. Subsequently, we showed that the defect in monocyte inflammation during tumour bearing was selective for monocytes and that there was no defect in PMN responses[10]. Using a tumour induced by 7,12-dimethylbenz(a)anthracene (DMBA) transplanted to syngeneic DA strain rats, peritoneal exudates were induced at different time periods during tumour growth (Figure 23.1). The yield of exudate-induced macrophages decreased progressively as the tumour grew to complete suppression of macrophage inflammation with advanced malignancy. In contrast, the yield of PMN was normal and even increased in late stages of tumour bearing. This latter finding argues against the abnormality in monocyte inflammation reflecting debilitation of the tumour-bearing host. The generalized nature of the defect in monocyte inflammation during tumour bearing has now been established. It has been observed in experimental peritonitis in rats, mice, and guinea pigs with both chemically and virally induced neoplasms[8-11]. In addition, the defect is present not only in the peritoneal cavity but also in the tissues (Table 23.1).

Table 23.1 Subcutaneous tumour bearing impairs monocyte inflammation both in the peritoneal cavity and at a tissue site remote to the tumour

Experimental animal	Subcutaneously inserted filters: macrophages/oil immersion field	Peritoneal exudates (macrophages $\times$ 10^6)
Normal rat	215 ± 16	26 ± 3
Tumour-bearing rat	89 ± 11 (-59%)	4 ± 1 (-85%)

Data obtained 16 days after transplantation of DMBA induced fibrosarcoma to syngeneic DA strain rats. Data reported as mean $\pm$ standard error of the mean. Cellulose nitrate filters were removed 18 h after insertion. Peritoneal exudates were obtained 3 days after intraperitoneal peptone injection and the data corrected for macrophage yield of unstimulated peritoneal cavity.

Patients with malignancy have decreased chemotaxis of their circulating monocytes[12-14]. Similarly, macrophages obtained from the stimulated peritoneum of rats and mice bearing transplanted neoplasms are less responsive than normal macrophages in chemotaxis tests[10,11]. While the studies with circulating blood monocytes are best explained on the basis of an intrinsic defect in the chemotactic behaviour of the cells, the studies with peritoneal exudates can be interpreted differently. The resident macrophage

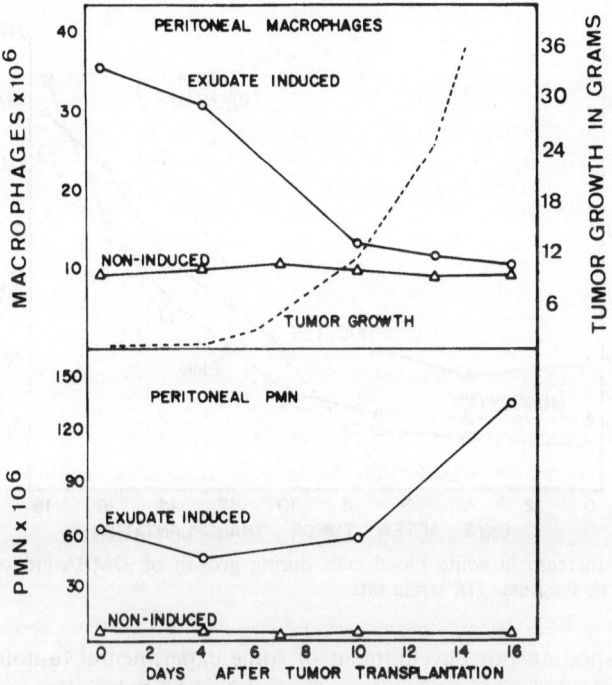

Figure 23.1 Yield of exudate-induced phagocytes during growth of DMBA induced sarcoma transplanted to syngeneic DA strain rats. Exudate-induced macrophages were harvested 3 days after intraperitoneal injection of sterile proteose peptone; exudate-induced PMN were obtained 9 h after sodium caseinate

population of the peritoneal cavity is not diminished by tumour bearing (Figure 23.1) and these cells are chemotactically a poorly responding population[10]. Accordingly, the decreased chemotactic response of macrophages harvested from tumour-bearing animals reflects a progressive shift in macrophage populations from one dominated by the high responding cells induced by inflammatory stimuli to one dominated by the relatively low responding resident cells.

Nevertheless, decreased chemotactic responsiveness of circulating blood monocytes appears to be a more plausible explanation for the decreased inflammatory response than sequestration of macrophages in the tumour[9]. In some but not all tumours, the defect can be demonstrated early after transplantation when the tumour is small (Figure 23.1) and in animals whose tumours contain relatively low numbers of macrophages[15]. In addition to the defect in blood monocyte chemotaxis demonstrated in human patients with malignancy, the decreased monocyte inflammatory response in experimental animals occurs despite an adequate and increasing number of monocytes in the blood (Figure 23.2). This monocytosis in experimental animals with transplanted malignancies[10,16,17] is unusual because such a phenomenon is not observed with most known human solid malignancies

305

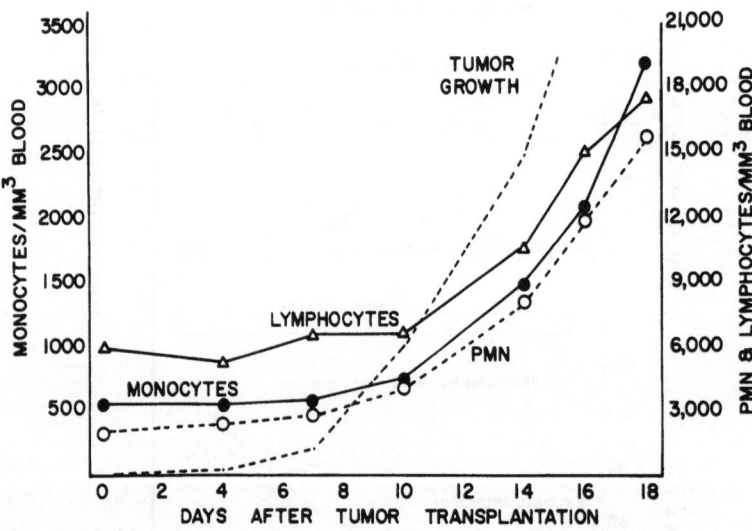

Figure 23.2 Increase in white blood cells during growth of DMBA-induced sarcoma transplanted to syngeneic DA strain rats

or during spontaneous development of some experimental tumours. Therefore, does the behaviour of monocytes in transplanted malignancies reflect that observed in spontaneous malignancies? Circulating monocytes in animals with transplanted malignancies do turn over faster than normal monocytes[8], but it is not certain why this should be so if the flux of monocytes into tumours has been compromised. Further evidence suggesting that circulating monocytes are altered during tumour bearing is the finding that tumour bearer sera are not defective in chemotactic attractants and such sera are not more inhibitory to monocyte chemotaxis than normal sera[10,15]. This latter observation does not exclude serum inhibitors to other monocyte functions. For example, North, Kirstein and Tuttle[18] report that sera of tumour-bearing mice do contain a low molecular weight factor which can be passively transferred to normal mice thereby inhibiting the capacity of the host macrophages to resist infection.

2. MONOCYTE INFLAMMATION AT THE TUMOUR SITE

If interactions between tumour cells and macrophages were to occur in tissues, then circulating monocytes present in the blood must be brought to the neoplasm. While division of macrophages may occur at the tissue level, evidence is overwhelmingly in favour of the proposition that most macrophages in inflammatory sites represent entering blood monocytes of bone marrow origin[19,20]. Our studies have shown that cultured tumour cells elaborate no factors which are chemotactic for macrophages although they produce weak attractants for PMN[21]. That thoracic duct drainage decreases the content of tumour macrophages[22] suggests that macrophages are attracted to the tumour by reaction of sensitized lymphocytes with tumour antigens. A lymphocyte dependent chemotactic factor for macrophages has been described[23].

While macrophages as well as lymphocytes exist in varying numbers (4–55%) around spontaneous autochthonous and transplanted syngeneic tumour masses[2,3], it is not clear whether these percentages were obtained during early or late stages of tumour growth. Accordingly, we have attempted to determine if the defect in macrophage inflammation in the peritoneal cavity correlated with a similar defect in the inflammatory response to the tumour.

For these experiments, we selected the methylcholanthrene (MCA) induced P-815 mastocytoma grown in ascites phase in syngeneic DBA/2 mice because the tumour and inflammatory cells could be obtained easily by washout of the peritoneal cavity. Figure 23.3 presents the yield of macrophages during tumour growth initiated by 5000 tumour cells. The macrophage yield increased during early tumour growth, reached a maximum

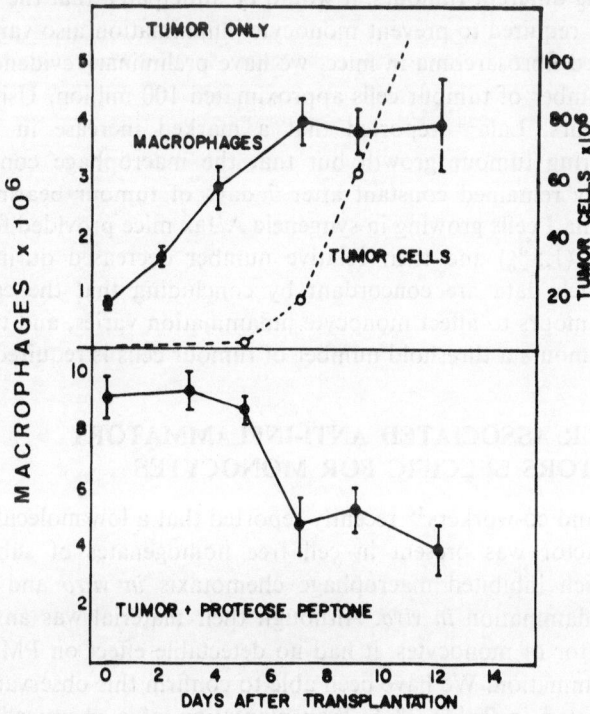

Figure 23.3 Yield of tumour associated macrophages during growth of P-815 mastocytomas compared to yield of macrophages in the tumour following injection of proteose peptone. Tumours were initiated by inoculating 5000 mastocytoma cells intraperitoneally into syngeneic DBA/2 mice

at day 7, and remained constant thereafter. When proteose peptone was injected into the peritoneal cavity during intraperitoneal growth of the tumour, a macrophage exudate was induced with the expected number of cells only during the first 5 days. By 7 days proteose peptone injection had no effect on the macrophage content of the growing tumour. When the inoculum was increased to 2 million tumour cells, growth of the tumour produced marginal macrophage inflammation and the response to proteose peptone was diminished by 3 days and completely suppressed by 5 days. Therefore, a defect in macrophage accumulation in the tumour did occur concurrently with the development of an impaired macrophage response to proteose peptone. Since impaired monocyte inflammation appeared related to the number of tumour cells transplanted, additional experiments established that the threshold number of tumour cells in this system was approximately 10 million.

If a threshold number of tumour cells must be achieved, the onset of impaired monocyte inflammation should vary with the size of the tumour inoculum. This was observed in the experiment with P-815 cells. Since the capacity of tumours to influence macrophage activities probably varies widely among different tumours, it would be anticipated that the number of tumour cells required to prevent monocyte inflammation also varies. In one MCA induced fibrosarcoma in mice, we have preliminary evidence that the threshold number of tumour cells approximated 100 million. Using Ehrlich ascites tumours, Lala[24] reported that a marked increase in leukocytes occurred during tumour growth but that the macrophage content while rising initially remained constant after 7 days of tumour bearing. Ascites phase Sarcoma I cells growing in syngeneic A/Jax mice provided few macrophages early (1.5%) and their relative number decreased during tumour growth[25]. Such data are concordant by concluding that the capacity of individual tumours to affect monocyte inflammation varies, and that within individual tumours a threshold number of tumour cells is required.

3. TUMOUR ASSOCIATED ANTI-INFLAMMATORY MEDIATORS SPECIFIC FOR MONOCYTES

Snyderman and co-workers[26] recently reported that a low molecular weight, dialysable factor was present in cell free homogenates of subcutaneous tumours which inhibited macrophage chemotaxis *in vitro* and depressed monocyte inflammation *in vivo*. Although their material was an extremely potent inhibitor of monocytes, it had no detectable effect on PMN chemotaxis or inflammation. We have been able to confirm this observation to the extent illustrated in Table 23.2. Transplantation of a chemically induced tumour in both rats and mice depressed macrophage inflammatory reactions in the peritoneum by approximately 70% and cell free homogenates of these tumours injected into non-tumour bearing animals were equally effective

Table 23.2 Effect on macrophage inflammatory response of tumour bearing compared to passive transfer of cell free tumour homogenate

	Peritoneal exudate (macrophages $\times$ 10^6)		
Subcutaneous tumour	Control	Tumour bearing	Tumour homogenate
DMBA induced fibrosarcoma (DA strain rat)	27	4 (-85%)	3 (-89%)
MCA induced fibrosarcoma (C5751/6 mouse)	9.7	3.1 (-68%)	2.4 (-75%)
MCA induced (P-815 mastocytoma (DBA/2 mouse)	8.2	9.9 $(+21\%)$	6.9 (-16%)

Peritoneal exudates were harvested 3 days after intraperitoneal (i.p.) injection of sterile proteose peptone. Tumour bearing animals were used 16–18 days after transplantation of 2×10^6 viable tumour cells to syngeneic animals. Tumour homogenates of similarly aged tumours were made using either sonication or mechanical disruption and were given intramuscularly at a dose equivalent of 50–150 million tumour cells 24 h prior to i.p. proteose peptone challenge. Data have been corrected for macrophage yield of the unstimulated peritoneal cavity.

in ablating the macrophage inflammatory response. On the other hand, P-815 mastocytoma cells which inhibited macrophage inflammation when transplanted intraperitenoally failed to do so when transplanted intramuscularly. Homogenates of this subcutaneous P-815 tumour also failed to inhibit monocyte inflammation. This latter observation underscores the limitations in our basic knowledge of the phenomenon and serves also to

Table 23.3 Inhibition of macrophage chemotaxis and inflammation by cell culture supernates*

	Inhibition of chemotaxis				Inhibition of inflammation§	
	Added to cells†		Added to attractant‡			
Culture supernate	% V/V	relative potency	Macrophages 4HPF	% Inhibition	Macrophages $\times$ 10^6	% Change
Medium only	1.56	1	501	—	41	—
3T3 fibroblasts	0.95	2	457	9	40	-2
SV-40 transformed 3T3 fibroblasts	0.029	54	375	25	not tested	
DMBA induced rat neoplasm	0.020	78	304	39	30	-39
Polyoma virus induced rat neoplasm	0.003	578	158	68	23	-64

* Data for 48 h cultures.

† Culture supernates were added directly to the cells just prior to placement in a chemotaxis chamber. Data reported as the lowest dilution in Medium 199 at which inhibition of macrophage chemotaxis was observed.

‡ Culture supernates were mixed in equal proportion with a strong chemotactic attractant and placed in the lower non-cell compartment of a chemotaxis chamber. Macrophage-rich rat exudate cells were placed in the upper cell compartment. Only cells migrating completely through the filters were counted in 4 high powered fields (HPF).

§ Culture supernates were injected intravenously at 1 ml/rat followed 60 min later with proteose peptone intraperitoneally. Macrophage yield was quantitated 3 days later.

point out that not all tumours growing in all sites produce anti-inflammatory effects.

An alternative approach which we have used to define further the mechanism by which tumours inhibit monocyte inflammation involves cell culture of normal and neoplastic cell lines. As summarized in Table 23.3, we have found that certain neoplastic cells which proliferate rapidly in culture elaborate factors into the culture supernate which inhibit the chemotactic migration of macrophages. The inhibitory agent was not toxic for macrophages and appeared to inhibit cellular migration by binding onto cell surfaces. When injected intravenously, certain of the culture supernates depressed macrophage accumulation to intraperitoneal peptone. These effects were specific for monocyte/macrophages because the culture supernates neither inhibited PMN chemotaxis *in vitro* nor decreased PMN inflammation *in vivo*.

However, Fauve *et al.*[27] have reported that the PMN response characteristic of acute inflammation is depressed by a low molecular weight substance contained in the culture supernate of teratocarcinoma cells. No data were reported on macrophage inflammation. As we have at no time seen depressed PMN responses, teratocarcinoma may be an exception rather than characteristic of the biologic effects of tumour bearing.

CONCLUSIONS

If macrophages are indeed major effector cells controlling the growth of cancer cells, it is appropriate to ask how tumours escape from growth regulation by macrophages. Compelling evidence has accumulated that a cell selective inhibition in monocyte inflammation occurs during tumour growth. However, the onset of this defect appears to require a threshold number of, tumour cells. Accordingly, tumour associated macrophages do increase during the early stages of tumour growth. In some instances a monocyte defect does not develop until the tumour reaches a relatively large size and in at least one tumour the defect did not develop at all. Consequently, the described monocyte defect does not seem to compromise immunosurveillance sufficiently early to account for the emergence of tumour cells.

If the defect in monocyte inflammation does not contribute to the emergence of tumours, what then is its biologic significance? Several investigators have reported an inverse relationship between the content of tumour macrophages and the capacity for metastasis[22,28]. In addition, host defence mechanisms involving macrophages appear to suppress growth of metastatic lesions, contribute to concomitant immunity, and determine the fate of latent tumour cells which remain viable but do not grow after surgical excision of the primary tumour[29-31]. That activated macrophages possess growth regulating activities over cancer cells seems a well established *in vitro* phenomenon[4-7]. Therefore, a defect in monocyte mobility might influence the tumour–host relationship in several ways. By limiting the number of tumour associated macrophages, it might contribute to progressive growth and to metastatic spread of the primary tumour. By altering the ratio of macrophages to tumour cells at a metastatic site, it might permit these cells to survive and actually facilitate their growth. Too few macrophages or too little immunity may actually stimulate tumour growth[5,32]. Compromised monocyte inflammation is a mechanism which could explain why infection becomes an important medical problem in the terminal stages of malignancy.

Some tumours do grow and kill despite an abundance of macrophages. While such tumours may not engender effective anti-inflammatory factors, the observation also suggests that tumours possess additional means to escape growth regulation by macrophages. One possibility is that the distribution of macrophages in the tumour is such that the close contact necessary for killing does not occur between the macrophage and its target cell. Alternatively, the tumour associated macrophages may not be appropriately activated or their cytostatic and cytocidal activities are in some way compromised. While macrophages isolated from tumours have been shown to be cytostatic for the homologous tumour cell[33,34], the isolation procedure may have altered the functional state of the cell.

The tumour bearing animal reacts to its tumour with opposing effects on macrophages: namely, enhanced numbers in blood but an inability to mobilize such cells to areas of inflammatory need. Are factors stimulating monocytosis during tumour growth separate from those inhibiting monocyte migration? What is the nature of such factors? Can they be produced by clones of cancer cells? What is the relationship, if any, between these factors inhibitory to macrophages and those described as interfering with lymphocyte functions? What is the role of locally produced lymphocyte derived pro-inflammatory effector agents (lymphokines) with respect to coping with anti-inflammatory tumour cell products?

Inhibition of macrophage chemotaxis by cell culture supernates is not restricted to neoplastic cells[21]. This observation raises the question if inhibition of macrophage inflammation is a unique property of neoplastic cells. Preliminary studies indicate that non-malignant but rapid cell proliferation such as occurs in regenerating livers influences monocyte function. Could this contribute to the accelerated growth of tumours transplanted to hepatectomized animals[35]? Is it possible that what we have observed with malignant cells reflects a more general biologic process that limits monocyte inflammation and regulates macrophage participation in cellular growth control?

Acknowledgements

This work was supported by National Institute of Health Grants HD–00384 and CA–15334, and by Swiss National Science Foundation Grant

3.600.75 and Hoffman-La Roche, Basel. This work is Tumor Biology Unit Publication number 122.

References

1. Currie, G. A. (1974). *Cancer and the Immune Response*. (Edinburgh: T. A. Constable Ltd.)
2. Evans, R. (1972). Macrophages in syngeneic animal tumors, *Transplantation*, **14**, 468
3. Gauci, C. L. and Alexander, P. (1975). The macrophage content of some human tumors, *Cancer Lett.*, **1**, 33
4. Keller, R. (1973). Cytostatic elimination of syngeneic rat tumor cells *in vitro* by non-specifically activated macrophages. *J. Exp. Med.*, **138**, 625
5. Keller, R. (1976). Cytostatic and cytocidal effects of activated macrophages. In: *Immunobiology of the Macrophage* (D. S. Nelson, ed.) p. 487. (New York: Academic Press)
6. Remington, J. S., Krahenbuhl, J. L. and Hibbs, J. B. (1975). A role for the macrophage in resistance to tumor development and tumor destruction. In: *Mononuclear Phagocytes in Immunity, Infection and Pathology* (R. van Furth, ed.) p. 869. (Oxford: Blackwell Scientific Publications)
7. Hibbs, J. B. (1975). Activated macrophages as cytotoxic effector cells. I. Inhibition of specific and non-specific tumor resistance by trypan blue. *Transplantation*, **19**, 77
8. Bernstein, I. D., Zbar, B. and Rapp, H. J. (1972). Impaired inflammatory response in tumor bearing guinea pigs. *J. Nat. Cancer Inst.*, **49**, 1641
9. Eccles, S. A. and Alexander, P. (1974). Sequestration of macrophages in growing tumors and its effect on the immunological capacity of the host. *Brit. J. Cancer*, **30**, 42
10. Normann, S. J. and Sorkin, E. (1976). Cell-specific defect in monocyte function during tumor growth. *J. Nat. Cancer Inst.*, **57**, 135
11. Snyderman, R., Pike, M. C., Blaylock, B. L. and Weinstein, P. (1976). Effect of neoplasms on inflammation: depression of macrophage accumulation after tumor implantation. *J. Immunol.*, **116**, 585
12. Boetcher, D. A. and Leonard, E. J. (1974). Abnormal monocyte chemotactic response in cancer patients. *J. Nat. Cancer Inst.*, **52**, 1091
13. Snydermann, R. and Stahl, C. (1975). Defective immune effector function in patients with neoplastic and immune deficiency diseases. In: *The Phagocytic Cell in Host Resistance* (J. A. Bellanti and D. H. Bayton, eds.) p. 267. (New York. Raven Press)
14. Hausman, M. S., Brosman, S., Snyderman, R., Mickey, M. R. and Faney, J. (1975). Defective monocyte function in patients with genitourinary carcinoma. *J. Nat. Cancer Inst.*, **55**, 1047
15. Normann, S. J. and Sorkin, E. (1977). Cell specific inhibition of monocyte inflammation and chemotaxis by tumor cells. *Proceedings First European Conference on Phagocytic Leukocytes, Trieste*. (In press)
16. Eccles, S. A., Brandlow, G. and Alexander, P. (1976). Monocytosis associated with the growth of transplanted syngeneic rat sarcomata differing in immunogenicity. *Br. J. Cancer*, **34**, 20
17. Gauci, C. L., Wrathmell, A. and Alexander, P. (1975). The origin and role of blood-borne monocytes in rats with a transplanted myelogenous leukemia. *Cancer Lett.*, **1**, 33
18. North, R. J., Kirstein, D. P. and Tuttle, R. L. (1976). Subversion of host defense mechanisms by murine tumors. I. A circulating factor that suppressed macrophage mediated resistance to infection. *J. Exp. Med.*, **143**, 559
19. Volkman, A. and Gowans, J. L., (1965). The production of macrophages in the rat, *J. Exp. Pathol.*, **46**, 50
20. Volkman, A. and Gowans, J. L. (1965). The origin of macrophages from bone marrow in rat. *Br. J. Exp. Pathol.*, **46**, 62
21. Normann, S. J. and Sorkin, E. (1977). Inhibition of macrophage chemotaxis by neoplastic and other rapidly proliferating cells *in vitro*. *Cancer Res.*, **37**, 705
22. Eccles, S. A. and Alexander, P. (1974). Macrophage content of tumors in relation to metastic spread and host immune reaction. *Nature (London)*, **250**, 667

23. Altman, L. C., Snyderman, R., Oppenheim, J. J. and Mergen-hagen, S. E. (1973). A human mononuclear leukocyte chemotactic factor. Characterization, specificity and kinetics of production by homologous leukocytes. *J. Immunol.*, **110**, 810
24. Lala, P. K. (1974). Dynamics of leukocyte migration into the mouse ascites tumor. *Cell Tissue Kinet.*, **7**, 293
25. Baker, P., Wieser, R. S., Jutilia, J., Evans, C. A. and Blandau, R. (1962). Mechanisms of tumor homograft rejection: the behavior of sarcoma I ascites tumor in the A/Jax and C57B1/6 mouse. *Ann. N.Y. Acad. Sci.*, **10**, 46
26. Snyderman, R. and Pike, M. C. (1976). An inhibitor of macrophage chemotaxis produced by neoplasms. *Science*, **192**, 370
27. Fauve, R. M., Brigitte, H., Jacob, H., Gaillard, J. A. and Jacob, F. (1974). Anti-inflammatory effects of murine malignant cells. *Proc. Nat. Acad. Sci. USA*, **71**, 4052
28. Wood, G. W. and Gillespie, G. Y. (1975). Studies on the role of macrophages in regulation of growth and metastasis of murine chemically induced fibrosarcomas. *Int. J. Cancer*, **16**, 1022
29. Fidler, I. J. (1974). Inhibition of pulmonary metastasis by intravenous injection of specifically activated macrophages. *Cancer Res.*, **34**, 1074
30. Eccles, S. A. and Alexander, P. (1975). Immunologically-mediated restraint of latent tumor metastases. *Nature (London)*, **257**, 52
31. Alexander, P., Evans, R. and Mikulska, Z. B. (1973). Relationship between concomitant immunity and metastasis—the role of macrophages in concomitant immunity involving the peritoneal cavity. In: *Chemotherapy of Cancer Dissemination and Metastasis* (S. Gorattini and G. Franchi, eds.) p. 177. (New York: Raven Press)
32. Prehn, R. T. (1972). The immune reaction as a stimulator of tumor growth. *Science*, **176**, 170
33. von Loveren, H. and den Otter, W. (1974). Macrophages in solid tumors. I. Immunologically specific effector cells. *J. Nat. Cancer Inst.*, **53**, 1057
34. Haskill, J. S., Proctor, J. W. and Yamamura, Y. (1975). Host responses within solid tumors. I. Monocyte effector cells within rat carcinomas. *J. Nat. Cancer Inst.*, **54**, 387
35. Pliskin, M. E. (1976). Depression of host versus graft immunity and stimulation of tumor growth following partial hepatectomy. *Cancer Res.*, **36**, 1659

Discussion 23

I. L. Bonta:
(The Netherlands)

I am very impressed by these experiments.

I am confident that Dr. Normann is aware that when two inflammations are produced at the same time in the same organism, there is an interaction between the two inflammatory responses. This phenomenon, known as counter-irritation, has been extensively investigated in the past. When a tumour is induced in the animals, there might be some inflammatory response around the tumour, and in addition, it appears that any kind of non-specific stimulus may trigger certain anti-inflammatory responses in the organism through the liver, or even through materials that are produced at the site of the inflammation.

Were the macrophage infiltration and the macrophage response also tested when an inflammatory response—not a tumour—but any kind of non-specific response was induced? It is possible that in the tumour-bearing animals, the counter-irritation phenomenon, where certain mechanisms such as complement inhibition or activation of the liver to the output of acute phase reactant proteins are operating, might have some relevance to Dr. Normann's experiments.

Normann:

In the P-815 mastocytoma experiment the tumour was growing in the peritoneal cavity and the inflammation was induced into the tumour site, into the bed of the tumour, by the injection of proteose peptone. In the one given the large tumour dose, the presence of the tumour cells alone did not produce an inflammatory response in its own behalf. Injection of proteose peptone in that instance did not induce an inflammatory response, even though the tumour itself had no inflammatory reaction.

The other aspect of that comment to which I can respond is the fact that the subcutaneous tumours, which we were using, contained very few macrophages. This was one of the things that surprised us. We were under the impression that we would find relatively large numbers. The subcutaneous tumour, the chemically-induced tumour in mice contained approximately 4–6% macrophages, instead of the 25–55% which had been reported elsewhere. In fact, the tumour growing subcutaneously in these experiments was not producing a large inflammatory effect.

Finally, the PMN response in these animals is normal. In fact it is increased. We have, in contrast, a defect in monocyte mobilization which appears to occur despite the blood levels having been increased.

P. C. Wilkinson:
(UK)

I wanted to ask about the possible problem of viruses. Viruses, and virus-infected cells, may release products that depress phagocyte function and one is always a little worried with tumour cells about their status relative to either virus induction, or else passenger viruses in the cells.

Normann:
Has Dr. Normann given that any thought?
We have been thinking about viruses. That is one of the candidates on which we have to speculate.

In the passive transfer experiments with tumour homogenates, the evidence is that this is due to a low molecular weight substance, something which is dialysable, something which has been given a molecular weight range between 1000 and about 15 000. This information would suggest that at least a virus as an entity is probably not the mediator, at least in those experiments. Additional work obviously needs to be done to define the mechanism by which this inhibition is brought about and until we have more information the viruses remain a viable explanation.

D. Sofia:
(USA)
Has any attempt been made to induce an inflammation, such as adjuvant arthritis, or carrageenan, in the tumour-bearing animals?

Normann:
We have not tried that particular approach. We have been concerned about the fact that inflammation in the peritoneal cavity might not be representative of inflammation in the tissues. To this extent we have been implanting, subcutaneously, polycarbonate filters and measuring the macrophage response on the filters. This is compromised in the tumour-bearing animal.

Sofia:
Is there any suggestion that adjuvant arthritis might be induced in the model?

Normann:
I do not know.

O. Voisin:
(France)
Dr. Normann must certainly be aware of work done at the Pasteur Institute published in the *Proceedings of the National Academy of Science* about two years ago. It was found that the supernatants of tumour cell cultures *in vitro* were inhibitory for macrophages, and that the macrophages, when cultivated together with the tumour cells, were not able to invade the tumour cells, at least for certain types of tumour.

It was found, too, that these tumours could not invade cultures of trophoblastic cells.

How would Dr. Normann relate his own findings to those findings?

Normann:
I am not sure that there is any conflict here, with the exception of one point, which is the fact that that work described PMN and comprised PMN inflammatory responses *in vivo* with the injection of these culture supernates from teratocarcinoma cells. There are two possible points to be kept in mind in relation to those experiments. The stimulus that they used for those experiments was the culture fluid because the normal serum would attract PMN. We are not sure, therefore, whether the exciting agent may have been altered by the culture conditions.

Secondly, it is quite possible that teratocarcinoma cells have this effect. However, at no time have we observed inhibition in PMN as part of actual tumour-bearing effects in an animal. This is the experience of other groups too, (Snydermann), with the four or five tumours that have been studied. We have to consider, perhaps, that tumour bearing in an animal might have a different effect than the growth of teratocarcinoma cells and culture. It may be, too, that perhaps teratocarcinoma is an exception, and that when there has been an opportunity to explore more tumours and types, this may emerge as part of the picture as well.

R. van Furth:
(The Netherlands)
A question on specificity. When the homogenate is injected intramuscularly, how specific is this for the inhibition of the inflammatory response at another site?

Secondly, if injections are given intramuscularly, is it then possible to transfer the inhibitory response by taking the serum and injecting into other mice?

Normann:
In answer to the first, the injection subcutaneously compromises the

315

inflammatory response in the peritoneal cavity of macrophage, but not of PMNs.

van Furth: Is that for the tumour or for the homogenate of the tumour?

Normann: The homogenate of the tumour placed subcutaneously compromises macrophage inflammation intraperitoneally, but does not compromise PMN inflammation intraperitoneally.

In all fairness we have been saying this is a cell-selective defect, but we have not demonstrated, or even analysed at this point, the effect this may have on lymphocytes. When we talk about cell selectivity we are talking about PMNs versus macrophages and no information has yet appeared on the effect on lymphocytes.

van Furth: I was speaking about selectivity for the inducing of inflammation. Inflammation can be induced in the peritoneal cavity by several means. How specific is it on that?

Normann: It has been induced with proteose peptone. The defect has been described with PHA induction (Snydermann). We have used PHA ourselves and the same effect has been observed. Another group, (Alexander), have done it with glycogen and have reported similar results. It therefore appears to be relatively non-specific with respect to the inflammatory stimuli.

24
Role of platelets and of prostaglandin synthetase on hypotensive effects of arachidonic acid and of carrageenan

BERNARDO B. VARGAFTIG AND JEAN LEFORT (France)

INTRODUCTION

The hypotensive effects of slow reacting substance C (SRS-C) and of the prostaglandin (PG) precursor arachidonic acid (AA) are inhibited by non-steroidal anti-inflammatory agents (NSAID)[1-4]. Since SRS-C and AA trigger the formation from isolated lungs and from blood platelet preparations, of a material which has been named rabbit aorta contracting substance (RCS), this formation being suppressed by NSAID[5-9], it has been hypothesized that hypotension is due to generation of RCS in vivo[10]. Rabbit aorta contracting activity is considered to be accounted for by the non-prostanoic AA-derivative Thromboxane A2 (TxA2), also held responsible for the platelet aggregating activity of AA[11].

The site of formation of TxA2 has not been determined in vivo and the hypothesis has been proposed that hypotension might be explained by its generation from circulating platelets, particularly when aggregates are trapped in smaller vessels, as in lungs, there undergoing the aspirin-sensitive release reaction[10]. We have examined this hypothesis and compared the effects of AA with those of the pro-inflammatory polysaccharide carrageenan. The latter induces aggregation of rabbit platelets[12-14], which is accompanied by generation of thromboxane-like activity; only the latter is inhibited by NSAID, in parallel to their activity against PG synthetase. Our results indicate that circulating platelets are not required for the hypotensive effects of AA.

METHODS AND MATERIALS

Platelet aggregation in platelet-rich plasma (PRP) and of washed platelets resuspended in Tyrode solution was studied by turbidimetry (Born's technique)[13-16]. Carotid blood pressure of pentobarbitone-anaesthetized rabbits (30 mg/kg, i.v.) was recorded. Platelets were counted in arterial blood at intervals after drug injection, using a Coulter Counter. Bioassay of thromboxane activity was performed with rabbit aorta and mesenteric artery strips[13,17]. Bronchoconstriction in guinea pigs was studied by the Konzett–Rössler method, as used by us before[18], animals being pre-treated with propranolol (2.5 mg/kg i.p. + 1 mg/kg i.v.) at the start of the experiment, to reduce adrenergic bronchodilatation[19]. Rabbits and guinea pigs were injected i.v. unless otherwise stated, drugs and sources being in References 13 and 14. Antiplatelet serum was raised in dogs injected with washed rabbit platelets emulsified with complete Freund's adjuvant[14].

RESULTS

Effects of arachidonic acid, salicylic acid and aspirin

Injections of 50–200 μg/kg of AA to rabbits was followed by hypotension (Figures 24.1 and 24.2). Platelet counts were unaffected or reduced very slightly, samples being collected at close intervals starting 10 s after the injection, up to 5 min. As also seen in Figure 24.1, 20 mg/kg of aspirin i.v. prevented hypotension by AA fully, but the inhibitory effect faded within 1–2 h. Injections of ADP at doses that induce less marked hypotension than AA were regularly followed by fall in platelet counts, which provided a control for aggregability of circulating platelets (Figure 24.2). The reduced importance of platelet aggregation for AA-induced hypotension in rabbits was confirmed since after immune platelet depletion animals responded fully—and even died—when injected with an appropriate dose of AA (Figure 24.1). Moreover, if rabbits were pre-treated with ADP (50 mg/kg i.m., Reference 20), they failed to respond with acute thrombocytopenia to further i.v. injections of ADP, and the accompanying hypotensive response was reduced (Table 24.1). Under these circumstances, hypotension by AA was even increased. Those results rule out platelets as site of action for the hypotensive effects of AA, which result from formation of PG-related substances and of thromboxanes in other tissues, particularly lungs, from where they reach vessels. Others[21] have shown that in rabbits made thrombocytopenic by irradiation, AA retains its hypotensive effects and we have also demonstrated that bronchoconstriction by AA is not suppressed in thrombocytopenic guinea pigs, whereas bronchoconstriction by ADP and by ATP are abolished[18].

Although the inhibitory effects of aspirin towards hypotension by AA faded within 1–2 h, if platelet-rich plasma was prepared from blood collected at intervals after aspirin administration, and challenged with AA, aggregation and generation of thromboxane were suppressed for up to 7 h (Figure

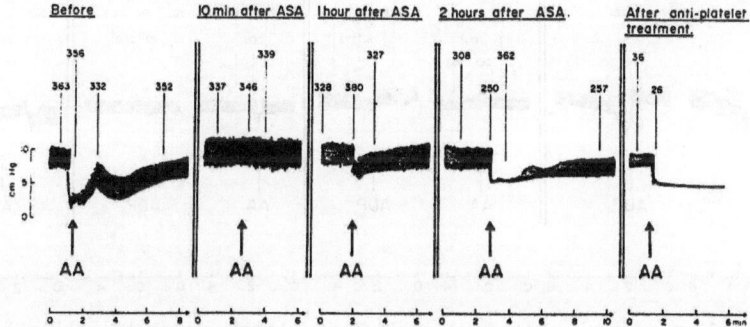

Figure 24.1 Arachidonic acid induces aspirin-sensitive hypotension in the rabbit without acute thrombocytopenia; interference of anti-platelet treatment. Recording of the arterial blood pressure of a rabbit injected with 100 μg/kg of arachidonic acid (AA) before and at various time intervals after the injection of 20 mg/kg of aspirin. Figures indicate platelet counts × 10^3 per μl before, 10 s, 1 and 6 min after AA was injected. Note that there is no significant drop in platelet content of arterial blood after AA and the reappearance of hypotensive response to AA one, and clearly two hours after administration of aspirin.

Reduction of platelet content to 10% of basal levels did not prevent AA from inducing irreversible hypotension

Vertical scale: arterial blood pressure in cmHg

Table 24.1 Interference of adenosine diphosphate with hypotension and acute thrombocytopenia induced by itself and by arachidonic acid administered intravenously to rabbits

Agonist	% drop in platelet counts						% hypotension	
	Before			After			Before	After
	10 sec	30 sec	60 sec	10 sec	30 sec	60 sec		
ADP	60.5	49	12.4	10.8*	12.9*	2.5	53.8	20.0*
	(16)	(20.5)	(17)	(5.7)	(9.8)	(2)	(19.9)	(13.0)
Arachidonic acid	11	5	4.6	6.5	5.5	2.4	64.2	88
	(10.4)	(3.7)	(4.3)	(3.9)	(2.5)	(2.6)	(16)	(19)

Arachidonic acid and ADP were infused in 30 s at 0.1 mg/kg and at 0.2 mg/kg respectively to six rabbits. Mean ± SD in parenthesis for drops in platelet counts at intervals indicated during and after cessation of infusion and for maximum extent of hypotension before and thirty minutes after a 50 mg/kg injection of ADP i.m. This treatment desensitizes to further effects, of ADP, but does not affect those of arachidonic acid

* Significant at $p < 0.05$

319

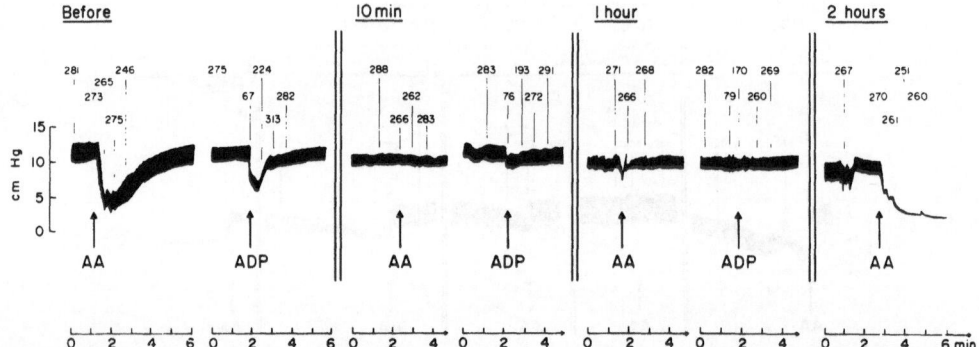

Figure 24.2 Arachidonic acid induces aspirin-sensitive hypotension in the rabbit without acute thrombocytopenia. Arterial blood pressure of a rabbit injected with 100 μg/kg of arachidonic acid (AA) or ADP before and after 5 mg/kg of aspirin. Figures indicate platelet counts $\times$ 10^3 per μl before 10, 30, 60 s and 2 min after AA or ADP injection. Observe that for a larger hypotensive response the administration of AA is not accompanied by thrombocytopenia, whereas ten seconds after ADP the blood platelet content drops. Observe recovery of the antagonistic effect of aspirin within 2 h. Legends as in Figure 24.1

INHIBITION OF ARACHIDONIC ACID-INDUCED
AGGREGATION OF RABBIT PLATELETS AFTER
IN VIVO INJECTION OF ASPIRIN

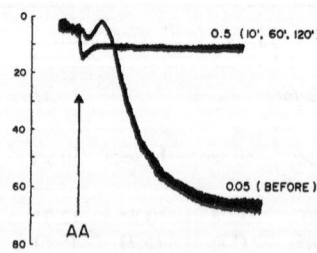

Figure 24.3 Inhibition of arachidonic acid-induced aggregation of rabbit platelets after *in vivo* injection of aspirin. Superimposed tracings of aggregation of rabbit platelets. Platelet-rich plasma was prepared from blood collected before or at the indicated intervals after a 5 mg/kg i.v. injection of aspirin. Even though the added concentration of AA was increased by ten times (from 0.05 to 0.5 mM, as indicated near each tracing), aggregation was irreversibly inhibited, for more than two hours, in this experiment
Vertical scale: % light transmission

24.3). The different time-course of inhibition of hypotension by aspirin, on one hand, and of aggregation of platelets and release of mediators, on the others, indicate that different mechanisms are responsible for the inhibitory activity of aspirin towards AA-induced hypotension (and bronchoconstriction in guinea pigs) and towards the platelet effects.

More evidence was collected by using salicyclic acid. The latter is equi-active with aspirin against carrageenan-induced rat paw oedema, but lacks significant activity against prostaglandin synthetase[22]. Salicyclic acid failed to interfere with hypotension due to AA, but prevented the inhibitory effect of aspirin[23]. Bronchoconstriction by AA is also unaffected by aspirin when the guinea pig is pre-treated with salicyclic acid (Figure 24.4). Furthermore, when platelet-rich plasma was prepared from blood collected from rabbits injected with salicyclic acid (200 mg/kg), followed within 30 min by aspirin (5 mg/kg), no inhibition of AA-induced aggregation nor of generation of thromboxane activity was seen.

Similar experiments were repeated *in vitro*: platelet-rich plasma was

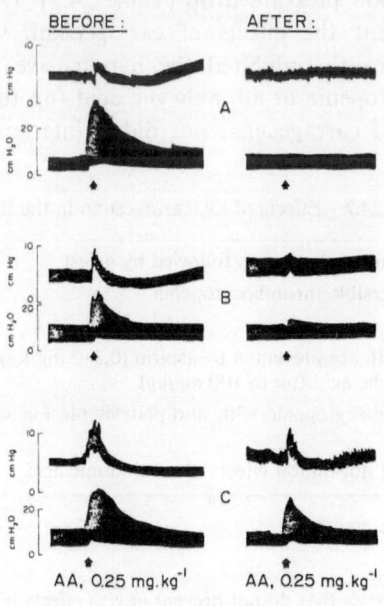

Figure 24.4 Interference of salicylic acid with aspirin-induced inhibition of bronchoconstriction due to arachidonic acid in the guinea pig. Arterial blood pressure (upper tracing) and bronchial resistance to inflation (lower tracing) were recorded in cmHg and in cmH$_2$O respectively. Arachidonic acid was injected before and after administration of salicylic acid (100, 150 and 200 mg/kg) to each of three pentobarbitone-anaesthetized guinea pigs. 30 min later, a fixed dose of 5 mg/kg of aspirin was given to each animal, amounting to a salicylic acid:aspirin ratio of 20, 30 and 40, respectively. Arachidonic acid was injected again. Observe that in the upper panel (ratio 20) bronchoconstriction is inhibited fully; that in the middle panel (ratio 30), inhibition is not complete, whereas in the lower panel (ratio 40), bronchoconstriction is not inhibited by aspirin

incubated with salicyclic acid (2 mM) for 30 min, then aspirin (50 μM) was added for 30 min as well. Platelets were thoroughly washed to remove the drugs, and resuspended either in Tyrode solution or in drug-free plasma[15]. Again salicylic acid prevented the expected aspirin-induced inhibition of aggregation and of generation of thromboxanes, whereas the drug solvent was inactive. Similar experiments repeated in absence of plasma (platelets being incubated with salicylic acid and with aspirin in a Tyrode-gelatin buffer), demonstrated that inhibition by salicyclic acid of aspirin-induced inhibition of platelets aggregation is independent of the suspension medium, and probably results from some sort of competition for binding to the membrane and/or to a more or less specific receptor/enzyme complex.

Effects of carrageenan on rabbits

Intravenous injections of 10 mg/kg of carrageenan to rabbits were followed by immediate hypotension, and by death[12,13]. Irreversible thrombocytopenia accompanied the blood pressure drop (Table 24.2). Drugs listed on Table 24.3 failed to prevent the effects of carrageenan, whereas aspirin and indomethacin significantly inhibited the hypotensive effect, but failed to influence thrombocytopenia at all. Salicylic acid (up to 100 mg/kg) did not prevent the effects of carrageenan, nor did it interfere with inhibition by

Table 24.2   Effects of i.v. carrageenan in the rabbit*

(a) hypotension, respiratory stimulation followed by arrest

(b) immediate and irreversible thrombocytopenia

(c) death within 5 min

(d) hypotension and death are prevented by aspirin (0.3–2 mg/kg), by indomethacin (5–10 mg/kg), but not by salicylic acid (up to 100 mg/kg)

(e) animals made thrombocytopenic with anti-platelet plasma were refractory to carrageenan

(d) platelet depletion did not inhibit effects of arachidonic acid

* Full discussion in Reference 14

Table 24.3   Drugs that do not prevent *in vivo* effects of carrageenan*

heparin—plasmin—epsilon aminocaproic acid

Arvin®—cyproheptadine—carboxypeptidase B

methysergide—reserpine—glycogen—metiamide†

Thus we may rule out intravascular coagulation, release of kinins, histamine and serotonin, and microvascular obstruction by platelet clumps.

* Doses and full description in Reference 14.

† 10 mg/kg i.v.

aspirin. Death due to carrageenan can thus be dissociated from the accompanying thrombocytopenia. Results that followed demonstrated that even though thrombocytopenia was present in aspirin or indomethacin-treated animals injected with carrageenan, the underlying release reaction, during which platelets extrude and/or generate vasoactive mediators, was completely suppressed. Indeed, when rabbit platelet-rich plasma was incubated with carrageenan at 37 °C (Table 24.4), thromboxane-like activity was generated

Table 24.4 Release of smooth muscle-contracting activities in incubates of rabbit platelet-rich plasma with carrageenan*

(a) incubation of carrageenan with PRP for 2–30 min is followed by the appearance of a contracting activity for the rabbit aorta strip, for the coeliac artery/mesenteric artery strip and for the rat stomach strip

(b) this activity was highly contaminated with 5HT, since use of PRP from reserpinized rabbits led to generation of a labile activity, that was nil within 5–8 min

(c) generation of the labile activity was inhibited by indomethacin (5–50 μM), by aspirin (50–100 μM), but salicylic acid was only active at 0.5–1 mM, thus dissociating release of substances from aggregation

(d) generation of the labile activity was inhibited also by catalase (500–1000 μg/ml), by dithiothreitol (0.2–1 mM) and by the two phospholipase A2 inhibitors mepacrine and bromophenacyl bromide

(e) generation of labile activity required platelet integrity, and was abolished by ultrasonication

* Full description in References 13 and 14.

and could be inhibited by indomethacin, and by aspirin (Figure 24.5). Salicylic acid was partially active at 0.5–1 mM. Furthermore, platelet-rich plasma prepared from blood collected from aspirin or indomethacin-treated rabbits also failed to generate the thromboxane A2 activity when challenged with carrageenan, as was the case when AA was used as the stimulating agent. This indicates that the mechanism through which platelets generate thromboxane activity was inhibited by NSAID, preventing the effects of AA and of carrageenan as well, and that the aggregating effect of the latter, although not of the former, is prostaglandin synthetase-independent.

It should be noted that when Tyrode-suspended platelets are used in place of platelet-rich plasma, the aggregating effect of carrageenan can be shown with concentrations down to 0.5–1 μg/ml, and that NSAID can inhibit it, provided they are left in the bath during the aggregation process. In contrast, when aspirin or indomethacin are incubated with platelet-rich plasma for an interval sufficient to suppress completely the aggregating effect of AA, and then platelets are washed and the inhibitors are removed from the suspension medium, carrageenan induces aggregation even though generation of thromboxane A2 by it and by AA is suppressed (Tables 24.5 and 24.6). Non-steroidal anti-inflammatory drugs inhibit mast cell histamine

INDOMETHACIN

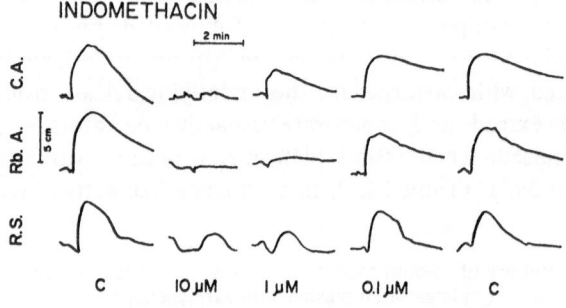

ASPIRIN

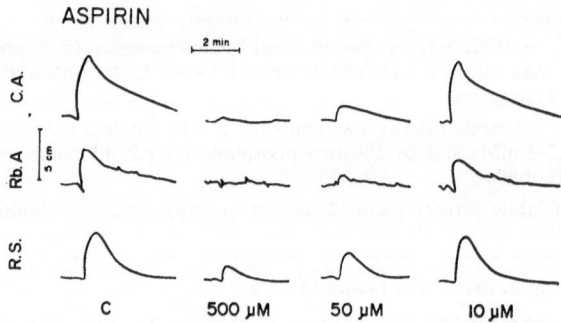

Figure 24.5 Inhibition by non-steroidal anti-inflammatory drugs of generation of pharmacological activity in incubates of platelet-rich plasma and carrageenan. Isolated strip of rabbit coeliac artery (C.A.), of rabbit aorta (Rb.A.) and of rat stomach (R.S.) were superfused. Samples of incubates of PRP with carrageenan (250 μg/ml) were bioassayed in absence (C, control), or in presence of indicated final concentrations of indomethacin or of aspirin, added to PRP one minute before carrageenan. Observe concentration-dependent inhibition of generation of pharmacological activities.

Table 24.5 Carrageenan-induced aggregation of rabbit platelets suspended in plasma*

(a) effective concentration of carrageenan: 50–1000 μg/ml

(b) aggregation is preceded by increased turbidity, accounted for by precipitation of plasma materials

(c) aggregation by threshold concentrations of carrageenan is prevented by salicylic acid, aspirin and indomethacin, used at 0.1–1 mM; inhibition of aggregation is surmounted by increasing the concentration of carrageenan

(d) aggregation is inhibited by EDTA, by n-ethylmaleimide and by adenosine

---

* Full description in References 13 and 14.

release possibly by interfering with Ca^{2+} movements across the membrane[24] and this may be how NSAID, including salicylic acid, interfere with carrageenan-induced aggregation of rabbit platelets irrespective of inhibition of prostaglandin synthetase.

Another explanation that might be proposed[30] is that carrageenan activates the kinin cascade, thus leading to release of vaso-depressor bradykinin-like polypeptides. This sort of effect has been described in rat and human plasma[25-27], but in our hands neither carrageenan nor cellulose sulphate

Table 24.6 Carrageenan-induced aggregation of rabbit platelets suspended in Tyrode*

(a) threshold concentration of carrageenan: 0.5–5 μg/ml

(b) aggregation is prevented by salicylic acid, aspirin and indomethacin, used at 0.05–1 mM; inhibition of aggregation is unsurmountable

(c) aggregation is *not* inhibited by heparin nor by tosylargininemethyl ester, which inhibit aggregation due to thrombin

(d) aggregation was not affected when platelets from reserpinized rabbits were used

(e) aggregation was inhibited by two phospholipase A2 inhibitors: mepacrine and bromophenacyl bromide, which also suppressed aggregation by thrombin

---

* Full description in References 13 and 14.

released kinin-like activity from rabbit plasma, in presence of various sorts of kininase inhibitors (EDTA, phenanthroline, bradykinin potentiating peptide 9; Reference 28). Although the effects of carrageenan on other species might thus involve kinins, this is not the mechanism by which it kills rabbits. The specificity of the effect of carrageenan is also indicated by its inability to trigger aggregation of rat[29] and of washed human platelets (J. Caen, personal communication; our unpublished results.)

The hypothesis has been raised (Reference 30 and Dr. A. Rothschild, Ribeirão Preto Medical Faculty, Brazil, personal communication) that carrageenan kills rabbits by releasing massive doses of histamine within the lungs and vessels, particularly since rabbit platelets recognizably are rich in histamine. Support to this hypothesis was given by experiments performed by Dr. F. Ruff (Faculté de Médecine Necker-Enfants Malades, Paris, to be published), which used an original method allowing the continuous monitoring of blood histamine. Histamine dropped immediately after carrageenan injections, which anyway indicates that platelet aggregates are retained within smaller vessels. Nevertheless, histamine fails to imitate the platelet effects of carrageenan, when injected at 1 mg/kg i.v. This dose is required to kill rabbits, which are known to be relatively refractory to its effects. Death is prevented by the anti-histaminic anti-serotonin agent cyproheptadine (1 mg/kg), and animals covered by this treatment resisted doses of histamine up to

10 mg/kg. Since cyproheptadine failed to inhibit the effects of carrageenan (Table 24.3) its effects are not due to *in vivo* histamine release.

CONCLUDING REMARKS

Platelets are not required for the hypotensive effects of arachidonic acid in the rabbit, nor for its inhibition by aspirin. Since the platelet effect of aspirin is prolonged, whereas the anti-hypotensive effect is relatively short-lived, both effects probably result from different mechanisms. The platelet effect may involve membrane acetylation[31,32], and access to the active site by aspirin may be hindered by salicylic acid[23]. In contrast, the anti-hypotensive effect may correspond to reversible non-acetylating inhibition of prostaglandin synthetase, which also occurs in perfused guinea pig lungs[6], where drug removal brings back the full activity of PG synthetase.

Carrageenan aggregates platelets by an unknown mechanism, and speculations on this mechanism are found in References 12 and 13. Although carrageenan aggregates washed rabbit platelets resuspended in Tyrode solution or in inactivated serum, a mechanism involving complement activation cannot be ruled out, since complement components are present within the platelet membrane, and participate in collagen-induced aggregation[33]. The effectiveness of aspirin against hypotension and death due to carrageenan, as compared to indomethacin and to salicylic acid, is reminiscent of its protective effect against adrenalin-induced kallikrein activation of rat mast cells[34], where the acetylating effect is directly involved. There is no parallelism between the ability of NSAID to inhibit aggregation or hypotension by carrageenan and their anti-inflammatory or anti-prostaglandin synthetase activity, and protection against carrageenan cannot be used as a procedure for detection of 'conventional' anti-inflammatory activity. Nonetheless, the mechanism of action of carrageenan *in vivo* is so sensitive to inhibition by aspirin, that a new property of the latter may well be involved.

References

1. Vargaftig, B. B., Miranda, E. P. and Lacoume, B. (1969). Inhibition by nonsteroidal anti-inflammatory agents of *in vivo* effect of 'slow reacting substance C'. *Nature (London)*, **222**, 883
2. Larsson, C. and Änggård, E. (1973). Arachidonic acid lowers and indomethacin increases the blood pressure of the rabbit. *J. Pharm. Pharmacol.*, **25**, 653
3. Rose, J. C., Johnson, M., Ramwell, P. W. and Kot, P. A. (1974). Effects of arachidonic acid on systemic arterial pressure, myocardial contractility and platelets in the dog. *Proc. Soc. Exp. Biol. Med.*, **147**, 652
4. Deby, C., Barac, G. and Bacq, Z. M. (1974). Action de l'acide arachidonique sur la pression artérielle du lapin avant et après héparine. *Arch. int. Pharmacodyn.*, **208**, 363
5. Piper, P. J. and Vane, J. R. (1969). Release of additional factors in anaphylaxis and its antagonism by anti-inflammatory drugs. *Nature (London)*, **223**, 29

6. Vargaftig, B. B. and Dao-Hai, N. (1971). Release of vasoactive substances from guinea pig lungs by slow reacting substance C and arachidonic acid. *Pharmacology*, **6**, 99
7. Palmer, M. A., Piper, P. J. and Vane, J. R. (1973). Release of rabbit aorta contracting substance (RCS) and prostaglandins induced by chemical or mechanical stimulation of guinea pig lungs. *Br. J. Pharmacol.*, **49**, 226
8. Vargaftig, B. B. and Dao-Hai, N. (1972). Interference of some thiol derivatives with the pharmacological effects of arachidonic acid and slow reacting substance C with the release of rabbit aorta contracting substances. *Eur. J. Pharmacol.*, **18**, 43
9. Vargaftig, B. B. and Dao-Hai, N. (1972). Selective inhibition by mepacrine of the release of 'rabbit aorta contracting substance' evoked by the administration of bradykinin. *J. Pharm. Pharmacol.*, **24**, 159
10. Vargaftig, B. B. (1974). Search for common mechanisms underlying the various effects of putative inflammatory mediators. In: *The Prostaglandins* (P. W. Ramwell, ed.) Vol. 2, p. 205. (New York: Plenum Press)
11. Hamberg, M., Svensson, J. and Samuelsson, B. (1975). Thromboxanes: A new group of biologically active compounds derived from prostaglandin endoperoxides. *Proc. Nat. Acad. Sci. USA*, **72**, 2994
12. Vargaftig, B. B. (1976). Effects of prostaglandin synthetase inhibitors and of other drugs on aggregation of plasma-free rabbit platelets by carrageenan and by thrombin. *Br. J. Pharmacol.*, **58**, 447P
13. Vargaftig, B. B. and Lefort, J. (1977). Acute hypotension due to carrageenan, arachidonic acid and slow reacting substance C in the rabbit: role of platelets and pharmacological antagonism. *Eur. J. Pharmacol.*, **43**, 125
14. Vargaftig, B. B. (1977). Carrageenan and thrombin trigger prostaglandin synthetase-mdependent aggregation of rabbit platelets: inhibition by phospholipase A$_2$ inhibitors. *J. Pharm. Pharmacol.*, **29**, 222
15. Vargaftig, B. B., Tranier, Y. and Chignard, M. (1974). Inhibition by sulphydryl agents of arachidonic acid-induced platelet aggregation and release of potential inflammatory substances. *Prostaglandins*, **8**, 133
16. Born, G. V. R. (1962). Aggregation of blood platelets by adenosine diphosphate and its reversal. *Nature (London)*, **194**, 927
17. Bunting, S., Moncada, S. and Vane, J. R. (1976). The effect of prostaglandin endoperoxides and thromboxane A$_2$ on strips of rabbit coeliac artery and certain other smooth muscle preparations. *Br. J. Pharmacol.*, **57**, 462
18. Lefort, J. and Vargaftig, B. B. (1975). Role of platelet aggregation in bronchoconstriction in guinea pigs. *Br. J. Pharmacol.*, **55**, 254P
19. Collier, H. O. J. (1966). Self-antagonism of bronchoconstriction induced by bradykinin and angiotensin. In: *Hypotensive Peptides* (E. G. Erdös, N. Back and F. Sicuteri, eds.) p. 305. (Berlin: Springer Verlag)
20. Busfield, D. and Tomich, E. G. (1968). Inhibition by adenosine diphosphate of the thrombocytopenia induced in rabbits by collagen or thrombin. *Nature (London)*. **217**, 376
21. Deby, C., Damas, J. and Bacq, Z. M. (1975). Un test in vivo de la synthèse des prostaglandines. *Bull. Acad. R. Med. Belg.*, **130**, 178
22. Vane, J. R. (1971). Inhibition of prostaglandin synthesis as a mechanism of action of aspirin-like drugs. *Nature New Biol.*, **231**, 232
23. Lefort, J. and Vargaftig, B. B. (1977). Salicylic acid prevents inhibition by aspirin of arachidonic acid-induced hypotension, bronchoconstriction and thrombocytopenia. *Br. J. Pharmacol.* (In press)
24. Whittle, B. J. R. (1976). Calcium and the inhibition of histamine release from rat peritoneal mast cells by non-steroid anti-inflammatory agents. *Br. J. Pharmacol.*, **58**, 446
25. Rothschild, A. M. and Gascon, L. A. (1966). Sulphuric esters of polysaccharides as activators of a bradykinin-forming system in plasma. *Nature (London)*, **212**, 1364
26. Rothschild, A. M. (1968). Some pharmacodynamic properties of cellulose sulphate, a kininogen-depleting agent in the rat. *Br. J. Pharmacol.*, **33**, 501
27. di Rosa, M. and Sorrentino, L. (1968). The mechanism of the inflammatory effect of carrageenan. *Eur. J. Pharmacol.*, **4**, 340
28. Giroux, E. and Vargaftig, B. B. (1977). Etudes récentes sur la composition, l'activation

et la pharmacologie des systèmes générateurs de kinines. In: *Actualites de Physiologie Pathologique* (Paris: Masson) (In press)

29. Zawilska, K., Giroud, J.-P., Timsit, J. and Caen, J.-P. (1973). Plaquettes et inflammation. I. Etude chez le rat des variations quantitatives et qualitatives des plaquettes au cours d'une réaction inflammatoire aiguë (Pleurésie à la carragénine). *Pathol. Biol.*, **21**, Suppl., 51

30. Rothschild, A. M. (1960). Alteraçoes farmacodinamicas provocadas por sulfato de celulose, polissacarídeo aniônico, no cão e no coelho. *Rev. Bras. de Pesqui. Med. Biol.*, **1**, 17

31. Rosenberg, F. J., Gimber-Phillips, P. E., Groblewski, G. E., Davison, C., Phillips, D. K., Goralnick, S. J. and Cahill, E. D. (1971). Acetylsalicylic acid: inhibition of platelet aggregation in the rabbit. *J. Pharmac. Exp. Ther.*, **179**, 410

32. Majerus, P. W. (1976). Why aspirin? *Circulation*, **54**, 357

33. Chater, B. V. (1976). The role of membrane bound complement in the aggregation of mammalian platelets by collagen. *Br. J. Haematol.*, **32**, 515

34. Rothschild, A. M., Castania, A. and Cordeiro, R. S. B. (1974). Consumption of kininogen formation of kinin and activation of arginine ester hydrolase in rat plasma by rat peritoneal fluid cells in the presence of 1-adrenaline. *Naunyn-Schmiedeberg's Arch. Pharmacol.*, **285**, 243

Discussion 24

H. Collier: (UK)	I was intrigued by the relative potency of indomethacin and aspirin in one of the later slides, against carrageenan. It reminded me of figures that we obtained years ago in the inhibition of bradykinin-induced bronchial constriction, where aspirin was seemingly more potent than indomethacin. In fact, for years I thought that it was. But recently we have been doing these experiments all over again, and we find that if indomethacin is given absolutely immediately on waking up, it is as potent as might be expected from other data, and much more potent than aspirin in inhibiting bradykinin-induced bronchial constriction. The indomethacin used in those tests years ago must have gone off. Has the possibility that the indomethacin might have lost potency before administration been explored?
Vargaftig:	We tried both arachidonic acid and carrageenan at various intervals after indomethacin injection: 5 minutes, 10 minutes, 1 hour, etc. What seems to be happening is that, particularly on platelets, aspirin has two known effects. One is what might be called the salicylic acid moiety—a very feeble anti-inflammatory agent. The other is the fact that it acetylates the protein. What we really see when we work with platelets is the acetylating effect which gives the wrong ratio with respect to indomethacin. This test does not really pick up a good anti-inflammatory agent from aspirin. It just shows its acetylation potency.
M. Dianzani: (Italy)	Arachidonic acid is the precursor of both prostaglandins and lipo-peroxides. If the production of prostaglandins is in some way prevented by indomethacin then a mild lipid peroxidation is to be expected. In Turin some of my colleagues have found that the lipo-peroxides produced from arachidonic acid, and also the lipohydroxy-peroxides, are able to produce increased vascular permeability.

Has lipid peroxidation been prevented by giving anti-oxidants, or do aspirin and the other anti-inflammatory substances used also have anti-oxidant properties? |
| **Vargaftig:** | We published two papers in 1972, using a variety of thiol agents and other anti-oxidants. They do block most of those reactions. This is not evidence for a specific role of lipoperoxides because they also block generation of thromboxane, and of PG-like activity.

What we are planning to do now, and are in the process of doing, is to use TRYA, which is known to block platelet lipoxygenase, and to see whether we still have a remaining effect, despite the treatment. But we have Professor Dianzani's point in view. |
| **Z. M. Bacq:** (Belgium) | We completely agree with Dr. Vargaftig when he says that platelets are not required for the hypotensive effect of arachidonic acid in the rabbit. We have studied, and published two years ago, that heavily irradiated rabbits in which platelets and white cells have been reduced to less than 5% of normal content in the blood, heavy irradiation does not prevent, does not change the effect of arachidonic acid on the blood pressure, and on the lungs. |

329

PERSPECTIVES IN INFLAMMATION

M. Smith: (UK)	Dr. Vargaftig has said that he regarded salicylate as a weak anti-inflammatory agent...
Vargaftig:	... With respect to indomethacin.
Smith:	Perhaps we should be quite clear on this point, and perhaps we are being led astray by the multiplicity of actions of acetylsalicylic acid as an acetylating agent, and perhaps we should distinguish these very clearly from the anti-inflammatory effect, because as far as I am concerned, at least, salicylate and aspirin are equivalent both in animal models and in human disease, and therefore we should distinguish between talking of those 'epi-potencies', and differences between them, in the variety of tests such as those described today.
Vargaftig:	I fully agree.

25

Evidence for a pivotal role of the endoperoxide, PGG₂, in inflammatory processes

F. A. KUEHL, Jr., J. L. HUMES AND R. W. EGAN (USA)

Since the reports by Vane[1] as well as Smith and Willis[2] that aspirin and indomethacin are potent inhibitors of prostaglandin synthetase, there has been a controversy concerning the role of such non-steroidal anti-inflammatory agents (NSAI) in inflammatory processes. Other studies demonstrated a reasonable correlation between the action of NSAI on PG synthetase and activity both in the rat paw carrageenan assay and the clinic[3-5]. Nevertheless, the failure of administered PGEs and PGFs to fully mimic the symptoms of inflammation did not foster this interpretation[6,7].

At the time of these initial studies, PGEs and PGFs, the primary prostaglandins, were the subject of attention. Although the endoperoxide intermediates PGG_2 and PGH_2 were believed to exist, and in fact, had been assigned the correct structures by Samuelsson in 1965[8], the possibility that such intermediates might be sufficiently stable to play a biological role was not then seriously considered. Figure 25.1 depicts the current concept of the oxygenation of arachidonic acid (AA) by PG-synthetase. New potential inflammatory mediators must now be considered, all of which are subject to the inhibitory action of NSAI. Both the endoperoxides, PGG_2 and PGH_2, as well as a new series, the thromboxanes, have now been isolated and, although relatively unstable, have been shown to have potent actions upon smooth muscle and in inducing platelet aggregation[9,10].

In the course of routine screening for NSAI using the carrageenan foot oedema assay of Winter, et al.[11], one compound was found to be a potent anti-inflammatory agent, yet devoid of activity in the PG synthetase assay[3]. This compound, MK-447 (2-aminomethyl-4-t-butyl-6-iodophenol), in addition to demonstrating activity in the rat paw assay, was found to synergize

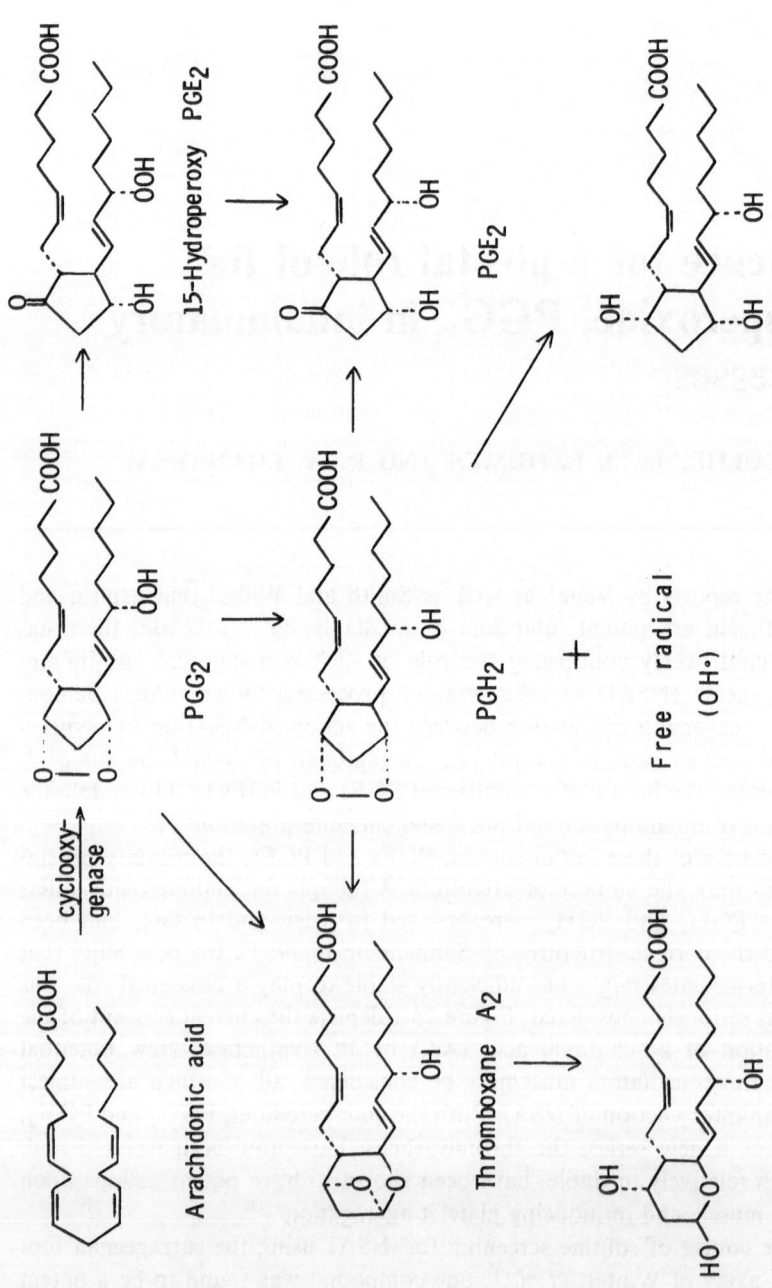

Figure 25.1 Enzymatic conversion of arachidonic acid to potential mediators of inflammation

the action of indomethacin[12]. In addition, it blunted the ulcerogenic action of high doses of indomethacin in the rat stomach[12]. Since coadministration of PGE$_2$ has been shown to neutralize the ulcerogenic action of indomethacin[13], it seemed possible that MK-447, apart from being a PG synthetase inhibitor, was, in fact, a stimulator of PG synthesis. In the sequence AA $\xrightarrow{a}$ X $\xrightarrow{b}$ PGs, in which a hypothesized intermediate, X, is derived from AA via the cyclo-oxygenase step (a) would be blocked by PG synthetase inhibitors. On the other hand, the MK-447 facilitated conversion of X to prostaglandins (PGs = PGEs + PGFs), step (b), would also depress levels of this intermediate coincident with increased synthesis of PGs. This working hypothesis was central to the studies reported here.

Utilizing a ram seminal vesicle preparation in the absence of artificial cofactors which is capable of measuring both inhibitors and stimulators of PG synthetase, MK-447 is seen (Table 25.1) to facilitate the conversion of

Table 25.1 Effects of non-steroidal anti-inflammatory agents on endoperoxides and prostaglandins derived from the enzymatic oxygenation of arachidonic acid

Product	Incubation time	No additions	MK-447 100 μM	Indomethacin 10 μM	Phenylbutazone 100 μM	Aspirin 100 μM
			nMol/mg protein			
AA	0.5 min	23	10	43	24	44
PGG$_2$	0.5 min	16	6	1	0	0
PGH$_2$	0.5 min	4	27	0	20	0
AA	5 min	7	7	44	22	44
PGG$_2$	5 min	13	0	0	4	0
PGH$_2$	5 min	5	18	0	11	0
PGs	5 min	8	15	0	7	0

AA to PGs in the 5 min incubation[14]. In the shorter 30 s period, the effect is seen to be one of stimulating the conversion of PGG$_2$ to PGH$_2$. A comparison with a number of NSAI reveals interesting differences. As expected of an inhibitor of cyclo-oxygenase, the initial enzymatic step in the oxygenation of AA, both indomethacin and aspirin blocked the formation of all products. Phenylbutazone less effectively inhibited the cyclo-oxygenase but, like MK-447, stimulated the conversion of PGG$_2$ to PGH$_2$. It is evident from these data that the effects of the NSAI studied differed widely. However, a consistent pattern in the action of all drugs examined was the depression of PGG$_2$ levels, despite various and even opposite effects on other enzymatic products including even a stimulation of PG formation by MK-447. This depression of PGG$_2$ levels by all NSAI, permitted the suggestion that this endoperoxide plays a pivotal role in inflammatory processes[14].

Earlier studies have shown that the manner by which phenol and related compounds stimulated the cyclo-oxygenase and overall PG synthesis is by preventing self-destruction of the cyclo-oxygenase[15]. More specifically, as shown in Figure 25.1, evidence was provided to show that the oxidizing equivalents released in the conversion of PGG_2 to PGH_2, generate radicals which may irreversibly oxidize the cyclo-oxygenase. There is little reason to doubt that the oxidation of certain susceptible organic substrates reported by Marnett et al. is effected by this radical[16]. MK-447, like phenol, has also been shown to stimulate both the conversion of PGG_2 to PGH_2 and overall PG synthesis by scavenging the radical[14]. In addition, a requirement for a free phenolic group for the anti-inflammatory action of MK-447 was also established[14]. Thus it was possible to conclude that the anti-inflammatory action of MK-447, concurrent with an increased synthesis of PGs, relates to its ability to stimulate the conversion of PGG_2 to PGH_2, implicating the radical.

Considering the oxygenation products derived from the action of PG synthetase on arachidonic acid, it is evident by the scheme represented in Figure 25.1 that there are many potential inflammatory mediators. Based upon the ability of MK-447 to increase the synthesis of PGE_2, $PGF_{2\alpha}$ and PGH_2, it is unlikely that these prostaglandins play important roles in acute inflammation represented by the rat paw assay. The pivotal role of PGG_2 suggested by the foregoing data would support a causal role of PGG_2 itself. Alternatively, and preferably, a non-prostaglandin product derived from PGG_2 such as thromboxane A_2 and/or the oxidizing radical could play the causal role.

Since the pathogenesis of acute inflammation may be divided into three major categories, vasodilation, pain and oedema, it is of interest to relate these symptoms to known properties of prostaglandins and their intermediates.

Vasodilation

This component of inflammation is well duplicated by administration of PGEs and thus it is reasonable to attribute the redness and heat of inflammation to PGE_2[17]. Unfortunately, the experimental models employed in our studies, the mouse ear and rat paw assays, are largely measures of oedema and thus not primarily representative of vasodilation.

Pain

Although pain may be produced by PGE_1 itself, simple hydroperoxy acids have been shown to be more effective pain inducers[18]. Again the model employed in our studies is not truly reflective of the pain of inflammation. However, since PGG_2 is in fact a hydroperoxy acid, the radical alluded to here is an attractive candidate for a pain inducing agent. It is of interest to note in this regard that the analgesic agent, paracetamol (p-acetamidophenol), like MK-447, has the ability to stimulate the conversion of PGG_2 to PGH_2 and thus is a potential free radical scavenger[19].

Oedema

This component of inflammation is most relevant to the studies noted here since both the mouse ear and rat paw assays are measures of oedema. Although it is possible that PGG_2 itself is a mediator of oedema, more likely a non-prostaglandin product derived therefrom is the true oedematous agent. As noted previously, the anti-inflammatory activity of MK-447 in these assays and the ability of this drug to stimulate the synthesis of PGE_2, $PGF_{2\alpha}$ and PGH_2, eliminate these as playing important roles in this component of inflammation. Thromboxane A_2 is a viable candidate for a causal role. Phenol, which has been shown to repress the weight gain in the mouse ear oedema assay[14] has been reported to inhibit the formation of thromboxanes from arachidonic acid[20]. Thromboxane B_2, the stable metabolite of thromboxane A_2, has also been shown to be synthesized by granuloma produced by administration of carrageenan into the rat paw[21].

The destructive nature of the oxidizing radical released in the conversion of PGG_2 to PGH_2 to both organic compounds and enzymes makes this a new and attractive candidate for involvement in the oedema of inflammation. This is evident by the actions of both phenol and MK-447 to neutralize the action of this radical *in vitro* and suppress oedema in the anti-inflammatory assays employed here. Support for this role is seen by the effect of aged but not recently purified eicosatrienoic acid to cause swelling when injected in the rat paw. As with arachidonic acid, on ageing eicosatrienoic acid spontaneously forms hydroperoxy acids. MK-447, but not indomethacin, was capable of suppressing the oedema induced by aged eicosatrienoic acid, implying involvement of the radical[12].

SUMMARY

In summation, with evidence that a stimulator of PG synthesis is capable of exhibiting anti-inflammatory activity it is possible to conclude that the primary PGs as represented by PGEs and PGFs are not the important mediators in these models of inflammation. The consistent depression of PGG_2 synthesis *in vitro* by all NSAI studied requires one to focus on this endoperoxide as a prime inflammatory mediator. However, instead of PGG_2 itself, a non-PG metabolite derived from it is more likely to be the actual inflammatory agent. A newly recognized component of the PG synthetase system, an oxygen dependent free radical released in the conversion of PGG_2 to PGH_2 is shown to be destructive to cyclo-oxygenase, thus limiting overall PG synthesis. Arguments are presented to suggest that this radical, a byproduct of the synthesis of prostaglandins, and thromboxanes may be the most important among the potentially numerous inflammatory mediators produced by the NSAI-sensitive oxygenation of PG precursor acids.

References

1. Vane, J. R. (1971). Inhibition of prostaglandin synthesis as a mechanism of action for aspirin-like drugs. *Nature New Biol.*, **231**, 232
2. Smith, J. B. and Willis, A. L. (1971). Aspirin selectively inhibits prostaglandin production in human platelets. *Nature New Biol.*, **231**, 235
3. Ham, E. A., Cirillo, V. J., Zanetti, M. E., Shen, T. Y. and Kuehl, Jr., F. A. (1972). Studies on the mode of action of non-steroidal antiinflammatory agents. In: *Prostaglandins in Cellular Biology* (P. W. Ramwell and B. B. Pharris, eds.) pp. 345–352. (New York: Plenum Press)
4. Tomlinson, R. V., Ringold, H. J., Qureshi, M. C. and Forchielli, E. (1972). Relationship between inhibition of prostaglandin synthesis and drug efficacy: Support for the current theory on mode of action of aspirin-like drugs. *Biochem. Biophys. Res. Commun.*, **46**, 552
5. Takeguchi, C. and Sih, C. J. (1972). A rapid spectrophotometric assay for prostaglandin synthetase: Application to the study of non-steroidal antiinflammatory agents. *Prostaglandins*, **2**, 169
6. Glenn, E. M., Bowman, B. J. and Rohloff, N. A. (1972). Pro-inflammatory effects of certain prostaglandins. In: *Prostaglandins in Cellular Biology* (P. W. Ramwell and B. B. Pharris, eds.) pp. 329–343. (New York: Plenum Press)
7. Moncada, S., Ferreira, S. H. and Vane, J. R. (1973). Prostaglandins, aspirin-like drugs and the oedema of inflammation. *Nature (London)*, **246**, 217
8. Samuelsson, B. (1965). On the incorporation of oxygen in the conversion of 8, 11, 14-eicosatrienoic acid to prostaglandin E_1. *J. Am. Chem. Soc.*, **87**, 3011
9. Hamberg, M. and Samuelsson, B. (1973). Detection and isolation of an endoperoxide intermediate in prostaglandin biosynthesis. *Proc. Nat. Acad. Sci. USA*, **70**, 899
10. Hamberg, M., Svensson, J. and Samuelsson, B. (1975). Thromboxanes: a new group of biologically active compounds derived from prostaglandin endoperoxides. *Proc. Nat. Acad. Sci. USA*, **72**, 2944
11. Winter, C. A., Risley, E. A. and Nuss, G. W. (1963). Antiinflammatory and anti-pyretic activities of indomethacin, 1-(*p*-chlorobenzoyl)-5-methoxy-2-methylindole-3-acetic acid *J. Pharmacol. Exp. Ther.*, **141**, 369
12. van Arman, C. G. and Risley, E. A. Unpublished observation
13. Roberts, A. (1973). Prostaglandins and the digestive system. In: *INSERM Seminar, The Prostaglandins* (E. Baubieu, ed.) pp. 297–315. (Paris: INSERM)
14. Kuehl, Jr., F. A., Humes, J. L., Egan, R. W., Beveridge, G. C. and van Arman, C. G. (1977). Role of prostaglandin endoperoxide PGG_2 in inflammatory processes. *Nature (London)*, **265**, 170
15. Egan, R. W., Paxton, J. and Kuehl, Jr., F. A. (1976). Mechanism for irreversible self-deactivation of prostaglandin synthetase. *J. Biol. Chem.*, **251**, 7329
16. Marnett, I. J., Wlodawer, P. and Samuelsson, B. (1975). Co-oxygenation of organic substrates by the prostaglandin synthetase of sheep vesicular gland. *J. Biol. Chem.*, **250**, 8510
17. Juhlin, L. and Michaelsson, G. (1969). Cutaneous vascular reactions to prostaglandins in healthy subjects and in patients with urticaria and atopic dermatitis. *Acta Derm. Venereol.*, **49**, 251
18. Ferreira, S. H. (1972). Prostaglandins, aspirin-like drugs and analgesia. *Nature New Biol.*, **240**, 200
19. Gale, P. H. Unpublished observation
20. Ho, P. P. K., Walters, P. and Sullivan, H. R. (1976). Biosynthesis of thromboxane B_2: assay, isolation and properties of the enzyme system in human platelets. *Prostaglandins*, **12**, 951
21. Chang, W.-C., Murota, S. and Tsurufuji, S. (1977). Thromboxane B_2 transformed from arachidonic acid in carrageenan-induced granuloma. *Prostaglandins*, **13**, 17

Discussion 25

H. Collier: (UK)	Does PGG$_2$ affect all the signs of inflammation? Dr. Kuehl dealt with oedema. Does it affect other signs of inflammation—pain, erethyma, and so on, in the same way?
Kuehl:	We feel that the vasodilation is well duplicated by prostaglandins of the E-type, and we know from other work that pain is induced partly by PGE$_2$, but better by bradykinin. Oedema is also elicited by PGE$_2$, but better by bradykinin in addition.
	We now know that bradykinin releases arachidonic acid, permitting the formation of lipoprostaglandin intermediates. We feel that the vasodilation now can be largely affected by the PGE$_2$, the pain by PGE$_2$ plus products derived from PGG$_2$, and the same for the oedema.
	It is obviously a very complicated picture, and one which we are only touching at present.
I. L. Bonta: (The Netherlands)	It appears that a complicated kind of shunting in the whole prostaglandin pathway is being tackled, where apparently the free radical formation is of great importance.
	I wonder whether free radical scavengers, such as pyrogallol or superoxide dismutase—and there are a number of others—might affect the whole shunting in a similar way to Dr. Kuehl's very interesting new compound.
Keuhl:	We used many free radical scavengers and they worked. Superoxide dismutase did not work and we feel that it may not get into the microsome envelope. We really think the free radical is superoxide, or more likely the hydroxy radical derived therefrom by the haemolysive reaction.

Discussion 24

26

Thiols and prostaglandin biosynthesis

C. DEBY, Z. M. BACQ AND P. VAN CANEGHEM (Belgium)

INTRODUCTION

The synthesis of PG may be studied on three main models: (1) *in vitro*, microsomes of bull or ram seminal vesicles with cofactors and arachidonic acid (AA) as substrate, (2) *in vivo*, temporary fall of blood pressure following intravenous injection of small amounts of AA in the anaesthetized rabbit or rat (for references, see [1]). The test used by Vargaftig[2], induction of platelet aggregation by injection of AA, indicates thromboxane formation after specific endoperoxidation of AA, (3) *in vitro* by addition of AA to the bath in which a sensitive smooth muscle (rat stomach strip) has been isolated. Generally speaking and according to the basic facts and ideas of Vane and his associates[3] there is good agreement between the results obtained with these three models; but there are some discrepancies useful to remember. For instance, heparine does not increase PG synthesis by the seminal vesicles microsomes but increases the response of the rabbit or rat blood pressure[4,1]; furthermore, certain substances which markedly inhibit the microsome system do not abolish the hypotension induced in the rabbit by AA injections[5,1]. Tryptophan added to the *in vitro* microsome system increases the yield of PG[6] and potentiates *in vivo* the hypotensive effect of AA in the rabbit[7].

Several pharmacological arguments strongly suggest that the oxygen utilized *in vivo* by the mixed oxygenase is not molecular oxygen ($^3O_2$) but a form of activated oxygen: the singlet oxygen $^1O_2$[8,9]. For instance, injection of the classical scavenger of singlet O_2, diphenylisobenzofurane (DPBF), temporarily inhibits the AA induced hypotension in the rabbit, while substances or systems which generate $^1O_2$ (paraquat, hypoxanthine + xanthine oxidase) increase this reaction, i.e. increase *in vivo* PG synthesis.

The importance of thiols in the synthesis of bioactive compounds derived from AA were for the first time observed by Samuelsson[10] and van Dorp[11] who demonstrated the favourable effect of glutathione on PG synthesis.

339

Vargaftig[12,13,2] has seen that mercaptoethanol and dithiothreitol inhibit arachidonic-acid-induced platelet aggregation, and responses of smooth muscles to this fatty acid.

In the present work, our purposes are:

(1) to compare the effects of different thiols on the AA induced hypotension in the rabbit, and on the response of rat stomach strips to AA;

(2) to try, on the same systems, the modifications eventually afforded by use of two thiol blocking agents;

(3) to see if the active thiols can modify the production of singlet oxygen.

Techniques

The carotid blood pressure is registered by the classical electronic equipment in rabbits (Fauve de Bourgogne, 2–2.7 kg, males) deeply anaesthetized by slow injection of urethane (20% in water) until disappearance of the corneal reflex. The rabbits are sensitized to AA by heparin (1 mg/kg), 1 h before the beginning of the experiment. AA injections in the jugular vein are such that they induce about 40% decrease of arterial pressure.

Stomach fundus strips (4 mm $\times$ 25 mm) with the epithelium carefully protected, from normally fed male rats ($\pm$ 180 g) are isolated in a 5 ml bath (Tyrode pH 7.6; t° 34 °C) automatically washed every 90 s. Injected arachidonic acid (AA) remains in contact with the strip for exactly 30 s. Drugs are also in contact with the preparation for 30 s; they are washed; AA is tested after a delay of 60 s.

The isotonic contractions are continuously registered (2 mm/min) with the sensitive apparatus previously described[14].

Solutions of AA (Sigma) are extemporaneously prepared from a 10 mg/ml solution in chloroform-hexane (1:2) stored under nitrogen at −60 °C. 0.1–0.5 ml of this solution are evaporated to dryness by a flow of N_2, taken in saline (rabbits) or Tyrode (stomach strips) and adjusted to pH 7.7. Sensitive chemical tests (gas–liquid chromatography and thiobarbiturate test) indicate the absence of peroxides in these solutions.

Chemiluminescence assays: Thiols have been tested as eventual singlet oxygen quenchers, in the Mallet reaction[15]

$$H_2O_2 + OCl^- \qquad {}^1O_2 + H_2O + Cl^- + h\nu$$

The appearance of a red luminescence shows that the liberated oxygen is in the singlet form[16]. 1 ml of sodium hypochloride is added with a syringe to 1 ml of hydrogen peroxide in a spectrophotometric cuvette, and the flash measured at its maximum with a photomultiplicator (SAFAS). Thiols were mixed to the H_2O_2 in the cuvette; the intensity of the flash is expressed in per cent of the controls.

Substances used

Mercaptoethanol, cysteine, glutathione (Merck); sodium cacodylate (BDH); D-penicillamine, lipoic acid, dithiothreitol and bismuthiol (Aldrich); N-ethylmaleimide, thioglycolate = mercaptoacetate (Fluka), cystamine (Labaz); crystalline cysteamine (Bracco) kept under argon. Absence of oxidation to S–S of cysteamine and glutathione is tested by amperometry.

Results

Table 26.1 summarizes our observations on the rabbit blood pressure. So far, only five of the substances mentioned in Table 26.1 have been tested on the rat stomach strip. Cysteine and glutathione in contact with the strip during 30 s at the concentration of 10^{-3}M increase the response to AA for 20 min despite the automatic washing every 90 s; the sensitization disappears progressively. On the contrary, mercaptoethanol at the same concentration, acting during the same time, completely desensitizes the preparation to AA during about 20 min; slow recovery may be observed and control

Table 26.1 Modifications of arachidonic acid (AA) hypotension in rabbits by thiols and thiol reagents

Substance	Dose (M/kg)	Number of animals	Coefficient*	Duration of effect (min)
Cysteine	8×10^{-5}	4	0.8–1	more than 120
	2×10^{-4}	4	0.6–0.8	more than 120
Glutathione	5×10^{-5}	6	0.5	more than 120
Cysteamine	5×10^{-4}	3	3	4–6
	1×10^{-3}	4	5–8	6–10
Cystamine	5×10^{-4}	4	2–2.5	7–10
Lipoic acid (thioctic acid)	2.4×10^{-5}	5	7–9	8–10
Mercaptoethanol	5×10^{-5}	4	1	
	1×10^{-4}	4	2–5	10–18
	2.5×10^{-4}	6	12–16	35–70
D-penicillamine	1×10^{-4}	2	1	
	2.5×10^{-4}	5	1	
Dithiothreitol	5×10^{-4}	4	4–5	4–6
Bismuthiol	5×10^{-4}	4	2	8–10
Thioglycolate	5×10^{-4}	4	1	
Na cacodylate	3×10^{-5}	6	0.5	20–30
	6×10^{-5}	8	0.3–0.4	90–130
N-ethylmaleimide	1×10^{-5}	5	0.3–0.4	more than 120 ·

* This coefficient is the number by which the dose of arachidonic acid must be multiplied in order to obtain the same decrease in blood pressure after injection of the substance. Thus a coefficient of 1 indicates no change; less than 1 = sensitization: more than 1 = inhibition.

response is reached after about 60 min. Lipoic acid similarly inhibits the response to AA, but recovery is more rapid and begins at 10 min. D-penicillamine 10^{-3}M does not alter the sensitivity of the strip to AA.

Reduced glutathione cysteine and mercaptoethanol at the concentration of 10^{-3}M do not alter the Mallet chemoluminescence; lipoic acid 10^{-3}M decreases it to 38% of the controls.

DISCUSSION

1. There is good agreement between the responses of the two biological tests: (1) mercaptoethanol and lipoic acid are inhibitory, (2) cysteine and glutathione sensitize, (3) penicillamine and thioglycolate are indifferent.

Numerous experiments of Vergaftig and associates on the modifying effects of thiol and thiol reagents[2] have been performed on platelets which react very much like smooth muscles. There is generally no difference between their results and ours but we insist on the fact that the drop of blood pressure induced by AA injections in the rabbit does not seem to be due primarily to release of PG by platelets in the plasma. We have seen that rabbits respond like normal animals to AA injections 9 days after heavy X-irradiation, i.e. when the concentration of platelets and white cells in the blood has been reduced to a few per cent of normal[1]. We believe that PG synthesis and subsequent metabolism in the blood vessel walls (for instance the formation of PGX) are more important for the changes in blood pressure than the events occurring in the platelets.

2. The desensitizing effect of mercaptoethanol, cysteamine and dithiothreitol might be correlated with the reduction to –SH of S–S functions of proteins[17,18], this reduction would increase the possibility of proteins to bind AA and consequently less substrate would become available. The fatty acid binding sites in proteins are located near the reduced sulphydryl groups[17]; this binding is altered by the oxidation of cysteinyl SH groups of plasma mercaptalbumins[18].

The sensitization by two –SH blocking agents (N-ethylmaleimide and cacodylate) agrees with this interpretation. The absence of effect of penicillamine and thioglycolate may be due to their lack of reducing action on S–S proteins. These two thiols do not act on the isolated rat liver mitochondria which react perfectly to glutathione and cysteine[19]. The chemiluminescence of Mallet reaction, proof of singlet oxygen generation, is significantly diminished by lipoic acid, a well known quencher of this excited form[20]. Thus, the inhibitory effect of lipoic acid on our two biological tests might be correlated with the same inhibitory action of other quenchers of singlet oxygen[8].

Other interpretations might be put forward of the effects of the thiols which do not correlate with any modification of singlet oxygen generation. Stimulating action of cysteine and GSH can be explained by the catalysing role of these thiols in lipid peroxidation[21-23] the importance of lipid peroxidation, as the first step in arachidonic acid conversion to prostanoid substances, is stressed in recent papers[24,25].

SUMMARY

Mercaptoethanol, cysteamine, dithiothreitol and lipoic acid inhibit the response to arachidonic acid (AA) of the isolated rat stomach strip and the hypotension of the anaesthetized heparinized rabbit. Cysteine and glutathione increase these actions of AA. Penicillamine and thioglycolate do not change them. The sensitizing effect of two –SH blocking agents (N-ethylmaleimide and cacodylate) may be correlated with the opposite effect of mercaptoethanol, cysteamine and dithiothreitol which by reduction of –S–S bonds of proteins, increase the binding of AA and decrease the availability of AA for PG synthesis. Lipoic acid is a quencher of singlet oxygen; these quenchers inhibit PG synthesis in vivo from AA. Other interpretations might be put forward.

References

1. Deby, C., Damas, J. and Bacq, Z. M. (1975). Un test in vivo de la synthèse des prostaglandines. Bull. Acad. Roy. Méd. Belg., 130, 178
2. Vargaftic, B. B., Tranier, Y. and Chignard, M. (1974). Inhibition by sulfhydryl agents of arachidonic acid-induced platelet aggregation and release of potential inflammatory substances. Prostaglandins, 8, 133
3. Flower, R. J. and Vane, J. R. (1974). Inhibition of prostaglandins biosynthesis. Biochemical Pharmacology, 23, 1439
4. Deby, C., Barac, G. and Bacq, Z. M. (1974). Action de l'acide arachidonique sur la pression artérielle avant et après héparine. Arch. Intern. Pharm. Ther., 208, 363
5. Deby, C., Descamps, M., Binon, F. et Bacq, Z. M. (1975). Inhibition de la biosynthèse in vitro de la PGE$_2$ par des substances anti-inflammatoires. Biochemical Pharmacology, 24, 1089
6. Miyamoto, T., Yamamoto, S. and Hayashi, O. (1974). Prostaglandin synthetase system. Resolution in oxygenase and isomerase components. Proc. Nat. Acad. Sci. USA, 71, 3645
7. Bacq, Z. M., Barac, G. and Deby, C. (1974). Potentiation by certain amino acids of hypotension induced by arachidonate. Brit. J. Pharmacology, 52, 111P
8. Deby, C. (1976). Action de piègeurs et d'un générateur d'oxygène singulet sur la synthèse in vivo des prostaglandines à partir d'acide arachidonique. Arch. Intern. Physiol. Bioch., 84, 867
9. Deby, C. (1900). Relation entre le métabolisme de l'oxygène et la biosynthèse des prostaglandines. Proc. Intern. Symp. on New Anti-inflammatory and Anti-rheumatic Drugs, Tirrenia 11 June 1976. In press in Tissue Reactions
10. Samuelsson, B. (1967). Biosynthesis and metabolism of prostaglandins. Progr. Biochem. Pharmac., 3, 59
11. Van Dorp, D. A. (1967). Aspects of the biosynthesis of prostaglandins. Progr. Biochem. Pharmacology, 3, 71
12. Vargaftig, B. B. and Dao-Hai, N. (1972). Interference of some thiol derivatives with the pharmacological effects of arachidonic acid and slow reacting substance C and with the release of rabbit aorta contracting substances. Europ. J. Pharmacol., 18, 43
13. Vargaftig, B. B. (1974). Search for common mechanisms underlying the various effects

of putative inflammatory mediators. In *The Prostaglandins* (P. W. Ramwell, ed.) vol. **2**, pp. 205–276. (New York: Plenum Press)

14. Deby, C., Espreux, G. and Topa, C. (1972). Appareil d'enregistrement électrique des contractions musculaires de faible amplitude. *Experientia*, **28**, 114
15. Mallet, L. (1927). Phénomènes de luminescence au cours de réactions oxydantes en solutions aqueuses. *C. R. Acad. Sci. Paris*, **185**, 352
16. Khan, A. U. and Kasha, M. (1964). Rotational structure in the chemiluminescence spectrum of molecular oxygen in aqueous systems. *Nature, London*, **204**, 241
17. Spector, A. A. (1975). Fatty acid binding to plasma albumin. *J. Lipid Res.*, **16**, 165
18. Fuller, Noel, J. K. and Hunter, M. J. (1972). Bovine mercaptalbumin and non-mercaptalbumin monomers. Interconversions and structural differences. *J. Biol. Chem.*, **247**, 7391
19. Neubert, D. and Lehninger, A. L. (1962). The effect of thiols and disulfides on water uptake and extrusion by rat liver mitochondria. *J. Biological Chemistry*, **237**, 952
20. Goda, K., Kimura, T., Thayer, A. L., Kees, K. and Schaap, P. (1974). Singlet molecular oxygen in biological systems: non-quenching of singlet oxygen-mediated chemiluminescence by superoxide dismutase. *Biophys. Biochem. Res. Comm.*, **58**, 660
21. Hoffsten, P. E., Hunter, F. E., Gebicki, J. M. and Weinstein, J. (1962). Formation of "lipid peroxide" under conditions which lead to swelling and lysis of rat liver mitochondira. *Bioch. Biophys. Res. Comm.*, **7**, 276
22. Hochstein, P. and Ernster, L. (1963). ADP-activated lipid peroxidation coupled to the TPNH oxidase system of microsomes. *Biochem. Biophys. Res. Comm.*, **12**, 388
23. Skrede, S. and Christophersen, B. O. (1966). Effects of cystamine and cysteamine on the peroxidation of lipids and the release of proteins from mitochondria. *Biochem. J.*, **101**, 37
24. Cook, H. W. and Lands, W. E. M. (1975). Evidence for an activating factor formed during prostaglandin biosynthesis. *Biochemical Bioph. Res. Comm.*, **65**, 464
25. O'Brien, P. J. and Rahimtula, A. (1976). The possible involvement of singlet oxygen in prostaglandin biosynthesis. *Biochem. Biophys. Res. Comm.*, **70**, 832

Discussion 26

B. Vargaftig: I want to confirm some of the topics raised by Professor Bacq.
(France)

With reduced glutathione, with cysteine, and with penicillamine as well—that is with three amino-thiols—a variety of effects of arachidonic acid on platelets could be potentiated both *in vivo* and *in vitro*. The interpretation is very difficult because there is, at least, the free radical hypothesis.

27

Interactions of non-steroidal anti-inflammatory drugs with substance P-like and gastrointestinal hormones-like polypeptides

J. P. FAMAEY, J. FONTAINE AND J. REUSE (Belgium)

INTRODUCTION

Prostaglandins (PGs) have been demonstrated to play a role in contractions of intestinal smooth muscle[1]. It has been shown by several authors that non-steroidal anti-inflammatory drugs (NSAID) inhibit PG-synthetases in various tissues[2]. NSAID were thus used in the guinea pig isolated ileum for further exploration of the functional significance of PGs in this model[3,4].

We have shown that at relatively high concentrations they reversibly inhibit contractions induced by acetylcholine (Ach), histamine (His), electrical stimulations and nicotine (Nic) in this order of increasing potency and that PGE_1, E_2 and $F_{2\alpha}$ largely overcome these inhibitions[5]. Similar observations were made on contractions to 5-hydroxytryptamine (5-HT)[6] and to angiotensine (Ang)[7]. In addition to the inhibitory effect on PG-synthesis we have suggested that these inhibitions could be due also to other NSAID effects such as those on biological membranes and on distribution of ions[5,8] well described by us and others in other models at similar concentrations[9]. Moreover we have recently shown that high concentrations of NSAID have also an inhibitory action on PG effects on the guinea pig ileum[10].

Anti-inflammatory steroids as well as chloroquine which both inhibit the prostaglandin production by acting on the phospholipase system have similar effects[8]. These might be also explained by biochemical effects on membranes and distribution of ions in addition to a reduction of the PG production. However it seems difficult to link our recent observation of a

347

similar activity produced by several sex steroids to an effect of these hormones on ileal PG metabolism and, in this case, a non-specific smooth muscle desensitization appears to be the most probable explanation[11].

From all these data we conclude that PGs must have a non-specific ileal smooth muscle sensitization property and that their reversal effect on NSAID inhibitions is partly specific and largely non-specific.

In order to obtain further support for this theory we have now investigated the capacity of other natural biological substances which have been described to sensitize the ileal smooth muscle to reverse these NSAID inhibitions.

Substance P sensitizes the guinea pig ileum to cholinergic contractions[12] and we have recently shown that the substance P-like polypeptide, physalaemin, extracted from the skin of the frog *Physalaemus fuscumaculatus* has very similar properties[13]. The gastrin-cholecystokinin-like polypeptide, caerulein, extracted from the skin of the frog *Hyla caerulea* seems to sensitize the guinea pig ileum not only to cholinergic contractions but also to contractions to non-cholinergic agonists[14].

We have thus tested various concentrations of caerulein and physalaemin for reversing properties on the inhibitions induced by several NSAID on contractions produced by Ach, His and Nic (and some preliminary experiments with 5-HT).

MATERIALS AND METHODS

Adult guinea pigs of either sex were stunned and bled and segments of ileum (4 cm) at least 10 cm from the caecum were set up in Krebs–Henseleit solution at 37 °C gassed with a mixture of 5% CO_2 and 95% O_2. Contractions to Ach (20 ng/ml), His (30 ng/ml) and Nic (0.5 µg/ml) were isotonically recorded as described elsewhere[5]. Inhibitions by NSAID were induced and recorded as described elsewhere[5]. After 1 to 3 contractions recorded in the presence of the inhibitory NSAID, according to the drug and the agonist tested, physalaemin (0.16–1.25 ng/ml) or caerulein (0.16–5 ng/ml) were added to the bath and one contraction at least was recorded in the presence of both NSAID and the polypeptide. In each experiment the ileum was finally challenged with the agonist after washing out both NSAID and the polypeptide. All the results were compared to control contractions obtained on the same ileal segments before adding the NSAID. The significance of the inhibitions and reversals was confirmed by Student's t-test for paired data.

RESULTS AND DISCUSSION

It appears that caerulein as well as physalaemin have no reversing properties on totally inhibitory NSAID concentrations but reverse quite well contractions which are partly (approximately 30–60% of control contractions) inhibited. This was also observed by us with PGs[5,8].

The concentrations of caerulein tested were increased from 0.16 ng/ml up to 5 ng/ml (Figure 27.1). These concentrations are known to induce ileal indirect contractions by themselves, probably mediated through nervous pathways[15]. Such contractions were observed (Figure 27.1) but they were less important than those induced by similar concentrations of caerulein in the absence of NSAID in the bath. These changes in ileal tone have not impaired observations at concentrations up to 5 ng/ml. It appears thus that in addition to a reversing effect of caerulein on NSAID inhibitions (which is better observed for concentrations from 0.63 ng/ml up to 5 ng/ml) there is an inhibitory action of NSAID on caerulein effects. We have currently undertaken a systematic investigation of these inhibitions which from our preliminary results appear also to be reversed by PGs.

The concentrations of physalaemin tested were increased from 0.16 ng/ml up to 1.25 ng/ml (Figure 27.2). These concentrations are known to induce ileal direct contractions by themselves[16]. Such contractions were observed (Figure 27.2). Even if they had sometimes a very high magnitude much more pronounced than those obtained when studying caerulein, they were less important than those induced by similar concentrations of physalaemin in the absence of NSAID in the bath. These changes in ileal tone have partly impaired observations at concentrations of 1.25 ng/ml and completely disturbed observations at higher physalaemin levels. It appears thus that in addition to a reversing effect of physalaemin on NSAID inhibitions (which

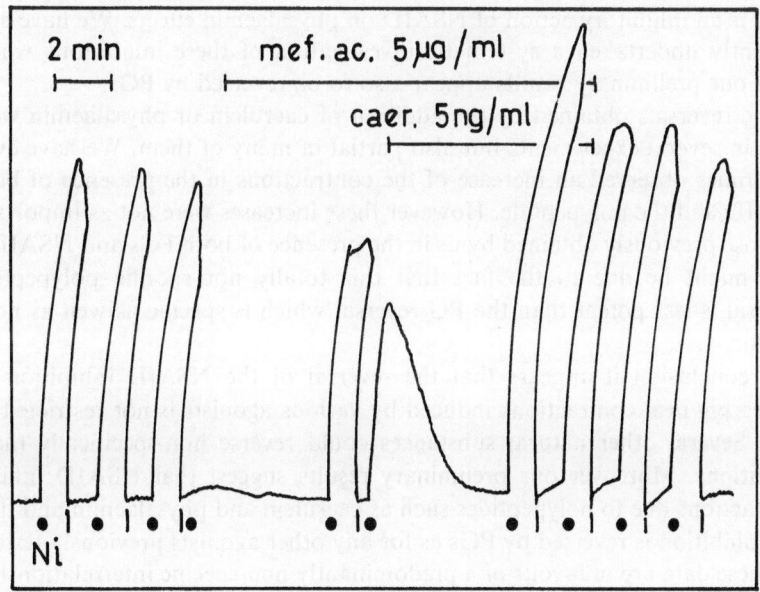

Figure 27.1 The reversal by caerulein (5 ng/ml) of the inhibition by mefenamic acid (5 μg/ml) of guinea pig isolated ileum contractions to nicotine (0.5 μg/ml)

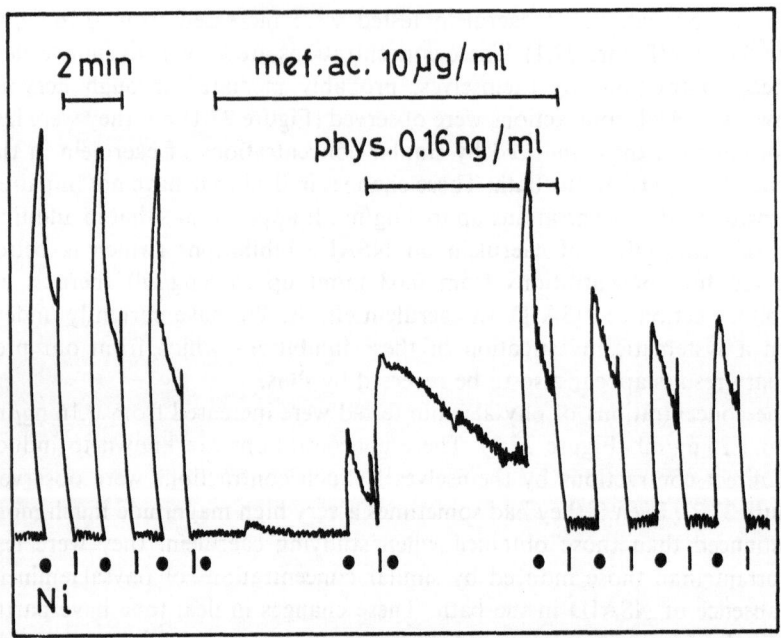

Figure 27.2 The reversal by physalaemin (0.16 ng/ml) of the inhibition by mefenamic acid (10 μg/ml) of guinea pig isolated ileum contractions to nicotine (0.5 μg/ml)

seems most easily observed at concentrations of 0.63 ng/ml, even if sometimes obtained at lower or higher concentrations from 0.16 ng/ml to 1.25 ng/ml) there is an inhibitory action of NSAID on physalaemin effects. We have also currently undertaken a systematic investigation of these inhibitions which from our preliminary results appear also to be reversed by PGs.

The reversals obtained by the addition of caerulein or physalaemin were total in several experiments but also partial in many of them. We have even sometimes observed an increase of the contractions in the presence of both NSAID and the polypeptide. However these increases were not as important as those previously obtained by us in the presence of both PGs and NSAID[5]. This might be due to the fact that this totally non-specific polypeptide reversal is less potent than the PG reversal which is specific as well as non-specific.

In conclusion it appears that the reversal of the NSAID inhibition of guinea pig ileal contractions induced by various agonists is not restricted to PGs. Several other natural substances could reverse non-specifically these inhibitions. Moreover our preliminary results suggest that NSAID inhibit contractions due to polypeptides such as caerulein and physalaemin and that this inhibition is reversed by PGs as for any other agonists previously tested. All these data are in favour of a predominantly non-specific interrelationship between NSAID and PGs effects on the guinea pig isolated ileum induced contractions.

350

Acknowledgements

The authors thank Mrs. J. Husson and C. Debruyne for their technical assistance, the Belgian 'Fonds National de la Recherche Scientifique' for financial support and Dr. Praga (Farmitalia, Italy) for the gift of caerulein and physalaemin.

References

1. Bergström, S., Eliasson, R., von Euler, U. S. and Sjövall, J. (1959). Some biological effects of two crystalline prostaglandins factors. *Acta Physiol. Scand.*, **45**, 133
2. Flower, R. J. (1974). Drugs which inhibit prostaglandins biosynthesis. *Pharmacol. Rev.*, **26**, 33
3. Bennett, A., Eley, K. G. and Scholes, G. B. (1969). Effects of prostaglandins E_1 and E_2 on human, guinea-pig and rat isolated small intestine. *Br. J. Pharmacol.*, **34**, 630
4. Bennett, A., Eley, K. G. and Stockley, H. L. (1975). The effects of prostaglandins on guinea-pig isolated intestine and their possible contribution to muscle activity and tone. *Br. J. Pharmacol.*, **54**, 197
5. Famaey, J. P., Fontaine, J. and Reuse, J. (1977). The effects of non-steroidal anti-inflammatory drugs on cholinergic and histamine-induced contractions of guinea-pig isolated ileum. *Br. J. Pharmacol.* (In press)
6. Famaey, J. P., Fontaine, J., Seaman, I. and Reuse, J. (1977). A possible role of prostaglandins in guinea pig isolated ileum contractions to serotonin. *Prostaglandins.* (Submitted for publication)
7. Famaey, J. P., Fontaine, J. and Reuse, J. (1977). Are prostaglandins involved in guinea-pig isolated ileum contractions to angiotensine? (In preparation)
8. Famaey, J. P., Fontaine, J. and Reuse, J. (1975). The inhibiting effect of morphine, chloroquine, non-steroidal and steroidal antiinflammatory drugs on the electrically induced contractions of guinea-pig ileum smooth muscle and the reversing effects of prostaglandins. *Agents Actions*, **5**, 354
9. Famaey, J. P., Brook, P. M. and Dick, W. C. (1975). Biological effects of non-steroidal antiinflammatory drugs. *Semin. Arthritis Rheum.*, **5**, 63
10. Famaey, J. P., Fontaine, J. and Reuse, J. (1977). Effect of high concentration of non-steroidal and steroidal antiinflammatory drugs on prostaglandin induced contractions of the guinea-pig isolated ileum. *Prostaglandins*, **13**, 107
11. Seaman, I., Famaey, J. P., Fontaine, J. and Reuse, J. (1977). Inhibitory effects of sexual hormones on the responses of the guinea-pig isolated ileum to acetylcholine and histamine. *Arch. Intern. Pharmacol. Ther.* (In press)
12. Hedqvist, P. and von Euler, U. S. (1975). Influence of Substance P on the response of guinea-pig ileum to transmural nerve stimulation. *Acta Physiol. Scand.*, **95**, 341
13. Fontaine, J., Famaey, J. P. and Reuse, J. (1977). Enhancement by physalaemin of the contractions induced by cholinergic stimulants in the guinea-pig ileum. *J. Pharm. Pharmacol.* (Submitted for publication)
14. Fontaine, J., Famaey, J. P. and Reuse, J. (1977). Sensitization of the contractions of the guinea pig isolated ileum to different agonist induced by caerulein. *Eur. J. Pharmacol.*, (Submitted for publication)
15. Del Tacca, M., Soldani, G. and Crema, A. (1970). Experiments on the mechanism of action of caerulein at the level of the guinea-pig ileum and colon. *Agents Actions*, **1**, 176
16. Bertaccini, G., Cei, J. M. and Erspamer, V. (1965). Occurrence of physalaemin in extracts of the skin of Physalaemus fuscumaculatus and its pharmacological actions on extravascular smooth muscle. *Br. J. Pharmacol.*, **25**, 363

Discussion 27

M. J. Parnham: In the light of Northover's findings, on the effects of indomethacin on
(The Netherlands)   calcium uptake in smooth muscle, and certainly the apparent non-
                 specificity of the effect of non-steroidal anti-inflammatory drugs on
                 Dr. Famaey's model, would it not seem reasonable that these effects
                 are mediated by the effect on calcium mobilization?

Famaey: That is a valuable hypothesis and we are currently undertaking
                 experiments by estimating the amount of calcium in the incubation
                 box to see if we could have the same kind of results and the same kind
                 of inhibition and reversing action of prostaglandin.

Parnham: Is there any indication of calcium in those experiments?

Famaey: For the moment we have only reduced half the amount of calcium.
                 The results are similar but we tend to reduce more.

28

Salicylic acid and proquazone: the differences in absorption and biodistribution explain their different profile of side-effects

ALAIN SCHWEITZER AND KAY BRUNE (Switzerland)

INTRODUCTION

It is now widely accepted that aspirin and related non-steroidal anti-inflammatory drugs (NSAID) cause side-effects in the stomach by direct interaction with mucosa cells of the stomach[1]. However, as to the molecular mechanisms which lead to decay of mucosa cells there is still controversy. On the one hand, it is believed that these drugs 'break the mucosa barrier' as proposed by Davenport[2] leading to back diffusion of protons from the gastric fluid into the mucosa cells which in turn get destroyed. On the other hand, one may follow Martin's concept[3]. He proposed, on the basis of the well accepted concepts of non-ionic diffusion of (acidic) drugs, that protonated aspirin (or other acids) may enter mucosa cells directly from the gastric fluid, get largely ionized and therefore trapped in the cell interior due to the neutral environment encountered, and destroy these cells by changing the intracellular pH together with the molality of the 'milieu interne'. This latter hypothesis was recently developed further by Rainsford and Brune[4] who, on the basis of clinical and histological findings, proposed that trapping of NSAID, especially salicylates, should preferentially occur and destroy parietal cells. These theoretical considerations were the starting point for the experiments to be reported. The absorption of salicylic acid and proquazone was monitored using biochemical and radioautographical methods. These drugs were chosen because the first one causes considerable gastric irritation and the latter one is a novel non-acidic anti-inflammatory drug which causes little gastric

353

damage[5]. By doing this we hoped to get proof for either one of the hypotheses described and, in addition, find an explanation for the low gastric irritancy of proquazone.

METHODS

All experiments were done using Sprague–Dawley rats bred in the Biocenter. Details of the morphological and biochemical methods used may be found in the legends of the figures.

RESULTS

Whole body radioautographical studies using young rats showed that both drugs (or their metabolites) accumulate in inflamed tissue and to some extent in the kidney (Figure 28.1a, b). However, although salicylic acid is accumulated in the wall of the non-glandular and glandular part of the rat stomach, proquazone remains in the lumen of the stomach for hours but it leaves the wall free of detectable radioactivity. This result was further confirmed by biochemical studies. In these experiments, either one of the tritium-labelled drugs was administered orally to rats in equimolar and therapeutic doses. After different time intervals the animals were killed, the stomachs removed, rinsed and gently cleaned with paper tissues. Samples taken from the mucosa and/or submucosa of the glandular and non-glandular part of the stomach were weighed, digested with protosol, counted and after correction for quenching and background, the results were expressed as dpm per mg tissue. In addition, blood obtained at the same times was processed correspondingly. The results are given in Figure 28.2a, b and c. They show that rapid absorption of salicylic acid occurs within the first minutes after administration in the glandular part of the rat stomach. In the non-glandular part activity continues to accumulate in the superficial layer of the mucosa for at least 1 h. However, proquazone is neither taken up in comparable quantities in the glandular nor in the non-glandular part of the rat stomach. These results were further confirmed by radioautographs of thin slices of the stomach wall obtained from deep-frozen specimens which were processed and exposed at $-25\ °C$. They show high concentrations of activity already one minute after administration of [³H]salicylic acid in the glandular part of the stomach. After 5 min, activity begins to disappear, however, in some areas of the glandular stomach, activity is retained in the parietal cells[6]. After 15 min, only small amounts of randomly distributed activity can be found. By contrast, in the non-glandular part of the stomach ³H-salicylic acid is slowly accumulating in the cornified surface layer of the mucosa reaching highest concentrations between 15 and 45 min after administration[6]. However, only minute amounts of activity can be found in the cells beneath the cornified surface layer of this 'mucosa'. As was to be expected from our biochemical studies, [³H]proquazone reached too low concentrations in all

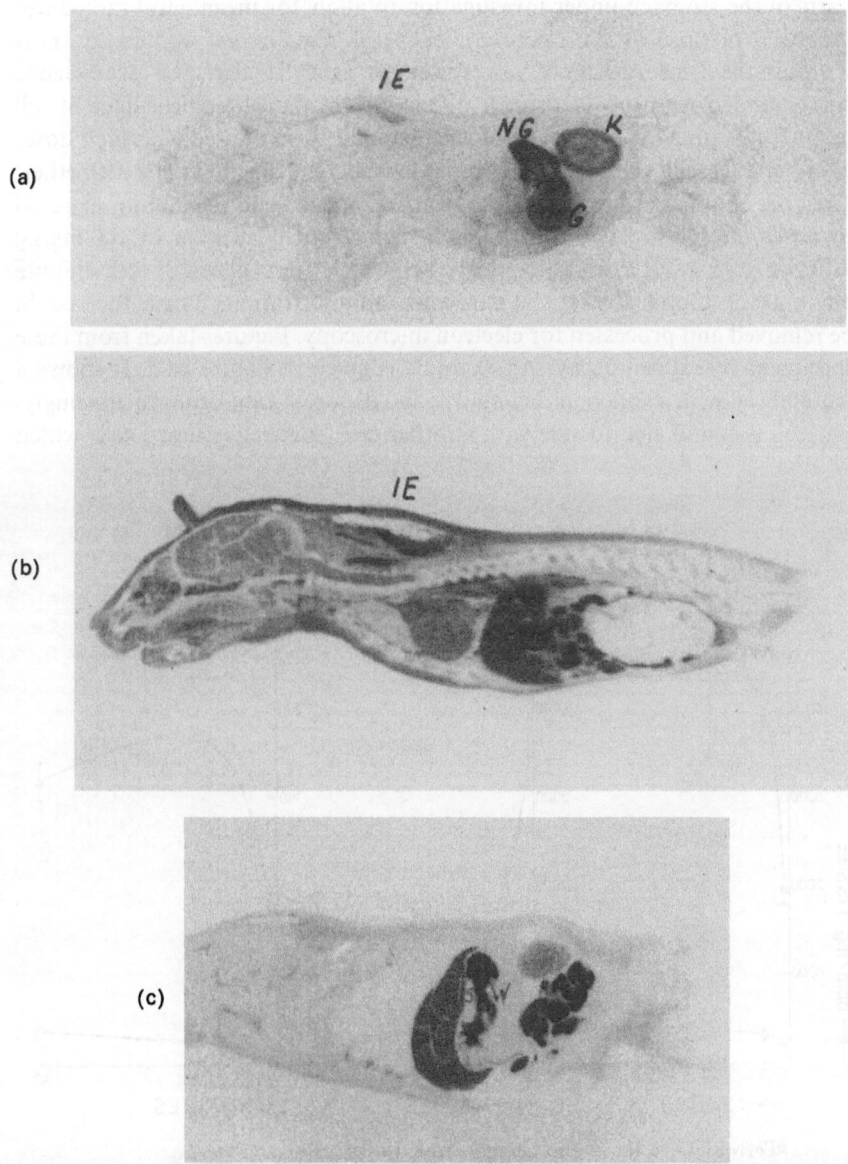

Figure 28.1 In young rats (40 g body weight) [^{14}C]salicylic acid (a) or [^{14}C]proquazone (b,c) was administered orally at 0-time (10 μCi/100 g). At the same time an inflammation was elicited by the injection of carrageenan (1 % w/v in saline) in the subcutaneous tissue of the neck. Three hours later the rats were killed, exsanguinated, deep frozen and cut for radioautography. Slices (100 μm thick) were lyophilized, then mounted on X-ray film and exposed for 3 weeks. The radioautograph obtained with [^{14}C]salicylic acid shows high activity in the glandular (GS) and non-glandular (NS) part of the stomach, the kidney and the inflammatory exudate (IE). Activity stemming from proquazone is clearly outside the stomach wall (SW), but some activity is seen in the fat pad of the inflamed tissue and in the kidney

parts of the stomach under investigation to allow for meaningful radioauto-graphical pictures at the microscopical level. Finally, we wanted to know whether the time course of absorption of salicylic acid and proquazone corresponded with the occurrence or the lack of morphological signs of cell decay in the glandular stomach of rats. Animals being dosed with high doses of either one drug were anaesthetized after different time intervals with ether. Then the abdomen was opened, the stomach opened and the interior exposed to observation with a dissecting microscope. Administration of 100 mg/kg salicylic acid caused microscopical foci which were covered with minute amounts of blood already 20 min after administration. These foci could be removed and processed for electron microscopy. Pictures taken from these specimens reveal cell decay. An example is given in Figure 28.3. It shows a parietal cell with swollen mitochondria and distorted canaliculi. Interestingly, this cell is found side to side with another cell (connective tissue cell) which

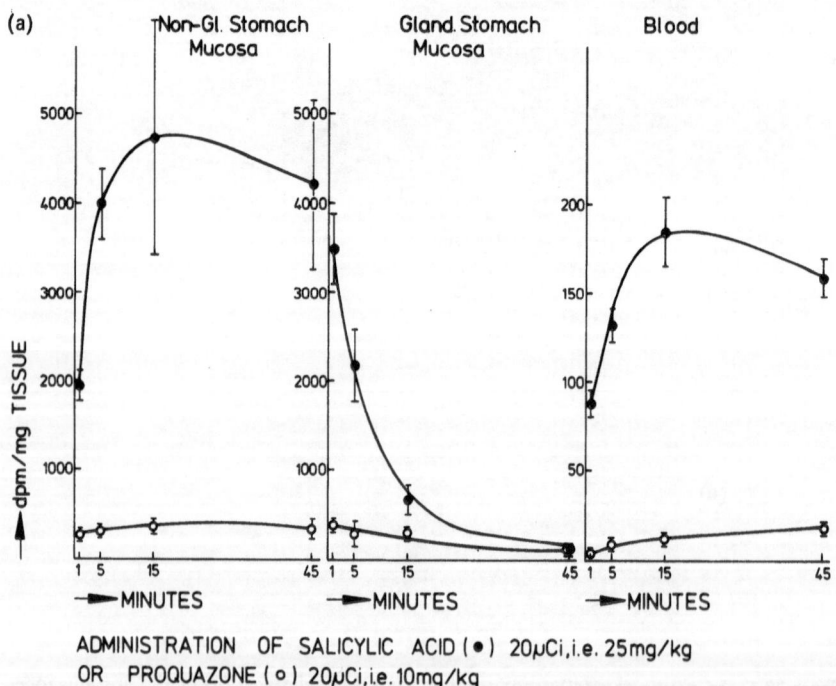

ADMINISTRATION OF SALICYLIC ACID (•) 20µCi, i.e. 25mg/kg
OR PROQUAZONE (○) 20µCi, i.e. 10mg/kg

Figure 28.2 Time course of [³H]salicylic acid and [³H]proquazone concentration in the glandular and non-glandular stomach and the blood of rats. Rats (100 g body weight) were fasted for 16 h, dosed with the drugs suspended in 0.5 ml saline by stomach tube and killed after different time intervals. The stomach was removed, rinsed with saline and gently cleaned with tissue paper. Samples from the parts of the stomach indicated, i.e. mucosa (a); submucosa (b) and whole stomach wall (c) were weighed, digested with Protosol and counted in a liquid scintillation spectrometer. The results were corrected for quenching and background and means ± SEs calculated from each time five experiments

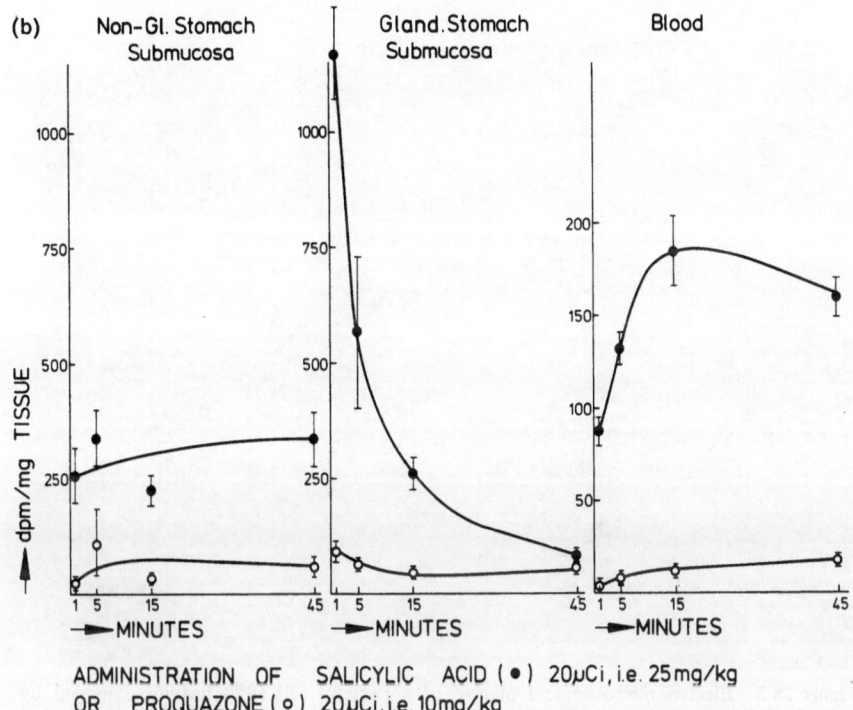

ADMINISTRATION OF SALICYLIC ACID (•) 20 μCi, i.e. 25mg/kg
OR PROQUAZONE (○) 20 μCi, i.e. 10mg/kg

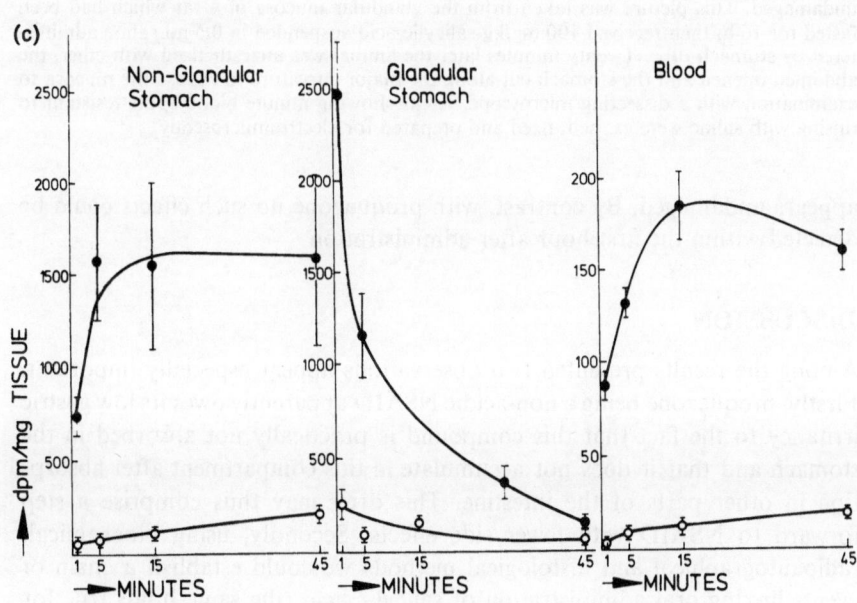

ADMINISTRATION OF SALICYLIC ACID (•) 20 μCi, i.e. 25mg/kg
OR PROQUAZONE (○) 20 μCi, i.e. 10mg/kg

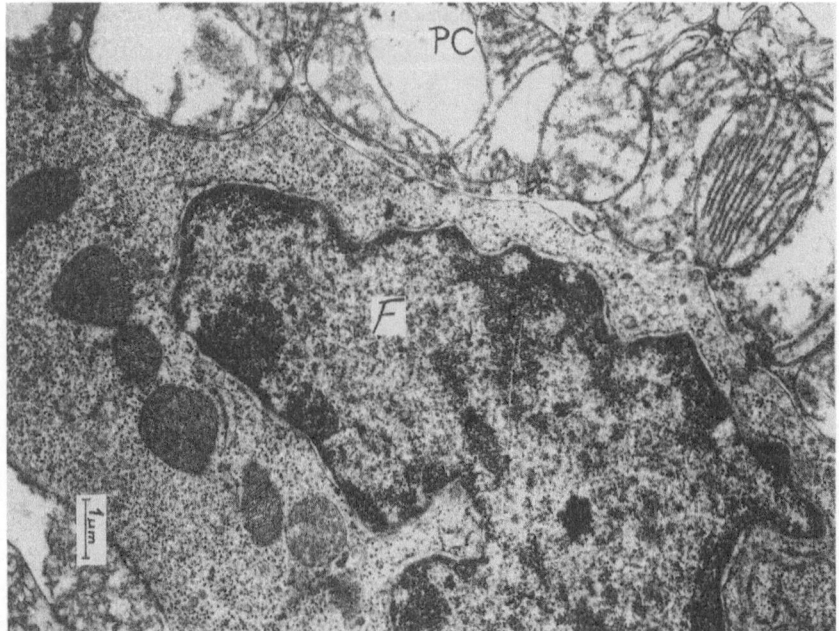

Figure 28.3 Electronmicroscopical picture of a parietal cell (PC) heavily damaged by administration of salicylic acid. This cell shows swollen and lysed mitochondria and distorted canaliculi. It was found in close vicinity of a connective tissue cell (F) appearing undamaged. This picture was taken from the glandular mucosa of a rat which had been fasted for 16 h, then received 100 mg/kg salicylic acid suspended in 0.5 ml saline administered by stomach tube. Twenty minutes later the animal was anaesthetized with ether, the abdomen opened and the stomach cut along the major curvature to expose the mucosa to examination with a dissecting microscope. Areas showing minute blood spots resistant to rinsing with saline were excised, fixed and prepared for electronmicroscopy

appears undamaged. By contrast, with proquazone no such effects could be detected within the first hour after administration.

DISCUSSION

Among the results presented two observations appear especially important. Firstly, proquazone being a non-acidic NSAID apparently owes its low gastric irritancy to the fact that this compound is practically not absorbed in the stomach and that it does not accumulate in this compartment after absorption in other parts of the intestine. This drug may thus comprise a step forward to NSAID with fewer side effects. Secondly, using biochemical, radioautographical and histological methods we could establish a chain of events linking oral administration of salicylic acid (the same holds true for aspirin), rapid absorption in the stomach, trapping in mainly parietal cells and decay of these cells together. These findings support the relevance of

Martin's[3] and our own concepts[4] of the molecular events causing gastric damage by NSAID especially salicylates. They are in good agreement with the observation that salicylates given in low doses in an acidic solution primarily inhibit ATP production (mitochondria!) and ion flux in the stomach wall and only secondarily cause back diffusion of protons[7]. These results are also relevant with respect to the proposed role of prostaglandins (PGs) in gastric damage due to NSAID[8]. Salicylic acid is almost devoid of PG-synthesis inhibition. Nevertheless it causes cell decay within minutes. Proquazone being a potent inhibitor of PG-synthesis, shows little gastric side effects[5]. These observations, however, do not rule out that pharmacological doses of prostaglandins or analogues[9] may influence absorption of salicylates and/or capillary blood flow in the stomach thus preventing cell decay. Lack of time prohibits discussing whether proquazone or its metabolites cause gastric irritation at later times and whether possible metabolites accumulate in the inflamed tissue[10]. These questions are under investigation at present.

References

1. Cooke, A. R. (1976). The role of the mucosal barrier in drug induced gastric ulceration and erosions. *Am. J. Dig. Dis.*, **21**, 2, 153
2. Davenport, H. W. (1967). Salicylate damage to the gastric mucosal barrier. *N. Eng. J. Med.*, **276**, 1307
3. Martin, B. K. (1963). Accumulation of drug anions in gastric mucosal cells. *Nature (London)*, **198**, 896
4. Rainsford, K. D. and Brune, K. (1976). Role of the parietal cell in gastric damage induced by aspirin and related drugs: Implications for safer therapy. *Med. J. Aust.*, **1**, 881
5. Takesue, E. I., Perrine, J. W. and Trapold, J. H. (1976). The anti-inflammatory profile of proquazone. *Arch. Int. Pharmacodyn.*, **221**, 122
6. Brune, K., Eckert, H. and Schweitzer, A. (1977). Parietal cells of the stomach trap salicylates during absorption and die. (Submitted for publication)
7. Kuo, Y. J. and Shenbour, L. L. (1976). Mechanisms of action of aspirin on canine gastric mucosa. *Am. J. Physiol.*, **230**, 762
8. Flower, R. J. and Vane, J. R. (1974). Inhibition of prostaglandin biosynthesis. *Biochem. Pharmacol.*, **23**, 1439
9. Lee, Y. H., Cheng, W. D., Bianchi, R. G., Mollison, K. and Hansen, J. (1973). Effects of oral administration of PG E_2 on gastric secretion and experimental peptic ulceration. *Prostaglandins*, **3**, 29
10. Van Ryzin, R. J., Bagdon, R. E., Hartman, H. A., Hrab, R. and Trapold, J. H. (1977). Animal safety evaluation studies on the anti-inflammatory quinazolinone, proquazone. *Toxicol. Appl. Pharmacol.* (In press)

Discussion 28

Whittle:
(UK)
Many non-steroid anti-inflammatory drugs—particularly indomethacin and aspirin—can cause gastric damage when they are administered
systemically, intravenously or subcutaneously, rather than intra-
gastrically. How does this fit in with the authors' hypothesis? Are they
suggesting that the gastric wall accumulates aspirin, or indomethacin,
in the bloodstream?

K. Brune:
(Switzerland)
We are well aware of these observations. However, we are also aware
of the limits of these observations. In administering salicylates by
routes other than the oral route, about 3–5 times the dose will be
needed to achieve some effects in the stomach. If our concept is
correct—and we are open to any suggestion that it might not be correct
—this will also lead to accumulation of the drug when the gradient
flux is from the blood to the stomach wall. It might well be indicated
that these high concentrations of salicylates necessary can, under these
conditions, also lead to damage in the stomach.

D. Sofia:
(USA)
I presume that these studies were done in normal rats. Have similar
studies been undertaken, or are there any plans for similar studies in
animals that are inflamed, such as the adjuvant-induced polyarthritic
rat? There may be changes. One of the suggestions was capillary flow
alterations. Might the same sorts of phenomena be seen in adjuvant-
induced polyarthritis?

Schweitzer:
(Switzerland)
All the experiments were done using Sprague–Dawley rats bred in the
Basel centre. We have plans to repeat the experiments using other rats
in order to correlate our results, but we are not yet so advanced.

29

Degradation of bovine nasal cartilage by a neutral protease from human leukocyte granules

D. KRUZE, P. SALGAM, K. FEHR AND A. BÖNI (Switzerland)

INTRODUCTION

It is generally believed that proteolytic enzymes from the lysosomes of polymorphonuclear leukocytes (PMN) participate in rheumatic inflammatory processes. One of the ways in which they act appears to be by damaging the articular cartilage. Cartilage consists of approximately 50% collagen and 50% chondromucoprotein[1,2].

PMN contain enzymes capable of hydrolysing these two main components. Lazarus et al.[3] isolated a leukocyte collagenase which solubilized reconstituted collagen fibrils. Ohlsson and Olsson[4] purified and characterized two collagenolytic enzymes from PMN. In the crude extract from the same cells, Kruze and Wojtecka[5] found a collagenase proenzyme which was activated by rheumatoid synovial fluid.

Another group of enzymes from PMN is able to degrade the chondromucoprotein of the cartilage matrix. Ziff et al.[6] demonstrated that extracts of human leukocytes reduce the viscosity of chondromucoprotein solutions. Using slices of rabbit ear cartilage as substrate, Ignarro et al.[7] showed that lysates of granules from human leukocytes released mucopolysaccharide degradation products into the incubation medium at pH 7.4. The same investigators[8] showed that the enzyme(s) degrading the non-collagenous matrix of cartilage are released from viable human peripheral leukocytes during the process known as non-phagocytic release. Recently, two neutral proteases purified from human PMN have been shown to degrade proteoglycan from rabbit articular cartilage slices and proteoglycan isolated from bovine nasal cartilage[9,10]. The present authors have purified and characterized a neutral protease from human PMN and have shown in preliminary experiments that it releases proteoglycan from human articular cartilage[11].

In a previous paper the effect of antirheumatic drugs on the activity of neutral protease against synthetic ester as substrate was reported[12]. In this study, bovine nasal cartilage was used as substrate. A satisfactory assay method using this tissue has been devised to quantify neutral protease activity and to measure the inhibitory effect of drugs.

MATERIALS AND METHODS

Drugs and reagents

The following drugs were tested: phenylbutazone, oxyphenylbutazone, sulfinpyrazone, diclofenac (Ciba-Geigy Limited, Basle, Switzerland*), gold sodium thiomalate (Byk Gulden GmbH, Constance, GFR), pyrazinobutazone (Dr. Wild & Co., Basle, Switzerland*), indomethacin (Merck Sharp & Dohme, Zurich, Switzerland*), hydroxychloroquine sulphate (Winthrop AG, Basle, Switzerland*), pentosan polysulphate (Benechemie GmbH, Munich-Sollin, GFR*), Arteparon (Luitpold-Werk, Munich, GFR*).

Hyaluronic acid and carbazole were obtained from Fluka AG, Buchs, Switzerland, N-t-BOC-L-alanine p-nitrophenyl ester (Z-Ala-NPh) from Sigma Chemical Co. St. Louis, Mo., USA, triple-crystallized bovine trypsin from Worthington Bioch. Corp., Freehold, New Jersey USA. Other chemical reagents and solvents were of analytical grade.

Enzyme

Neutral protease from human leukocytes was purified as described by Kruze et al.[11]. After the last purification step the final concentration of the pooled enzyme was 0.27 mg/ml. The esterolytic activity of the purified enzyme was measured against Z-Ala-NPh: 2.7 μg of the enzyme in 3 ml of 50 mM Tris buffer pH 7.4 containing 0.1 M NaCl at 25 °C increased the absorbance at 347.5 mM to 0.06 units per minute (1 cm light path).

Preparation of cartilage

Bovine nasal cartilage was freed from surrounding tissues, cut into small pieces about 7×7 mm in size, washed briefly with water and lyophilized. The dried cartilage was then ground in a coffee-mill and sieved (0.63 mm sieve). The pulverized cartilage was incubated in 0.1 M Tris buffer pH 7.4 containing 0.5 M NaCl (150 ml buffer per 10 g cartilage) for 3 h at 36 °C, washed thoroughly four times with water and centrifuged. This was followed by a second lyophilization, grinding and sieving. The procedure resulted in a yield of 13 g of dry pulverized material from 80 g wet cartilage. Uronic acid

*We wish to thank these firms for kindly supplying pure samples of the drugs named

was determined by Dische's reaction as modified by Bitter and Muir[13], using hyaluronic acid as standard.

Method of assay

20 mg of previously prepared cartilage was suspended in 5 ml of 50 mM Tris–HCl buffer pH 7.4 containing 0.1 M NaCl, pre-incubated in a shaking water-bath for 60 min at 36 °C, and then centrifuged for 20 min at 24 000 g. The supernatant was discarded and the pellet suspended in 2 ml of the same buffer. Appropriate amounts of neutral protease or trypsin in a volume of 25 μl were then added. The suspension was incubated in a shaking water-bath for 40 min at 36 °C and the reaction stopped by cooling in ice. After centrifuging twice for 10 min at 24 000 g, 0.5 ml of completely clear supernatant was taken for Dische's reaction. A blank was prepared in the same way but without enzyme.

Effect of drugs

The effect of drugs on neutral protease activity was studied by means of the above method of assay. An appropriate amount of the drug concerned was dissolved in 50 mM Tris–HCl buffer pH 7.4 + 0.1 M NaCl, after which 2 ml of this solution was added, together with 0.05 μg of neutral protease in a volume of 25 μl, to the washed pellet of cartilage from the pre-incubation step. In the event that the drug concerned was insoluble in this buffer, dimethyl sulphoxide (final concentration 0.5%) was added. The rate of inhibition was calculated in relation to the activity in an experiment conducted in the same way but without the drug. Previous experiments had shown neither an effect of the 0.5% solvent on neutral protease nor of the test concentration of the drug on Dische's reaction.

RESULTS

Complete digestion of bovine cartilage

In order to characterize the prepared cartilage, it was completely digested with an excess of neutral protease. In the course of a 5 h incubation, 0.304 μg of neutral protease released the whole of the digestible chondromucoprotein matrix from 5 mg of cartilage (Figure 29.1). Increasing the amount of the enzyme did not increase the rate of digestion. From this experiment it was calculated that the prepared cartilage contained the equivalent of about 31% hyaluronic acid.

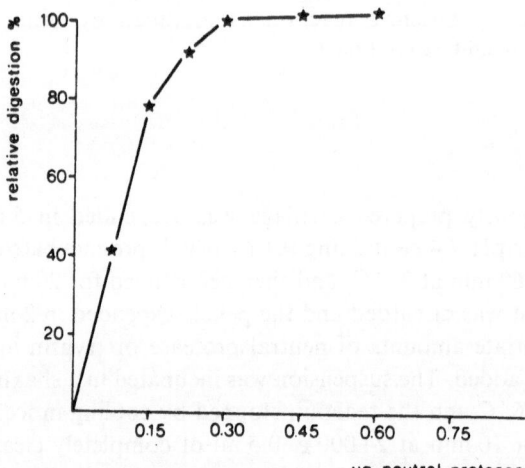

Figure 29.1 Exhaustive digestion of bovine nasal cartilage by human neutral protease from leukocytes. 5 mg cartilage was incubated for 5 h at 37 °C in 2 ml of 50 mM Tris–HCl buffer pH 7.4 + 0.1 NaCl with various amounts of leukocyte neutral protease. The rate of digestion is shown as the percentage of the total uronic acid released from the cartilage into the incubation medium

Effect of pH

The pH value for optimum activity of leukocyte neutral protease in respect of nasal bovine cartilage was found to be 7.4 (Figure 29.2). This pH was chosen for the assay method.

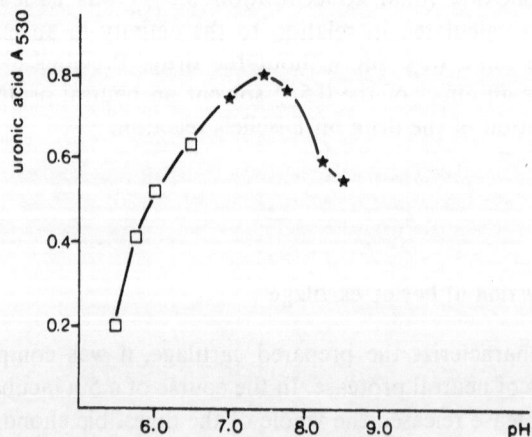

Figure 29.2 Effect of Ph on the activity of human leukocyte neutral protease using nasal bovine cartilage as substrate. 0.075 μg of neutral protease was used. The other conditions were as described in the assay method. The activity was measured by determining the amount of uronic acid released. Buffers were Tris–HCl (□—□—□) and phosphate (★—★—★), both at 50 mM concentration containing 0.1 M NaCl

Dependence on incubation time and amount of enzyme

The linearity of the enzyme assay with time when amounts of 0.05 μg neutral protease and 0.03 μg trypsin are used is shown in Figure 29.3. For neutral protease and for trypsin the linearity remains constant for over 60 and 40 min respectively, corresponding to an absorbance of more than 0.7. The control sample, incubated without enzyme, reaches its maximum in about 15 min, after which its value remains almost unchanged. In order to obtain

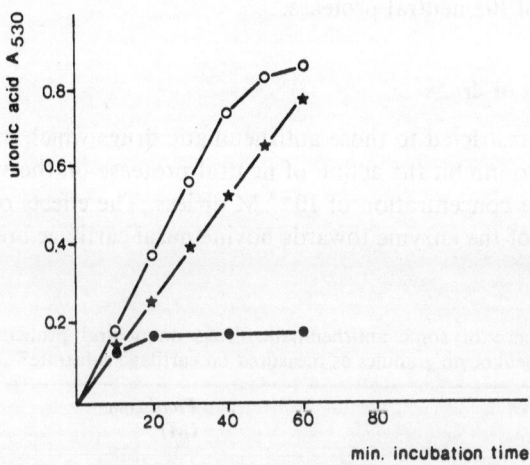

Figure 29.3 Effect of incubation time on the degradation of bovine nasal cartilage by human neutral protease and trypsin. 0.05 μg of neutral protease ★—★—★ and 0.03 μg of trypsin O—O—O were used. Blanks ●—●—● consisting of buffer alone were used as controls

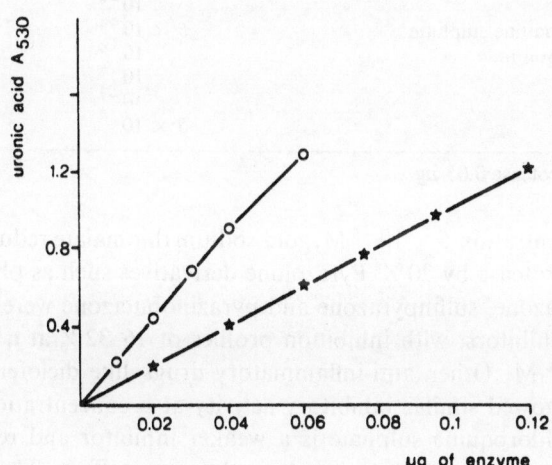

Figure 29.4 Comparison of the activities of human neutral protease and trypsin in the degradation of bovine nasal cartilage. Neutral protease ★—★—★, trypsin O—O—O. The conditions were as described in the assay methods.

satisfactory precision, a 40 min incubation time was chosen for all the subsequent experiments. Under these conditions the amount of enzymatically released uronic acid was about three times greater than that in the control.

The relationship between uronic acid release and the amount of neutral protease is shown in Figure 29.4. The linearity holds for amounts up to 0.12 μg neutral protease and also for an amount of enzyme less than 0.01 μg. For trypsin the relationship is also linear, but as shown in Figure 29.4, trypsin releases about twice as much uronic acid from the cartilage as the same amount of the neutral protease.

Inhibitory effect of drugs

The study was restricted to those antirheumatic drugs which had previously been shown[12] to inhibit the action of neutral protease on the synthetic ester Z-Ala-NPh at a concentration of 10^{-4} M or less. The effects of these drugs on the activity of the enzyme towards bovine nasal cartilage are summarized in Table 29.1.

Table 29.1 Influence of some antirheumatic drugs on neutral protease from human leukocyte granules as measured on cartilage substrate*

Drug	Final conc. (M)	Inhibition (%)
Gold sodium thiomalate	5×10^{-5}	20
Phenylbutazone	2×10^{-4}	26
Oxyphenbutazone	2×10^{-4}	32
Sulfinpyrazone	2×10^{-4}	17
Pyrazinobutazone	2×10^{-4}	16
Diclofenac	10^{-4}	26
Indomethacin	10^{-4}	24
Hydroxychloroquine sulphate	5×10^{-4}	23
Pentosan polysulphate	10^{-6}	60
SP-54	10^{-7}	18
Arteparon	10^{-7}	56
	5×10^{-8}	18

* Neutral protease 0.05 μg

At a concentration 5×10^{-5} M, gold sodium thiomalate reduces the activity of neutral protease by 20%. Pyrazolone derivatives such as phenylbutazone, oxyphenbutazone, sulfinpyrazone and pyrazinobutazone were also found to be potent inhibitors, with inhibition profiles of 16–32% at a concentration of 2×10^{-4} M. Other anti-inflammatory drugs like diclofenac and indomethacin, showed similar inhibitory activity at a concentration of 10^{-4} M.

Hydroxychloroquine sulphate is a weaker inhibitor and required a fivefold higher concentration to produce the same effect. The most potent inhibitors of neutral protease, on a molar basis, were the two sulphonated polysaccharides Arteparon and pentosan polysulphate; at a concentration of 10^{-7} M these substances brought about 56% and 18% inhibitions respectively. Even at half this concentration Arteparon had a significant effect.

DISCUSSION

The results of the study reported here show that purified neutral protease from human PMN digests bovine nasal cartilage at physiological pH. Since the purified neutral protease lacks collagenolytic and hyaluronidase activity (unpublished data) this process consists solely of proteolysis of the proteoglycan of cartilage. Further study is necessary to determine more exactly which of the protein constituents, the core protein or proteoglycan link proteins, or both, are degraded. The rapidity of the degradation, the similarity to digestion by trypsin (Figures 29.3 and 29.4) which is known to yield peptide fragments containing 1–10 chondroitin sulphate chains[14,15]—and the ready solubility of the released fragments in the incubation medium all suggest that neutral protease cleaves proteoglycan at many of its amino acid residues and that at least the proteoglycan subunit core protein is involved in this process. Keiser et al.[10] analysed the digestion products of isolated cartilage proteoglycan with two cationic proteases from PMN and found that two protein constituents were degraded.

Exhaustive digestion with neutral protease released an amount of uronic acid from the pulverized cartilage corresponding to about 15% of its initial weight (Figure 29.1). In view of the known amount of keratan sulphate present and the fact that chondromucoprotein consists of about 70% sulphated polysaccharides and 30% protein[1] it can be concluded that neutral protease is capable of solubilizing almost the whole of the proteoglycan contained in cartilage.

The activity of neutral protease against the proteoglycan of cartilage as substrate is nearly a half of that of trypsin (Figure 29.4), and is thus of considerable importance. 1 μg of neutral protease releases the equivalent of 0.17 mg of hyaluronic acid per min. Allowing for the proportions of keratan sulphate and collagen in cartilage, this corresponds to the damage of about 0.37 mg of native cartilage.

In order to quantify the inhibitory effect it was necessary to devise a satisfactory assay method. Existing methods used by many investigators, like sedimentation coefficient assay and viscosimetric measurement, or the method recently devised by Sapolsky et al.[16], use isolated and solubilized proteoglycan from cartilage.

With fresh slices of cartilage, the relationship between release of digested products and time of incubation is not linear[9]. Moreover, as we found in preliminary experiments in this laboratory, the blank values with fresh slices were too high for a quantitative method. Two-stage incubation, once before lyophilization and again just before digestion, removed readily extractable material and probably also proteolytic enzymes capable of interfering with the enzyme assay[16,17]. In the method described in this paper, the relationship of the amount of uronic acid released with time and with enzyme concentration are linear. Thus linearity is a prerequisite for measurement of the activity of an unknown sample or of the activity of a proteolytic enzyme in an inhibitor mixture. The sensitivity of the method is very high: satisfactorily accurate assays are possible with less than 15 ng of neutral protease. It is not as time-consuming as viscosimetric or sedimentation coefficient measurements and thus is suitable for assaying large numbers of samples, for example during purification procedures. Since pulverized whole cartilage is used, the method is applicable to the study of the simultaneous action of proteolytic enzyme and of collagenase or a glycosidase.

All the typical anti-inflammatory or antirheumatic drugs tested caused marked inhibition of neutral protease (Table 29.1). Most effective in this respect were the two sulphonated polysaccharides Arteparon and pentosan polysulphate. The former is used in the treatment of degenerative joint diseases[18], while in animal experiments the latter has proved to be a potent anti-inflammatory drug[19]. A very interesting finding was that the widely used drug gold sodium thiomalate, which is a very effective inhibitor of cathepsin B_1[20], is also a potent inhibitor of neutral protease. This is in agreement with the observations by Perper and Oronsky[21] that this drug inhibits some of the cartilage-degrading enzymes present in leukocyte granule lysate. Other potent anti-inflammatory agents, like the pyrazolone derivatives, diclofenac and indomethacin, had a distinct inhibitory action at a concentration of 2×10^{-4} M. Such a concentration in plasma is reached under the therapeutic regimens usual with some pyrazolone derivatives[22-24], but exceeds that obtainable with diclofenac or indomethacin[25,26]. As has been shown for indomethacin[27], however, the possibility of their accumulation in the synovial tissue cannot be excluded.

The inhibitory effect of some drugs against cartilage as substrate was smaller than against synthetic ester[12]. It was very marked for the gold salt and for the two sulphonated polysaccharides. It is possible that these drugs become bound to cartilage and that in this way their inhibitory activity is reduced[28]. It should be noted that natural conditions are more exactly reproduced by the assay method using cartilage than by assay with a synthetic substrate. The effect of drugs was studied in the light of the hypothesis that therapeutically effective antirheumatic agents would inhibit neutral protrease. The results reported support this assumption and may to some extent explain the clinical effectiveness of these substances.

SUMMARY

A purified neutral protease from human leukocyte granules degrades bovine nasal cartilage by releasing digestion products of proteoglycan at physiological pH. 1 μg of this enzyme releases the equivalent of 0.17 mg of hyaluronic acid per minute. A photometric method of assay has been devised for the quantitative measurement of the digestion, based on the determination of the amount of uronic acid released from suitable prepared cartilage. The sensitivity of the method allows measurement of less than 10 ng of trypsin and of about 15 ng of neutral protease with satisfactory precision. Of the drugs tested, two sulphonated polysaccharides, Arteparon and pentosan polysulphate, are the most potent inhibitors of neutral protease when calculated on a molar basis. They are effective at concentrations of 10^{-8} M and 10^{-7} M respectively. The pyrazolone derivatives diclofenac and indomethacin inhibit at a concentration of 2×10^{-4} M, gold sodium thiomalate at a concentration of 5×10^{-5} M. These results support the assumption that the neutral protease concerned plays an important role in the pathological process of joint destruction.

Acknowledgements

The authors wish to thank Mr. E. G. Boyce and Miss E. Feller for help in preparing the manuscript.

This work was supported in part by research grants from 'Eidgenössische Rheumakommission' of the Swiss Public Health Service and from 'Schweizerischer Nationalfonds zur Förderung der wissenschaftlichen Forschung', grant No. 3.027–073 and No. 3.419–0.74.

References

1. Sapolsky, A. J., Woessner, Jr., J. F. and Howell, D. S. (1975). A photometric assay for protease digestion of the proteoglycan subunit. *Anal. Biochem.*, **67**, 649
   Shatton, J. and Schubert, M. (1954). Isolation of mucoprotein from cartilage. *J. Biol. Chem.*, **211**, 568
2. Malawista, J. and Schubert, M. (1958). Chondromucoprotein; new extraction method and alkaline degradation. *J. Biol. Chem.*, **230**, 535
3. Lazarus, G. S., Daniels, J. R., Brown, R. S., Bladen, H. A. and Fullmer, H. M. (1968). Degradation of collagen by a human granulocyte collagenolytic system. *J. Clin. Invest.*, **47**, 2622
4. Ohlsson, K. and Olsson, J. (1973). The neutral proteases of human granulocytes. Isolation and partial characterization of two granulocyte collagenases. *Eur. J. Biochem.* **36**, 473
5. Kruze, D. and Wojtecka, A. (1972). Activation of leukocyte collagenase proenzyme by rheumatoid synovial fluid. *Biochim. Biophys. Acta*, **285**, 436
6. Ziff, M., Gribetz, H. J. and LoSpalluto, J. (1960). Effect of leukocyte and synovial membrane extracts on cartilage mucoprotein. *J. Clin. Invest.*, **39**, 405
7. Ignarro, L., Oronsky, A. and Perper, R. (1973). Breakdown of noncollagenous chondromucoprotein matrix by leukocyte lysosome granule lysates from guinea pig, rabbit and human. *Clin. Immun. Immunopathol.*, **2**, 36
8. Oronsky, A., Ignarro, L. and Perper, R. (1973). Release of cartilage mucopolysaccharide degrading neutral protease from human leukocytes. *J. Exp. Med.*, **461**, 138
9. Janoff, A., Feinstein, G., Malemud, C. J., and Elias, J. M. (1976). Degradation of cartilage proteoglycan by human leukocyte granule neutral proteases—A model of joint injury. I. Penetration of enzyme into rabbit articular cartilage and release of $^{35}SO_4$-labelled material from the tissue. *J. Clin. Invest.*, **57**, 615

10. Keiser, H., Greenwald, R. A., Feistein, G. and Janoff, A. (1976). II. Degradation of isolated bovine nasal cartilage proteoglycan. *J. Clin. Invest.*, **57**, 625
11. Kruze, D., Menninger, H., Fehr, K. and Böni, A. (1976). Purification and some properties of neutral protease from human leukocyte granules and its comparison with pancreatic elastase. *Biochim. Biophys. Acta*, **438**, 503
12. Kruze, D., Fehr, K., Menninger, H. and Böni, A. (1976). Effect of antirheumatic drugs on neutral protease from human leukocyte granules. *Z. Rheumatol.*, **35**, 337
13. Bitter, T. and Muir, H. M. (1962). A modified uronic acid carbazole reaction. *Anal. Biochem.*, **4**, 330
14. Heinegard, D. and Hascall, V. C. (1974). Characterization of chondroitin sulfate isolated from trypsin-chymotrypsin digests of cartilage proteoglycans. *Arch. Biochem. Biophys.*, **165**, 427
15. Keiser, H. and deVito, J. (1974). Immunochemical studies of fragments of bovine nasal cartilage proteoglycan subunit. *Connect. Tissue Res.*, **2**, 273
16. Sapolsky, A. J., Howell, D. S. and Woessner, Jr., J. F. (1974). Neutral proteases and cathepsin D in human articular cartilage. *J. Clin. Invest.*, **53**, 1044
17. Dziewiatkowski, D. D., Tourtellotte, C. D. and Campo, R. D. (1968). In: *Chemical Physiology of Mucopolysaccharides* (G. Quintarelli, ed.) pp. 63–79. (Boston: Little, Brown)
18. Hofer, H. and Zimmerebner, O. (1972). Spätergebnisse der medikamentösen lokalen Langzeittherapie bei Arthrosen. *Wien. Klin. Wochenschr.*, **84**, 190
19. Kalbhen, D. A. (1973). Pharmacological studies on the anti-inflammatory effect of a semi-synthetic polysaccharide (pentonen polysulfate). *Pharmacology*, **9**, 74
20. Kruze, D., Fehr, K. and Böni, A. (1976). Effect of antirheumatic drugs on cathepsin B_1 from bovine spleen. *Z. Rheumatol.*, **35**, 95
21. Perper, R. J. and Oronsky, A. L. (1974). Enzyme release from human leukocytes and degradation of cartilage matrix. *Arthr. Rheum.*, **17**, 47
22. Burns, J. J., Rose, R. K., Chenkin, T., Goldman, A., Schubert, A. and Brodie, B. B. (1953). The physiological distribution of phenylbutazone (Butazolidin) in man and a method for its estimation in biological material. *J. Pharm. Exp. Ther.*, **109**, 346
23. Wilhelmi, E. (1965). In: *Symposium über die posttraumatische Entzündung und ihre Behandlung*, Davos 1964. pp. 62–67. (Basel and New York: S. Karger)
24. Inaka, T., Besley, M. E. and Chow, E. J. (1975). Determination of sulfinpyrazone in serum by high performance liquid chromatography. *J. Chromatogr.*, **104**, 165
25. Riess, W., Stierlin, H., Geiger, U. P., Gerardin, A., Schmid, K., Wagner, J. and Theobold, W. (1975). Presented at the Symposium 'Die chronischen Polyarthritiden' in Torremolinos
26. Hucker, H. B., Zacchel, H. G., Cox, S. V., Brodie, D. A. and Cantwell, N. H. (1966). Studies on the absorption, distribution and excretion of indomethacin in various species. *J. Pharm. Exp. Ther.*, **153**, 237
27. Langkilde, M. (1966). Distribution of indomethacin on the soft tissue. In: *Indomethacin Symposium* p. 69
28. Greiling, H. and Kaneko, M. (1973). Die Hemmung lysosomaler Enzyme durch ein Glykosaminoglykanpolysulfat. *Arzneim. Forsche.*, **23**, 593

30

Inhibition of experimental ocular inflammation by topical application of non-steroidal anti-inflammatory drugs (NSAID)

P. GAUTHERON, Ph. CONQUET, AND J. C. LEDOUAREC
(France)

INTRODUCTION

There is now ample evidence suggesting the involvement of prostaglandins (PGs) in some form of experimental ocular inflammation. Detectable amounts of PGs of the E and F types were found in aqueous humour of rabbit eyes injured either by paracentesis of the anterior chamber[1,2], scratching the iris[3] or non-perforating trauma[4]. The inflammatory response to such physical stimuli, such as blood aqueous barrier disruption, hyperaemia, miosis and intraocular pressure (IOP) elevation[5,6], could be mimicked by local application or intracameral injection of PGs or arachidonic acid (AA)[7-11].

Non-steroidal anti-inflammatory drugs given topically or by other routes of administration proved effective in different experimental models in the rabbit. Inhibition of protein leakage into aqueous humour, induced by paracentesis or other trauma, was achieved with aspirin, indomethacin, pirprofen, indoprofen, and to a lesser extent, by oxyphenbutazone[3,12-15]. Similarly, blood aqueous barrier disruption and IOP rise following AA instillation were prevented or reduced by aspirin, indomethacin, indoxole and other non-steroid anti-inflammatory agents[16-20]. Indomethacin and indoxole were among the most active agents in this respect.

The presence of PG synthesis in ocular tissues was confirmed by *in vitro* studies. Microsomal fractions from rabbit anterior uveal tissues (iris +

371

ciliary body) and from conjunctiva generated PG-like activity after AA administration[21]. The effect of drugs was also demonstrated in the *in vitro* situation; indomethacin, indoprofen and indoxole strongly inhibited PG-synthetase, whereas oxyphenbutazone and aspirin presented little or on activity[15,22].

In the present study, the anti-inflammatory activity of indomethacin, indoxole, aspirin and oxyphenbutazone was compared in three rabbit models of ocular inflammation in which PG-release is likely; paracentesis, non-perforating trauma of the cornea and AA-instillation. Differences of potency observed with drugs under study seem to be related to their capability to reach the appropriate site of PG-synthesis.

MATERIALS AND METHODS

Albino rabbits of either sex weighing 2.5–3.0 kg were used throughout this study. Paracentesis and non-perforating trauma were performed with local anaesthesia. Unless otherwise stated, drugs were suspended in 0.5% hydroxy-ethylcellulose (HEC) in water, and administered in a single 50 μl instillation in both eyes of animals 30 min before the injury. In each experiment, three groups of four rabbits were used for IOP determination and three groups of six rabbits were employed in the other models; one control group receiving the vehicle and two groups being treated.

1. Paracentesis

Paracentesis was performed twice at 30 min intervals with a 25-gauge needle using a special gun. Direct trauma of the iris or the lens was avoided. In a preliminary study, this time interval was shown to be sufficient to allow refilling of the anterior chamber by newly formed aqueous humour. Proteins in the aqueous were determined in the primary and secondary samples. Hyperaemia of the iris was graded according to an arbitrary scale of 0 to 3, including half scores.

2. Non-perforating trauma

This type of injury was performed with a special spring-powered device consisting of a steel rod to one end of which a plastic ball was appended. An adjustable part of this instrument was firmly applied to the edge of the orbit, thus giving a constant distance between the ball and the cornea. The injury was produced by a blow to the centre of the cornea. 30 min after trauma, iris hyperaemia was scored and aqueous humour collected for protein determinations.

3. Arachidonic-acid instillation

Iris hyperaemia and protein determinations in the aqueous humour were determined in a separate group of animals from those in which IOP measurements were made. In the first series, 50 μl of 2% AA (Sigma, Grade 1) in triacetin was instilled in both eyes of rabbits. Iris hyperaemia and proteins were determined 30 min later. In the second series, IOP was indirectly measured by applanation tonometry using a Bausch and Lomb pneumatic tonometer previously calibrated by manometry in the anaesthetized rabbit. Animals were accustomed to restraint in wooden boxes for 2 days during which IOPs were determined several times a day[23]. Following this pretest period, 50 μl of an 0.5% AA solution in triacetin was instilled in both eyes of the test animals. IOP was measured without anaesthesia just before AA application, and then every 15 min for 1 h. Drugs were instilled 30 min before AA. The percentage of inhibition was calculated by comparing the area under the curve of increased IOP (ΔP) of treated versus controls from $t = 0$ to $t - 60$ minutes.

4. Protein determination

Proteins were routinely estimated by the refractive index of aqueous humour determined with the Bausch and Lomb refractometer and by comparison with a standard curve established with the Lowry technique[24].

Data in tables are given as per cent inhibition of treated series versus controls. Statistical analysis was made with the student's t-test.

RESULTS

Figure 30.1 represents the ocular response to the different types of injury. The protein content in aqueous humour, 30 min after paracentesis (3800 mg/100 ml) was 5 times greater than after trauma (750 mg/100 ml) and 3.5 times that after AA instillation (1080 mg/100 ml). By contrast, the intensity of iris hyperaemia was in the same range for the three models. The IOP response to AA took place rapidly. The maximal effect was reached after 15 min, followed by a return to initial value (Figure 30.2).

1. Effect of drugs in paracentesis (Table 30.1)

The large protein leakage in aqueous humour induced by paracentesis was reduced in a dose-related manner by aspirin, indomethacin and oxyphenbutazone. Aspirin was very active in this test with a 54% inhibition at 5% concentration (ED50 = 750 μg/eye), whereas the maximal inhibitory effect exhibited by indomethacin was 45% at 0.01%. Nevertheless, this drug was significantly active at a concentration as small as 0.001% (0.5 μg/eye). The

Table 30.1 Anterior chamber paracentesis. Effect of drugs on proteins in aqueous humour
—percentage of inhibition

	Concentration %					
	0.001	0.01	0.1	1.0 (d)	5.0	10.0
Indomethacin in						
Ph.V. (a)	8	48 (b)	62 (b)	52 (b)		
Indomethacin in HEC	22 (b)	45 (b)	38 (b)	42 (b)		
Indoxole in Ph.V. (a)			+8 (c)	0		
Aspirin in HEC		12 (b)	27 (b)	55 (b)	54 (b)	
Oxyphenbutazone in HEC		11 (b)	1	14	25 (b)	45 (b)

Drugs suspended either in Ph.V. or in HEC were instilled (50 μl) once 30 min before
paracentesis.

(a) Pharmaceutical vehicle containing polysorbate 1.5 mg/ml (see p. 373).

(b) Significant for $P < 0.05$.

(c) Proteins in A.H. were increased.

(d) Corresponds to 500 μg/eye.

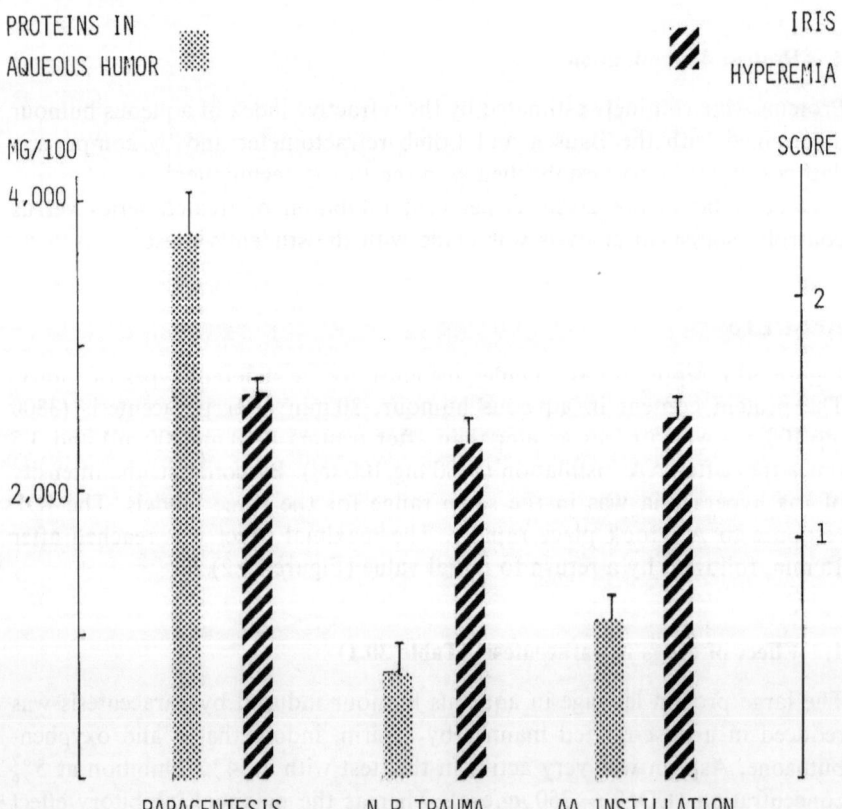

Figure 30.1 Proteins in aqueous humour and iris hyperaemia induced by various types of
injury in the rabbit eye. Data are given with SD

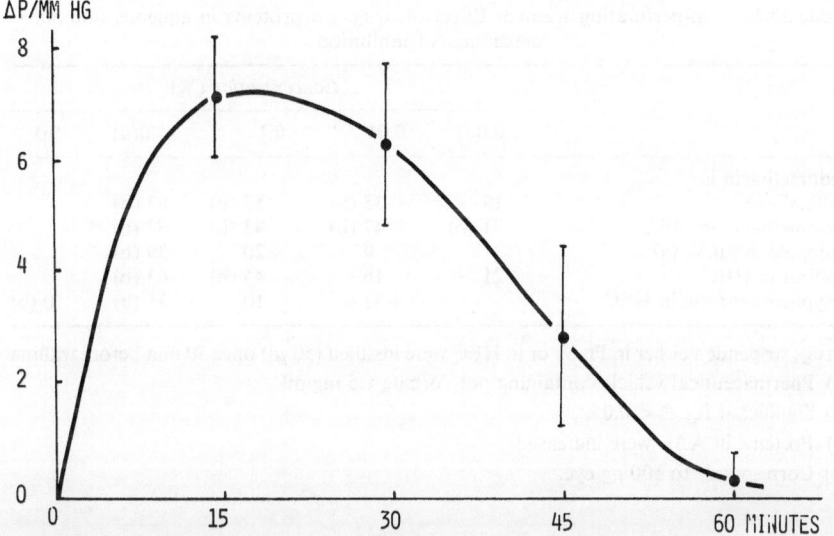

Figure 30.2 Intraocular pressure (IOP) elevation induced by instillation of arachidonic acid 0.5% in the rabbit eye. Data are given with SD

use of a pharmaceutical vehicle* containing 1.5 mg/ml polysorbate, greatly improved the potency of indomethacin; the maximal inhibition reaching 62% with an ED50 of 50 μg/eye. Oxyphenbutazone was the least active drug since at 10% concentration proteins were reduced only by 45%. Indoxole was found inactive at 0.1 and 1% either suspended in hydroxyethylcellulose or the pharmaceutical vehicle, or solubilized in triacetin.

2. Effect of drugs in non-perforating trauma

The inhibition of protein leakage induced by drugs is shown in Table 30.2. The drugs appeared slightly more active in this model since ED50s for indomethacin, aspirin and oxyphenbutazone were 85, 115 and 2300 μg/eye, respectively, When suspended in the pharmaceutical vehicle, indomethacin exhibited a greater inhibitory effect. Protection of the blood aqueous barrier with this drug attained 87% with an ED50 of 18 μg/eye. In the same vehicle, indoxole was found inactive at 0.01% and 0.1% concentration, but significantly reduced proteins in aqueous humour by 39% at 1% concentration.

* Vehicle composition: 0.02 g lecithin, 0.25 g phenylethyl alcohol, 0.25 g benzyl alcohol, 0.02 g benzalkonium HCl, 0.05 g disodium edetate, 0.2 g sodium disulphite, 0.6 g sodium chloride, 1 g sorbitol solution, 0.15 g polysorbate 80, 0.15 g hydroxyethylcellulose, water for injection qs ad 100 ml.

Table 30.2 Non-perforating trauma. Effect of drugs on proteins in aqueous humour—percentage of inhibition

	Concentration (%)				
	0.001	0.01	0.1	1.0(d)	5.0
Indomethacin in Ph.V. (a)	19	35 (b)	53 (b)	87 (b)	
Indomethacin in HEC	31 (b)	47 (b)	43 (b)	57 (b)	
Indoxole in Ph.V. (a)		0	+20	39 (b)	
Aspirin in HEC	21	16	45 (b)	63 (b)	
Oxyphenbutazone in HEC		+23 (c)	10	31 (b)	50 (b)

Drugs suspended either in Ph.V. or in HEC were instilled (50 μl) once 30 min before trauma
(a) Pharmaceutical vehicle containing polysorbate 1.5 mg/ml.
(b) Significant for $P < 0.05$.
(c) Proteins in A.H. were increased.
(d) Corresponds to 500 μg/eye.

3. Effect of drugs on AA-induced protein leakage in aqueous humour

Except for oxyphenbutazone, test compounds were found extremely active in this model (Table 30.3). Indomethacin (1 %) and aspirin (5 %) were able to reduce proteins in aqueous humour by about 70 % with ED50s of 0.45 and 77 μg/eye, respectively. Indoxole, suspended in the pharmaceutical vehicle, was found more potent (ED50 = 6 μg/eye) than aspirin, but less than indomethacin either suspended in hydroxyethylcellulose or in the pharmaceutical

Table 30.3 Arachidonic acid (AA) instillation. Effect of drugs on proteins in aqueous humour—percentage of inhibition

	Concentration (%)								
	0.000 001	0.000 01	0.000 1	0.001	0.01	0.1	1.0 (d)	5.0	10.0
Indomethacin in Ph.V. (a)	+20 (c)	50 (b)	42 (b)	82 (b)	88 (b)	92 (b)	91 (b)		
Indomethacin in HEC		+23 (b)	37 (b)	63 (b)	70 (b)	68 (b)	71 (b)		
Indoxole in Ph.V. (a)			+ 9	29 (b)	65 (b)	69 (b)	90 (b)		
Aspirin in HEC				17	14	76 (b)	78 (b)	72 (b)	
Oxyphenbutazone in HEC				+ 8	12	22 (b)	21 (b)	34 (b)	

Drugs suspended either in Ph.V. or in HEC were instilled (50 μl) once 30 min before AA (50 μl–2 % in triacetin) instillation.
(a) Pharmaceutical vehicle containing polysorbate 1.5 mg/ml.
(b) Significant for $P < 0.05$.
(c) Proteins in A.H. were increased.
(d) Corresponds to 500 μg/eye.

vehicle (ED50 = 0.09 μg/eye). Blood aqueous barrier disruption was almost completely prevented by indomethacin and indoxole suspended at 1% in pharmaceutical vehicle. However, indomethacin exhibited a greater potency since significant reduction was obtained for concentrations as low as 0.000 01 per cent corresponding to a topical application of 0.005 μg/eye.

4. Effect of drugs on AA-induced IOP elevation

All test compounds were found very active in a dose-related manner in this assay (Table 30.4). Indoxole and indomethacin at 1% were able to inhibit the

Table 30.4 Arachidonic acid (AA) instillation. Effect of drugs on intraocular pressure (IOP) elevation—percentage of inhibition

	Concentration (%)					
	0.001	0.01	0.05	0.1	0.5	1
Indomethacin in Ph.V. (a)	23	54		55		85 (b)
Indomethacin in HEC		41		46 (b)		68 (b)
Indoxole in Ph.V. (a)	28	36		54		78 (b)
Aspirin in HEC		5	43	73 (b)		69 (b)
Oxyphenbutazone in HEC		23		24	33	69 (b)

Drugs suspended either in Ph.V. or in HEC were instilled (50 μl) once 30 min before AA (50 μl–0.5%) instillation (t0)

Percentages of inhibition were calculated in comparing area under curves of treated *vs* controls from t0 to t + 60 min after AA application.

(a) Pharmaceutical vehicle containing polysorbate 1.5 mg/ml.

(b) Significant for $P < 0.05$.

AA-induced IOP elevation by 78% and 85%, respectively. Oxyphenbutazone and aspirin, at the same concentration, both inhibited this reaction by 69%. It is to be pointed out that indomethacin, suspended in hydroxyethylcellulose, appeared to be less active than when suspended in the pharmaceutical vehicle. The following ED50s were obtained: indomethacin (in HEC) (45 μg/eye), indomethacin (in pharmaceutical vehicle) (10 μg/eye), indoxole (20 μg/eye), aspirin (50 μg/eye) and oxyphenbutazone (350 μg/eye).

5. Effect of test compounds on iris hyperaemia

As shown in Table 30.5, the inhibitory effect of the test compounds was less marked on iris hyperaemia than on the other parameters, protein and IOP. Maximal reduction of iris vasodilatation, achieved by any compound, was 45%. Indomethacin, however, was active at much smaller concentrations than the other agents. Contrary to other parameters, the effect of a drug on iris hyperaemia did not appear to depend on the type of injury, except for oxyphenbutazone which was more effective in trauma.

377

Table 30.5 Inhibition by NSAID of iris hyperaemia induced by various injuries maximal and minimal significant inhibitions (in %)

		Paracentesis		Non-perforating trauma		Arachidonic acid instillation	
Indomethacin in HEC	Maximal inhibition (d)	28	(1.0)(c)	46	(1.0)	59	(1.0)
	Minimal inhibition	12	(0.001)	37	(0.01)	8	(0.000 1)
Indomethacin in Ph.V. (a)	=	42	(1.0)	39	(1.0)	43	(0.1)
		9	(0.001)	16	(0.01)	15	(0.001)
Indoxole in Ph.V. (a)	=	(b)		(b)		38	(1.0)
						7	(0.01)
Aspirin in HEC	=	41	(5.0)	41	(1.0)	54	(5.0)
		30	(1.0)	29	(0.1)	31	(0.1)
Oxyphenbutazone in HEC	=	12	(10.0)	47	(5.0)	9	(10.0)
		11	(5.0)	21	(1.0)	9	(10.0)

(a) Pharmaceutica! vehicle containing polysorbate (1.5 mg/ml).

(b) Inactive.

(c) Drug concentration (in %).

(d) Drugs were tested at intermediate concentrations—Data are not given.

DISCUSSION

This study confirms that topically applied non-steroid anti-inflammatory drugs inhibit inflammatory responses of the eye following trauma. However, few studies have appeared comparing their effectiveness in different models of traumatic inflammation. As far as the blood aqueous barrier is concerned, the ocular response seems quantitatively different according to the type of injury. Barrier disruption appeared more severe after paracentesis than after AA application or trauma. Using fluorescein angiography, Bhattacherjee and Hammond[25] observed a larger disruption, as visualized by entry of the dye in the anterior chamber, after paracentesis than after AA instillation. 30 min after paracentesis, the anterior chamber was entirely refilled with plasmoid humour, whereas after application of AA or after non-perforating trauma, the newly formed plasmoid humour was diluted with about $200 \mu l$ of protein-free aqueous humour. This explains why less proteins were present in aqueous humour after AA instillation or trauma. Our values for protein in aqueous humour after paracentesis or AA instillation are in the range of those reported in the literature, i.e. about 4000 mg/100 ml and 1000 mg/ml, respectively[6,15,17,18].

Non-steroid anti-inflammatory drugs do not completely protect the blood eye barrier from the disruption induced by paracentesis; about 30% is resistant to drug. This relative failure has been previously observed for aspirin, indomethacin or pirprofen given topically or by other routes of administration[6,12,25]. The following explanations might be proposed:

(1) Drugs did not penetrate in the eye in sufficient amounts. Indirect

378

evidence was given in this study of the influence of the vehicle on indo-methacin effect. Direct evidence of an enhanced penetration of indomethacin through use of a tensio-active vehicle has been demonstrated[26].

(2) Mediators, other than PGs, might be implicated in the permeability changes of the blood aqueous barrier[6,25,27].

Most of the authors have reported dilatation of iris vessels following various eye traumas, but very few have studied its inhibition by non-steroid anti-inflammatory drugs. This is probably due to lack of useful objective techniques. Although the scale we used is subjective, it seems that a great part of iris hyperaemia, induced by either injury, is not inhibited by such agents. This confirms the observations of Ohtsuki et al.[28] and of Whitelocke and Eakins[29]. However, hyperaemia, induced by post-ganglionic sympathetic denervations, seems to be prevented by pretreatment with indomethacin[30]. Mediators, other than prostaglandins, may be involved in iris vasodilation induced by physical or chemical trauma.

Our data (Table 30.6), on the relative potency of drugs, are in keeping with previous studies. Thus, indomethacin is one of the most powerful anti-inflammatory agents either in vivo[18,20] or in vitro[15]. However, indomethacin was reported less effective than indoxole on microsomal fractions from uveal or conjunctival tissues[18], but more active on AA-induced IOP rise[20]. When suspended in the same vehicle (containing polysorbate), we found that indomethacin was twice as active as indoxole on IOP elevation induced by AA, and 66 times in reducing protein after AA application. In this latter test, topical application of 0.000 01 % indomethacin was able to significantly reduce protein leakage by 50%. Indoxole was completely inactive at this concentration. Aspirin was reported to be weakly active in vitro on PG-synthesis using eye microsomal fraction[15,18]. Our in vivo study, as well as others[2,12,17], indicates that this drug is very active against the rupture of the blood aqueous barrier induced by various injuries as well as on IOP elevation following AA application.

Table 30.6 Inhibition by NSAID of protein leakage in aqueous humour and of IOP rise induced by various injuries—ED 50 (μg per eye)

	Paracentesis	Non-perforating trauma	Arachidonic acid instillation	
			Effect on protein	Effect on IOP
Indomethacin in HEC	>500	85	0.45	45
Indomethacin in Ph.V. (a)	50	18	0.090	10
Indoxole in Ph.V. (a)	(b)	(c)	6	20
Aspirin in HEC	750	115	77	50
Oxyphenbutazone in HEC	>2500	2300	>2500	350

(a) Pharmaceutical vehicle containing polysorbate (1.5 mg/ml).

(b) Inactive.

(c) Significantly active only at 1%.

When suspended in hydroxyethylcellulose, indoxole was ineffective against the disruption of the blood aqueous barrier induced by paracentesis or non-perforating trauma, whereas a significant reduction of protein in aqueous humour was observed after trauma by changing hydroxyethylcellulose for a pharmaceutical vehicle containing polysorbate. The protective effect of indoxole on paracentesis-induced blood aqueous barrier disruption was not reported except by Bhattacherjee and Hammond[25] who estimated protein leakage by fluorescein angiography and used a vehicle containing 30 times more polysorbate than ours. Nevertheless, that study, as well as the present work, seemed to indicate that indoxole did not easily penetrate into the ocular tissues. Podos and Becker[20] and Bhattacherjee and Eakins[18] have shown that indoxole potency in AA-induced IOP changes could be increased (by 60 and 5 times respectively) by the use of polysorbate containing vehicles. Since indoxole inhibited the effects of AA but not those of paracentesis or non-perforating trauma because of a lack of penetration, it is hypothesized that the site of PG-synthesis is not the same in both cases; one of them being more readily accessible than the other. Thus, it is likely that AA, topically administered, is transformed in PGs in the conjunctiva, whereas paracentesis stimulates synthesis in the iris, also known as a site of PG synthetase activity. Non-perforating trauma could trigger PG synthesis both in iris and conjunctiva.

In conclusion, penetration into ocular tissues is critical for the pharmacological effect of topical agents and should be studied accordingly. Penetration studies are in progress to compare the penetration of the drugs investigated above after topical application in the rabbit eye.

Acknowledgements

The skilful technical assistance of Mrs. G. Courtadon, D. Alix and L. Coulbault is gratefully acknowledged.

References

1. Ambache, N., Kavanagh, L. and Whitting, J. (1965). Effect of mechanical stimulation on rabbits' eyes: Release of active substance in anterior chamber perfusates. *J. Physiol.* (*London*), **175**, 378
2. Miller, J. D., Eakins, K. E. and Atwal, M. (1973). The release of PGE$_2$-like activity into aqueous humor after paracentesis and its prevention by aspirin. *Invest. Ophthal.*, **12**, 939
3. Cole, D. F. and Unger, W. G. (1973). Prostaglandins as mediators for the responses of the eye to trauma. *Exp. Eye Res.*, **17**, 357
4. Dray, F., Charbonnel, B., Bechetoille, A., Nou, B. and Sarraux, H. (1974). Prostaglandines E$_2$ et F$_{2a}$ dans l'humeur aqueuse au cours de l'hypertension oculaire post-contusive précoce chez le lapin. *Arch. Ophthal.* (*Paris*), **34**, 899
5. Neufeld, A. H. and Sears, M. L. (1973). The site of action of prostaglandin E$_2$ on the disruption of the blood-aqueous barrier in the rabbit eye. *Exp. Eye Res.*, **17**, 445
6. Unger, W. G., Cole, D. F. and Hammond, B. (1975). Disruption of the blood-aqueous barrier following paracentesis in the rabbit. *Exp. Eye Res.*, **20**, 255

7. Beitch, B. R. and Eakins, K. E. (1969). The effects of prostaglandins on the intraocular pressure of the rabbit. *Br. J. Pharmacol.*, **37**, 158
8. Starr, M. S. (1971). Further studies on the effect of prostaglandin on intraocular pressure in the rabbit. *Exp. Eye Res.*, **11**, 170
9. Green, K. and Kim, K. (1975). Pattern of ocular response to topical and systemic prostaglandin. *Invest. Ophthalmol.*, **14**, 36
10. Meyers, R. L., Shabo, A. L. and Maxwell, D. S. (1975). Effect of prostaglandin on the blood aqueous barrier in the rabbit ciliary process. *Prostaglandins*, **9**, 167
11. Szalay, J., Goldberg, R. and Klug, R. (1976). The effect of prostaglandin on iridial blood vessel permeability. *Acta Ophthal. (Kbh)*, **54**, 731
12. Neufeld, A. H., Jampol, L. M. and Sears, M. L. (1972). Aspirin prevents the disruption of the blood-aqueous barrier in the rabbit eye. *Nature (London)*, **238**, 158
13. Unger, W. G., Cole, D. F. and Hammond, B. (1975). The ocular response to paracentesis in the rabbit. *Exp. Eye Res.*, **20**, 177 (Abstracts)
14. Bechetoille, A., Chabanais, J. L., Jallet, G. and Saraux, H. (1976). Indomethacine locale et réaction oculaire post-contusive précoce chez le lapin *Arch. Ophtal. (Paris)*, **36**, 419
15. Ku, E. C., Signor, C. and Eakins, K. E. (1976). Anti-inflammatory agents and inhibition of ocular prostaglandin synthetase. In: *Advances in Prostaglandin* and *Thromboxane research*. (B. Samuelson and R. Paoletti, eds.) Vol. 2, pp. 819–823. (New York: Raven Press)
16. Podos, S. M., Becker, B. and Kass, M. A. (1973). Indomethacin blocks arachidonic acid-induced elevation of intraocular pressure. *Prostaglandins*, **3**, 7
17. Podos, S. M., Becker, B. and Kass, M. A. (1973). Prostaglandin synthesis inhibition and intraocular pressure. *Invest. Ophthalmol.*, **12**, 426
18. Bhattacherjee, P. and Eakins, K. E. (1975). Inhibition of the ocular effects of sodium arachidonate by antiinflammatory compounds. *Prostaglandins*, **9**, 175
19. Conquet, Ph., Plazonnet, B. and Le Douarec, J. C. (1975). Arachidonic acid-induced elevation of intraocular pressure and antiinflammatory agents. *Invest. Ophthalmol.*, **14**, 772
20. Podos, S. M. and Becker, B. (1976). Comparison of ocular prostaglandin synthesis inhibitors. *Invest. Ophthalmol.*, **15**, 841
21. Bhattacherjee, P. and Eakins, K. E. (1974). Inhibition of the prostaglandin synthetase systems in ocular tissues by Indomethacin. *Br. J. Pharmacol.*, **50**, 227
22. Bhattacherjee, P. and Eakins, K. E. (1974). A comparison of the inhibitory activity of compounds on ocular prostaglandin biosynthesis. *Invest. Ophthalmol.*, **13**, 967
23. Vareilles, P., Conquet, Ph. and Le Douarec, J. C. (1977). A method for the routine intraocular pressure (IOP) measurement in the rabbit. Range of IOP variations in this species. *Exp. Eye Res.*, **24**, 369
24. Lowry, O. H., Rosenbrough, N. J., Farr, A. L. and Randall, R. J. (1951). Protein measurement with the Folin phenol reagent. *J. Biol. Chem.*, **193**, 265
25. Bhattacherjee, P. and Hammond, B. R. (1975). Inhibition of increased permeability of the blood-aqueous barrier by non-steroidal anti-inflammatory compounds as demonstrated by fluorescein angiography. *Exp. Eye Res.*, **21**, 499
26. Plazonnet, B. and Schmitt, C. Ocular penetration of indomethacin in the rabbit. (In preparation)
27. Jampol, L. M., Neufeld, A. H. and Sears, M. L. (1975). Pathways for the response of the eye to injury. *Invest. Ophthalmol.*, **14**, 184
28. Ohtsuki, K., Mizuno, K. and Sears, M. L. (1975). Disruption of the blood aqueous barrier demonstrated by histofluorescence microscopy. *Jpn. J. Ophthalmol.*, **19**, 153
29. Whitelocke, R. A. F. and Eakins, K. E. (1973). Vascular changes in the anterior uvea of the rabbit produced by prostaglandins. *Arch. Ophthalmol.*, **89**, 495
30. Neufeld, A. H., Chavis, R. M. and Sears, M. L. (1973). Degeneration release of norepinephrine causes transient ocular hyperemia mediated by prostaglandins. *Invest. Ophthalmol.*, **12**, 167

31

Potentiation of acenocoumarin-induced anticoagulation by a new anti-inflammatory agent in man *(Abstract)*

I. CARUSO, M. FUMAGALLI, F. MONTRONE, M. B. DONATI, R. LATINI, G. BIANCHETTI AND L. CARRATELLI, (Italy)

Ed: Unfortunately the complete manuscript was not received in time for publication.

A single-blind study was performed in six healthy volunteers on long-term acenocoumarin treatment to study the possible interactions with a new salicylate derivative, endowed with anti-inflammatory and analgesic activity (MK-647, 2(hydroxy)-5(2; 4-difluorphenil) benzoic acid, Merck Sharp & Dohme, N. J., U.S.A.). The subjects were anticoagulated during at least three weeks before administration of MK-647 and one week after its interruption. During the whole study period the acenocoumarin dosage was constant and no other medication was administered. Blood collections were performed at two-day intervals during anticoagulation alone and daily during the association of the two drugs. Plasma levels of acenocoumarin were measured with a new method based on gas-liquid chromatography-electron capture detection, which was found to be of higher specificity and sensitivity than the previously available spectrophotometric methods. Treatment with MK-647 (375 mg twice a day for 4–7 days) resulted in a marked decrease in the prothrombin complex activity and in the levels of factors II, VII and X. In two cases this interaction led to prothrombin complex activities judged of potential haemorrhagic risk for the patients: accordingly the MK-647 treatment was interrupted before completion of the study period. Plasma levels of acenocoumarin dropped in four of the six patients and were almost unchanged in the two others. Upon withdrawal of MK-647, the prothrombin complex activity reverted to the initial values whereas the acenocoumarin levels were found to increase in only one patient, at least during the time interval studied. Studies are in progress to establish whether the observed potentiation of acenocoumarin-induced anticoagulation by MK-647 is to be ascribed to displacement of acenocoumarin from binding to plasma proteins.

Discussion 31

J.-P. Giroud: (France)	Is there any reason to believe that this drug interaction does not take place, as usual, simply by competition for the binding sites on the albumin?
Latini:	The main importance, the initial importance, was the competition of the binding with all the anticoagulant drugs. But now, with these bindings, we must question that first hypothesis. Perhaps there could be an interaction at metabolic elimination level of acenocoumarin. We need further studies, perhaps under more controlled conditions, in order to determine the real level of the interaction. Moreover, we shall be doing some studies of drug binding interaction *in vitro*. Even this experiment could not say exactly at what level the interaction occurs. Perhaps we could develop some hypothesis.
Giroud:	Obviously it would be of greater interest if some anti-inflammatory drug that did not act that way could be found. That is one of the problems in giving anti-vitamin K.
Latini:	Yes. It is. We tried all the drugs interacted with the acenocoumarin drug. At the moment we are trying to see if there is any interaction between MK–647, and other long-acting anticoagulant drugs. Preliminary data lead us to believe that there are two drugs which should not interact together—but I do not have the data here.

32

In vitro methods for assessing anti-inflammatory drug activity (*Abstract*)

A. TURSI, M. P. LORIA, G. SPECCHIA AND L. BONOMO (Italy)

Ed: Unfortunately the complete manuscript was not received in time for publication.

The need for reliable and reproducible parameters of the activity of anti-inflammatory drugs (AID) is well recognized. In this paper we have studied the effect of a number of steroidal and non steroidal AID on some cellular mechanisms of inflammation by using the following *in vitro* methods: lymphocyte blast transformation; leukocyte phagocytosis (investigating both the ingestive and the killing phase of phagocytosis); phagocyte spontaneous and oriented motility. The results obtained show that the methods employed could be a reliable probe of the AI activity, particularly those based on the phagocytic and motion functions of the macrophages and neutrophil granulocytes. Furthermore the AID studied show partially different behaviours with respect to the various methods of study, probably depending on their different mechanisms of action. These studies may provide some parameters of the *in vivo* activity of AID and could afford new methods for the *in vitro* study of inflammation.

Discussion 32

J.-P. Giroud: (France)	Quite high concentrations of these drugs—I would assume in the range of 10^{-3} and 10^{-4} molarity—have been used. Were there no problems in getting phenylbutazone and indomethacin into solution under these conditions? Was it necessary to use a detergent?
Tursi:	Some of the drugs were used in water solution and some in organic solvents. We have already done a control study with these solvents and they did not affect the cells.
K. Brune: (Switzerland)	What about the motility of the cells?
Tursi:	Movement of granulocytes? There was no interference from the solvents on the movement of the granulocytes.
	So far as chemotaxis is concerned, we have studied the spontaneous motility of the granulocytes. I did not show the results. Results were not reproducible for all the drugs studied.
P. Davies: (USA)	How did Professor Tursi and his colleagues check for the lack of toxicity of the drugs in their experiments?
	Secondly, how did they distinguish between the attachment phase and the ingestion phase in the phagocytosis experiments?
Tursi:	On the second point, we used the method of phagocytosis of latex particles, or yeast granules. We did not distinguish between the attachment phase. We only studied the ingestion phase, counting the particles or the granules ingested into the granulocytes.
	We checked for lack of toxicity with extrusion of blue dye from the cells. Until the dose reached 100 μg/ml there was no mortality in the cells and they were viable.
Davies:	It is notoriously difficult to distinguish between ingestion and attachment using particles for phagocytosis experiments. This is something that one should be warned against. In order to do phagocytosis experiments properly, it is almost essential to do proper kinetic measurements, with measurement of particle uptake in relation to any specific period of time.
D. Gwyn Williams: (UK)	Were these experiments, particularly the chemotaxis and phagocytosis, performed in the presence of serum, or in its absence?
Tursi:	We used the serum of the donors—the ten healthy donors. We made a pool of their serum.
Gwyn Williams:	Have any other steroid drugs been studied? Looking at the literature, there is obviously a great variation in action, not only in chemotaxis, phagocytosis, but bacterial killing, candicidal killing, and other types of neutrophil tests. We have been looking at prednisolone, *in vitro* and *in vivo*, and have failed to demonstrate any effect of this drug, either *in vitro* or *in vivo*, on any form of neutrophil function.
Tursi:	We did not get the same results with all the drugs. Some drugs did not inhibit the chemotaxis.
A. Raz: (Israel)	I want to comment on the hydrocortisone and phagocytosis. We measured the effect of hydrocortisone on phagocytosis of yeast cells

388

to peritoneal macrophages and we found that for up to 90 minutes there is a marked inhibition of the hydrocortisone, but that at the 90-minute point there is no difference of the phagocytosis of yeast cells to peritoneal macrophages that are normally hydrocortisone treated. It seems that the hydrocortisone effect is not on the adsorption phase, but on the ingestion phase of the yeast into the macrophages.

Tursi: We have observed that hydrocortisone did not inhibit the ingestion phase. We have seen an inhibition on the killing phase of the bacteria.

Section V
General Aspects   II

CHAIRMAN: G. P. Velo

CO-CHAIRMAN: J. Sondergaard

33
Potentiation of antibody formation by proteases *in vivo*

THOMAS L. VISCHER (Switzerland)

INTRODUCTION

The importance of proteases in inflammation seems well established: neutral proteases of various specificities are involved in coagulation, fibrinolysis, the complement cascade, the generation of kinins and in tissue destruction, all facets of inflammation[1]. In addition, immune processes play a role in many types of inflammation. In fact, infiltrates of lymphocytes, plasmocytes and macrophages accumulate in many inflammatory sites, and similar lesions can be induced by immunological means. In the following, some recent results from our laboratories about the effect of proteases on lymphocytes will be discussed.

RESULTS

All neutral proteases tested stimulate *in vitro* murine and human lymphocytes to transform into blast-like cells, to divide and to incorporate [³H]thymidine[2-5]. Table 33.1 gives the results obtained with some commercial proteases. The effect of these enzymes can be inhibited by appropriate inhibitors as reported in Table 33.1 for aprotinin and ovomucoid. Together with Drs. U. Bretz and M. Baggiolini, we obtained similar results with two proteases isolated from the granules of human polymorphonuclear leukocytes[6]: cathepsin G, a chymotrypsin-like enzyme, and an elastase (see Table 33.2). In the mouse all these enzymes stimulate B-lymphocytes only. As seen in Table 33.3, immunoglobulin containing cells appear in the cultures during the course of stimulation induced by trypsin and the leukocyte proteases. In collaboration with Drs. R. Gisler and P. Dukor, using the Mishell-Dutton system, we have demonstrated an increase in both specific and non-specific plaque forming cells against sheep erythrocytes. In cultures lacking

T-cells, large numbers of plaque-forming cells only developed in the presence of LPS or trypsin. One experiment is given in Table 33.4. Aprotinin inhibited this response[7].

Table 33.1 Stimulation of mouse spleen cells by various proteases ([³H]thymidine incorporation—c.p.m.)

		No inhibitor	Aprotinin 50 KIU	Ovomucoid
No stimulant		2918	2014	3798
PHA P	(0.1 μl)	83 283	53 034	64 203
Trypsin	(0.25 μg)	46 911	2809	4532
Chymotrypsin	(0.5 μg)	28 976	3292	8884
Pronase	(0.25 μg)	41 718	10 201	8163
Elastase	(1 μg)	14 625	9166	4586
Collagenase	(25 μg)	21 018	7940	16 085
Plasmine	(8 mU)	22 025	6700	14 725

1×10^6 mouse spleen cells were cultured in 0.2 ml serum-free RPMI 1640 medium. Stimulants and inhibitors were added at the beginning of the cultures. [³H]thymidine was added at 32 h and the cultures harvested at 48 h.

Table 33.2 Stimulation of [³H]thymidine incorporation in mouse spleen cells by neutral proteases from human leukocyte granules

	[³H]thymidine (c.p.m.)
No stimulant	4796
Phytohaemagglutinin	145 556
Trypsin (pancreas)	57 927
Cathepsin G (granulocytes)	25 616
Elastase (granulocytes)	22 573

5×10^6 Balb/c spleen cells were cultured for 27 h in 1 ml serum-free medium. [³H]thymidine was added áfter 58 h and the cultures ended at 72 h. Stimulants were added in optimal amounts as determined from a response curve. For details of preparation of cathepsin G and elastase see Reference 6.

Table 33.3 Cells containing intracellular immunoglobulin after stimulation*

Mitogens	Cells with intracellular Ig† (% ± SD)
None	1.0 ± 1.73
LPS	23.7 ± 3.0
PUM	6.7 ± 2.9
Trypsin	19 ± 6.8

* 5×10^6 spleen cells cultured for 4 days in 1 ml serum-free RPMI 1640.

† Smears were prepared with a cytocentrifuge, fixed in methanol and stained with an anti-mouse immunoglobulin antibody. All samples contained similar numbers of viable cells.

Table 33.4 Effect of trypsin on primary antibody production
in T-cell deprived (nu/nu) spleen cell cultures

	pfc/culture
T-cell deprived	440
T-cell deprived + T-cells	2840
T-cell deprived + trypsin	2555

8×10^6 spleen cells in 1 ml RPMI 1640 medium (with 8% fetal calf serum and 3×10^6 sheep erythrocytes) were cultured for 4 days according to the method of Mishell & Dutton. Irradiated lymphnode cells from nu^+ mice function as T-cells. Trypsin was added after 16 h of culture. (For details see Reference 7).

DISCUSSION

Neutral proteases from various sources stimulate B-lymphocytes, at least in the mouse. Immunoglobulin-containing and antibody-producing cells increase, and proteases substitute for the T-helper cell effect, at least *in vitro*.

In chronic inflammation, proteases are produced by macrophages[8], released from granulocytes[9] and generated, e.g. during complement activation[10]. Lymphocytes in tissues might become activated by these proteases and even get immunized in the absence of T-helper cells. Thus auto-immune responses, often implicated during chronic inflammations, could be mediated by such a mechanism. A similar effect has been discussed for LPS[11]. In addition, increased antibody production might potentiate humoral reactions involved in the pathogenesis of certain types of inflammation. However, the biological implications of these findings remain speculations as long as they are not confirmed in an appropriate *in vivo* situation.

References

1. Reich, E., Rifkin, D. B. and Shaw, E. (1975). *Proteases and Biological Control.* (Cold Spring Harbor Laboratory, Cold Spring Harbor)
2. Vischer, T. L. (1974). Stimulation of mouse B-lymphocytes by trypsin. *J. Immunol.*, **113**, 58
3. Kaplan, J. G. and Bona, C. (1974). Proteases as mitogens. *Exp. Cell Res.*, **88**, 388
4. Chen, L. B., Teng, N. N. H. and Buchanan, J. M. (1976). Mitogenicity of thrombin and surface alterations on mouse splenocytes. *Exp. Cell Res.*, **101**, 41
5. Vischer, T. L. and Bertrand, L. (1976). Stimulating effect of neutral proteases on cells *in vitro. Agents Actions*, **6**, 180
6. Vischer, T. L., Bretz, U. and Baggiolini, M. (1976). *In vitro* stimulation of lymphocytes by neutral proteinases from human polymorphonuclear leukocyte granules. *J. Exp. Med.*, **144**, 863
7. Gisler, R. H., Vischer, T. L. and Dukor, P. (1976). Trypsin increases *in vitro* antibody synthesis and substitutes for helper T-cells. *J. Immunol.*, **116**, 1354
8. Gordon, S., Unkeless, J. C. and Cohn, Z. A. (1974). Induction of macrophage plasminogen activator by endotoxin stimulation and phagocytosis. *J. Exp. Med.*, **140**, 995
9. Weissmann, G. and Dukor, P. (1970). Role of lysosomes in immune responses. *Adv. Immunol.*, **12**, 283
10. Cooper, N. R. and Ziccardi, R. J. (1976). The nature and reactions of complement enzymes. In: D. W. Ribbons and K. Brew, *Proteolysis and Physiological Regulation*

PERSPECTIVES IN INFLAMMATION

(Miami Winter Symposium) (D. W. Robbins and K. Brew, eds.) Vol. 11, p. 167. (New York: Academic Press)
11. Primi, D., Hammarstroem, L., Smith, C. I. E. and Moeller, G. (1977). Characterization of self-reactive B-cells by polyclonal B-cell activators. *J. Exp. Med.*, **145**, 21

Discussion 33

P. C. Wilkinson: (UK)
This is obviously very important. Are the neutral proteases, which monocytes must contain, likely to have any influence on the transformation of blood lymphocytes in the transformation assays that we do all the time? We have mixtures of monocytes and lymphocytes whenever we do these cultures, and presumably there must be neutral proteases there. Is this important in the interpretation of such experiments?

Vischer:
It is difficult to say. We tried to inhibit the influence of macrophages on lymphocytes by protease inhibitors, but all work with protease inhibitors in such systems is extremely tricky because most of the substances are toxic for the cells, so we do not know what we would get finally.

I. Ginsburg: (Israel)
22 μg enzyme were used and 13 μg cathepsin-G. How is this translated to numbers of cells and to the amount of these proteases in real exudates? Is it a ton of exudate, or a litre, or what?

Vischer:
These were complicated preparations and purifications. I cannot relate the amount of proteases used here to the amount contained in one leukocyte.

Secondly, I do not believe that we have any data about amounts of proteases in exudate for the simple reason that exudates contain a lot of inhibitors. However, we have some data on synovial fluid, but we cannot compare it. It was casein digestion and we cannot translate it to these purified preparations here. A different method was used.

G. A. Voisin (France)
The problem of activation of lymphocytes by proteases is one of the current important problems. It has been studied in our laboratory, but working with a somewhat different system—the plasminogen–plasmin system. In order to see whether this could be physiological, the capacity of the spleen cells to activate plasminogen into plasmin was studied first, and it was found that this was done by adherent cells. We then found that lymphocytes have receptors for plasmin and it has now been shown that this plasmin is able to activate the lymphocytes, and presumably the B-lymphocytes—although the experiments for this have yet to be completed—and that this resulted in an increase of fivefold, or tenfold, in the number of plaque-forming cells in this system.

Finally there is some preliminary evidence that this can play a role in *in vivo* experiments.

A. Bryceson: (UK)
There are certain clinical situations in infectious diseases where overproduction of immunoglobulin is of clinical importance. I am thinking particularly of trypanosomiasis and of malaria. In trypanosomiasis, for example, the over-production of IgM may be so great that natural antibody production is actually impaired because of the abnormal production.

There is no understanding at all as to why these diseases give rise

Vischer:

to such enormous immunoglobulin production. Is there any information on, for example, protease production by any of these organisms? We have very little information available on protease production in inflammatory situations. It is again the problem of the inhibitors because proteases are probably produced, might react, and get inactivated, or blocked, by the inhibitors. Esterase substrates, which are often used, are very non-specific and get cross-reactivity.

34

Triggers of prostaglandin release from macrophages

MARCUS GLATT, KÄTHY WAGNER AND KAY BRUNE
(Switzerland)

INTRODUCTION

At present, macrophages are believed to play a key role in chronic inflammation[1]. Support for this assumption comes from the observation that these cells accumulate in the rheumatoid synovium[2], and that they are, when activated, efficient liberators of hydrolytic enzymes but also of prostaglandins (PGs)[3]. Hence they may mediate both, the vascular symptoms of inflammation and pain but also continuing tissue destruction. Due to the work of Allison, Davies and others[4,5] we know much about the mechanisms underlying enzyme release from these cells. On the other hand, little is known about the events which trigger PG release from macrophages. It was the aim of our investigation to describe some events which trigger PG release from these cells.

METHODS

Experimental design: 10^6 Mouse peritoneal cells grown overnight in 35 mm petri dishes were rinsed and exposed for 4 h to Dulbeccos modified Eagle medium (DMEM) containing either pure particles, serum factors or particles coated with serum factors. Then, the supernatant was harvested, centrifuged and assayed for PGE_2 by a direct radioimmunoassay. Of each group of five culture plates, two were used for fixation and staining of the cell layers for assessment of phagocytosis[6]. Two other cultures were exposed to Trypan Blue in order to assess viability.

Particles: Latex beads (SERVA) 1.1 μm in diameter were added to the cultures to give a final bead to cell ratio of 20:1. Zymosan (SIGMA) was added at a 1:1 ratio after boiling and washing according to Weissman *et al.*[7]. From Sephadex G-50 (Farmacia) previously boiled for 1 h a 50% (v/v) suspension was prepared in Ringer solution. To the culture dishes 0.2 ml of this suspension was given. Chicken red blood cells (CHRBC) washed in Tris–EDTA–Saline were formalinized before use. The ratio of CHRBC to macrophages was 10:1.

Sera: Anti CHRBC-Serum was raised in mice by standard methods. It was heat inactivated before use. Human serum was freshly prepared for each experiment.

Coated particles: Latex and Sephadex beads were treated with human serum according to Knapp[8]. To 10^8 CHRBC/ml, heat inactivated anti-CHRBC-serum was added to a final concentration of 1:80 and incubated for 15 min at 37 °C. Control CHRBC were treated with non-immune serum.

RESULTS

The effects of phagocytosis on PG release

Four hours after exposure of macrophages to particles we found that some caused PG release and others did not (Table 34.1A). Besides Sephadex which is too large to be ingested all particles were phagocytosed. Among the particles which induce the release of PG, zymosan decreased the vitality of the macrophages. It was therefore excluded from further experimentation. On the other hand, Sephadex alone resulted only in a moderate increase in PG release when compared with controls. This was especially useful because Sephadex adsorbs selectively C3 or a split product of $C3^{8,9}$.

The influence of C3 on PG release

In Allison's *et al.*[5] experiments C3b was found a potent trigger of lysosomal enzyme release from macrophages. In a further experiment therefore macrophages were exposed to Sephadex and Sephadex coated with C3. The results are given in Table 34.1B. It turned out that the PG release was increased 4.2 and 11 times respectively when Sephadex or serum treated Sephadex were used. These findings indicated that C3 components may serve as trigger for PG release, however, it does not rule out that other potent triggers exist.

The influence of other serum factors on PG release

In further experiments we coated latex or chicken erythrocytes with different sera.

Some results of these experiments are compiled in Table 34.1C. Most striking among these results are the ones obtained with chicken erythrocytes coated with specific antibodies. Although chicken erythrocytes incubated

Table 34.1 Release of PGE_2 by macrophages exposed to different particles

	% of cells phagocytosing	PGE_2*	P < †
(A) Latex	68	0.9 ± 0.3	NS
CHRBC	45	0.7 ± 0.2	NS
Zymosan	62	24.1 ± 5.4	0.01
(B) Sephadex	Adherence	4.2 ± 1.7	0.05
Sephadex + serum	Adherence	11.5 ± 4.6	0.01
(C) Latex + serum	70	5.6 ± 1.7	0.05
CHRBC + serum	52	2.6 + 0.4	0.05
CHRBC + anti-serum	88	25.1 ± 4.7	0.01

* Data are expressed as fractions of controls (mean ± SE).
Controls and experimental sets always consisted of 5 or more cultures.
Values for controls are ranging between 1 and 4 μg PGE_2/ml.
† Student's *t*-test.

with mouse serum from non-immunized animals did not act as a trigger of PG release despite ingestion, chicken erythrocytes incubated with serum from sensitized mice caused a 25 times increase in PG release without change in cellular viability compared with controls. This effect was further investigated in a time course study. It showed that PG release by this trigger occurs within the first hour after exposure. The amount of PG release remains stable thereafter for at least 4 h. It may be added that during this time no measurable metabolism of PGE_2 in our macrophage cultures took place.

DISCUSSION

Among the results presented two appear especially important. Firstly, it is obvious that phagocytosis alone is no sufficient trigger for prostaglandin release as the results using uncoated latex beads or erythrocytes have shown. It is striking, however, that particles like zymosan or Sephadex beads which spontaneously induce PG release, are both potent activators of complement[8-10]. Macrophages synthesize and secrete complement components, mainly C3[11,12]. Therefore the possibility cannot be ruled out from our experiments that even under serum free culture conditions zymosan or Sephadex interact with cellular complement factors. Additionally, C3 components attached to Sephadex beads were found to enhance PGE_2 production. This finding indicates a correlation between C3b-induced macrophage activation and PG release. Secondly, we found ingestion of antibodies attached to their receptors on erythrocytes to be another potent trigger for PG release from macrophages. Since antibody coated erythrocytes were prepared in heat inactivated serum it is unlikely that reactive complement factors were adherent to the antigen–antibody complexes. Hence antigen–antibody complexes appear to comprise a further potent trigger of complement release.

From results presented it is concluded that PG release is an early and measurable sign of macrophage activation. That this activation can be efficiently triggered by ingestion of antigen–antibody complexes appears especially relevant to the understanding of the processes in chronic inflammation, e.g. rheumatoid arthritis. The continuing formation of antigen–antibody complexes, especially in rheumatoid joints, is likely to cause constant release of PGE_2 from macrophages which in turn can perpetuate the inflammatory symptoms of this disease.

Supported by the Swiss National Science Foundation (Grant 3.588–0.75).

References

1. Allison, A. C. and Davies, P. (1974). Mechanisms underlying chronic inflammation. In: *Future Trends in Inflammation* (G. P. Velo, D. A. Willoughby and J.-P. Giroud, eds.) p. 449. (Padua: Piccin Medical Books)
2. Ishirawa, H. and Ziff, M. (1976). Electron microscopic observations of immunoreactive cells in the rheumatoid synovial membrane. *Arthritis Rheum.*, **19,** 1
3. Gordon, D., Bray, M. A. and Morley, J. (1976). Control of lymphokine secretion by prostaglandins. *Nature (London)*, **262,** 401
4. Davies, P., Page, R. C. and Allison, A. C. (1974). Changes in cellular enzyme levels and extracellular release of lysosomal acid hydrolases in macrophages exposed to group A streptococcal cell wall substance. *J. Exp. Med.*, **139,** 1262
5. Schorlemmer, H. U. and Allison, A. C. (1976). Effects of activated complement components on enzyme secretion by macrophages. *Immunology*, **31,** 781
6. Boyle, W. (1968). An extension of the ^{51}Cr-release assay for the estimation of mouse cytotoxins. *Transplantation*, **6,** 761
7. Weissmann, G., Dukor, P. and Zurier, R. B. (1971). Effect of cyclic AMP on release of lysosomal enzymes from phagocytes. *Nature New Biol.*, **231,** 131
8. Brade, V., Nicholson, A., Bitter-Suermann, D. and Hadding, U. (1974). Formation of the C3-cleaving properdin enzyme on zymosan. Demonstration that factor D is replaceable by proteolytic enzymes. *J. Immunol.*, **113,** 1735
9. Knapp, W. (1975). Interactions of the third component of complement (C3) with cross-linked dextran. II. Demonstration of an alternate pathway activation as binding mechanism of C3 to cross-linked dextran. *Z. Immunol., Forsch.*, **149,** 69
10. Knapp, W. (1975). Interactions of the third component of complement (C3) with cross-linked dextran. III. Isolation and characterization of interacting components after enzymatic digestion of complement coated cross-linked dextran. *Z. Immun. Forsch.*, **149,** 389
11. Einstein, P., Schneeberger, E. E. and Colten, H. R. (1976). Synthesis of the second component of complement by long-term primary cultures of human monocytes. *J. Exp. Med.*, **143,** 114
12. McClelland, D. B. L. and van Furth, R. (1976). *In vitro* synthesis of $\beta_1 C/\beta_1 A$ globulin (the C3 component of complement) by tissues and leukocytes of the mice. *Immunology*, **31,** 855

Discussion 34

G. P. Velo: (Italy)	Would Dr. Glatt comment on the difference between polymorphs and macrophages in the release of prostaglandins during phagocytosis. It is just a speculation.
Glatt:	I did not mention the effects of phagocytosis on polymorphonuclear leukocytes. We have several times tried to induce prostaglandin release by these cells. For this purpose we have used chicken polymorphonuclear leukocytes, and we never got convincing results.
P. Davies: (USA)	As I think we agreed earlier on in the course of the meeting, Dr. Glatt's data, and our own, complement each other rather well. There are one or two points where we do not agree and that is in the situation with the latex, where it is coated with serum, and a certain increase in prostaglandin biosynthesis and secretion results.
	I was not quite clear about the time course experiment with the chicken red cells. Was Dr. Glatt's baseline level, where he showed serum only, simply a case of putting antiserum in without the chicken red cells, or was it a case of coating chicken red cells with normal serum not containing any antibody?
Glatt:	The baseline was produced with chicken red blood cells treated with normal mouse serum from non-immunized animals.
Davies:	Would Dr. Glatt then comment as to the difference here, where our chicken red cells coated with serum give no release of prostaglandin, whereas latex coated with serum does give release. Was the latex, for example, free of endotoxin?
Glatt:	I cannot answer that question. The latex preparation was a standard preparation purchased by ourselves and washed extensively in a sterile Ringer's solution. We did not check for contamination of pyrogens, or endotoxin, but we used hospital-made sterile Ringer's solution which should be free of these components. In fact, I have no good explanation of the effects of serum-treated latex particles. I would be happy if nothing would have happened there. But I do not think that it is easy to explain these serum factors in one way or the other. Everybody would like to have C3 or C3b as the single and the all-resolving factor but it is not so. We have tried to elute C3 components from Sephadex. But, the C3 components, once bound to Sephadex, cannot be eluted without completely destroying them.
D. Roos: (The Netherlands)	Having said that phagocytosis was not enough to give release of prostaglandins, has Dr. Glatt correlated the release of the prostaglandins with the amount of phagocytosis?
	Secondly, Dr. Glatt says that complement is necessary. Has he measured the amount of complement on his particles?
Glatt:	The phagocytosis of latex particles was always optimal; i.e. more than 90% of the cells had taken up more than five particles per cell.
Roos:	But how would one know that it is uptake? Why is it not binding?
Glatt:	These cells have been extensively washed.

Roos:	And is Dr. Glatt sure that there is none on the outside?
Glatt:	Yes.
Roos:	How does he know?
Glatt:	The uptake of latex particles is a standard technique. From EM pictures, for example, it was shown that latex particles are spontaneously taken up by these cells.
	On the second point, concerning the binding of C3. I have no method for measuring it. It has been shown in studies with immunofluorescent labelled antibodies that Sephadex beads are coated with C3 components selectively and there is no IgG, IgM or IgA binding to these particles.
Roos:	I completely disagree. I am absolutely sure that there is IgG binding when zymosan is added to normal serum.
Glatt:	I did not say anything about zymosan. Zymosan was always added in a serum-free medium. All these experiments were done in a serum-free environment.
G. A. Voisin: (France)	I have not followed the procedures that were used to eliminate or to antagonize complement, particularly C3, in these experiments.
Glatt:	Antagonize what?
Voisin:	In order to suppress the increase in prostaglandin release has any attempt to eliminate complement from the fresh serum, or to antagonize it, been made?
Glatt:	We used potassium bromide-treated serum or heat-inactivated serum where the effects are reduced.
G. Higgs: (UK)	The data would look a lot more convincing if an index of phagocytosis for each of the cell situations was included. Is phagocytosis measured?
Glatt:	The phagocytosis of chicken red blood cells was measured.
Higgs:	Was it measured for all the situations that have been reported?
Glatt:	Boyle. *Transplantation VI*—published 1968. The attached cells are lysed by trace ammonium treatment prior to staining.
Higgs:	For comparative purposes, which is essentially what this data is all about, phagocytosis should be measured in every situation.
Glatt:	Yes. Rates of phagocytosis with chicken red blood cells and antiserum ranged from 85 to 90% of the cells taking up two or more red blood cells, whereas, as a rule, chicken red blood cells treated only with non-specific serum have an index of 5–10% less. But, there is no correlation between this decreased uptake of about 5–10% and the huge increase in PG production.
M. Bray: (UK)	Might I inject a slight note of confusion. When we do our guinea pig peritoneal exudate macrophage cultures we find that in the absence of serum over a 24-hour culture we get low levels of prostaglandin production. In the presence of fetal calf serum this is greatly increased, and this would fit in with what Dr. Glatt says. However, if the serum is heated to 56 °C for half an hour, the usual inactivation process, we find that we can increase the prostaglandin generation even more—which would seem to be the opposite to what is being suggested.
	Secondly, could Dr. Glatt give some idea of the amounts of prostaglandin being generated in his cultures.
Glatt:	On the first point. Following heating, either the serum must be put through a sterile filter, or else ultra-centrifugation has to be used, because there is always a slight complex formation, particularly if the sera are frozen. As soon as these cells are exposed to protein aggregates an increased PG production results.
	On the second point, I have said that the basal level of PG production was from 0.8 to 2.0 ng PGE-like material per plate.

35

Biological, chemical and pharmacological induction of the properdin-mediated pathway of complement activation *in vitro*

T. DI PERRI, A. AUTERI, F. LAGHI PASINI AND F. MATTIOLI
(Italy)

The role of the complement system, either in acute or in chronic inflammation, although formally accepted, is not completely understood. It is generally accepted that the complement is involved in many reactions of the humoral immunological response[1], but it has been observed that it plays an important role in the acute inflammation even if an immunological mechanism is not operating[2]. Recently a role for the complement in the chronic immunological processes has been hypothesized suggesting a specific activity of C3 either on the stimulation of the T-lymphocytes activation or on the T-dependent antibody synthesis and macrophage functions[3,4].

The molecular bases of the complement activation have been rather profoundly studied: several alternative pathways which lead to the C3 activation shunting the activation of the earlier components were identified. The best known of these methods is the properdin-dependent one which appears also to be the most important from the biological point of view. This pathway differs from the classic pathway either for the trigger mechanisms, or for the cationic requirement or for the initial sequence of the activation process.

As regards the first point, the alternate properdinic pathway may be triggered either by several chemical and bacterial polysaccharides, or by the IgA, while IgG and IgM cannot activate this sequential chain[5].

Secondly the electrolyte requirement of the properdin way is also different from that of the classic way: the latter needs the presence of Ca^{2+} for the activation of C1 and of Mg^{2+} for the activation of C4, while the properdinic pathway requires only Mg^{+2} which can be considered also a triggering factor.

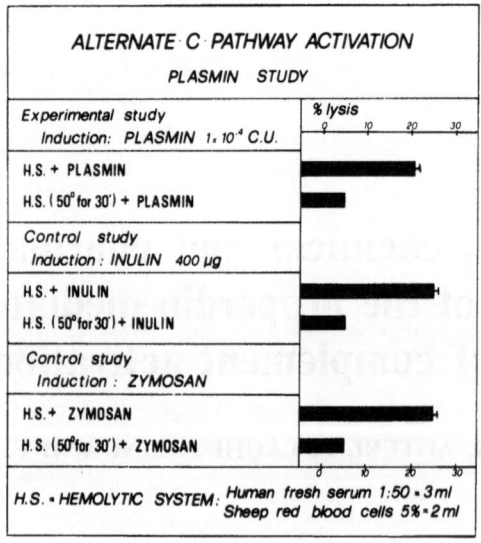

Figure 35.1 Plasmin activation of alternate complement pathway. *In vitro* assay

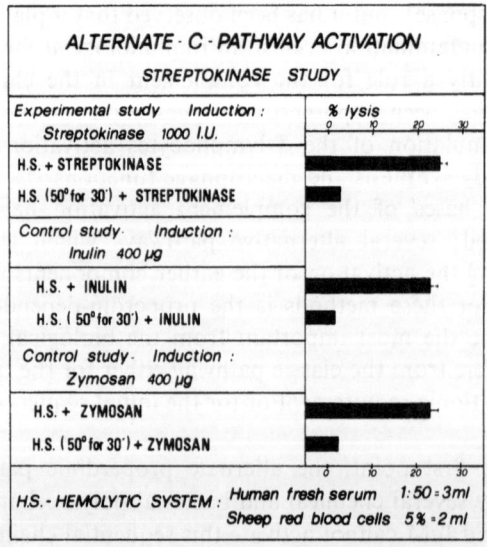

Figure 35.2 Streptokinase activation of alternate complement pathway. *In vitro* assay

It is also admitted that an increase of Ca^{2+} concentration may counteract the Mg^{2+} role at some level of the properdinic sequence, introducing the hypothesis of a reciprocal control of the two ions on the regulation of some steps of the biological processes[6].

As regards the last aspect, the sequential chain begins with the activation of the properdin and the so-called factor B, followed by the formation of a particular convertase (PC3bBb) specifically cleaving C3[7]. The classic and the properdin pathway of activation appear closely interdependent *in vitro* as well as *in vivo* since the breakdown of C3 is followed by the formation of the cleavage fragment C3b which shows a specific activating power on the component B of the properdin system.

This positive feedback can initiate a self-perpetuating process of recruitment dependent on the formation of C3b which is cleaved from C3 either by the classic or by the alternate pathway activation. The C3b activity is in turn regulated by the action of a specific inactivator, the C3b inactivator (C3b INA) which appears as the pivotal mechanism modulating the recruitment loop.

It is not known if there are other factors involved in the regulation of the complement activation which is theoretically stimulated only to participate in the inflammatory reaction according to the general homeostasis of the living tissues.

The meaning of the evaluation of the biological activity of the whole system or of the circulating concentration of the single factors is limited by the impossibility of stating the underlying anabolic and catabolic component, since the serum concentration of each component and its biological activity derives from the algebraic sum of the synthesized and the catabolized amount.

The mechanisms which regulate the cellular system are not known, therefore a comprehensive judgement of the behaviour of the system both in normal and abnormal situations is now rather impossible.

Moreover the short loop of the interrelationships between the classical and alternate properdinic pathways must be considered from an enlarged and integrated point of view: several reciprocal, either activating or inhibiting, influences with the other humoral systems: coagulation, kinin-forming system and fibrinolysis, were identified and the single steps of these biological processes are now under analytical investigation.

Another group of interrelationships has been proposed with the membrane activity of some cells either strictly related to the immunological system, like lymphocytes, or transformed cells, which present a surface activator of factor B thus initiating the properdin sequence of complement[8].

The possibility of influencing the biological activity of the system has been studied, and from the pharmacological point of view many drugs inhibiting the activation of one or more components of complement have been selected. The drugs which inhibit the activation of the earlier components do not modify the haemolytic reaction induced by inulin or zymosan, i.e. do not

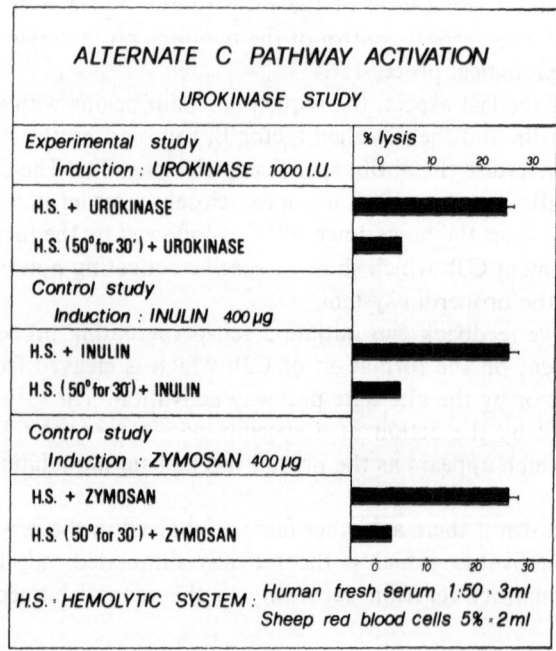

Figure. 35.3 Urokinase activation of alternate complement pathway. *In vitro* assay

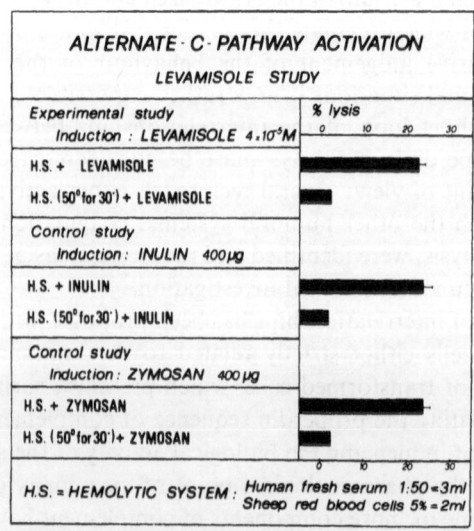

Figure 35.4 Levamisole activation of alternate complement pathway. *In vitro* assay

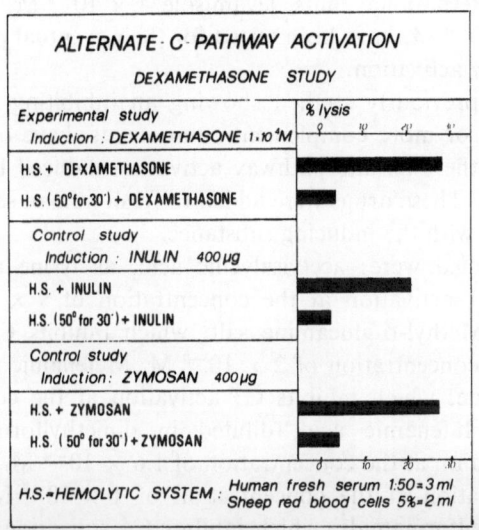

Figure 35.5 Dexamethasone activation of alternate complement pathway. *In vitro* assay

inhibit the properdin-dependent pathway but only the classic pathway. On the contrary the drugs which inhibit the activation of the third component, show a blocking action on both the classic and the properdin pathway[9-12]. Subsequently the possibility of inducing the complement activation by pharmacological means has been considered.

The aim of this paper concerns this question and is focused on studying the eventual action stimulating the properdin-dependent pathway of some drugs theoretically related either to the complex interrelationships of the complement system or to some functions of the immunocompetent system.

MATERIALS AND METHODS

The haemolytic system to assay the complement alternate pathway was formed by sheep red cells diluted in Veronal buffer (pH 7.4; ionic strength 0.050) to the final concentrations of 2.5×10^5 and human fresh serum (1:50 in Veronal buffer).

The system was incubated at 37 °C for 30 min with the inducing substance and the haemolysis of the supernatant phase is photometrically evaluated at 540 nm after centrifugation. The amount of the haemolysis was calculated as per cent lysis according to Kabat and Mayer[13].

Inulin (400 μg) or zymosan (400 μg) were used as inductors of alternate pathway activation.

Highly purified human plasmir (Kabi) containing 15 casein units (CU) per mg of protein, according to Sgouris *et al.*, at the concentration of 1×10^{-4} CU, streptokinase (Hoechst) 1000 international units, urokinase

(Serono) 1000 international units, levamisole 4×10^{-5} M, dexamethasone phosphate 1×10^{-4} M, have been tested for their eventual power to induce alternate pathway activation.

Several drugs previously studied showing an inhibiting activity on the activation of one or more complement components, have been studied for the influence on the alternate pathway activation induced by all the mentioned substances. These drugs were added to fresh human serum before the incubation phase with the inducing substance.

The drugs studied were: acetylsalicylic acid, as lysine acetylsalycilate, which inhibits C1 activation at the concentration of 9×10^{-4} M. Indomethacin, as N-Methyl-D-glucamine salt, which inhibits C2, C4 and C3 activation at the concentration of 2×10^{-3} M. Mefenamic acid, diluted in dimethylformamide, which inhibits C3 activation at the concentration of 1.2×10^{-4} M. Flufenamic acid, diluted in dimethylformamide, which inhibits C3 activation at the concentration of 1.6×10^{-4} M. Heparin which inhibits C3 activation at the concentration of 1×10^{-3} M. Cinnarizine, diluted in dimethylformamide, which inhibits C4 activation at the concentration of 7×10^{-5} M by a Mg^{2+} dependent mechanism. Dypiridamole which inhibits C1 and C4 activation at the concentration of 4×10^{-4} M.

The alternate pathway localization of the inducing substance has been controlled inhibiting the properdin haemolytic process by heating the serum at 50 °C for 30 min.

Every group of assays has been performed on the same fresh human serum with a controlled normal complement immunohaemolytic activity.

RESULTS

The results are summarized in the Figures. All the values are the mean $\pm$ SD of five determinations.

The substances tested for their power to induce haemolysis *in vitro* by the activation of the properdin-dependent pathway showed an inducing activity of the same degree as that shown by the two control inductors, inulin and zymosan. The human plasmin proved active at the concentration of 10^{-4} CU, streptokinase and urokinase at the concentration of 1000 IU, levamisole at the concentration of 4×10^{-5} M and dexamethasone phosphate at the concentration of 10^{-4} M.

The inhibition of the haemolytic reaction by heating the system at 50 °C for 30 min has been assumed as a method to control the specificity of the alternate pathway, since it is known that at this temperature the C3-activator appears inhibited. In every group of assays the preheating inhibited the induction of haemolysis.

The pretreatment of the haemolytic system showed that either the plasmin or the urokinase or the streptokinase induction are inhibited by heparin

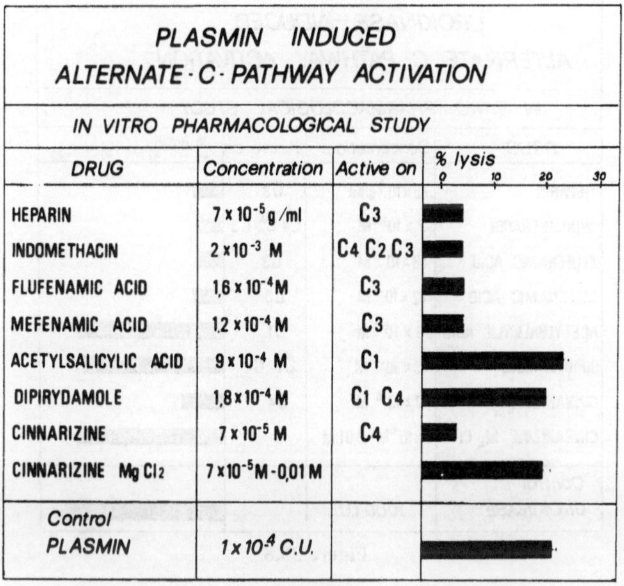

PLASMIN INDUCED ALTERNATE-C-PATHWAY ACTIVATION

IN VITRO PHARMACOLOGICAL STUDY

DRUG	Concentration	Active on	% lysis
HEPARIN	7×10^{-5} g/ml	C_3	
INDOMETHACIN	2×10^{-3} M	$C_4\,C_2\,C_3$	
FLUFENAMIC ACID	1.6×10^{-4} M	C_3	
MEFENAMIC ACID	1.2×10^{-4} M	C_3	
ACETYLSALICYLIC ACID	9×10^{-4} M	C_1	
DIPIRYDAMOLE	1.8×10^{-4} M	$C_1\,C_4$	
CINNARIZINE	7×10^{-5} M	C_4	
CINNARIZINE $MgCl_2$	7×10^{-5} M $- 0.01$ M		
Control PLASMIN	1×10^{-4} C.U.		

Figure 35.6

Figures 35.6–35.10 *In vitro* pharmacological study of the action of some drugs on the alternate complement pathway activation induced by plasmin, streptokinase, urokinase, levamisole, dexamethasone

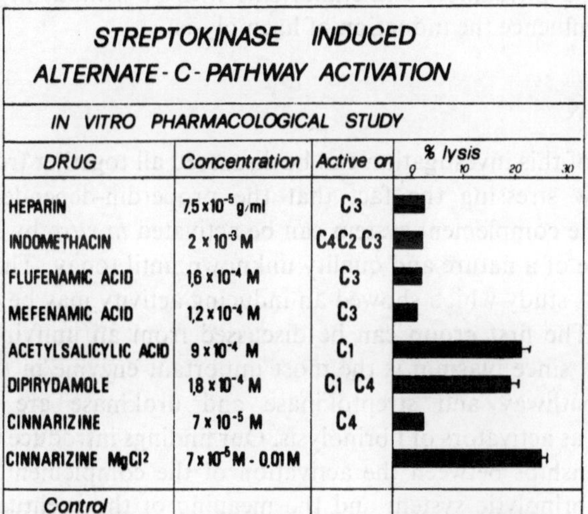

STREPTOKINASE INDUCED ALTERNATE-C-PATHWAY ACTIVATION

IN VITRO PHARMACOLOGICAL STUDY

DRUG	Concentration	Active on	% lysis
HEPARIN	7.5×10^{-5} g/ml	C_3	
INDOMETHACIN	2×10^{-3} M	$C_4\,C_2\,C_3$	
FLUFENAMIC ACID	1.6×10^{-4} M	C_3	
MEFENAMIC ACID	1.2×10^{-4} M	C_3	
ACETYLSALICYLIC ACID	9×10^{-4} M	C_1	
DIPIRYDAMOLE	1.8×10^{-4} M	$C_1\,C_4$	
CINNARIZINE	7×10^{-5} M	C_4	
CINNARIZINE $MgCl_2$	7×10^{-5} M $- 0.01$ M		
Control STREPTOKINASE	1000 I.U.		

Figure 35.7

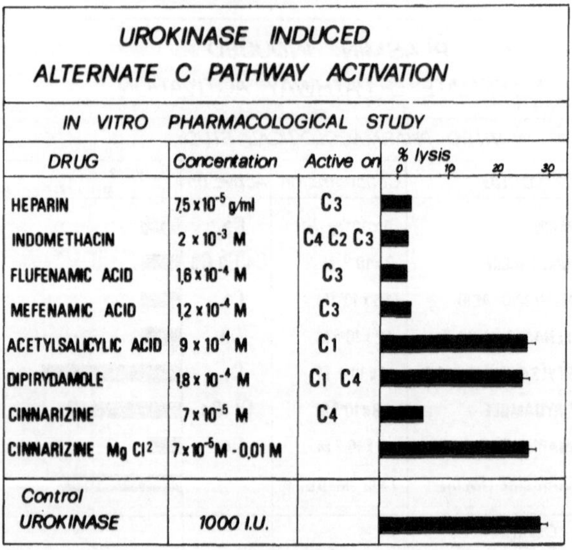

UROKINASE INDUCED ALTERNATE C PATHWAY ACTIVATION			
IN VITRO PHARMACOLOGICAL STUDY			
DRUG	Concentration	Active on	% lysis
HEPARIN	7.5×10^{-5} g/ml	C3	▬
INDOMETHACIN	2×10^{-3} M	C4 C2 C3	▬
FLUFENAMIC ACID	1.6×10^{-4} M	C3	▬
MEFENAMIC ACID	1.2×10^{-4} M	C3	▬
ACETYLSALICYLIC ACID	9×10^{-4} M	C1	▬▬▬▬▬▬▬
DIPIRYDAMOLE	1.8×10^{-4} M	C1 C4	▬▬▬▬▬▬▬
CINNARIZINE	7×10^{-5} M	C4	▬
CINNARIZINE Mg Cl²	7×10^{-5} M - 0.01 M		▬▬▬▬▬▬▬
Control *UROKINASE*	*1000 I.U.*		▬▬▬▬▬▬▬

Figure 35.8

(7×10^{-5} g/ml) or indomethacin (2×10^{-3} M) or flufenamic acid (1.6×10^{-4} M) or mefenamic acid (1.2×10^{-4} M) or cinnarizine (7×10^{-5} M).

The inhibitory effect of cinnarizine was cancelled by $MgCl_2$ 0.01 M. Acetylsalicylic acid (9×10^{-4} M) and dypiridamole (1.8×10^{-4} M) did not show any effect on the induction of haemolysis.

The inducing action either of levamisole or of dexamethasone was inhibited by heparin or indomethacin or flufenamic and mefenamic acids while acetyl-salicylic acid, dypiridamole and cinnarizine with or without $MgCl_2$ did not appreciably influence the induction of haemolysis.

DISCUSSION

The findings of this investigation can be discussed all together from a general point of view stressing the fact that the properdin-dependent alternate pathway of the complement system can be activated *in vitro* by some inductors which are of a nature and quality unknown until today. The substances assayed in this study which showed an inducing activity may be divided into two groups. The first group can be discussed from an unifying biological point of view, since plasmin is the most important enzyme in the activated fibrinolytic pathway and streptokinase and urokinase are biologically characterized as activators of fibrinolysis. Our findings introduce the question of the relationships between the activation of the complement system and that of the fibrinolytic system and the meaning of the eventual reciprocal influence. In previous papers from our laboratory the activity on the induction of the properdin-dependent pathway of complement displayed by

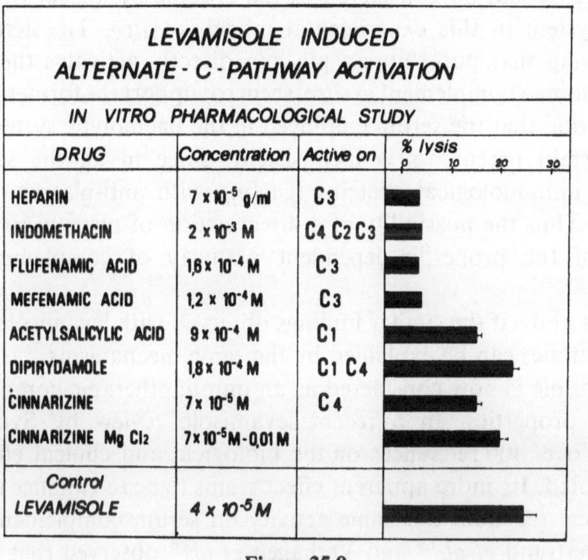

LEVAMISOLE INDUCED ALTERNATE · C · PATHWAY ACTIVATION

IN VITRO PHARMACOLOGICAL STUDY

DRUG	Concentration	Active on	% lysis
HEPARIN	7×10^{-5} g/ml	C_3	
INDOMETHACIN	2×10^{-3} M	$C_4\ C_2\ C_3$	
FLUFENAMIC ACID	1.6×10^{-4} M	C_3	
MEFENAMIC ACID	1.2×10^{-4} M	C_3	
ACETYLSALICYLIC ACID	9×10^{-4} M	C_1	
DIPIRYDAMOLE	1.8×10^{-4} M	$C_1\ C_4$	
CINNARIZINE	7×10^{-5} M	C_4	
CINNARIZINE $Mg\ Cl_2$	7×10^{-5}M - 0.01 M		
Control LEVAMISOLE	4×10^{-5} M		

Figure 35.9

DEXAMETHASONE INDUCED ALTERNATE · C · PATHWAY ACTIVATION

IN VITRO PHARMALOGICAL STUDY

DRUG	Concentration	Active on	% lysis
HEPARIN	7.5×10^{-5} g/ml	C_3	
INDOMETHACIN	2×10^{-3}	$C_4\ C_2\ C_3$	
FLUFENAMIC ACID	1.6×10^{-4} M	C_3	
MEFENAMIC ACID	1.2×10^{-4} M	C_3	
ACETYLSALICYLIC ACID	9×10^{-4} M	C_1	
DIPIRYDAMOLE	1.8×10^{-4} M	$C_1\ C_4$	
CINNARIZINE	7×10^{-5} M	C_4	
CINNARIZINE $Mg\ Cl_2$	7×10^{-5}M - 0.01M		
Control DEXAMETHASONE	1×10^{-4} M		

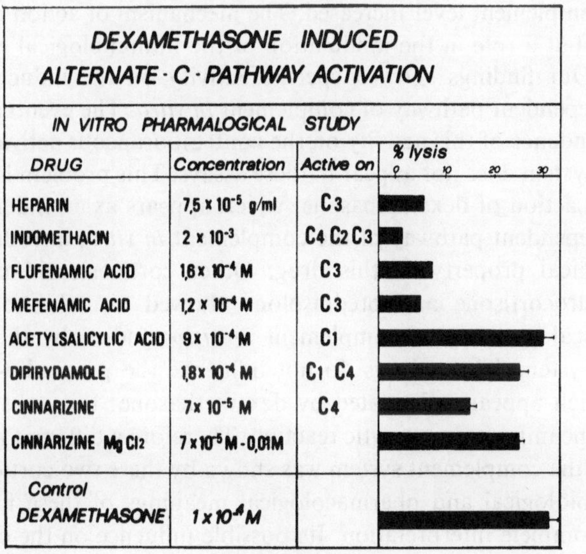

Figure 35.10

streptokinase and urokinase was shown, and these findings were discussed in terms of a possible mediated mechanism leading to the activation of plasmin which could be considered as the specific biological trigger of the properdin system in this experimental model *in vitro*. The actual results, clearly showing that pure human plasmin directly activates the properdin pathway of human complement *in vitro*, seem to support the former hypothesis.

The objection that the serum employed in the haemolytic system does not contain plasmin precursors is inconsistent, since in all the samples the presence of immunological proteins reacting with anti-plasmin serum has been found. Thus the possibility of a direct action of plasmin to induce the activation of the properdin-dependent pathway of complement can be admitted.

We do not know if the similar findings observed with levamisole and dexamethasone studies can be explained by the same mechanisms.

The levamisole is now considered as an immunotherapic component with anti-anergic properties. In a recent levamisole review by Symoens and Rosenthal[14] over 400 references on the biological and clinical effect of this drug were noted. Its more apparent effect seems to be to enhance the delayed immunological reaction, but some activity on serum complement has been described. Bertrand et al.[15] and Verhagen et al[16] observed that in patients in whom the total haemolytic complement was increased the administration of levamisole resulted in a fall of the values to normal. De Cock et al.[17] observed that in elderly people treated with levamisole for less than 2 months the serum complement level increased. The mechanism of action of the drug is unknown but a role in the modulation of the immunological processes is supported. Our findings show a specific activity on the induction of the properdin-dependent pathway of complement *in vitro*. The eventual relationship or dependence of this activity on the contemporaneous activation of the fibrinolytic system does not appear in these assays. This problem is still open.

Lastly the action of dexamethasone, which appears as an inductor of the properdin-dependent pathway of the complement *in vitro*, introduces a new pharmacological property of this drug. Other corticosteroid compounds such as hydrocortisone and prednisolone showed an inhibitory activity of the classical pathway of complement *in vitro* studied by the immuno-haemolytic system. These drugs do not influence the properdin-dependent pathway which appears stimulated by dexamethasone; this substance does not modify the immunohaemolytic reaction. Therefore a different mechanism of action on the complement system was shown by these two corticosteroidal drugs. The biological and pharmacological meanings of these findings are far from a complete interpretation. Its possible influence on the cooperative mechanism of the humoral and cellular components of the immune system may be theoretically postulated, stressing the recent evidence of a complement dependence of some functions of lymphocyte and macrophage.

The last part of our study was focused on the action of some drugs on the haemolysis induced by the tested substances. In previous papers from our laboratory a specific inhibition of the activation of one or more components of the complement shown by several drugs was described. In this study the drugs inhibiting the C3 activation showed also an inhibiting power on the activation of the properdin-dependent pathway, whichever was the inductor employed, either the classical known inductors such as inulin and zymosan or the substances assayed in this study such as plasmin, streptokinase, urokinase, levamisole and dexamethasone. The drugs inhibiting C3 activation and the alternate pathway tested were heparin, indomethacin, flufenamic and mefenamic acids. Other drugs such as acetylsalicylic acid, which inhibits the activation of C1, and dypiridamole, which inhibits the activation of both C1 and C4, do not show any influence on the properdin-dependent haemolysis induced by all the substances tested in this study. These findings agree with our knowledge on the different sequential reactive chain of the classic and properdin-dependent pathway of activation. In the former the C3 activation requires the precedent activation of C1, C4 and C2, while in the latter the C3 activation occurs bypassing the early components. Therefore the drugs inhibiting specifically the activation of C1, C4 and C2 but not of C3, do not influence the properdin-dependent pathway, which, on the contrary, is inhibited by the drugs specifically blocking the activation of C3.

The action of cinnarizine must be considered separately since this drug inhibits specifically the activation of C4 but it proves active also to inhibit the properdin pathway. Its activity seems related to the Mg^{2+} role in the process of activation, since the addition of Mg^{2+} salts cancels the inhibitory effect of cinnarizine. The known Mg^{2+} dependence of both the activation processes, the C4 and the C3A, may explain the apparently paradoxical effect of this drug.

In conclusion plasmin, streptokinase, urokinase, levamisole and dexamethasone show an inducing activity on the properdin-dependent pathway of the human complement system *in vitro*. It seems premature to make a critical interpretation from the biological point of view, stressing only the evidence of a relationship between the plasmin system and the complement system and the possibility of introducing a new pharmacological component on the modulation of the complement biological activity.

References

1. Ward, P. A., Cochrane, C. G. and Mueller Eberhard, H. J. (1965). The role of serum complement in chemotaxis of leukocytes *in vitro*. *J. Exp. Med.*, **122**, 327
2. Willoughby, D. A. and DiRosa, M. A. (1971). A unifying concept for inflammation: A new appraisal of some mediators. In: *Immunopathology of Inflammation*. (Amsterdam: Excerpta Medica)
3. Pepys, M. B. and Butterworth, A. E. (1974). Inhibition by C3 fragments of C3 dependent rosette formation and antigen induced lymphocyte transformation. *Clin. Exp. Immunol.*, **18**, 273
4. Dukor, P. and Hartman, K. (1973). Bound C3 as the second signal for B cells activation. *Cell. Immunol.*, **7**, 385

5. Osler, A. G. (1976). Complement. In: *Mechanisms and Functions*. (Englewood Cliffs, New Jersey: Prentice-Hall Inc.)
6. May, J. E., Rosse, W. and Frank, M. M. (1973). Paroxysmal nocturnal hemoglobinuria. Alternate-complement-pathway-mediated lysis induced by magnesium. *N. Engl. J. Med.*, **289**, 14, 705
7. Fearon, D. T., Austen, K. F. and Ruddy, S. (1974). Properdin factor D. *J. Exp. Med.*, **140**, 426
8. McConnell, I. (1976). Lymphocyte markers. *Proc. R. Soc. Med.*, **69**, 657
9. DiPerri, T. and Auteri, A. (1974). On the anticomplementary action of some non-steroidal anti-inflammatory drugs. In: *Future Trends in Inflammation I* (G. P. Velo, D. A. Willoughby and J.-P. Giroud, eds.) (Padua: Piccin Medical Books)
10. DiPerri, T., Auteri, A., Laghi Pasini, F. and Mattioli, F. (1977). Interrelationship between the fibrinolytic and the complement systems *in vitro*. Activation of the properdin alternate pathway by streptokinase and urokinase. In: *International Symposium on New Antiinflammatory and Antirheumatic Drugs*. Tirrenia (Italy) 11–12 June 1976. (In press)
11. DiPerri, T., Auteri, A., Laghi Pasini, F. and Mattioli, F. (1977). Action of human plasmin, streptokinase and urokinase on the activation of the properdin alternate pathway of complement. *In vitro* study. In: *Third International Conference on Synthetic Fibrinolytic Thrombolytic Agents. Progress in Fibrinolysis*. Glasgow 28–30th September 1976. (In press)
12. DiPerri, T., Auteri, A., Laghi Pasini, F. and Mattioli, F. Action of Cinnarizine on properdin dependent activation of complement. Evidence of a Mg^{++} dependent activity. *Arch. Int. Pharmacodyn*. (In press)
13. Kabat, A. E. and Mayer, M. M. (1971). *Experimental Immunochemistry*. (Springfield, Illinois: Charles C. Thomas & Co.)
14. Symoens, J. and Rosenthal, M. (1977). Levamisole in the modulation of the immune response. The current experimental and clinical state. *Clinical Research Report on Levamisole* (Janssen Pharmaceutica)
15. Bertrand, J., Renoux, G., Renoux, M. and Palat, A. (1974). Maladie de Crohn et levamisole. *Nouv. Presse Méd.* **3**, 2265
16. Verhaegen, H., DeCock, W. and De-Cree, J. (1974). The effect of levamisole on serum complement in patients with neoplastic disease. *Clinical Research Report on Levamisole*, No 17 (Janssen Pharmaceutica)
17. DeCock, W., DeCree, J. and Verhaegen, H. (1974). The effect of levamisole on serum complement in healthy subjects above 50 years of age. In: *Clinical Research Report on Levamisole*, No 18 (Janssen Pharmaceutica)

Discussion 35

J. P. Famaey:
(Belgium)
The anti-inflammatory drug, indomethacin, in the concentration used here has been described in work done elsewhere (Mitsushima *et al.*) to stabilize erythrocyte membranes against any kind of haemolysis.

Is that not a non-specific property of this drug in this case, instead of a specific property?

di Perri:
Every drug alone lacks any action on the system alone—on erythrocytes alone. We have controlled this.

36

Immune reactions of lymphocytes eluted from rheumatoid inflammatory tissue

T. G. ABRAHAMSEN, S. S. FRØHLAND, J. B. NATVIG AND
J. PAHLE (Norway)

The synovial tissue of patients with rheumatoid arthritis and juvenile rheumatoid arthritis is usually infiltrated by mononuclear cells including plasma cells and lymphocytes[1,2]. Immunological characterization of these cells may reveal pathogenic mechanisms in the local rheumatoid inflammation. Previous investigations have mainly focused on the plasma cells and their relation to the humoral immune response[1]. Until very recently the lymphocytes have received less attention.

We have eluted lymphocytes from rheumatoid tissues according to a procedure previously described[3]. Briefly, the specimens were collected during synovectomy of different joints, and dissociated by treatment with crude collagenase and DNase. The resulting cell suspensions were inoculated in tissue culture flasks and incubated overnight. Cells which did not attach to the surface of the flasks, were harvested, and the lymphocytes separated by the Isopaque–Ficoll gradient centrifugation method[4]. Up to 86×10^6 lymphocytes could be obtained by this procedure. The viability of the cells was about 80% as assessed by the Trypan Blue exclusion test. Judged by cytocentrifuge smears 75–85% of the cells were lymphocytes, 15–20% macrophage-like cells and the rest was more undefined cells. In some tissues variable proportions of granulocytes or cells with the histological appearance of plasma cells were eluted. It could be demonstrated that T-lymphocytes, determined by the sheep erythrocyte rosette assay, were predominant in the eluted cell suspensions, whereas B-lymphocytes, detected by staining with a FITC conjugated anti-F(ab')$_2$ antiserum, and Fc-receptor-bearing lymphocytes, determined by rosette-formation with sensitized human erythrocytes were found in small proportions. This lymphocyte population profile was found in cell suspensions both from rheumatoid arthritis patients and juvenile rheumatoid arthritis patients, as described previously[3,5,6].

We wanted to study *in vitro* functions of these eluted lymphocytes. This report deals with the stimulatory effect of various lymphocyte mitogens, including antigens and mitomycin-treated allogeneic lymphocytes, on the cells. Furthermore, we have used these cells as effector cells in antibody-dependent cell-mediated cytotoxicity.

LYMPHOCYTE TRANSFORMATION ASSAY

The non-specific mitogens phytohaemagglutinin (PHA), pokeweed mitogen (PWM) and concanavalin A (Con A) were used. The antigens were purified protein derivative of tuberculin (PPD) and *Candida albicans* antigen and also mitomycin-treated allogeneic lymphocytes which were always obtained from the same donor. Usually cultures stimulated with non-specific mitogens contained 20% fetal calf serum and were harvested at day 4 whereas the antigen-stimulated cultures and the one-way MLC were supplemented with 20% human AB-serum and terminated at day 6. Unstimulated control

Table 36.1 Lymphocyte transformation assay in rheumatoid arthritis patients[1]

	Sources of lymphocytes								
	Cell suspensions eluted from rheumatoid tissue			Peripheral blood					
				Patients operated:			Patients not operated:		
	n^2	Mean	Range	n	Mean	Range	n	Mean	Range
PHA	17	187 (18.8	12–501 1.3–53.2)	7	32 (14.1	3–87 2.3–56.6)	12[3]	174 (77.7	34–612 4.6–339.0)
PWM	10	74 (10.9	22–218 1.8–55.7)	3	25 (9.8	21–31 2.9–20.5)	11[3]	61 (20.1	13–206 2.7–45.5)
Con. A	5	202 (10.7	36–524 2.2–23.0)	1	31 2.9		11[3]	36 (13.1	11–111 1.6–38.8)
PPD₁[4]	12	278 (19.5	53–448 3.6–75.2)	6 5	63 (7.3	10–160 0.5–17.1)	12	70 (12.5	7–186 0.8–43.9)
PPD₂[4]	4	350 (22.0	287–480 14.5–30.8)	3 2	81 (10.9	49–124 7.6–14.1)		Not tested	
Candida antigen	10	43 (1.5	6–113 0.6–3.3)	5 4	19 (2.0	6–39 0.8–5.1)	4	20 (2.9	7–29 1.0–5.6)
Allogeneic[5] cells	3	51 (3.4	47–55 1.7–4.9)	3 2	39 (5.9	31–50 5.3–6.5)		Not tested	

[1] The results are presented as disintegration per minute (DPM) × 10³ and as the calculated transformation index (TI). The latter values are given in brackets.

[2] Number of patients tested.

[3] These cultures were harvested after 3 days.

[4] PPD₁ was purchased from Veterinaerinstituttet, Oslo, Norway and PPD₂ was purchased from Statens Seruminstitut, Copenhagen, Denmark.

[5] Mitomycin C-treated cells always from the same donor.

Table 36.2 [³H]thymidine incorporation on mitogen stimulation of lymphocytes eluted from synovial tissues of juvenile rheumatoid arthritis patients

Patient	Control (4 days)	PHA		PWM		Con A		Control (6 days)	PPD		Candida antigen	
	DPM	DPM	TI²	DPM	TI	DPM	TI	DPM	DPM	TI	DPM	TI
M.N. (Aug. 1975)	10.4	113	10.1	37	3.5	n.t.³	n.t.	n.t.	n.t.	n.t.	n.t.	n.t.
M.N. (March 1976)	11.7	119	10.2	n.t.	n.t.	n.t.	n.t.	52.5	28	0.5	n.t.	n.t.
G.M. (Oct. 1975)	7.2	33	4.5	26	3.6	n.t.	n.t.	17.0	23	1.4	n.t.	1.4
G.M. (Feb. 1976)	26.6	•772	29.1	516	19.4	372	14.0	68.0	84	1.2	102	1.5
M.R.	18.2	43	2.4	200	11.0	n.t.	n.t.	19.4	65	3.4	54	2.8
A.M.O.	5.0	43	8.6	49	9.7	32	6.4	9.0	12	1.3	11	1.2

¹ DPM × 10³.
² Calculated transformation index.
³ Not tested.

cultures were always included. Incorporation of [³H]thymidine was used to measure the DNA-synthesis.

A variable but consistent stimulation of the lymphocytes was obtained with the non-specific mitogens, thus showing that the eluted lymphocytes were functionally viable. The results of the lymphocyte transformation assay are summarized in Table 36.1. PHA usually gave the highest transformation index, but PWM reached a comparable magnitude in several experiments. Similar responses have previously been reported for purified T-lymphocyte suspensions[7]. These results are thus compatible with the predominance of T-lymphocytes in the eluted cell suspensions. Studies of the dose–response and the kinetics of the lymphocyte transformation were consistent with patterns previously reported for peripheral blood lymphocytes both for the non-specific mitogens[8] and PPD[9]. However, the response of the eluted lymphocytes to two different PPD preparations was remarkably high and of the same magnitude as the transformation induced by PHA. This pattern was not found for peripheral blood lymphocytes obtained post-operatively from the patients or patients which had not been operated. No response was commonly obtained with *Candida* antigen, and only weak responses in the one-way MLC. In cell suspensions obtained from juvenile rheumatoid arthritis patients results similar to adult patients were obtained with non-specific mitogens whereas PPD and *Candida* antigen usually caused no transformation (Table 36.2).

The difference between adult and juvenile rheumatoid arthritis patients in the PPD-response is probably due to lack of previous sensitization to PPD or cross-reacting antigens in the latter group. The increased transformation of the eluted lymphocytes obtained by PPD compared to peripheral blood lymphocytes may be explained by trapping of antigen-sensitive cells in an inflammatory site induced by a different antigen[10] or by differences in antigen-specific suppressor or helper cell activity. Normal peripheral blood lymphocytes treated as the rheumatoid tissue did not show this transformation pattern.

ANTIBODY-DEPENDENT CELL-MEDIATED CYTOTOXICITY

Chromium-labelled chicken erythrocytes sensitized with a rabbit antiserum were used as target cells. Usually the effector cell/target ratio was 12.5:1 and the incubation time was 20 h. The results are presented as the corrected cytotoxic index[11].

Significant cytotoxic activity of the eluted cells was demonstrated both for rheumatoid arthritis and juvenile rheumatoid arthritis patients. However, the observed activity was always less than in the patient's blood (Table 36.3). Further depletion of adherent cells by fractionation on nylon columns usually increased the cytotoxicity (Table 36.4). B-lymphocytes were largely

Table 36.3 Antibody-induced cytotoxic activity of cells eluted from synovial tissues and lymphocytes separated from peripheral blood of rheumatoid arthritis patients

		Source of effector cells						
		Synovial tissue CI		Peripheral blood CI				Days after operation
Patient	Disease[1]			Preoperative		Postoperative		
		Antiserum[2]	Medium[3]	Antiserum	Medium	Antiserum	Medium	
R.K.	RA+	24.7	9.2	47.9	3.7	38.5	10.4	1
G.L.	RA+	32.8	4.7	41.8	2.0	51.2	3.5	1
A.M.N.	RA+	17.4	5.9	n.t.[4]	n.t.	30.0	7.2	9
L.R.	RA+	13.3	2.1	n.t.	n.t.	34.2	5.1	15
E.K.	RA+	19.9	1.1	n.t.	n.t.	24.8	5.0	1
E.S.	RA+	14.5	6.4	n.t.	n.t.	18.4	1.7	8
O.L.	RA+	12.5	11.1	n.t.	n.t.	31.2	3.3	13
T.G.	RA−	11.5	17.8	n.t.	n.t.	15.7	3.7	8
T.G.	JRA	37.4	6.8	n.t.	n.t.	40.1	7.0	10
H.B.	JRA	19.4	4.4	n.t.	n.t.	32.9	5.0	11
Normal blood donors	(n = 10)	35.5 (20.5–60.5)	5.4 (1.2–10.3)	(n = 2)45.1 (42.8–47.4)	4.9 (4.2–5.5)	(n = 7)36.3 (20.2–60.5)	5.8 (3.0–10.3)	

[1] RA+, seropositive rheumatoid arthritis; RA−, seronegative rheumatoid arthritis; JRA, juvenile rheumatoid arthritis.
[2] Corrected cytotoxic index; antiserum dilution 1:10⁴.
[3] Cytotoxic index; control cultures with medium instead of antiserum.
[4] Not tested.

removed (Table 36.4) and the proportion of non-lymphoid cells as determined on stained cytocentrifuge smears, was reduced. Similar results have previously been reported for peripheral blood lymphocyte suspensions[11].

The cytotoxic patterns observed with different dilutions of the anti-chicken erythrocyte serum and with varying effector cell/target cell ratios were similar to results in the control experiments with normal peripheral blood lymphocytes performed on the same day. However, the kinetics of the

Table 36.4 Nylon column fractionation of cell suspensions eluted from synovial tissues of patients with rheumatoid disease: Effect on antibody-induced cytotoxicity and lymphocyte populations

		Before nylon column fractionation					After nylon column fractionation				
Patient	Disease[1]	Cytotoxic activity		Lymphocyte populations			Cytotoxic activity		Lymphocyte populations		
		Antiserum[2]	Medium[3]	E-RFC[4]	Ig-C[5]	EA-RFC[6]	Antiserum	Medium	E-RFC	Ig-C	EA-RFC
O.Ø.	RA+	20.5	9.1	75	5	8	30.6	7.5	84	<1	3
I.I.	RA+	11.9	8.7	75	n.t.[7]	3	21.2	10.0	80	n.t.	1
R.K.	RA+	24.7	9.2	73	n.t.	n.t.	23.5	12.4	n.t.	n.t.	n.t.
M.H.	RA+	8.5	4.1	n.t.	4	1	8.8	9.4	n.t.	<1	<1
K.J.	RA+	12.1	4.4	n.t.	3	n.t.	4.4	16.9	n.t.	<1	3
E.D.	RA+	17.3	4.9	n.t.	5	3	10.4	8.1	n.t.	<1	3
E.K.	RA+	19.9	1.1	n.t.	n.t.	4	25.3	5.6	n.t.	<1	1
V.H.	RA−	14.3	5.3	70	6	2	19.4	4.9	55	1	3
Normal blood donors	(n=7)	35.0 (24.4–46.3)	6.9 (1.2–12.9)								

[1] RA+, seropositive rheumatoid arthritis; RA−, seronegative rheumatoid arthritis.
[2] Correction cytotoxic index; antiserum dilution 1:10⁴
[3] Cytotoxic index; control cultures with medium instead of antiserum.
[4] Percentage of lymphocytes forming rosettes with sheep erythrocytes (e.g. T-lymphocytes
[5] Percentage of lymphocytes showing membrane staining with a FITC-conjugated anti-F(ab′)₂ serum (e.g. B-lymphocytes).
[6] Percentage of lymphocytes forming rosettes with IgG-sensitized human erythrocytes (e.g. Fc-receptor-bearing lymphocytes)
[7] Not tested.

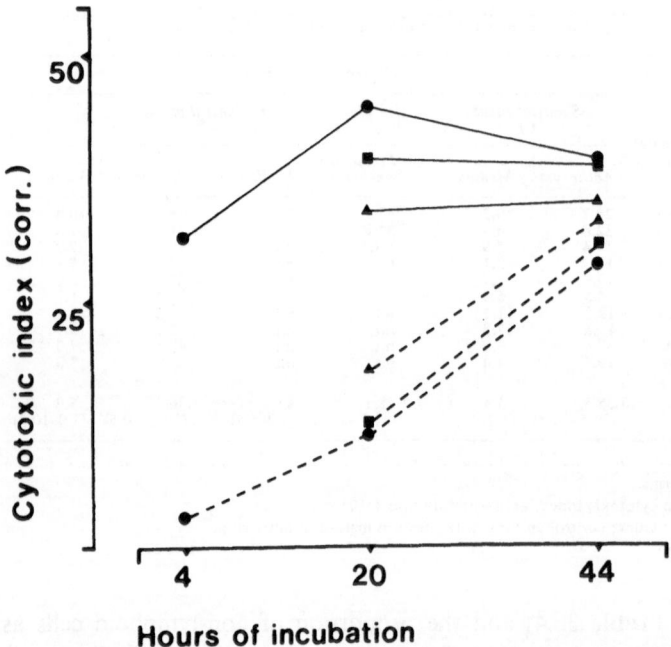

Figure 36.1 Time course of the antibody-dependent cytotoxicity mediated by cells eluted from rheumatoid synovial tissue (- - - - - - - - -) and normal peripheral blood lymphocytes (——————). Identical symbols represent experiments performed on the same day

cytotoxicity showed a much more pronounced increase for the eluted cells than for the controls (Figure 36.1). This may show that the number of cytotoxic cells in the eluted cell suspensions is small. Furthermore, monocyte-derived macrophages and granulocytes are reported to cause a more rapid cytotoxic reaction[12]. A gradual recovery of the cytotoxic cells from damage caused by the elution procedure is possible, but normal peripheral blood lymphocytes did not significantly change in their cytolytic ability after treatment as the rheumatoid tissue. These data suggest that the observed cytotoxicity has a similar effector mechanism as in peripheral blood where the Fc-receptor-bearing lymphocytes seem to be the main effector cell[13]. However, the activity in the EA-RFC depleted cell suspensions did not consistently decrease. This may be due to contamination with EA-rosetting and phagocytic adherent cells in the preparations[14]. Our data do not permit the exclusion of B- and T-lymphocytes as effector cells. The cytotoxic mechanisms operating in the rheumatoid tissue may be quite different from peripheral blood and perhaps include true antigenic specificity against IgG-sensitized target cells. These data are presented in detail elsewhere[15].

Further investigations are needed to clarify the probable *in vivo* involvement of antibody-dependent cell-mediated cytotoxicity in the rheumatoid inflammation.

References

1. Zvaifler, N. J. (1973). Immunopathogenesis of rheumatoid joint inflammation. *Adv. Immunol.*, **16**, 265
2. Bywaters, E. G. L. and Ansell, B. M. (1965). Monoarticular arthritis in children. *Ann. Rheum., Dis.*, **24**, 116
3. Abrahamsen, T. G., Frøland, S. S., Natvig, J. B. and Pahle, J. (1975). Elution and characterization of lymphocytes from rheumatoid inflammatory tissue. *Scand. J. Immunol.*, **4**, 823
4. Bøyum, A. (1968). Separation of leukocytes from blood and bone marrow. *Scand. J. Clin. Invest.*, **21**, Suppl., 97
5. van Boxel, J. A. and Paget, S. A. (1975). Predominantly T-cell infiltrate in rheumatoid synovial membranes. *N. Engl. J. Med.*, **293**, 517
6. Abrahamsen, T. G., Frøland, S. S., Natvig, J. B. and Pahle, J. (1977). Lymphocytes eluted from synovial tissue of juvenile rheumatoid arthritis patients. *Arthritis Rheum.* (In press)
7. Chess, L., MacDermott, R. P. and Schlossman, S. F. (1974). Immunologic functions of isolated human lymphocyte subpopulations. I. Quantitative isolation of human T and B cells and response to mitogens. *J. Immunol.*, **113**, 1113
8. Douglas, S. D. (1972). Electron microscopic and functional aspects of human lymphocyte response to mitogens. *Transplant. Rev.*, **11**, 39
9. Blomgren, H. (1975). Role of B cells in the expression of the PPD response of human lymphocytes *in vitro*. *Scand. J. Immunol.*, **4**, 499
10. McGregor, D. D. and Logie, P. S. (1974). The mediator of cellular immunity. VII. Localization of sensitized lymphocytes in inflammatory exudates. *J. Exp. Med.*, **139**, 1415
11. Wisløff, F. and Frøland, S. S. (1973). Antibody-dependent lymphocyte-mediated cytotoxicity in man: No requirement for lymphocytes with membrane bound immunoglobulin. *Scand. J. Immunol.*, **2**, 151
12. Perlmann, P. and Perlmann, H. (1970). Contactual lysis of antibody-coated chicken erythrocytes by purified lymphocytes. *Cell. Immunol.*, **1**, 300
13. Wisløff, F., Frøland, S. S. and Michaelsen, T. E. (1974). Antibody-dependent cytotoxicity mediated by human Fc-receptor-bearing cells lacking markers for B- and T-lymphocytes. *Int. Arch. Allergy*, **47**, 139
14. Abrahamsen, T. G., Johnson, P. M. and Natvig, J. B. (1977). Membrane characteristics of adherent cells dissociated from rheumatoid synovial tissue. *Clin. Exp. Immunol.* (In press)
15. Abrahamsen, T. G. Froland, S. S., Natvig, J. B. and Pahle, J. Antibody-dependent cytotoxicity mediated by cells elected from synovial tissues of patients with rheumatoid arthritis and juvenile rheumatoid arthritis. (Submitted for publication)

Discussion 36

G. Loewi:
(UK)

I did the same sort of work three years ago and I got much the same results as Dr. Abrahamsen. The secret of the whole thing is to incubate the cells after eluting them with enzymes. If PHA, or concanavalin A, are added straight away, then nothing. They have to be incubated.

Abrahamsen:
We incubate overnight.

Loewi:
One has to. I have tried without and it did not work. If they are incubated for something like 12 h then there is the same sort of response as for peripheral blood cells.

Abrahamsen:
Also, because of the enzyme treatment it is wise to incubate overnight. There may be an effect from the enzymes, as we heard.

Loewi:
The average of T-cells was 80%.

Abrahamsen:
We get 75%, both for adult and juvenile rheumatoid arthritis.

G. A. Voisin:
(France)

We have heard that the cells had to be incubated for several hours in order to obtain the reaction. This seems to be an important point. Many years ago work was done on immunological tolerance transferred by cells from tolerant animals into irradiated animals. The tolerance was successfully transferred, but when cells that had been incubated overnight were used, the transfer of immunological tolerance failed. Since then several experiments have been done to show that if cells are incubated then the results will be either a disappearance of the suppressive properties of suppressor cells—not the disappearance of suppressor cells, but the disappearance of their suppressive properties; or, alternatively, the stimulation of cells that would not otherwise have been stimulated in the absence of *in vitro* incubation.

The precise mechanism is not yet known, but it is nevertheless an important phenomenon.

37

Attempts at producing immune complexes *in vitro* between isolated macroglobulins and purified IgGs

NANNA SVARTZ (Sweden)

The rheumatoid factor (RF) is by many authors considered to be one of the components of immune complexes occurring in rheumatoid arthritis (RA)[1,2]. These immune complexes have been said to be the primary cause of the disease[3,4]. If this was true, the RF must, of course occur earlier than the onset of other symptoms of RA. In order to disentangle this, it seemed necessary to

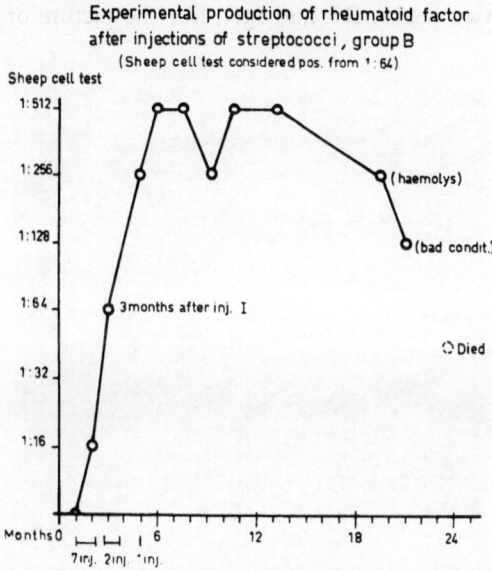

Figure 37.1 Experimental production of RF by injections of streptococci, group B (and nothing else). The Waaler Rose test became definitely positive after 3 months

determine the time of the occurrence of RF in relation to the time for the onset of other symptoms of the disease. This was possible in cases with an acute onset. The observations showed that the RF did not appear earlier than 3 weeks after the onset of clinical symptoms and often much later[5]. The same was the case as to arthritis experimentally provoked in rats by injections[6,7] of streptococci, group B (Figure 37.1).

The facts here referred to, seemed to speak against the theory that immune complexes were the origin of RA. In spite of that, immune complexes are probably of great value for the continued course of the disease. In order to come further into this problem it seemed desirable to do some new types of research. We decided to attempt to make immune complexes *in vitro*. For this purpose RF, isolated by cryoprecipitation and chromatography, was used and in addition various IgGs, purified by the same methods. First, the RF was mixed in the ratio 1:1 with an IgG isolated from common human γ-globulin. The mixture was kept at 37 °C for 2 h. Figure 37.2 demonstrates ultracentrifugation (UC) on the mixture. Two peaks are seen, the RF and the IgG. No complex could be observed. Figure 37.3 shows the same components in ratio 1:3. There are still two peaks in the mixture. However, the IgG peak is somewhat larger than in Figure 37.2. Otherwise, the two pictures are identical. It should be added that the influence of dilution was always considered.

The next step was experiments of adding a 'specific' IgG, obtained by immunizing rabbits with RF and isolating the active principle from the anti-RF serum, produced in rabbits. Figure 37.4 shows UC on a mixture 1:1 of RF and the 'specific' IgG, called IgRheumatoid, abbreviated IgR[7]. The UC shows two peaks, RF and IgR, like the picture of RF:IgG. But a

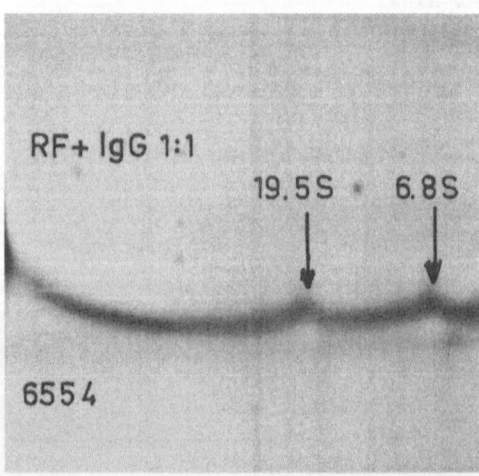

Figure 37.2 Ultracentrifugation (UC) of a mixture of isolated RF and common IgG. Two peaks are seen. No complex

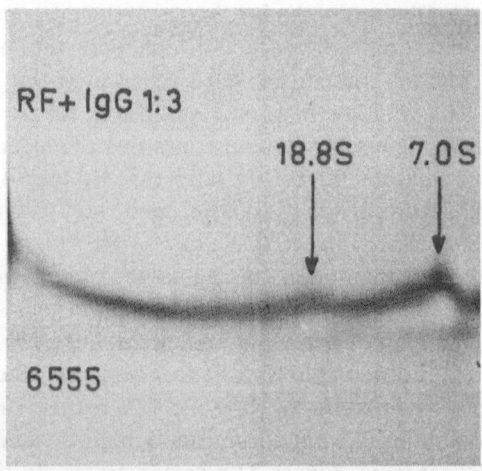

Figure 37.3 UC of a mixture of RF and IgG in ratio 1:3. Two peaks as in Figure 37.2, but the IgG peak is somewhat larger

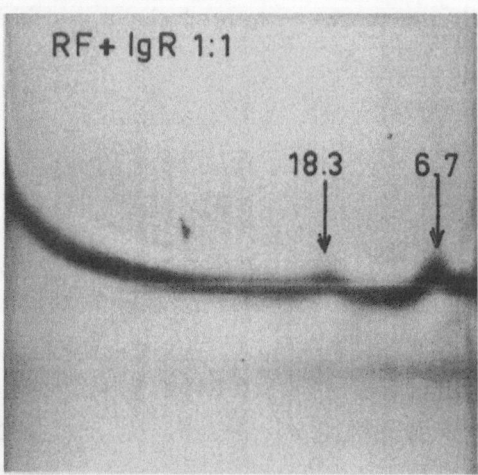

Figure 37.4 UC of a mixture of RF and its specific antibody IgR in ratio 1:1. Same result as in Figure 37.2

completely different picture was obtained when mixing RF and IgR in the ratio 1:3 or more (Figure 37.5) UC no longer shows any macroglobulin. There is only one peak and this has a sedimentation constant of only about 7S, like common IgG. Obviously, the IgR has caused a decomposition of RF. The new 7S compound does not react with common antibodies (anti-γM, anti-γA, anti-γG). The experiment has been repeated 40–50 times with the same result. Thus, an addition *in excess* of IgR to RF is followed by a decomposition of RF. Figure 37.6 demonstrates this change in immunoelec-trophoresis (IE) on a mixture RF/IgR in ratio 1:3. No macroglobulin could be observed in this mixture. It was, of course, important to find out whether other macroglobulins behaved in the same way as RF. First, the result was experienced in a disease that often has a macroglobulin with rather low S-value, i.e. SLE. An anti-SLE was produced in rabbits and isolated. Figure 37.7 shows, in IE, the effect when SLE was mixed with anti-SLE in excess. No macroglobulin was observable on IE. Consequently, the same change was obtained as with the mixture RF/IgR 1:3. Thereafter, the reaction was proved on a macroglobulin having an unusually high S-value, i.e. 28S in a case of reticulumcell-sarcoma. Figure 37.8 demonstrates, on IE, the effect of adding to 28S an excess of anti 28S. No macroglobulin could be observed. As far as I know, this effect of adding an *excess* of a specific antibody to its antigen is not earlier described.

What is now the nature and significance of this new macro-IgG-compound? It is not known yet. It is not a complex in the meaning that this term has been used. In a complex the components have still the property of reacting with antibodies. Our MI-compound does not react with common antibodies against proteins. We are on the way to producing a specific antibody to the

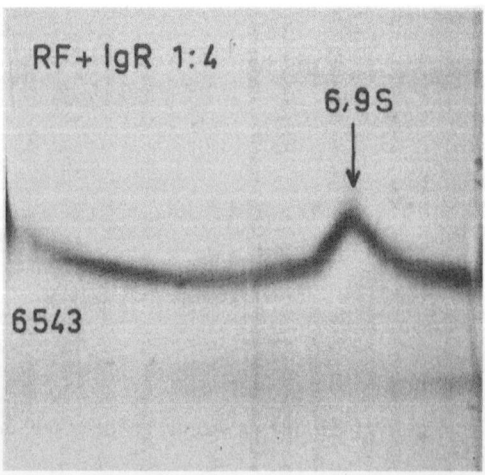

Figure 37.5 UC of a mixture of RF and IgR in ratio 1:4. Only one peak is seen, and this has an S-value of only 7S. No macroglobulin is observable. It had been brought to de-composition, when IgR was added *in excess*

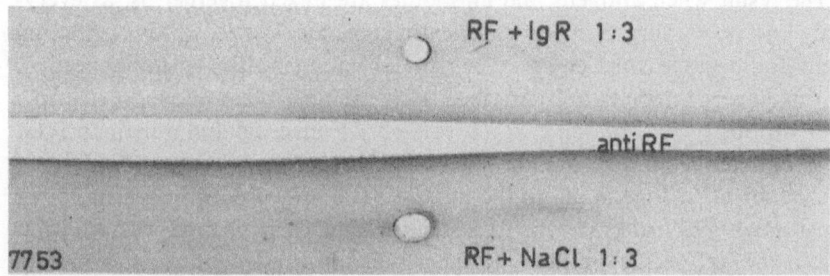

Figure 37.6 Immunoelectrophoresis (IE) on the same kind of mixture as in Figure 37.5. No macroglobulin is seen in the upper half

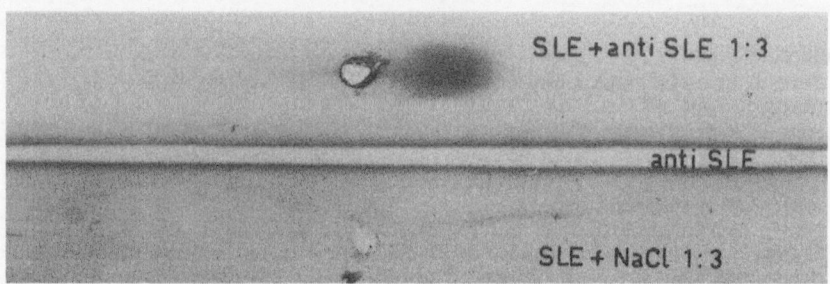

Figure 37.7 IE of a mixture of SLE and anti-SLE in excess. No macroglobulin is seen in the upper half

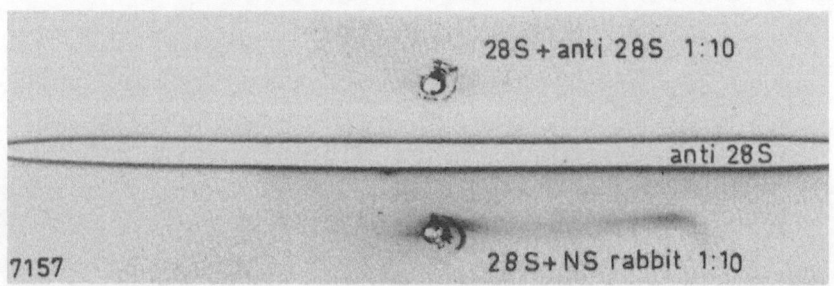

Figure 37.8 IE of a mixture of 28S (from reticulumcell sarcoma) and anti-28S in excess. No macroglobulin is seen. It has been decomposed by anti-28S

actual compound. As mentioned above, the S-value of the compound is about 7S, like the S-value of a common 7S globulin. It is possible that some animal experiments, started recently, may better explain the phenomenon.

The result when antigens and antibodies are mixed together, is, as everybody knows, varying. Sometimes an extra substance is needed for combining them (for instance complement or enzyme). Heating is also sometimes needed. In this paper, attempts are described of combining macroglobulins *in vitro* with various IgGs. Mixing, e.g., an isolated RF macroglobulin with an IgG, isolated from common human γ-globulin provokes only an insignificant change, or no change at all, in the mixture. The only procedure which in our experiments *in vitro* gave rise to a definite and clear change was addition *in excess* of a 'specific' antibody to the actual antigen. In our trials we mostly used macroglobulins, and their antibodies. No real complex was formed, but instead of it, a new compound[2] showing a sedimentation constant of only 7S, but it did not react as a common 7S γ-globulin. On the whole, the compound, here discussed, did not react with any of the usual antibodies against 7S γ-globulins.

References

1. Turk, J. L. (1974). Mechanism of immunological tissue damage. *Front. Intern. Med.* (Basle: Karger) 280
2. Allison, A. C., Cardella, C. and Davis, P. (1975). *Rheumatology, Immun. Aspects*, 231, (Basle: Karger)
3. Ziff, M. (1974). Immune complexes in rheumatoid synovitis. *Proc. XII Int. Congress Internal Medicine. Abstracts*, 31
4. Natvig, J., Munthe, E. and Pahle, J. (1975). *Rheumatology, Immun. Aspects*, 6, 167
5. Svartz, N. (1976). Late appearance of the rheumatoid factor and reaction with anti-rheumatoid factor IgG. *IRCS Medical Science*, 4, 112
6. Svartz, N. (1966). Hemagglutinating factor experimentally produced with pleomorphic diplococci of the Streptococcus agalactiae group, *Acta Med. Scand.*, 167, 77
7. Svartz, N. (1975). The origin of rheumatoid arthritis. Symp. on Immunol. Aspects of Rheumatoid Arthr., Montpellier 1974. *Rheumatology*, 6, 322

Discussion 37

G. Loewi: (UK)	What does Professor Svartz mean by antibody to SLE? I did not understand that.
Svartz:	We have injected antigen into rabbits and have obtained this antibody. We have tried to fix the ratio in this way. We have looked at the mixture in ultra-centrifugation and we have seen that the peaks are too isolated, and we have found that when there is an excess of the antibody there is only one-peak in ultra-centrifugation. There seems to be some rule that if there is an excess of the antibody then the antigen can be made to disappear.
R. Turner: (USA)	Professor Svartz's system seems to involve a rheumatoid factor that is not truly human in that it is raised in rabbits. Has she any data to show that this rheumatoid factor, used in her experiments, is comparable to the human rheumatoid factor seen in rheumatoid arthritis?
Svartz:	The rheumatoid factor was isolated completely, and that is necessary for the results. The antibody is also isolated by cryoprecipitation and chromatography. The ratio can then be measured by means of ultra-centrifugation and immune electrophoresis.
Turner:	But the rheumatoid factor is not truly from humans. It is from rabbits. It is raised in rabbits by injecting with bacteria. In what ways is it comparable to human rheumatoid factor in, say, a disease like rheumatoid arthritis?
Chairman:	This might be better discussed later.
I. Ginsburg: (Israel)	I have a general comment on the appearance of rheumatoid-like factors in laboratory animals subjected to infections with micro-organisms.

We have repeated some of Professor Svartz's results with rabbits and found that we constantly get beautiful chronic arthritis in rabbits injected intravenously with living Group B streptococci. We could also repeat it with Group A.

I want to quote two very interesting studies and to raise some questions on the possible role played by bacterial enzymes in the modification of the IgG molecule.

In the UK, several years ago, there was a very interesting paper (Mackintosh). γ-globulin was taken from rabbits and put into a test tube with Group A streptococci. The IgG was then re-isolated and injected back into the rabbit, and a beautiful nephritis—but not arthritis—followed. Precipitates of IgG and anti-IgG could be demonstrated in the kidneys. The author of that work believes that Group A streptococci produces an enzyme, or a group of enzymes, which is capable of removing the hexosamines and sialic acid from the IgG, thus probably exposing new immunogenic determinants that then elicit the formation of antibodies to the altered IgG.

Recently we read about studies that showed that *Streptococcus sanguis*—an oral streptococcus of the viridans group—can cleave IgA molecules specifically.

433

I believe that some of the controversies over experimental arthritis induced by bacteria can be explained, perhaps, by the capacities of certain bacteria to alter IgG to form auto-antigen.

Finally, anybody working with infectious diseases, such as syphilis, knows about the appearance of rheumatoid factors in the serum. However, there is no arthritis similar to rheumatoid arthritis, and so this is a very difficult question.

Svartz: What about different IgG? It is very interesting that the common IgG from human gamma globulin does not react in the same way as that which is produced by injecting rheumatoid factor into animals. There are now other IgGs that are also of interest, e.g. the IgG that reacts with SLE has about the same effect as that obtained in the rheumatoid factor.

It would be interesting to study the different IgGs. They do not, as has been postulated, have the same end groups. The end groups are different, and I believe that that is what determines the reaction with the rheumatoid factor.

38

Behaviour of some inflammation parameters in plasma and synovial fluid in some rheumatic diseases (*Abstract*)

R. NUMO AND V. PIPITONE (Italy)

A contemporaneous evaluation of some inflammation parameters was carried out in synovial fluid and plasma in three groups of patients with different rheumatic diseases.

(1) RA patients;

(2) Osteoarthrosis patients;

(3) Miscellanea (in this group were included SLE, rheumatic fever, reactive arthritis cases, etc.).

All the patients were without any treatment when the investigations were carried out. The following parameters were evaluated: alpha-1-antitrypsin, alpha-2-macroglobulin, fibrinogen and leucinoaminopeptidase (LAP).

A significant difference in plasma and synovial fluid levels for alpha-1-antitrypsin ($a1AT$) in patients with RA was observed, whilst no correlation was noted in the osteoarthrosis group, and a negative correlation was obtained in the miscellanea group.

The behaviour of fibrinogen, alpha-2-macroglobulin, and alpha-1-AT indicates that the levels of these molecules in synovial fluid express the degree of inflammation in synovium. Moreover a good correlation was found for LAP/$a1AT$ ratio in rheumatoid synovial fluid. Finally, the differences for $a1AT$, fibrinogen and $a2M$ in osteoarthrosis and miscellanea group as well, revealed not significant.

Discussion 38

G. P. Velo:	I should like to know something more about the significance of the
(Italy)	data. The slides are not too clear.
Numo:	The basic idea is that when the degree of inflammation increases, high

molecular weight proteins are able to go through the vessel and to be found in the synovial space. But not all of this is true. Sometimes—for instance for a-2-macroglobulins—low levels can be found. This was covered in the last part of my paper. It is true only because a-2-macroglobulins after this action have been the molecules—the enzyme, plasmin, elastase, and so on, and so to some extent they are macerated and not detectable.

Not for the fibrinogen. Fibrinogen has no aptitude to lean, to bend or to uptake other molecules—mainly enzymes.

39

Some applications of quantitative two-dimensional immunoelectrophoresis in the study of the systemic acute-phase reaction of the rat

R. SCHERER, M. ABD-EL-FATTAH AND
G. RUHENSTROTH-BAUER (Germany)

RESULTS AND DISCUSSION

By means of two-dimensional immunoelectrophoresis according to the method of Clarke and Freeman[1] it is possible to determine quantitatively at least 30 immunologically distinct rat serum proteins[3]. Fifteen of these proteins were identified by specific staining methods, physicochemical parameters or biochemical functions (Table 39.1).

Table 39.1 Identification of 15 individual rat serum proteins after separation by 2-dimensional immunoelectrophoresis

Precipitate no.	Identity	Method of identification
1	Prealbumin	electrophoretic mobility
2	Albumin	electrophoretic mobility
4	α-Lipoprotein	oil red O staining
5	α_1-macroglobulin	column chromatography[3]
7	α_1-acid-glycoprotein	column chromatography[3]
9	α_1-antitrypsin	trypsin binding[3]
10	cholinesterase	indoxylacetate staining
11	coeruloplasmin	p-phenylene-diamine staining
17	haptoglobin	benzidine staining
20	hemopexin	benzidine staining
23	$\beta_1 - A$	C3-conversion, specific antiserum[3]
26	transferrin	binding of $^{59}FeCl$, autoradiography[3]
27	$\beta_1 - C$	C3-conversion, specific antiserum[3]
28	β-lipoprotein	oil red O staining
30	IgG	monospecific antiserum

Kinetics of the acute-phase protein changes after inflammatory stimulation

It is known from previous experimental work[2,3] that the injection of irritants such as carrageenan and endotoxic lipopolysaccharide causes a systemic acute-phase response in the rat. The resulting plasma protein changes, especially the increase of circulating alpha- and beta-globulins, have been demonstrated by conventional cellulose acetate electrophoresis in a rather unspecific way. Applying the technique of quantitative immunoelectrophoresis we were able to follow the specific serum concentration changes of 30 immunologically defined proteins after either intraperitoneal injection of endotoxic lipid A or injection of 0.2 ml of a 2% carrageenan suspension into each hind paw of the rat. Despite the different types of inflammatory stimulants and the different routes of application, a rather uniform acute-phase response could be observed in each set of experiments. Seventeen individual rat plasma proteins reacted with an increase, 6 plasma proteins with a decrease of their respective serum concentration. The serum concentrations of only 8 plasma proteins were not affected by the systemic inflammatory response. The time course of changes in the serum levels of those proteins which were most affected by the acute-phase reaction is illustrated in Figures 39.1 and 39.2. All plasma protein determinations were performed with pooled serum from three rats for each time interval. The control animals were injected with sterile, pyrogen-free saline solution. In those rats treated with carrageenan the inflammatory response reached peak values after 24 h, while in the lipid A injected rats the response was more extended and reached the maximum only during the second day after the inflammatory stimulation. The decrease of concentration (Figure 39.2), which was most pronounced with prealbumin, albumin, cholinesterase, transferrin and the unidentified peak No. 12 seems to be a counter-regulatory phenomenon. It is caused in some instances by a selective decrease of the hepatic synthesis rate of these proteins,[4] in other instances the decrease of the circulating amount of these proteins might be due to local binding at the site of inflammation and an accelerated catabolism of these proteins. The initial increase of the serum concentrations of a number of proteins, which was observed in the lipid A injected rats (Figure 39.2), is most probably caused by a temporary increase of vascular permeability and subsequent hemoconcentration.

Effect of phenylbutazone treatment on the acute-phase response

One hour before inflammatory stimulation with lipid A or carrageenan phenylbutazone was injected subcutaneously in the region of the scapulae at a dose of 200 mg/kg body weight of the rats. This dose proved to be sufficient to suppress almost completely oedema formation in the rat paws injected with carrageenan. Surprisingly the anti-inflammatory therapy did not

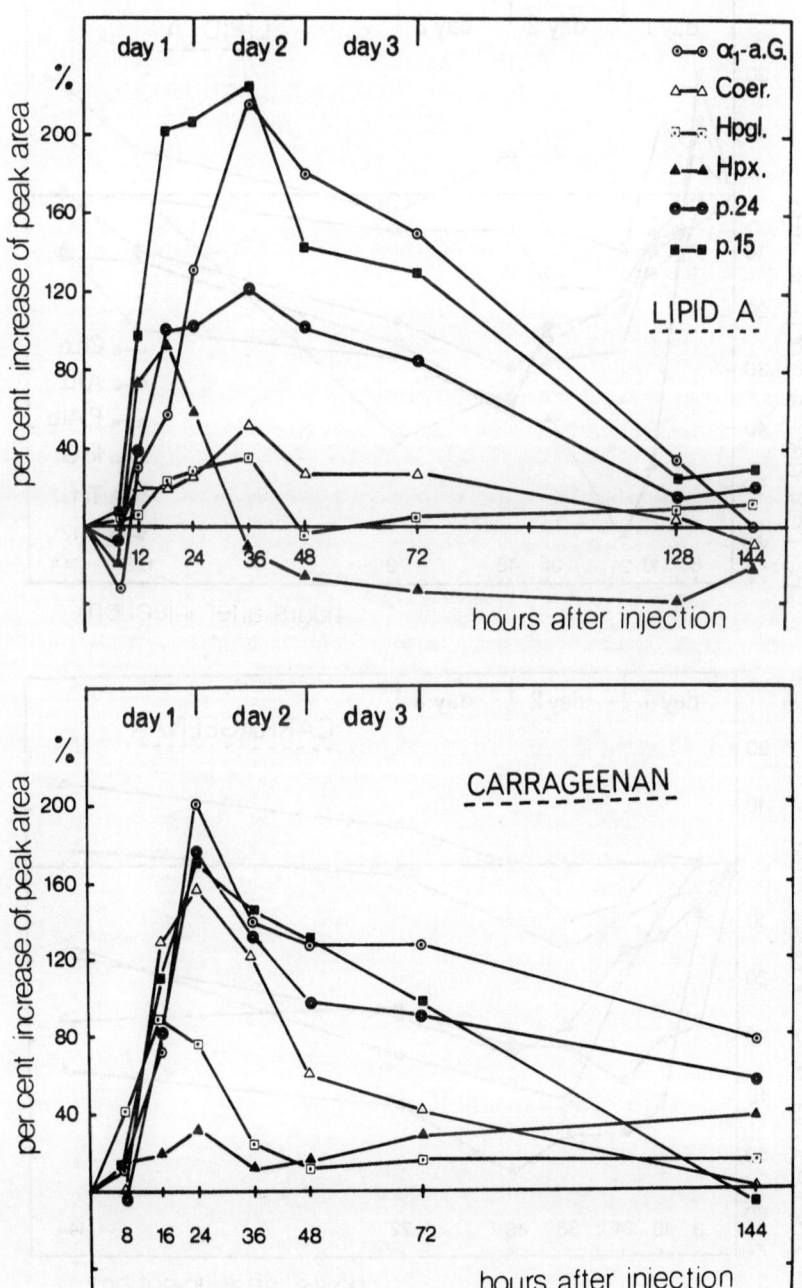

Figure 39.1 Kinetics of the increase in serum concentration of 6 plasma proteins after inflammatory stimulation either with endotoxic lipid A or with carrageenan Abbrev.: α_1−a.G.: α_1-acid-glycoprotein, Coer.: coeruloplasmin, Hpgl.: haptoglobin, Hpx.: hemopexin, p.24: peak 24, p.15: peak 15

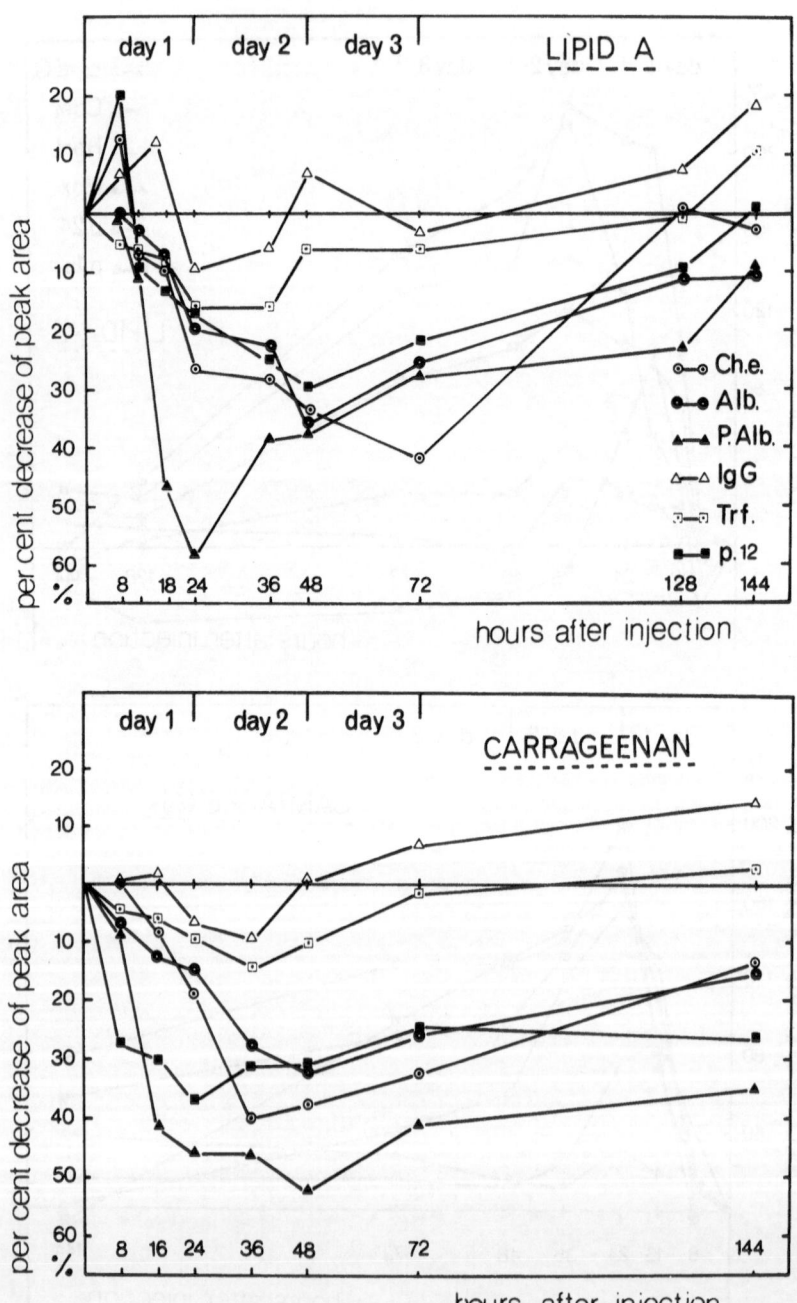

Figure 39.2 Kinetics of the decrease in serum concentration of 6 plasma proteins after inflammatory stimulation either with endotoxic lipid A or with carrageenan. Abbrev.: Ch.e.: cholinesterase, A.b.: albumin, P.Alb.: prealbumin, IgG: immunoglobulin G, Trf.: transferrin, p.12: peak 12

at all reduce the systemic acute-phase response. On the contrary phenyl-butazone treatment seemed to enhance the acute-phase protein changes despite its local anti-inflammatory activity (Figures 39.3, 39.4 and 39.5). Phenyl-butazone treatment alone in the absence of inflammatory stimulation did not

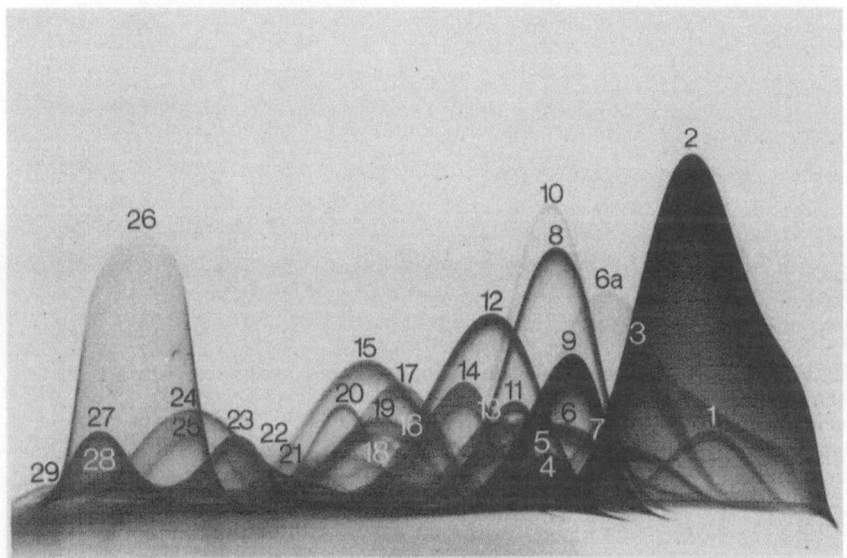

Figure 39.3 Two-dimensional immunoelectrophoresis of pooled serum from healthy control rats injected with sterile 0.9 % saline solution

induce a significant change of the rat plasma protein profile. Another un-expected observation, which we cannot explain as yet, was a remarkable delay of complement activation in those rats receiving antiphlogistic therapy. Injection of lipid A as well as carrageenan usually induces complement activa-tion, which can be monitored by the conversion of B_1C- into B_1A-globulin. The single dose therapy with phenylbutazone apparently inhibited comple-ment activation until after 20–30 h the level of phenylbutazone, which is eliminated in the rat with a half-life of 6 h, dropped below a critical value.

Induction of a systemic acute-phase response in the rat by leukocytic endogenous mediators (LEM)

LEM was prepared according to established method[5,6]: rabbits were infused intraperitoneally with a sterile saline solution containing 0.2 % shell-fish glycogen (Mann Research Laboratories, New York). After 14 h the

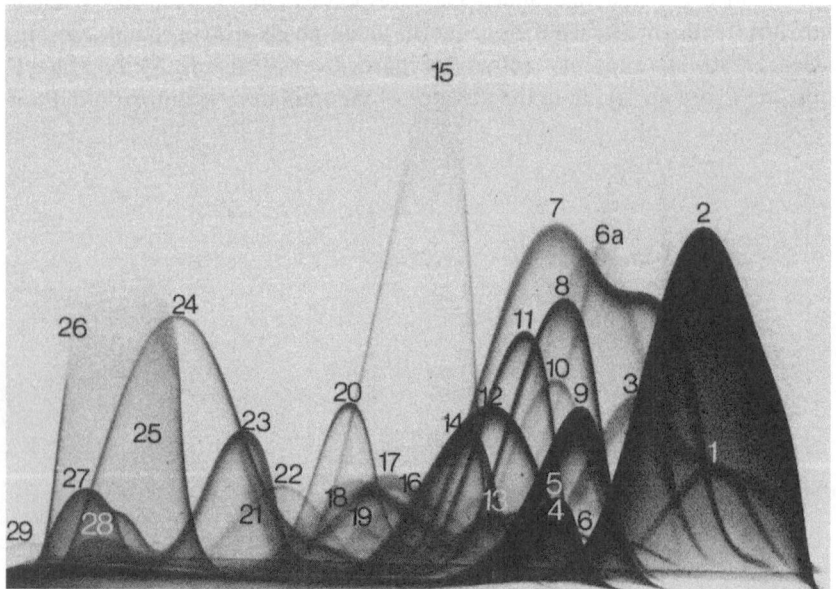

Figure 39.4 Two-dimensional immunoelectrophoresis of pooled serum from rats injected with carrageenan

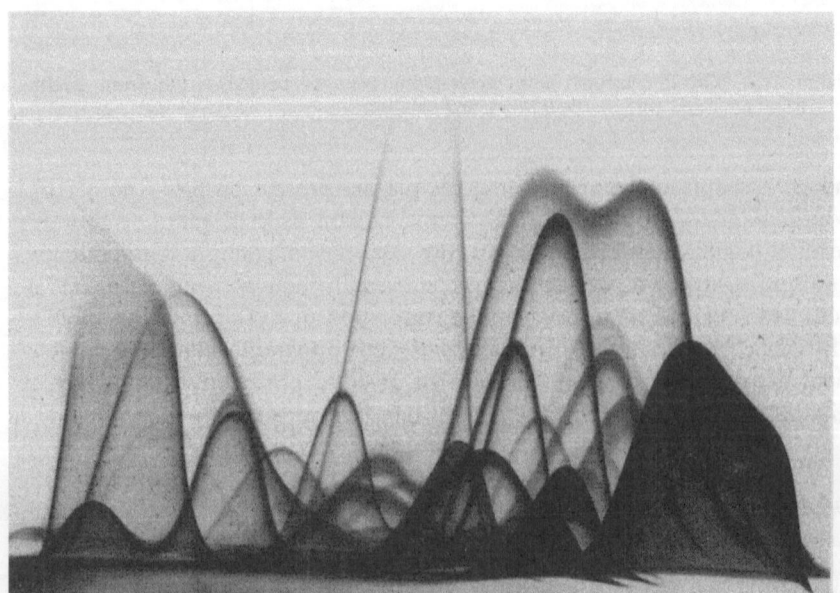

Figure 39.5 Two-dimensional immunoelectrophoresis of pooled serum from rats injected with carrageenan after treatment with therapeutical doses of phenylbutazone

peritoneal leukocytes were harvested, washed twice with saline solution and were then incubated at 37 °C for 2 h. LEM released by the stimulated polymorphonuclear leukocytes (PMN) was obtained in the cell-free supernatant after centrifugation. In order to remove contaminating high molecular weight proteins the crude LEM-solution was passed through an Amicon XM-100 filter and was finally concentrated by means of pressure filtration with an Amicon PM-10 filter. The LEM-preparation was injected intraperitoneally into perfectly healthy rats at a dose corresponding to the amount of LEM secreted by 4.5×10^7 PMN. Serum obtained only 12 h after treatment revealed a fully developed acute-phase protein pattern. This is in accordance with findings of other investigators, who looked upon the LEM-induced increase of individual acute-phase proteins such as fibrinogen[7], haptoglobin[7], a_2-acute-phase protein[8] and coeruloplasmin[9].

We think that LEM is not a single mediator protein, but a whole group of low molecular weight proteins regulating the hepatic synthesis rates of different plasma proteins. If this is so, two-dimensional quantitative immunoelectrophoresis will be an excellent tool, discriminating the different mediators after separation by further purifying the as yet crude LEM-preparation.

In order to assess the physiological relevance of LEM, we depleted rats of their white blood cells by a combined treatment with methotrexate (3 daily i.p. injections of 2.5 mg/kg body weight) and a single 400 R irradiation. The agranulocytoxic rats were then challenged with a subplantar injection of carrageenan into the hind paws. Immunoelectrophoretic analysis of the rat sera 24 h after inflammatory stimulation revealed a significant reduction of the systemic acute-phase response. Further analysis after 48 h showed that by then a fully developed acute-phase protein profile had appeared in the agranulocytotic rats. This might be explained by the finding that cells other than granulocytes, e.g. reticuloendothelial cells, also produce and release LEM[10]. Injection of LEM instead of carrageenan into the agranulocytoxic rats evoked a rather normal systemic acute-phase response, which confirms that the delayed reponse to carrageenan is in fact due to the lack of circulating granulocytes.

Although we do not know the individual function of many acute-phase proteins, the acute-phase response as a whole can be considered to be a beneficial and desirable physiological reaction. It seems to be directed at preventing a spread of local inflammatory tissue damage and at the induction of tissue repair processes. In view of these beneficial effects, the possibility of manipulating the acute-phase response as it has been shown in the reported experiments may be of considerable therapeutical value in the future.

References

1. Clarke, M. H. G. and Freeman, T. (1968). Quantitative immunoelectrophoresis of human serum proteins. *Clin. Sci.* **35**, 403.

2. DiRosa, M. D. (1972). Biological properties of carrageenan. *J. Pharm. Pharmacol.*, **24**, 89
3. Abd-El-Fattah, M., Scherer, R. and Ruhenstroth-Bauer, G. (1976). Application of quantitative two-dimensional immunoelectrophoresis in the study of the acute-phase reaction following injection of the lipid A component of bacterial lipopolysaccharides in rats. *J. Mol. Med.* **1**, 211.
4. Billingham, M. E. and Gordon, A. H. (1975). The role of the acute phase reaction in inflammation. In: *Future Trends in Inflammation II* (J.-P. Giroud, D. A. Willoughby and G. P. Velo, eds.) pp. 195–200. (Basel and Stuttgart: Birkhäuser Verlag)
5. Pekarek, R., Wannemacher, R., Powanda, M., Abeles, F., Mosher, D., Dintermann, R. and Beisel, W. (1974). Further evidence that leukocytic endogenous mediator (LEM) is not endotoxin. *Life Sci.*, **14**, 1765
6. Pekarek, R., Wannemacher, R. W., Chapple, F. E., Powanda, M. C. and Beisel, W. (1972). Further characterization and species specificity of leukocytic endogenous mediator (LEM). *Proc. Soc. Exp. Biol. Med.*, **141**, 643
7. Kampschmidt, R. F. and Upchurch, H. F. (1974). Effect of leukocytic endogenous mediator on plasma fibrinogen and haptoglobin. *Proc. Soc. Exp. Biol. Med.*, **146**, 904
8. Eddington, C. L., Upchurch, H. F. and Kampfschmidt, R. F. (1972). Quantitation of plasma α-2-AP globulin before and after stimulation with leukocytic extracts. *Proc. Soc. Exp. Biol. Med.*, **139**, 565
9. Pekarek, R. S., Powanda, M. C. and Wannemacher, R. W. (1972). The effect of leukocytic endogenous mediator on serum copper and coeruloplasmin concentrations in the rat. *Proc. Soc. Exp. Biol. Med.*, **141**, 1029
10. Beisel, W. R. (1975). Metabolic response to infection. In: *Annual Review of Medicine* (W. P. Creger, C. H. Coggins and E. W. Hancock, eds.) Vol. 26, pp. 9–20

40

Restoration of the neutrophil chemotactic responsiveness by levamisole treatment in patients with recurrent infections, eczema and hyperimmunoglobulinaemia E

R. S. WEENING, Liesbeth STRICKER, D. ROOS, J. L. MOLENAAR, L. J. DOOREN AND R. K. B. SCHUURMAN (The Netherlands)

Abbreviations

PMN – polymorphonuclear leukocytes

INTRODUCTION

In 1972 Buckley et al.[1] described a syndrome in two adolescents, in which an undue susceptibility to infections was associated with hyper-immuno-globulinaemia E. These patients suffered from chronic dermatitis and from recurrent subcutaneous, pulmonary, and joint abscesses. Repeatedly, *Staphylococcus aureus* and *Candida albicans* could be cultured from these lesions. One year later, Clark et al.[2] described a similar syndrome and found this condition to be associated with a defect in the neutrophil chemotactic responsiveness. Since then, high IgE titres in combination with a predisposition to bacterial infections and defective PMN chemotaxis have been reported in a variety of other defects (for review, see Discussion of Reference 3). In most instances these conditions were accompanied by depressed cellular and humoral immunity.

Levamisole, an anthelminthic drug, has been reported to exert—besides various immunostimulating properties—an enhancing effect on neutrophil chemotaxis of normal cells *in vitro*[4]. The effect of long-term treatment *in vivo* with levamisole on chemotaxis, however, has hardly been investigated. We have studied neutrophil chemotaxis in four patients with defective chemo-taxis, recurrent pyogenic infections, eczematous dermatitis, and hyper-immunoglobulinaemia E before and during long-term treatment with levamisole.

CASE REPORTS

Case 1

J.S., a boy, born April 15, 1960, was the first child of healthy parents. The family history was unremarkable. Pregnancy, delivery, and perinatal period were uneventful. From the age of a few weeks he suffered from 'seborrhoic dermatitis' with pyoderma and recurrent lymphadenitis. He also showed chronic blepharitis, rhinitis, sinusitis, and external otitis. Despite local treat-ment and courses of antibiotics, incision of lymph gland abscesses in the neck, axillae and groins was frequently necessary. From skin lesions and lymph glands *Staphylococcus aureus* was cultured. Other organ systems, e.g. the lower respiratory tract, were never seriously infected. Viral infections ran a normal course, fungal infections were never noted, and vaccinations were without complications (no smallpox vaccination was performed). The boy showed a normal physical and psycho-motor development. Laboratory investigation showed no eosinophilia (<600 eosinophils/mm^3). Extensive examination *in vivo* and *in vitro* of humoral and cellular immune capacities showed no abnormalities, except a very high serum IgE level of 5000–6000 IU/ml. Radio-allergo-sorbent tests showed specific IgE antibody activity against house dust, house mites, egg protein, and cat hair. Lymph gland biopsy showed a picture of chronic inflammation, but no granulomas were seen. In June 1976, treatment with levamisole (2.5 mg/kg body weight orally on 3 successive days of each week) was started. Since then the skin lesions have gradually improved and diminished. Abscesses have no longer developed and all other treatment was discontinued. Regular control of peripheral blood values and serum chemistry showed no abnormalities.

Case 2

D.M., born April 7, 1962, was the first child of apparently healthy parents. He was born after a normal pregnancy and delivery. There was no family history of recurrent infections, skin disease, or allergy. He suffered from recurrent, *Staphylococcus aureus* infected pyoderma and otitis media since he was 3 weeks old. He also suffered from a balanitis. When he was 4 years old he had a lobectomy for a lung abscess complicated by pyopneumothorax. From the abscess *Staphylococcus aureus* was cultured. Since then he was treated repeatedly with local and systemic antibiotics for chronic skin infec-tions. At 12 years of age he developed abscesses in his scrotum and his left leg. Despite adequate drainage of the abscesses and treatment with anti-biotics, the abscess in his leg fistulated. Moreover, he developed a chronic osteomyelitis of his left femur. Surgical excision of the fistula and the abscess finally resulted in a complete recovery.

Laboratory investigations showed a variable eosinophilia (up to 1495 eosinophils/mm³). Serum IgE levels were elevated with a positive radio-allergo-sorbent test for house dust. He was treated with levamisole (2.5 mg/kg body weight orally, on 3 successive days of each week) starting May 1976. All other therapy was stopped. After 8 months of treatment he is for the first time in his life practically free of skin lesions.

Case 3

R.L., a Maroccan boy, born October 16, 1974, had eczema from birth. Skin diseases nor other defects are known in his family. Many periods of fever and malaise were caused by severe infections of the skin. A coagulase positive *Staphylococcus aureus* was always cultured from the lesions. Severe episodes of this impetigo were treated with systemic antibiotics. At the age of one year he was admitted to hospital with a severe bronchitis, impetigo, and acute otitis media. Five months later he developed abscesses on his head, in the axillae, and in the buttocks. These abscesses and a lobular pneumonia which did not improve with systemic antibiotic treatment led the patient to be sent to the Sophia Children's Hospital in Rotterdam. With intravenous antibiotic treatment for 10 weeks the persistent pneumonia resolved but he was left with several large lung cysts. Surgical incision and drainage was needed for the dermal abscesses and axillary lymph node abscesses. During this hospital stay maxillary sinus drainage was performed many times because of recurrent sinusitis. He also had many bouts of acute otitis media.

Laboratory investigation showed a persistent eosinophilia (up to 1080 eosinophils/mm³). A slight anaemia persisted although he was treated with vitamins and iron. High levels of immunoglobulins without restricted hetero-geneity and normal antibody levels against different viruses, red blood cell antigens A and B, and bacterial vaccines suggested a normal antibody response. Antibodies against staphylolysins were always absent. IgE levels were very high (>2000 IU), with positive radio-allergo-sorbent tests for house dust, house mites, cat hair, milk, and egg protein. Histopathology of the skin showed the picture of impetigo. Treatment with levamisole (2.5 mg/kg body weight orally, on 3 successive days of each week) was started in July 1976. Since then the patient has not needed any antibiotic treatment, although he developed minor recurrencies of impetigo. There have been no recurrencies of his pneumonia.

Case 4

R.v.d.W., a Dutch boy, was born on March 3, 1973. He was one of a non-identical twin and was admitted to the Sophia Children's Hospital because of prematurity (34 weeks). On the third day he developed conjunctivitis and dermatitis. The dermatitis was complicated by extensive exfoliation, starting from the palms of the hands and the soles of the feet. The dermatitis was treated with variable success by systemic and locally applied antibiotics and bathing in chlorohexidine. Bacterial cultures from the skin almost always gave a growth of *Proteus mirabilis*, sometimes haemolytic streptococcus (different types) and the last years also a penicillin-resistant *Staphylococcus aureus*. In the beginning he suffered from diarrhoea with a tendency to dehydration. However, from January 1974 on he has had moderate to severe constipation. His growth is retarded, especially of the lower extremities and pelvis. Neither his twin sister nor other family members have had any dermatological or other illnesses. The dermal infections caused a persistent lymphadenopathy which once needed surgical intervention because of lymphadenitis of the neck with abscess formation. A further hospital admission was necessary for suppurating inguinal lymph nodes.

Laboratory investigations showed a persistent eosinophilia (up to 1950 eosinophils/mm^3). The IgE level was normal on the first day of birth but later on became higher than 2000 IU/ml with highly positive radio-allergo-sorbent tests for house dust and egg proteins. The histological diagnosis was *Eczema seborrhoica psoriatiforme*. Further investigations showed higher than normal amounts of mast cells in the lymph nodes and the skin. Large amounts of IgE were seen by immunofluorescence on the membranes of these mast cells. Further immunological investigations (lymphocyte transformation, antibodies, autoantibodies against dermis, basement membranes, etc. and bone marrow fluorescence) showed no abnormalities. Starting July 1976, he was treated with levamisole (2.5 mg/kg body weight orally, on 3 successive days of each week) without any clinical improvement so far.

MATERIALS AND METHODS

Levamisole

Levamisole (kindly provided by Janssen Pharmaceutica, Beerse, Belgium) was dissolved in phosphate-buffered saline (pH 7.2) in final concentrations of 10^{-3}–10^{-6} M for the studies *in vitro*.

Isolation of granulocytes

Granulocytes were prepared from fresh defibrinated blood with a modification of the Bøyum technique, as described elsewhere[5]. The final cell suspensions contained more than 95% granulocytes.

Chemotaxis

Chemotaxis was determined with the 'leading front' method[6]. In this assay, cell penetration into a millipore filter with a thickness of 100–150 μm and a pore size of 3 μm was measured. The chemotaxis chambers consisted of sawn-off syringe barrels from 1 ml disposable syringes, to the lower end of which the filter was glued. The syringe barrel was suspended in a small beaker containing 10 ml Earle's balanced salt solution fortified with 25 mM HEPES (pH 7.2 at 37 °C), penicillin (200 U/ml), and streptomycin (50 μg/ml). To the upper compartment (the syringe barrel) 0.2 ml of cells was added in a final concentration of 1×10^6 granulocytes/ml in the same medium. To the lower compartment 1 mg casein per ml was added as the chemotactic stimulus. After incubation at 37 °C for 70 min, the upper compartments were emptied by inversion and the cells which had penetrated into the filters were fixed in absolute ethanol for 10 min and stained with Harris haemotoxylin. The filters were mounted under a cover slip with Canada balsam and examined with a microscope. A micrometer reading was taken at the plane in which the nuclei of two or more cells that had penetrated the farthest into the filter were in focus. Another reading was taken at the top of the filter. Thus, the distance between the leading front and the top of the filter was measured. This procedure was repeated at 5 different places in the filter and the mean of these values was calculated. Each test was performed with five separate filters. The standard deviation of the test was 9 % ($n = 25$).

Phagocytosis

The uptake of ^{14}C-labelled *Staphylococcus aureus* was measured by counting the radioactivity in the PMN after lysis of non-ingested bacteria with lysostaphin.

Opsonization

The opsonic activity of the patients' sera was measured by comparing the rate of phagocytosis by normal control cells in pooled human AB serum versus the uptake in the patients' sera.

Bactericidal activity

The intracellular killing of *Staphylococcus aureus* by PMN was measured using a method described by Solberg[7].

Immunoglobulins

IgE levels were measured by a radioimmunometric method[8]. IgA, IgM, and IgG levels were determined using radial immunodiffusion techniques.

Lymphocyte reactivity *in vitro*

This was measured by ^{3}H-thymidine incorporation after stimulation by various mitogens and antigens[9].

RESULTS AND DISCUSSION

In all patients, serum immunoglobulin concentrations were normal, except for marked increased serum IgE levels (see Table 40.1). Normal antibody responses against viruses and bacterial vaccines were observed in three patients. In patient R.L., however, staphylolysins were always absent. The severe skin lesions in all patients made estimation of delayed type hypersensitivity *in vivo* by intradermal skin tests impossible. The number of circulating T- and B-cells, determined with E and EAC rosette formation, was in the normal range. No abnormalities were found in the lymphocyte reactivity *in vitro* (stimulation with PHA, pokeweed, Concanavalin A, anti-lymphocyte serum, PPD, diphtheria, tetanus, mumps, candida, and allogeneic cells). The serum concentrations of the complement components C2, C3, C5 and $C1_q$ were within the normal range. The opsonic indices of the patients' sera were also normal. Absolute numbers of granulocytes were repeatedly within the normal range. During infections an appropriate leukocytosis developed. Although none of the patients had clear allergic manifestations, there was an eosinophilia up to 10–30% in three patients. The PMN of the patients showed a normal uptake and intracellular killing of *Staphylococcus aureus*. Moreover, the normal stimulation of the oxygen uptake during phagocytosis indicated a normal metabolic stimulation of these cells. However, *in vitro* studies of the chemotactic responsiveness of the patients' granulocytes showed a consistent defect (Table 40.1).

Table 40.1 Serum IgE levels and PMN chemotaxis of patients with recurrent infections, eczema and hyper-immunoglobulinaemia E

Patients	Serum IgE (IU/ml)	Chemotaxis (µm)
1. J.S.	5000–6000 ($n = 2$)	42–46 ($n = 4$)
2. D.M.	2100 ($n = 1$)	45–47 ($n = 2$)
3. R.L.	10 400 ($n = 1$)	47 ($n = 1$)
4. R.v.d.W.	1525 ($n = 1$)	38–44 ($n = 3$)
Controls	<500 ($n = 30$)	61–84 ($n = 30$)

These findings suggest that the high susceptibility for bacterial infections of these patients might be based upon the chemotactic defect. Our patients resemble the cases reported by Hill *et al.*[10].

Family studies were restricted to the parents of the patients. Apart from the slightly depressed chemotactic responsiveness of the PMN of the father of patient R.L., we found neither abnormalities in neutrophil chemotaxis nor in serum IgE levels of these family members (Table 40.2).

Anderson *et al.*[4] recently reported that levamisole in concentrations of 10^{-3} or 10^{-4} M increased chemotaxis of normal neutrophils *in vitro*. In our hands, however, no stimulatory effect on normal PMN was found. In fact, in some instances we found an inhibition of the chemotaxis at all concentrations

Table 40.2 Serum IgE levels and chemotaxis of the parents of patients with recurrent infections, eczema and hyperimmunoglobulinaemia E

	Serum IgE (IU/ml)*	Chemotaxis (μm)*
Father J.S.	<100	75
Mother J.S.	<100	70
Father D.M.	<100	69
Mother D.M.	<100	64
Father R.L.	<100	55
Mother R.L.	<100	63
Father R.v.d.W.	<100	80
Mother R.v.d.W.	<100	68
Controls	<500	61–84

*IgE levels and chemotaxis of family members were determined once
Control values are range of 30 experiments

tested (Table 40.3). The effect of levamisole on the patients' granulocytes, however, showed a somewhat different pattern. In contrast to normal cells, levamisole at concentrations of 10^{-4} or 10^{-5} M never caused a significant decrease in the chemotactic responsiveness of the patients' cells (see Table 40.3).

The effect of treatment *in vivo* with levamisole on chemotaxis is shown in Figure 40.1. The patients were treated with 2.5 mg levamisole/kg body weight

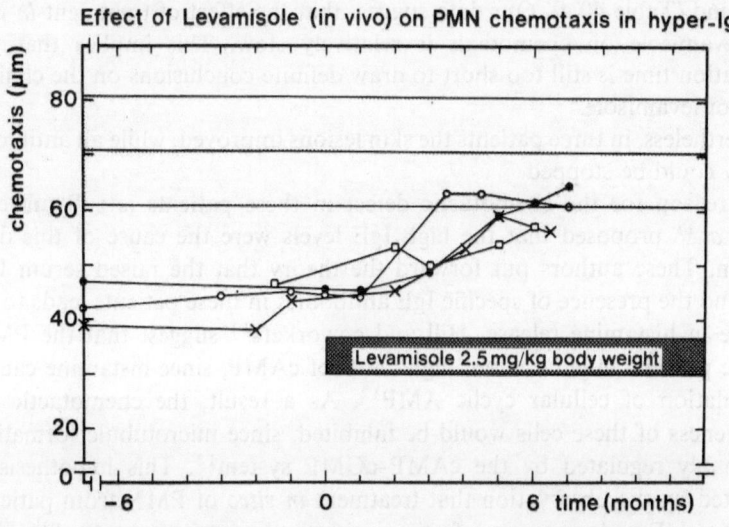

Figure 40.1 Effect of treatment *in vivo* with levamisole on chemotactic responsiveness of PMN from patients with recurrent infections, eczema and hyperIgE. Chemotactic response (vertical axis) of normal PMN is given as mean (71 μm) ± 2 SD (*n* = 30) (shaded area). Chemotactic response of patients' PMN is shown before and after onset of levamisole treatment (2.5 mg/kg body weight orally, on 3 successive days of each week). Levamisole treatment was started at *t* = 0. ○-○, case 1; ●-●, case 2; □-□, case 3; ×-×, case 4

Table 40.3 Effect of levamisole on PMN chemotaxis *in vitro*

Additions	Pat. J.S. (n = 2)	Pat. D.M. (n = 1)	Pat. R.L. (n = 1)	Pat. R.v.d.W. (n = 2)	Controls (n = 3)
None	43–45	45	47	38–44	63–74
10^{-3} M levamisole	40–56	43	33	48–49	31–63
10^{-4} M levamisole	43–63	42	42	49–53	37–71
10^{-5} M levamisole	50–60	44	53	44–51	46–71
10^{-6} M levamisole	45–56	42	42	42–45	44–54 (n = 2)

Table 40.4 Serum IgE levels before and during levamisole treatment

Patients	Serum IgE (IU/ml)	
	before	>6 months levamisole
1. J.S.	5000–6000 (n = 2)	5900–11 000 (n = 2)
2. D.M.	2100 (n = 1)	1800 (n = 1)
3. R.L.	10 400 (n = 1)	22 000 (n = 1)
4. R.v.d.W.	1525 (n = 1)	4100 (n = 1)
Controls	<500 (n = 30)	n.t.

orally, on 3 successive days of each week. After 6 months treatment a significant increase in the chemotactic response was found in all patients. In one patient a complete normalization of neutrophil chemotaxis was already observed after 3 months treatment. However, no effect on serum IgE levels was found (Table 40.4). Our data suggest that the effect of treatment *in vivo* with levamisole on chemotaxis is relatively slow. This implies that the observation time is still too short to draw definite conclusions on the clinical effects of levamisole.

Nevertheless, in three patients the skin lesions improved, while all antibiotic therapy could be stopped.

The reason for the chemotactic defect in these patients is still unclear. Hill *et al.*[11] proposed that the high IgE levels were the cause of this dysfunction. These authors put forward the theory that the raised serum IgE levels and the presence of specific IgE antibodies in these patients leads to an increase in histamine release. Hill and coworkers[11] suggest that the PMN of these patients might contain high levels of cAMP, since histamine causes accumulation of cellular cyclic AMP[12]. As a result, the chemotactic responsiveness of these cells would be inhibited, since microtubule formation is probably regulated by the cAMP–cGMP system[13]. This hypothesis is supported by the observation that treatment *in vitro* of PMN from patients with hyperIgE and recurrent infections with the histamine receptor blocking agent burimamide significantly increased the chemotactic responsiveness[11].

Several points in this theory are either unproven or seem to be in contradiction with other findings, however. First, neither elevated serum histamine levels nor increased PMN cAMP levels have been measured in these patients.

Second, Hill et al.[11] found no chemotactic defect in other atopic patients with high serum IgE levels. And third, our results with levamisole treatment indicate that persisting high IgE levels do not prevent normalization of the chemotactic responsiveness of the patients' neutrophils. However, since levamisole has been shown to increase the cGMP levels in normal PMN[4], the underlying defect in the chemotactic dysfunction in these patients might still be an elevated cAMP:cGMP ratio, albeit not caused by the high serum IgE levels.

Acknowledgements

We thank Dr. P. Th. A. Schellekens and co-workers for performing the lymphocyte transformation tests, and Dr. R. C. Aalberse for measuring IgE levels and performing radio-allergo-sorbent tests.

References

1. Buckley, R. H., Wray, B. B. and Belmaker, E. Z. (1972). Extreme hyperimmuno-globulinemia E and undue susceptibility to infection. Pediatrics, 49, 59
2. Clark, R. A., Root, R. K., Kimball, H. R. et al. (1973). Defective neutrophil chemotaxis and cellular immunity in a child with recurrent infections. Ann. Intern. Med. 78, 515
3. Vanheule, R., de Cree, J. Adriaenssens, K., et al. (1976). Levamisole therapy for cellular immunologic deficiency with high IgE values. Acta Paediatr. Belg. 29, 41
4. Anderson, R., Glover, A., Koornhof, H. J. et al. (1976). In vitro stimulation of neutro-phil mobility by levamisole: maintenance of cGMP levels in chemotactically stimulated levamisole-treated neutrophils. J. Immunol. 117, 428
5. Weening, R. S., Roos, D. and Loos, J. A. (1974). Oxygen consumption of phagocytizing cells in human leukocyte and granulocyte preparations: A comparative study. J. Lab. Clin. Med., 83, 570
6. Zigmond, S. H. and Hirsch, J. G. (1973). Leukocyte locomotion and chemotaxis. New methods for evaluation and demonstration of cell-derived chemotactic factor. J. Exp. Med., 137, 387
7. Solberg, C. O. (1972). Protection of phagocytized bacteria against antibiotics. A new method for the evaluation of neutrophil granulocyte functions. Acta Med. Scand., 191, 383
8. Stallman, P. J. and Aalberse, R. C. Estimation of basophil bound IgE by quantitative immunofluorescence microscopy. Int. Arch. Allergy (in press)
9. Du Bois Ria, A. Meinesz, Bierhorst-Eijlander, A. et al. The use of microtiter plates in mixed lymphocyte cultures. Tissue Antigens, 4, 458
10. Hill, H. R. and Quie, P. G. (1974). Raised serum IgE levels and defective neutrophil chemotaxis in three children with eczema and recurrent bacterial infections. Lancet, 183
11. Hill, H. R., Estensen, R. D., Hogen, N. A. et al. (1976). Severe staphylococcal disease associated with allergic manifestations, hyperimmunoglobulinemia E, and defective neutrophil chemotaxis. J. Lab. Clin. Med., 88, 796
12. Bourne, H. R., Melmon, K. L. and Lichtenstein, L. M. (1971). Histamine augments leukocyte adenosine 3′, 5′-monophosphate and blocks antigenic histamine release. Science, 173, 743
13. Hill, H. R., Estensen, R. D., Quie, P. G. et al. (1975). Modulation of human neutrophil chemotactic responses by cyclic 3′, 5′-GMP and cyclic 3′, 5′-AMP. Metabolism, 24, 447

Discussion 40

J. Sondergaard: Were the patients that were presented selected cases? The atopic group
(Denmark) is a very vast group and it may be of major importance to know the
more basic mechanisms in this large category of patients.

Weening: This group of patients was a selected group of patients. In atopic
patients there is no defect in chemotaxis. This is a special group of
patients with very high susceptibility to infection, and there are some
atopic manifestations, but less than we observed in the atopics.

C. da Rocha-Afodu: Which recurrent infections were referred to in the presentation and
(Italy) which microbes were isolated in them?

Weening: Most patients suffered from *Staphylococcus aureus* bacteria, and there
was one instance of *Candida albicans*.

41

Rheumatoid-like joint lesions in rabbits injected intravenously with foreign serum

A. R. POOLE (Canada) AND R. R. A. COOMBS (UK)

In man, serum sickness can produce a clinically characterized polyarthritis involving large and medium-sized joints[1,2]. Experimental studies of serum sickness have concentrated mainly on lesions of the kidney, heart and blood vessels: no detailed descriptions of synovial lesions can be traced[3,4] except for a brief mention by Klinge[5] and by Hawn and Janeway[6]. We have recently observed that synovial lesions, closely resembling those seen in early rheumatoid arthritis, can be produced in rabbits which have received intravenous injections of a multiplicity of antigens in the form of bovine serum[7].

New Zealand White rabbits always received a primary intravenous (i.v.) injection of 5 ml of serum per kg body weight: sometimes, additional i.v. injections of 1.0–1.5 ml/kg were given over a period of up to 7 weeks when the knee (stifle) joints were examined.

In our earlier work we observed that approximately 20% of all injected rabbits exhibited rheumatoid-like synovial lesions, regardless of the secondary injection schedule employed. These changes were characterized by lining cell hyperplasia, sometimes with villous formation. Hyperplasia was invariably closely associated with the appearance of many lymphocytes and/or plasma cells under the lining cell layer. Lymphocytes appeared first in peri-vascular sites (around capillaries or venules) and often formed large focal collections. These changes were sometimes accompanied by fibroplasia which spread from under the lining layer into the capsular tissue, with much deposition of collagen. In about one third of animals showing gross lesions, pannus formation was noted. Cartilage proteoglycan was severely depleted in the area close to the invading pannus tissue (as indicated by a marked loss of Toluidine Blue staining). This pannus was always in continuity with the synovium and was always very vascular. Increased vascularity was frequently a feature of many inflamed synovia.

In some more recent studies we have observed that these synovial changes are associated with an elevated polymorphonuclear leukocyte (PMN) count in the joint fluid[8,9]: these leukocytes were rarely observed in the synovium, as is the case in established rheumatoid synovial lesions in man.

Immunohistochemical examinations of synovia[10] and cartilage[11] in rheumatoid joints in man have revealed the presence of immune complexes. Using fluorescein-labelled antibodies to rabbit IgG, Fab, and C3 we have observed staining in cytoplasmic vacuoles of synovial living cells and in the superficial cartilage of the patella in joints of animals where lesions have been observed histologically and where PMN counts are elevated. Uninjected rabbits display none of these histological changes or immunohistochemical staining patterns indicative of the presence of immune complexes. It is likely then that immune complexes are lodging in the joints of some rabbits in significant amounts and creating a local allergic response leading to synovial and joint fluid changes that are associated with cartilage destruction.

More recently we have observed that commercial colonies of New Zealand White rabbits produce a variable 'incidence' of gross joint lesions. Whereas in two colonies only 13% of all the rabbits injected in each case developed extensive lesions, 50% of those animals in a third colony displayed marked changes.

This study, which is continuing with other antigens, e.g. bacterial, provides a further animal model for investigating rheumatoid arthritis without any direct injection into the joint. It is hoped that it will be of use in future work concerned with the development and persistence of this disease.

References

1. Boots, R. H. and Swift, H. F. (1923). The arthritis of serum sickness. *J. Am. Med. Assoc.*, **80**, 12
2. Shulman, L. S. and Harvey, A. M. (1972). Polyarteritis and other arteritic syndromes. In *Arthritis and Allied Conditions. A textbook of rheumatology.* Eighth edition. (J. L. Hollander and D. J. McCarty, eds.), p. 918. (Philadelphia: Lea and Febiger)
3. Dixon, F. J. (1963). The role of antigen–antibody complexes in disease. *Harvey Lect.*, **58**, 21
4. Cochrane, G. G. and Koffler, D. (1973). Immune complex disease in experimental animals and man. *Adv. Immunol.*, **16**, 185
5. Klinge, F. (1929). Die eiweissüberempfindlichkeit (Gewebsanaphylaxie) der gelenke. Experimentelle pathologisch-anatomische studie zur pathogenese des gelenk-rheumatismus. *Beith Path. Anat.* **83**, 185
6. Hawn, C. V. Z. and Janeway, C. A. (1977). Histological and serological sequence in experimental hypersensitivity. *J. Exp. Med.*, **85**, 571
7. Poole, A. R. and Coombs, R. R. A. (1977). Rheumatoid-like joint lesions in rabbits with serum sickness. *Int. Arch. All.* (In press)
8. Poole, A. R., Oldham, G. and Coombs, R. R. A. (1977). (In preparation)
10. Bonomo, L., Tursi, A., Trizo, D., Gillardi, U. and Dammacco, F. (1970). Immune complexes in rheumatoid synovitis: a mixed staining immunofluorescence study. *Immunology*, **18**, 557
11. Cooke, T. D., Hurd, E. R., Jasin, H. E., Bienenstock, J. and Ziff, M. (1975). Identifications of immunoglobulin and complement in rheumatoid articular collagenous tissues. *Arth. Rheum.*, **18**, 541

Discussion 41

S. Wong: (USA)	The antigens used have not been specified.
Poole:	I did specify them. We used a multiplicity of antigens, in the form of bovine serum, simply because we wanted to try for all sorts of immune complexes, because whether or not immune complexes lodge in certain situations seems to depend on their size, the antigens and the antibodies involved in their formation. We gave ourselves initially the best possible chance of getting immune complexes which we hoped would produce a response within the joint.
Wong:	Was the bovine serum albumin modified in any way?
Poole:	It was just bovine serum. We did not modify it in any way, except to heat it at 56 °C for 30 min as a matter of course, and then to spin it afterwards to take out any aggregated material.
G. Vaes: (Belgium)	Has Dr. Poole any idea of the mechanism by which immune complexes are trapped inside the cartilage?
Poole:	Obviously this aggregated material cannot diffuse on its own. If it produces a size which can be seen with a light microscope, that cannot possibly get in. In this situation the IgG can diffuse in because it is fibrocartilage, and we know of situations where there is a predominance of type 1 collagen with the associated protein polysaccharides. We have a fairly permeable matrix, whereas in the articular hyaline cartilage only the superficial area is free. I would imagine that the immunoglobulin, and possibly the antigen, in the bovine serum, is diffusing in freely, in the form of soluble complex, or the antigen/antibody is diffusing in on its own, and there forming complexes within the cartilage. We are at a loss at the moment to know what these complexes contain, because we cannot demonstrate bovine antigens within them. It may be because there might be a minor component in their bovine serum, which is actually responsible for forming these complexes. We cannot allow the complexes to bind, or get them to bind bovine serum proteins which have been suitably labelled to detect binding. I would imagine that they form, as they seem to form in human rheumatoid disease, by the mechanisms that I have suggested, but this is pure conjecture.
Vaes:	Work done in our laboratory, has shown that collagen could bind immunoglobulins IgG under some conditions, exactly as IgG combines with C'1q, which has collagen-like segments. We are now investigating a possible way of binding immune complexes to collagen through the same mechanism.
Poole:	That is very interesting. We became aware of the collagen binding when we were trying to purify antibodies to collagenase, and so we had non-immune IgG bound to collagen. This may well be an important feature in the lodgment, the other limiting factor being the question of permeability.

That is very relevant.

A. Doble:
(UK)

This paper is extremely important. In the classical Dumonde–Glynn model a really chronic lesion necessitates the animals being immunized with antigen in Freund's complete adjuvant. If Dr. Poole has produced a chronic lesion without using Freund's complete adjuvant, I would be interested to know if he has looked for evidence of cell-mediated immunity to the horse serum, how often the injections of antigen were given, and how chronic the disease was after the last antigen injection?

Poole:

We are in the process at the moment of investigating the question of cell-mediated immunity to the antigen. Clearly there are a lot of antibodies being made and a lot of immune complexes. It is a difficult system to work with because there is a multiplicity of antigens. On the one hand there is the chance to get a result, but on the other hand, the interpretation of the result is complicated, but that we are doing at this moment.

As far as persistence of the lesion is concerned, there is evidence to believe that they will persist for many weeks, but we are still studying the persistence and factors responsible for its persistence.

I would imagine, from the data that we have at the moment, and from the experiments that we have been doing, that lesions will persist for many weeks afterwards—up to 5 or 6 weeks, and probably longer. We have not gone longer than that, as yet. The key point is the development of the auto-immune response within the joint, but this is my own personal feeling and that of my colleague, Professor Coombs. I have some ideas on this and this is what we are really looking at at the moment.

Primary synovitis in man can either clear, or it can heal, or it can progress to a rheumatoid condition, and I think that that again is related to the development of auto-immune reactions.

D. A. Willoughby:
(UK)

Has the possibility of transferring viruses been excluded?

Poole:

We have not absolutely excluded it because all that we have done is to remove bacteria. There is always the possibility that there could be viruses present in the serum. But even if there were viruses present, let us not forget that only a certain proportion of the rabbits in any one colony develop a response. This in itself is interesting. There is always the possibility that there is a virus there, as in all sorts of animal work, and this is something which has to be thought about and to have attention paid to it. We are paying attention to it right now. It is a question of excluding one thing at a time and sorting out the various problems.

We have looked at the kidneys and the heart. We have done most of the work on the kidneys, because most of the work on serum sickness has been done in kidneys. We have glib references to joint lesions which were never properly documented. We find that there is no correlation between the production of lesions in the joints, and the kidneys, and in all of our animals that have been injected with one or other, of a multiplicity of injections, we see kidney changes, mainly in the form of extra-glomerular lesions. The glomerular lesions are not too well defined, but we always see those lesions to varying degrees. Sometimes they are very marked. Occasionally, rabbits appear to be dying from kidney failure. However, in some animals we have seen a very gross kidney lesion indeed, but no joint lesion whatsoever.

I might add that in some of these animals, some groups, the lesions are produced bilaterally; in others unilaterally.

We have also only concentrated on these joints, because of the question of analysing so many rabbits. But, there are no parallels between kidney and joint lesion production.

A. Cats: **(The Netherlands)**	Did Dr. Poole look for anti-ITT antibodies in the animals that were treated?
Poole:	Yes, we did, but when one works with bovine gamma globulin in bovine serum this complicates any study of that kind.

Using a total rabbit-antibody rabbit-antigen system, we have found evidence of productions of low levels of rheumatoid-like factor, but only a very low titre, which we do not consider to be very significant. We have evidence for immuno-conglutinant formation and also plenty of homo reactant being produced—the antibody to the papain-prepared fab in the rabbit. It is difficult to evaluate, because of cross-reaction of antibodies to the bovine immunoglobulin with the animal's own.

We have tended to look at these things, but with a rather sceptical eye, because of the problems of attaching any real significance to it, which is why we are moving away from these systems wherever we can, to work with antigens which do not include immunoglobulins.

G. A. Voisin: **(France)**	In 1945 there was work done on experimental serum sickness with the involvement of the kidneys, the heart, the arteries, and so forth. Yet since then, only the kidney is extensively studied. This model is a very rich model that should be exploited. It is nice to see somebody interested in exploiting it in that direction.

42

Anti-inflammatory activity of some bacterial immunostimulants. Relation with macrophage migration

P. LALLOUETTE AND A. SCHWARTZ (France)

In 1968 we described the non-specific immunostimulating activity and the anti-inflammatory activity of a somatic antigen which we extracted from the *Bacillus subtilis* PT strain[1]. This antigen was obtained using the method outlined in Table 42.1. The main activity of this fraction is the increase of the non-specific resistance against bacterial infections in mice. This protection is more effective against Gram negative than against Gram positive bacteria. In the following Tables are shown the results obtained in assays of 360 mice infected by *E. coli* and receiving, 24 h before the infection by i.p. route, an injection of the antigen. These assays show a 'dose–effect' relationship and allow the determination of the 50% protective dose in treated animals (Table 42.2). This protective effect is due to the increase of phagocytosis by the reticulo-endothelial system which can be studied through the bacteriaemiae, according to the method which we previously described[2]. Tables 42.3 and 42.4 report the results obtained in controls and treated animals.

The antigen also increases the resistance of mice weakly immunized by a killed 'foot and mouth' vaccine and challenged with a virulent virus. The percentage of protection of the animals treated by the antigen is 50% higher than that of controls receiving the killed vaccine alone.

The antigen reverses the aggravating effect of cyclophosphamide on an experimental infection in mice, without modifying either the leukopenic effect of this substance or its blocking effect on the synthesis of SRBC antibodies[3].

On the other hand, this antigen does not increase the delayed hypersensitivity and does not act against grafted cancers in mice and rats such as P-815, T-2633, T-8, T-58.

Table 42.1

SUBMERGED CULTURE
↓
CENTRIFUGED
↓
ACETONE:20 VOLUMES
(4 °C–24 h)
↓
DIETHYL ETHER:10 VOLUMES
(4 °C–24 h)
↓
↓
DRIED BACTERIAL POWDER
(10 mg/ml WATER)
↓
LYSOZYME 80 μg/ml
(37 °C–1 h)
↓
TRYPSIN 80 μg/ml
(37 °C–1 h)
↓
HEATED 15 min 115 °C
↓
DIALYSED AGAINST WATER 24 h
↓
LYOPHILIZATION— CRUDE ANTIGEN
↓
SOLUBILIZED IN LIQUID PHENOL
↓
PRECIPITATED BY DIETHYL ETHER

Table 42.2

Controls : 100% Lethality

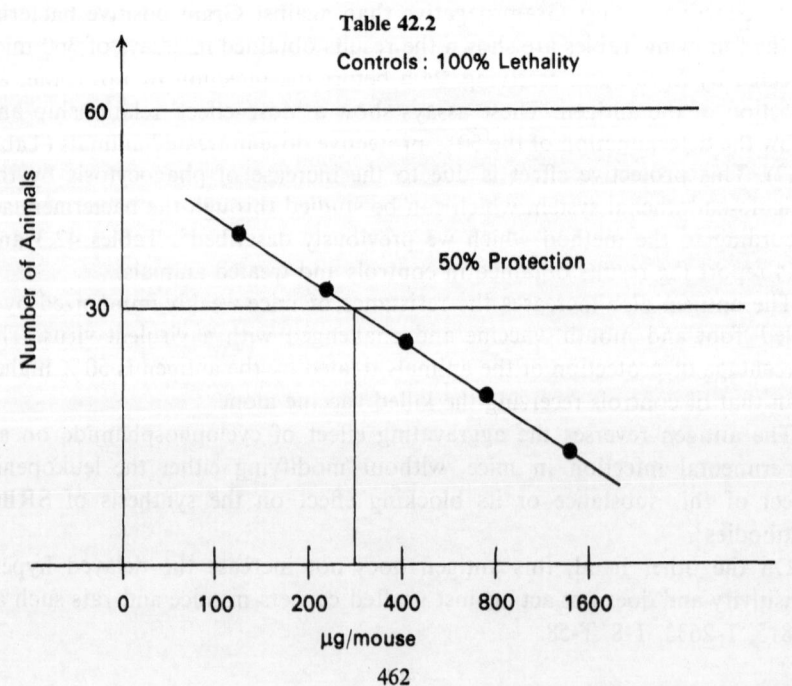

50% Protection

Table 42.3 Bacteriaemiae in mice

Time after inoculation	Control	Treated
0	0	0
15 min	135	148
1 h	206	102
2 h	550	9
4 h	70	2.5
8 h	105	0.2
16 h	1600	0

Groups of 28 animals
Treatment: 1 mg per animal parenteral route
Measure: counting of colonies on agar medium:
24 h 37 °C average on 4 assays

Table 42.4 Bacteriaemiae in mice—3rd hour

Mice	Control	Treated
1	445	1
2	565	4
3	500	34
4	907	1
5	254	1
6	167	0
7	114	0
8	111	0
9	437	3
10	32	1

The anti-inflammatory activity of the antigen was studied (in collaboration with R. Richou) in rats, guinea pigs, and mice in acute and subacute models using phenylbutazone as the control substance. We used as inflammatory agents: kaolin; carrageenan; saponin; abrin and α-staphylotoxin which we still use in screening, following the method which we reported in 1964[4].

The activities of these two non-steroidal products differed according to the models used. For instance, in rats, both products were very efficient against kaolin, carrageenan and α-staphylotoxin (Table 42.5). In guinea pigs, the phenylbutazone reduced the oedema reaction induced by abrin and the antigen was inefficient. Conversely, the antigen reduced the oedema produced by saponin more than the phenylbutazone (Table 42.6). In mice, the activity of the two products was comparable (Table 42.7).

Furthermore, using the same process of preparation, we compared the activity of fractions obtained from other strains of *Bacillus subtilis* from our own collection and from the 'Laboratoire Central de Recherches Vétérinaires' collection (L.P.; 7640; Byline; Jouanno; Avoco). Each of these preparations showed both immunostimulant activity and anti-inflammatory effect in the tests reported above, but we did not observe a constant parallelism between these activities.

Table 42.5 Anti-inflammatory activity in rats

Inflammatory substance	Phenylbutazone	Antigen of B. subtilis
Kaolin	38%	47%
Carrageenan	33%	33%
α-Staphylotoxin	37%	42%

Groups of 10 rats Wistar 150 g ± 10 g
Inflammation in foot pad measured at 24 h
Treatment: i.p. route: phenylbutazone, 300 mg/kg; antigen, 60 mg/kg

Table 42.6 Anti-inflammatory activity in guinea pigs

Inflammatory substance	Phenylbutazone	Antigen of B. subtilis
Carregeenan	26%	30%
Saponin	20%	45%
Abrin	50%	0%
Perfringens A toxin	0%	20%
α-Staphylotoxin	30%	16%

Groups of 10 guinea pigs 350–400 g
Inflammation in foot pad measured at 24 h
Treatment i.p. route: phenylbutazone, 300 mg/kg; antigen, 60 mg/kg

Table 42.7 Anti-inflammatory activity in mice

Inflammatory	Phenylbutazone	Antigen of B. subtilis
Kaolin	9%	53%
Carrageenan	21%	53%
α-Staphylotoxin	15%	22%

Groups of 20 animals 20 g ± 1 g
Inflammation in foot pad measured at 24 h
Treatment: i.p. route: phenylbutazone, 150 mg/kg; antigen, 30 mg/kg

Table 42.8 Migration of peritoneal macrophages on agar plates

Assays No.	Control animals		Treated animals (*)	
	Agar	Agar + antigen*	Agar	Agar + antigen*
1	64	60	38	32
2	30	32	21	26
3	24	25	14	12
4	25	25	15	17
	35	35	22	22

* Intramuscular route 1 mg of antigen 48 h before collecting the peritoneal macrophages

As this fraction was the most efficient, we used the somatic antigen of *Bacillus subtilis* PT when studying the macrophage migration on gel from treated and control animals. For mouse peritoneal macrophages, we adapted the migration inhibition test on agar plates described by Salvin and Nishio and modified by de Kozack and collaborators for the study of retinal antigens[5]. In Table 42.8 are reported the results obtained in four different assays. The mice were treated 48 h before the macrophage collection with 1 mg of antigen i.m. The migration inhibition test was done on agar plates both with and without antigen.

The result for each assay was determined by five readings for each group.

The comparison of the results of each group in each assay were statistically significant. The presence of the antigen in the agar medium does not play any part either with control or treated animal macrophages. The macrophage migration of the treated animals was 37% less than the migration of the macrophages of the control animals. The rate of inhibition of macrophage migration depends on the dose of antigen used. In these experimental conditions no activity was observed for a dose under 100 μg.

On the other hand, in collaboration with B. Bizzini and M. Raynaud we described in 1974[6] the immunostimulant activity of fractions extracted from *Corynebacterium granulosum*, using the process described in Table 42.9.

These fractions showed both immunostimulant and anti-inflammatory activities. The main difference between these fractions and the *B. subtilis* antigen is the induction of delayed hypersensitivity. The fractions from *Corynebacterium granulosum*, as well as the fractions from BCG, induce

Table 42.9

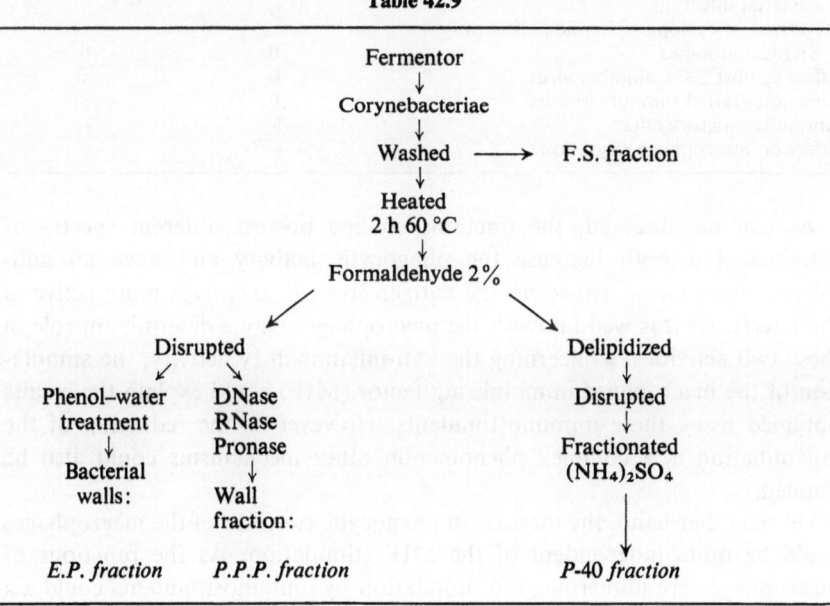

delayed hypersensitivity type reaction and also show activity in grafted tumours. On the other hand, the fractions from *B. subtilis* do not increase the delayed hypersensitivity type reaction in the same experimental conditions and do not act on the grafted tumours in mice and rats. Among the fractions from *Corynebacterium granulosum*, the more interesting one was the P-40 fraction which showed curative activity on the P-815 tumour grafted in mice. We have now used this tumour for 14 years on syngenic and non-syngenic lines of mice and have actually more than 500 linear transplantations in each group. We use this tumour which was kindly supplied, at that time, by D. M. Potter himself, with J. L. Parrot in our study of the specific histidine decarboxylase activity of this mastocytoma.

In Table 42.10 we compared the results obtained with the antigen from *B. subtilis* PT and the fractions extracted from *Corynebacterium granulosum*, in the same experimental conditions.

Table 42.10

Tests	Somatic antigen of B. subtilis PT	Fraction of Corynebacterium granulosum
Increase of resistance against bacterial infections	+ +	+
Increase of granulopexic activity	+ +	+ +
Increase of phagocytosis	+ +	+
Stimulating effect on SRBC antibodies	0	+ +
Stimulating effect on toxoids antibodies	0	+ +
Induction of delayed hypersensitivity	0	+ +
Reversion of cyclophosphamide effect on bacterial infection	+ +	+
Reversion of cyclophosphamide effect on SRBC antibodies	0	+
Effect against SK Columbia virus	0	0
Effect on grafted tumours in mice	0	+ +
Anti-inflammatory effect	+ +	+
Effect on macrophage migration	+ +	+

As can be observed, the fractions studied possess different spectra of activities, but both increase the phagocytic activity and have an anti-inflammatory effect. However, the antigen from *B. subtilis* is more active in these tests. As it is well known[7], the macrophages play a determinant role in these two activities. Concerning the anti-inflammatory activity, the stimulation of the macrophage immobilizing factor (MIF) could explain the results obtained using these immunostimulants. However as the reduction of the inflammation is a complex phenomenon other mechanisms could also be implied.

On the other hand, the increase in phagocytic function of the macrophages could be quite independent of the MIF stimulation. As the functions of macrophages are numerous, the stimulation by immunostimulants could act more or less on the diverse functions of these cells and, thus, explain certain dissociated results observed during our studies.

References

1. Lallouette, P. (1969). Etude sur un antigène somatique isolé d'une souche de B. Subtilis. *Rev. d'Immunol.*, **32**, 105
2. Lallouette, P. (1969). Etude de l'activité phagocytaire du système réticulo-endothélial par mesure de la bactériémie chez la souris infectée avec *E. coli* 111 B4—Activité de l'antigène isolé d'une souche de B. subtilis. *Soc. Biol.*, **163**, 2296
3. Lallouette, P., Schwartz, A. and Dhennin, L. (1976). Réversion du pouvoir dépresseur de la cyclophosphamide envers la défense anti-infectieuse de la souris au moyen d'un antigène somatique de Bacillus subtilis. *Soc. Biol.*, **170**, 765
4. Lallouette, P., Richou, R., Schwartz, A. and Richou, H. (1968). Recherches sur le pouvoir anti-inflammatoire d'une fraction somatique de Bacillus subtilis. *Rev. d'Immunol.*, **32**, 151
5. Lallouette, P., Schwartz, A. and Dhennin, L. (1976). Etude de l'action d'un antigène somatique de Bacillus subtilis sur la migration des macrophages de souris. *Soc. Biol.*, **170**, 769
6. Lallouette, P., Bizzini, B. and Raynaud, M. (1974). Pouvoir immunostimulant de fractions isolées de Corynebactérium granulosum. *Nouv. Gen. Med. (Paris)*, **6**, 13
7. Pillot, J. (1976). Les processus cellulaires de défense contre les agents infectieux. *Rev. Med.*, **32**, 1657

Discussion 42

Arrigoni-Martelli: (Denmark) What route of administration is used to estimate the anti-inflammatory activity of this bacterial adjuvant? Was administration oral, subcutaneous, or what?

Lallouette: The substances were administered intraperitoneally and the inflammatory substance was injected in the paw.

Arrigoni-Martelli: In that case could any non-specific counter-irritant effect, which could well explain the anti-inflammatory activity of cells, be excluded?

Lallouette: Yes. That is a possibility.

43

Inflammatory exudates and mitogenic activity

O. M. ADOLPHE, J. FONTAGNE, M. PELLETIER,
D. BLONDELON, P. LECHAT AND J. P. GIROUD (France)

It has been shown that rat peritoneal macrophages in culture were modified following treatment with inflammatory cell-free exudates induced by intra-pleural injection of dextran[1-2]. The main results are summarized in Table 43.1. They were obtained with non-inbred (Sprague–Dawley), and inbred strain of rats (Lewis, WAG). A similar effect, although less intense, was found following treatment of mouse peritoneal macrophages with rat exudates. Similar results were obtained by Wynne et al.[3] using exudates obtained from chronic inflammatory lesions. The induction of DNA synthesis and division of macrophages in culture were related to the release of a mitogenic factor in these particular inflammatory exudates.

Certain questions remained unanswered.

(1) Could the induction of DNA synthesis of macrophages be stimulated with other types of

(a) acute non-immunological

(b) immunological inflammatory exudates?

Table 43.1 Modifications of macrophages in culture after treatment with dextran exudate

Morphological modifications	
	—Increase of spreading of cells
	—Increase of size of nuclei
Metabolic modifications	
	—Increase of total number of cells
	—Increase of cells incorporating tritiated thymidine
	—Increase of mitotic index

For this purpose, the effects of cell-free pleural exudates of non-immunological reactions (induced by λ carrageenan, κ carrageenan, calcium pyrophosphate) and of immunological reactions (reverse passive Arthus reaction and delayed hypersensitivity pleurisy) were compared to the dextran reaction.

(2) Was the mitogenic activity found in inflammatory exudates specific to macrophages, or could it also produce the division of another type of cell such as the fibroblast? For this purpose, the stimulation of DNA synthesis of quiescent fibroblasts with calf serum was compared with that induced by dextran exudate.

MATERIALS AND METHODS

Production of pleural exudates

Pathogen-free Sprague–Dawley rats were used for all experiments.

Non-immunological exudates

1 ml of 6% dextran (40 000 Daltons), 0.15 ml of 1% λ carrageenan, 0.15 ml of 1% κ carrageenan (Satia), 1 ml of 1% calcium pyrophosphate suspension[4] were injected intrapleurally under sterile conditions. The exudates were harvested 4 h later at 4 °C and treated as previously described[2].

Immunological exudates

The reverse passive Arthus reaction was performed using the technique described by Yamamoto[5]: an intravenous injection of bovine serum albumin (BSA) followed 20 min later by anti-BSA intrapleural injection. The pleural exudate was harvested after 4 h (as above).

In delayed hypersensitivity pleurisy, the animals were sensitized to a suspension of *Bacillus pertussis* in incomplete Freund's adjuvant. 3 weeks later, they were challenged intrapleurally with 0.1 ml *B. pertussis*. The pleural exudate was harvested at the peak of the reaction which occurred 18 h after intrapleural injection (as above)[6].

Macrophage cultures

All the experiments were performed on cultures of non-activated rat peritoneal macrophages as previously described[2]. After 3 days of culture, the medium was replaced by 199 medium containing pleural exudate (50% concentration) and supplemented with 20% heat-inactived calf serum.

Fibroblast cultures

All the experiments were performed using BHK 21/13 cell line cultured in BHK medium[7]. To obtain quiescent cultures, 2×10^5 cells were seeded in

Leighton tubes in medium containing 10% calf serum. Two days later, the medium was removed and replaced by fresh medium containing 0.5% calf serum for one day. On the third day, this medium was replaced by:

(1) fresh medium containing 0.5% calf serum as a non-stimulation control,

(2) fresh medium containing 10% calf serum as a stimulation control,

(3) fresh medium containing 0.5% calf serum and 50% dextran cell-free exudate.

14, 16 and 20 h after addition of each particular medium, the labelling of cells was performed.

DNA synthesis

DNA synthesis was studied by incubating with 3 μCi/ml tritiated thymidine (3 h for macrophages, 1 h for fibroblasts). After autoradiography by the dipping technique, the labelling index (‰) was calculated by counting 2×10^3 cells in duplicate samples.

RESULTS

Macrophage experiments

(A)—Study of acute non-immunological inflammatory exudates
The numbers of cells in DNA synthesis were estimated on the 3rd and 4th day after treatment of rat macrophages with λ carrageenan, κ carrageenan, Ca pyrophosphate cell-free exudates and compared with dextran cell-free exudates (Figure 43.1 and 43.2).

The results showed an increase of the labelling index following treatment with each type of acute non-immunological exudate. By the third day, exudates induced by λ and κ carrageenan and Ca pyrophosphate were more effective than dextran exudate. By the fourth day, the stimulation was similar to that of all types of exudate. This may suggest that exudates induce semi-synchronous DNA synthesis.

(B)—Study of acute immunological inflammatory exudates
The exudates obtained with reverse passive Arthus (RPA) and delayed hyper-sensitivity reaction (DH) provoked also an induction of DNA synthesis of rat macrophages in culture on the 3rd and 4th day after treatment. For example, on the 3rd day, the labelling index of RPA treated cells was 130‰ and 97‰ for DH treated cells. By the 4th day, the mitogenic effect of both these exudates had fallen to 70‰.

Fibroblasts experiments

To determine whether the mitogenic activity found in inflammatory exudates was or was not specific to macrophages, fibroblast cell line BHK 21/13 was

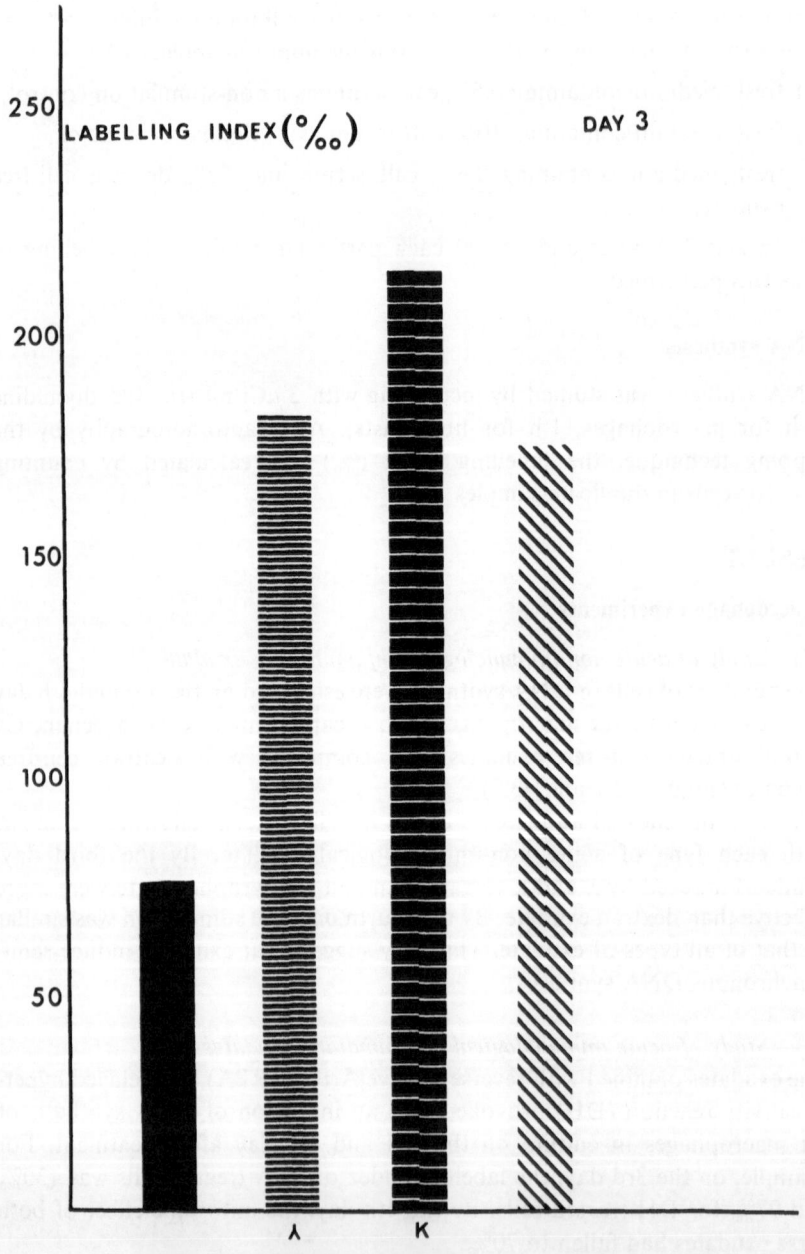

Figure 43.1 Labelling index (after tritiated thymidine incorporation for 3 h) in rat non-activated peritoneal macrophage culture, 3 days after treatment with different types of acute non-immunological inflammatory cell-free exudate harvested in rats 4 h after the intrapleural injection

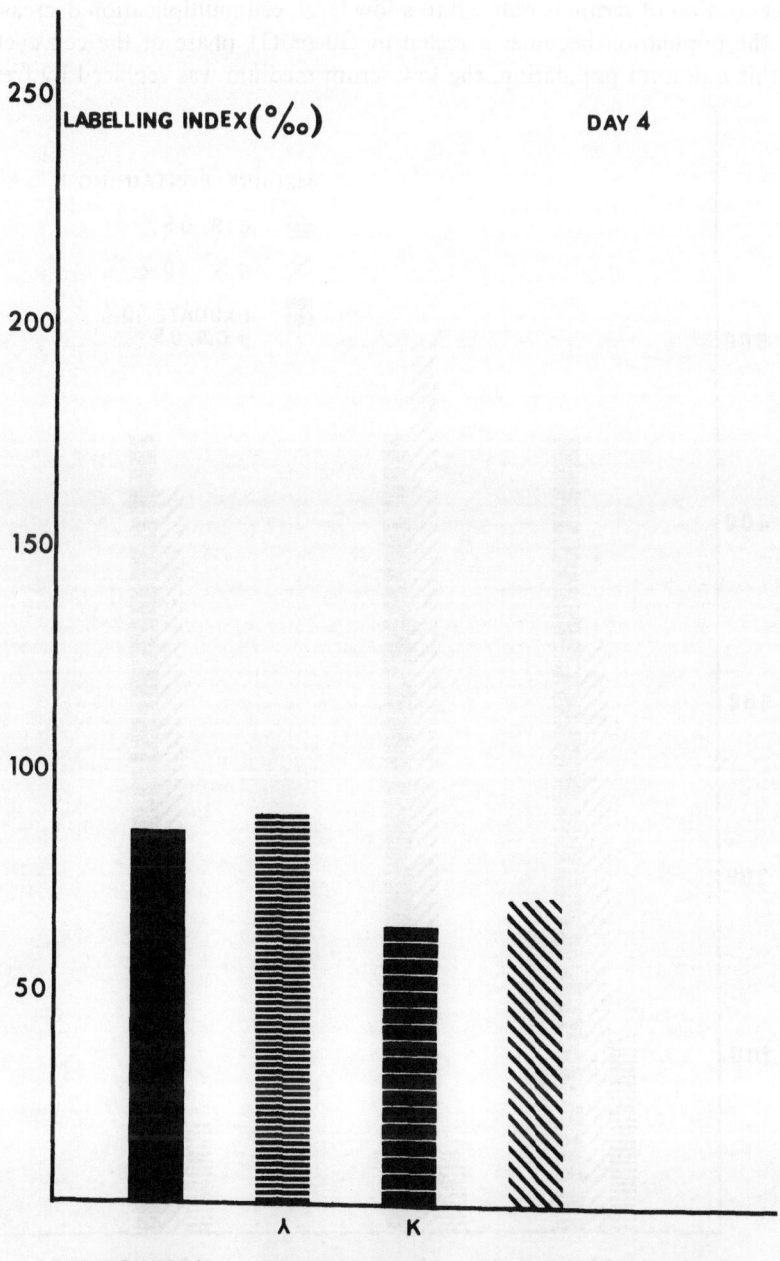

Figure 43.2 Labelling index (after tritiated thymidine incorporation for 3 h) in rat non-activated peritoneal macrophage cultur , 4 days after treatment with different types of acute non-immunological inflammatory cell-free exudate harvested in rats 4 h after the intrapleural injection.

maintained in a low serum medium to obtain quiescent cells. Indeed when the concentration of serum is reduced to a low level, cell multiplication decreases and the population becomes arrested in G0 or G1 phase of the cell cycle. On this quiescent population, the low serum medium was replaced by fresh

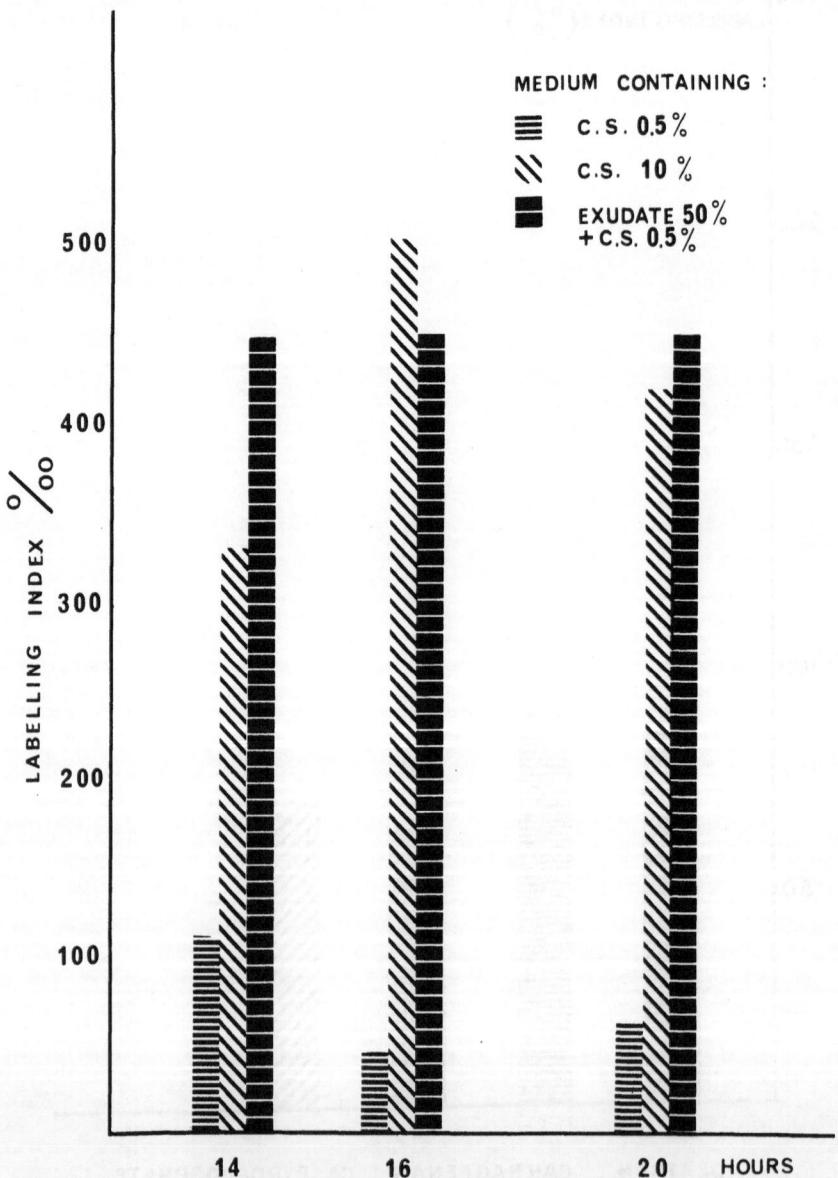

Figure 43.3 Labelling index (after tritiated thymidine incorporation for 1 h) in quiescent culture of fibroblasts (BHK 21/13), 14, 16, 20 h after the replacement of low serum medium by fresh medium containing 10% calf serum as stimulation control ⧄, fresh medium containing 0.5% calf serum as non-stimulation control ≡, and fresh medium containing 0.5% calf serum and 50% dextran culture exudate, ▬

medium containing 0.5% calf serum as non-stimulation control, 10% calf serum as stimulation control and 0.5% calf serum plus 50% dextran exudate; DNA synthesis was studied at intervals after these changes.

The results (Figure 43.3) showed that the replacement of old medium with

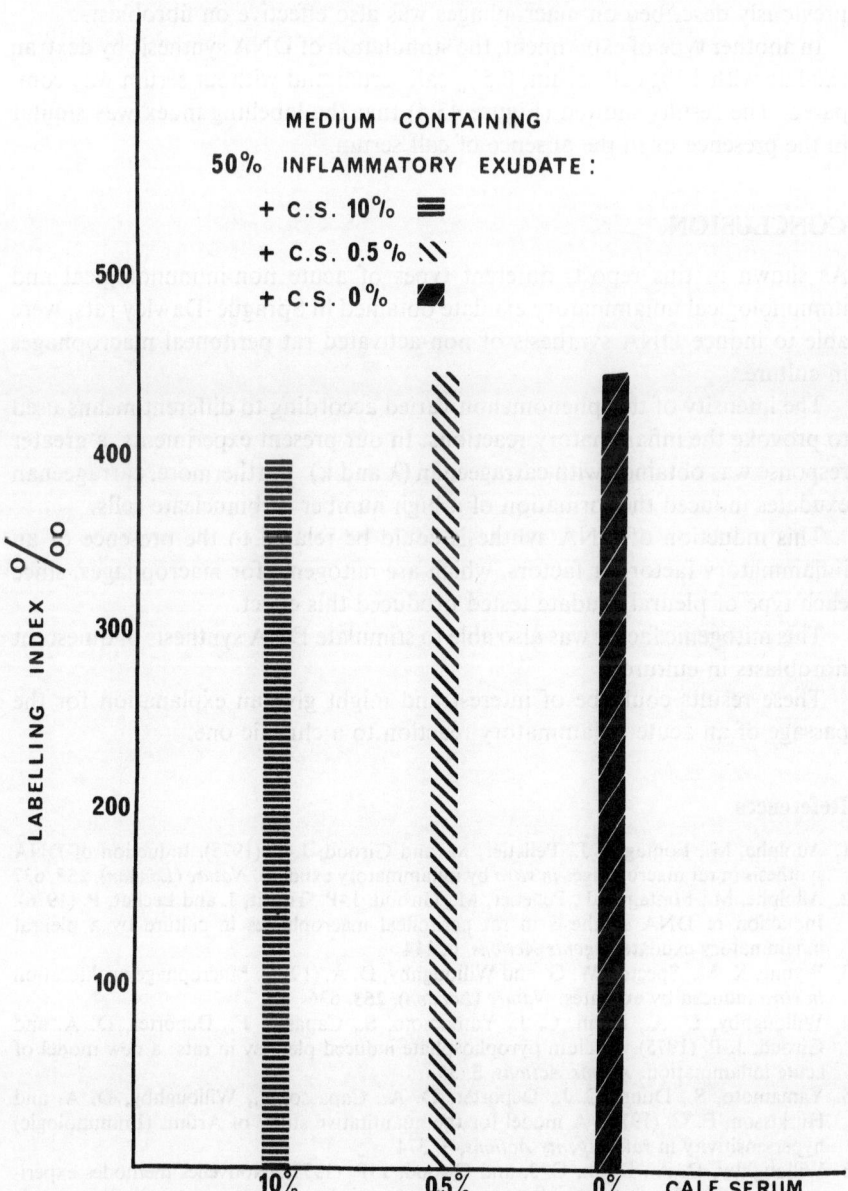

Figure 43.4 Labelling index (after tritiated thymidine incorporation for 1 h) in quiescent culture of fibroblasts (BHK 21/13) 16 h after the replacement of low serum medium by fresh medium containing 50% dextran cell-free exudate supplemented with 10% calf serum ≡ ,0.5% calf serum \\\ , and without serum ▟

fresh medium containing 0.5% calf serum was inefficient on DNA synthesis whereas an increase of the labelling index occurred at its maximum 16 h after stimulation with 10% calf serum; the same degree of stimulation was obtained with 50% pleural exudate. So the mitogenic activity of dextran exudate previously described on macrophages was also effective on fibroblasts.

In another type of experiment, the stimulation of DNA synthesis by dextran exudate with 10% calf serum, 0.5% calf serum and without serum was compared. The results showed (Figure 43.4) that the labelling index was similar in the presence or in the absence of calf serum.

CONCLUSION

As shown in this report, different types of acute non-immunological and immunological inflammatory exudate obtained in Sprague–Dawley rats, were able to induce DNA synthesis of non-activated rat peritoneal macrophages in culture.

The intensity of this phenomenon varied according to different means used to provoke the inflammatory reactions. In our present experiments, a greater response was obtained with carrageenan (λ and κ). Furthermore, carrageenan exudates induced the formation of a high number of binucleate cells.

This induction of DNA synthesis could be related to the presence of an inflammatory factor, or factors, which are mitogenic for macrophages, since each type of pleural exudate tested produced this effect.

This mitogenic factor was also able to stimulate DNA synthesis of quiescent fibroblasts in culture.

These results could be of interest and might give an explanation for the passage of an acute inflammatory reaction to a chronic one.

References

1. Adolphe, M., Fontagné, J., Pelletier, M. and Giroud, J.-P. (1975). Induction of DNA synthesis in rat macrophages *in vitro* by inflammatory exudate. *Nature (London)*, **253**, 637
2. Adolphe, M., Fontagné, J., Pelletier, M., Giroud, J.-P., Timsit, J. and Lechat, P. (1976). Induction of DNA synthesis in rat peritoneal macrophages in culture by a pleural inflammatory exudate. *Agents Actions*, **6**, 114
3. Wynne, K. M., Spector, W. G. and Willoughby, D. A. (1975). Macrophage proliferation *in vitro* induced by exudates. *Nature (London)*, **253**, 636
4. Willoughby, D. A., Dunn, C. J., Yamamoto, S., Capasso, F., Deporter, D. A. and Giroud, J.-P. (1975). Calcium pyrophosphate induced pleurisy in rats: a new model of acute inflammation. *Agents Actions*, **5**, 35
5. Yamamoto, S., Dunn, C. J., Deporter, D. A., Capasso, F., Willoughby, D. A. and Huskisson, E. C. (1975). A model for the quantitative study of Arthus (Immunologic) hypersensitivity in rats. *Agents Actions*, **5**, 374
6. Willoughby, D. A., Dunn, C. J. and Giroud, J.-P. (1977). Nouvelles méthodes expérimentales d'études des anti-inflammatoires et anti-rhumatismaux, *Actual Pharmacol.*, **29e**, 25
7. MacPherson, I. A. and Stoker, M. G. P. (1962). Polyoma transformation of hamster cell clones—An investigation of genetic factors affecting cell competence. *Virology*, **16**, 147

8. Giroud, J.-P., Fontagne, J., Blowdelon, D., Adolphe, M., Dunn, C. J., Willoughby, D. A. and Lechat, P. (1977). Stimulation of macrophage DNA synthesis in culture by different types of acute non-immunological inflammatory exudates. *Bioméd Express (Paris)*, **27**, 19

Discussion 43

G. P. Velo: (Italy)	Was an extraction of these substances tried? If so, can we hear more about the chemistry of them.
Adolphe:	We tried, but we had a lot of difficulty. It is a protein, but it is resistant to freezing, and to heating as well. I cannot give further information.
R. van Furth: (The Netherlands)	What has been shown is the incorporation of Tritiated Thymidine. Was there really DNA synthesis and has the DNA content of the cells been measured? To demonstrate the mitotic factor a doubling, at least, of DNA is necessary. Secondly, has cell proliferation been seen? If there really is mitosis one would need to end up with more cells.
Adolphe:	In answer to the second question, with these other types of exudate we do not measure the mitotic index. With dextran exudate we showed —at the 1975 meeting—an increase in the mitotic index, which is very important. We also studied the action of this factor on the haemato-poietic cells in culture in methyl cellulose, and we have obtained a growth of the different clones of cells, so that it is really a mitogenic effect.
van Furth:	I am saying that in contrast to others you found that your factor induces proliferation in bone marrow cells, where the colony stimu-lating factor usually used for the bone marrow cultures does not affect . . .
Adolphe:	Yes, it is interesting, because it is not really the same perhaps.
van Furth:	But you indicate more or less, as the answer, that you get proliferation.
G. Macpherson: (UK)	I should like to know more about the way in which the macrophages were prepared and about the purity of the population of macrophages used. If a normal rat peritoneal cell population was used, there are a fair number of other cell types in that, and how is the possibility of other cell types in the macrophage population controlled?
Adolphe:	It is peritoneal macrophage with the classic technique of selection—spreading in glass vessels. We confirm its role as a macrophage by phagocytosis.
G. Vaes: (Belgium)	My question is related to the question asked by Professor van Furth but it concerns fibroblasts. With just 50% exudate is it possible to completely suppress serum out of the culture of fibroblasts and get them growing and get them to confluent monolayers as one would normally get after seeding?
Adolphe:	With serum we obtained a classic stimulation, but we also obtained a classic picture without serum. I do not know about proliferation because we did not try it another time.
Vaes:	It was labelled Thymidine incorporation, not cell number-count?
Adolphe:	No. Only Thymidine incorporation.
Vaes:	Are any inhibitors of proteases present in the exudate? Is a-2-macro-globulin present, for instance?
Adolphe:	I do not know. I suppose that there are.

T. L. Vischer: (Switzerland)	If one adds serum to a fibroblast culture which is quiescent, they will go on multiplying, incorporating Thymidine and everything. Dr. Adolphe added 50% serum, and gets labelling indexes of 40% which would correspond to a new logarithmic growth phase, if it is growth, not incorporation, which could as well be obtained with 50% serum to any quiescent culture—even one with contact inhibition.
Adolphe:	This experiment was done to find out whether the presence of co-factor serum is useful to the proliferation of fibroblasts. In macrophage culture the presence of serum is useful for the stimulation of DNA synthesis.
Honor Fell: (UK)	Perhaps relevant to this discussion is some work by Fritz Jacoby in England—published a good many years ago now. Like others he found that mammalian macrophages in culture, could be maintained alive for long periods, but would not divide. Then he succeeded in inducing mitosis, by feeding them on conditioned medium from a fibroblast culture instead, and they grew then quite well.
M. Soria: (Italy)	Have protease inhibitors been added to the system? Proteases are known in some cells, and I was wondering about the BHK 21 cells—to increase DNA synthesis.
Adolphe:	We have not tried it.

44

Secretory activity of epithelioid cells

N. MOKHTAR AND W. G. SPECTOR (UK)

INTRODUCTION

Epithelioid cells are a main feature of granulomatous inflammation. Their ultrastructural features are characteristic[1] and it has been possible to obtain from mice peritoneal macrophages a homogenous culture of cells having similar ultrastructural characteristics[2]. The epithelioid cell ultrastructure suggests that these cells may be more active in secretion than phagocytosis. The present investigation was devised to compare the enzyme secretory activities of cells with the ultrastructural features of epithelioid cells with other types of macrophages.

MATERIALS AND METHODS

Adult male mice of average weight 25 g were injected intraperitoneally with 0.5 ml newborn calf serum (Flow Labs) 2 days prior to experiment, others were injected with 0.75 ml of thioglycollate medium[3] 4 days prior to experiments. A third group received no treatment prior to harvesting the macrophages.

Macrophages were harvested by peritoneal washing with medium 199 containing 10 IU of heparin/ml. Cells were centrifuged, resuspended in medium 199 plus 20% newborn calf serum decomplemented by heating at 56 °C for 30 min plus 100 U/ml penicillin plus 100 μg/ml streptomycin. Cells were then cultured in a volume of about 5 ml in tissue culture flasks at 37 °C in the presence of 5% CO_2 at a density of 1×10^6 cell/ml.

For cell lysates, cells were collected by scraping with the aid of a plastic policeman and incubated in 0.2% w/v Triton X-100 on ice for 1 h with frequent shaking.

Cell pellets for electron microscopy were obtained by scraping as above, fixing in cold 25% glutaraldehyde in 0.2 m sodium cocodylate for 1 h then washing in cocodylate sucrose buffer for 1 h. Second fixation was done with 2% OsO_4. Finally the cell pellet was embedded in Araldite mixture and left to polymerize overnight at 80 °C. Enzyme assays were performed photometrically. Lysozyme was measured against a *Micrococcus lysodeikticus* suspension[4]. L-aspartate and α-oxoglutarate were used as substrates in measuring GOT[5]. *p*-nitrophenyl phosphate was used as a substrate for measuring acid phosphatase at a pH of 4.8 and a wavelength of 505 nm[6,7]. Haemoglobin substrate was used for measuring acid cathepsins at a pH of 3.0[8]. Neutral cathepsins were assayed by using azocasein and azocoll as substrates at a pH of 7.5[9].

RESULTS

Cell morphology

Newborn calf serum (CS)-stimulated macrophages
These cells are large and polygonal with slender short ectoplasmic pseudopodia. The cells are close together but only a few processes unite. The nucleus is oval with a thin band of peripheral heterochromatin. The cytoplasm is abundant and contains many mitochondria and lysosomes of different sizes. The rough endoplasmic reticulum is prominent. The Golgi apparatus is large and situated near the nucleus.

CS stimulated cells after 2 days of in vitro *culture*
More cells are joined by their longer slender pseudopodia. The nucleus is more elongated. Cytoplasmic contents are more numerous.

CS stimulated cells after 6 days of culture (Figure 44.1)
Cells have now joined up on a large scale to produce the typical epithelioid syncytium. The nucleus is long and narrow with a very thin peripheral rim of hetero-chromatin, the remaining chromatin being finely dispersed. Nucleoli are prominent. The cytoplasm contains abundant strands of endoplasmic reticulum running at random. Mitochondria are numerous and large and their matrix is denser than the cytoplasmic ground substance. Some small endocytic vacuoles are present, sometimes containing small bits of solid material. Most of the Golgi apparatus is present between the nucleus and the cell surface. Lysosomes are numerous (Figure 44.2).

Thioglycollate stimulated cells
These are large, rounded or slightly elongated cells most of which are separate. The nucleus is big and rounded and occupies most of the cell cytoplasm. Dense lumpy heterochromatin lines the nuclear membrane. The cytoplasm is filled with big phagocytic vacuoles, some containing undigested debris. Many lipid vacuoles are also present. Mitochondria are numerous but

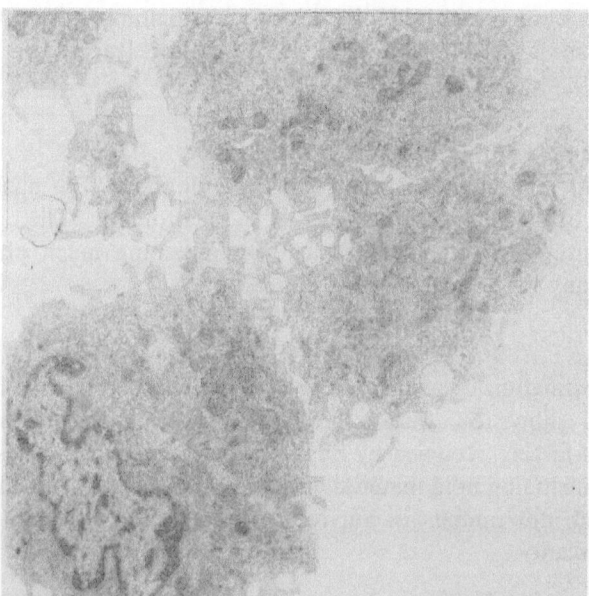

Figure 44.1 Three NBCS-stimulated macrophages in close proximity, their long slender pseudopods in contact. Nucleus and cytoplasm have the ultrastructural features of epithelioid cells. EM ×6300

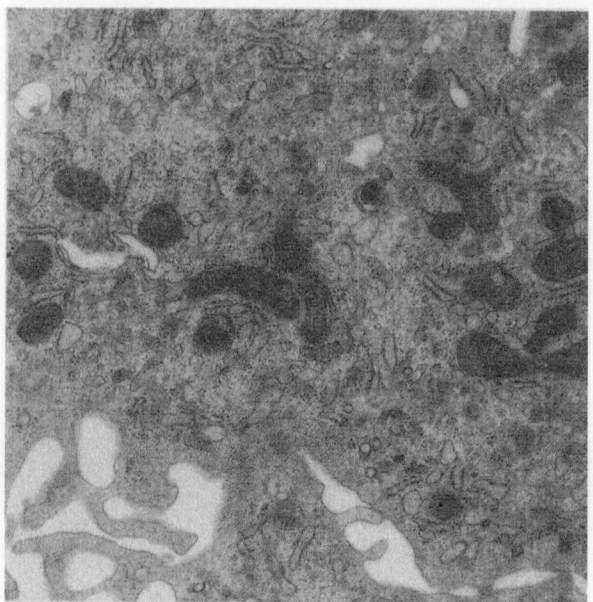

Figure 44.2 NBCS-stimulated macrophage. The cytoplasm shows a striking number of mitochondria. The rough endoplasmic reticulum is prominent and randomly distributed in the cytoplasm. Many lysosomes and Golgi vesicles are seen. EM ×16 000

small in size. Lysosomes and Golgi sacs are few in number. Rough endoplasmic reticulum is detectable usually in the perinuclear region but is not abundant.

TG stimulated cells after 2 days of in vitro culture

Cells are still separate with a few short pseudopodia. The nucleus is big, rounded or oval with dense peripheral heterochromatin. The cytoplasm is distended with large phagocytic vacuoles containing much phagocytosed material. Many lipid vacuoles are still present.

TG stimulated cells after 6 days of culture (Figure 44.3)

Some approximation of neighbouring cells is present on a small scale. The nucleus still shows the thick clustered peripheral heterochromatin. The cytoplasm is largely occupied by huge phagocytic vacuoles. These are filled with debris including lipid material and lysosomal ghosts. Mitochondria and lysosomes are now numerous but rough endoplasmic reticulum and Golgi vesicles are scanty.

Unstimulated macrophages

The cells are separate but many have interlacing pseudopodia. The shape of the cell and nucleus is variable. The cytoplasm contains well formed rough

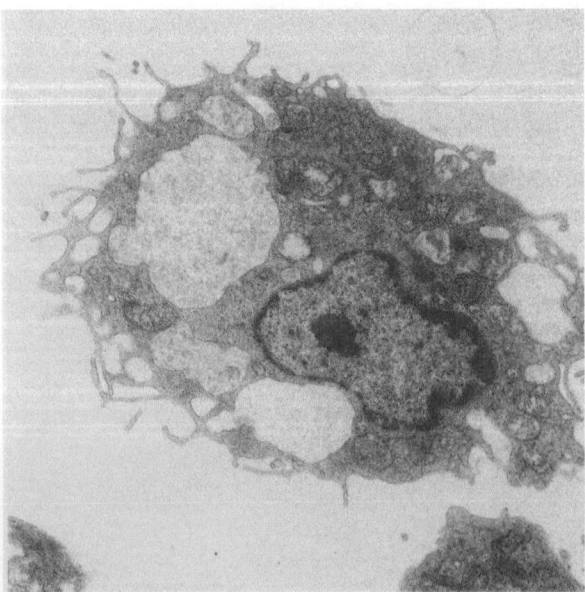

Figure 44.3 Thioglycollate-stimulated macrophage with phagocytic vacuoles filling the cytoplasm. Many small-sized mitochondria are seen. Rough endoplasmic reticulum is visible but not abundant. Few lysosomes and Golgi vesicles are seen. EM × 6300

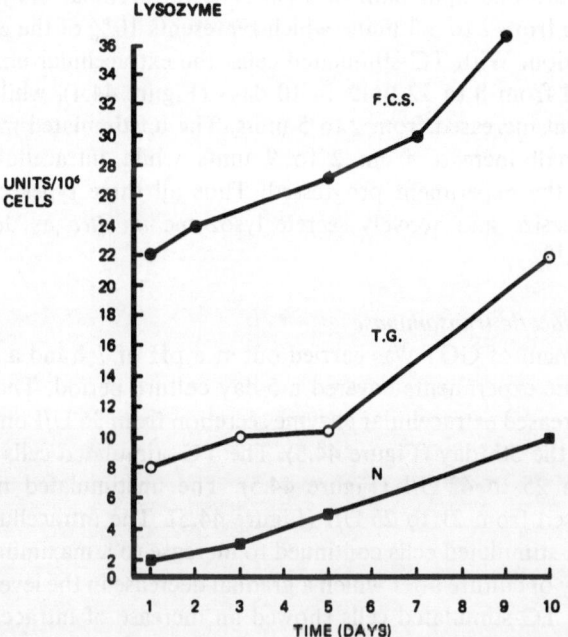

Figure 44.4 The extracellular concentration of lysozyme at various times after culture of FCS-stimulated macrophages, TG-stimulated macrophages and unstimulated macrophages

endoplasmic reticulum and a few small phagocytic vacuoles and mitochondria. There are very few lipid vacuoles, lysosomes and Golgi vesicles.

Unstimulated macrophages after 6 days of in vitro *culture*
The cells are bigger in size and some are in contact. The cytoplasm is more abundant and all cytoplasmic structures are increased in number but not to the same extent as in CS-stimulated cells.

Enzyme secretion

Lysozyme
Lysozyme was measured by determining the initial rate of lysis of a *Micrococcus lysodeikticus* suspension. Cells were cultured for 10 days and each day culture flasks were taken for assay of the supernatant medium. All experiments were repeated three times and the results given represent the mean values.

The extracellular lysozyme secretion into the medium by CS-stimulated macrophages was shown to increase from 22 to 37 units (Figure 44.4). One unit is defined as that amount of enzyme which will cause a ΔOD 450 of

0.001 in a *Micrococcus lysodeikticus* suspension in 1 min at pH 6.24 in 2.6 ml reaction mixture and light path of 1 cm. The intracellular enzyme content increased also from 2 to 5.3 units, which represents 10% of the extracellular enzyme secretion. With TG-stimulated cells, the extracellular enzyme secretion increased from 8 to 22 units in 10 days (Figure 44.4), while the intracellular content increased from 2 to 5 units. The unstimulated macrophages showed a small increase from 2 to 9 units while intracellular content decreased as the experiment progressed. Thus all three types of cell were able to synthesize and actively secrete lysozyme *in vitro* as described by Gordon *et al.*[10]

Glutamic oxalacetic transaminase

The measurement of GOT was carried out at a pH of 7.4 and a wavelength of 546 nm. The experiments covered a 5-day culture period. The CS-stimulated cells increased extracellular enzyme secretion from 36 U/I on the 1st day to 56 U/I on the 5th day (Figure 44.5). The TG-stimulated cells showed an increase from 25 to 42 U/I (Figure 44.5). The unstimulated macrophage values increased from 21 to 25 U/I (Figure 44.5). The intracellular enzyme content in CS-stimulated cells continued to increase to a maximum of 10 U/I on the 3rd day of culture after which a gradual decrease in the level of enzyme was detected. TG-stimulated cells showed an increase of intracellular GOT content but the decline of enzyme level started on the 2nd day of culture. Unstimulated macrophages gave a constant value till the 3rd day after which values diminished rapidly (Figure 44.5).

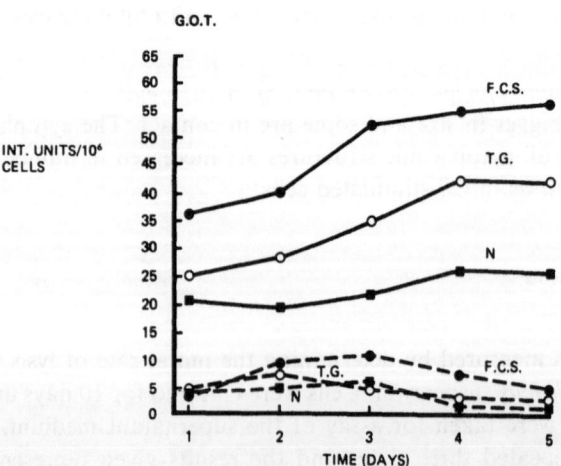

Figure 44.5 The extracellular and intracellular concentration of GOT at various times after culture of FCS-stimulated macrophages, TG-stimulated macrophages and unstimulated macrophages

——————— extracellular enzyme level

– – – – – – – intracellular enzyme level

Acid phosphatase

Cells were cultured for 6 days. Medium in which CS-stimulated cells have been maintained showed the greatest increase of about 5.5 U/I during the period of culture. Medium from the TG-stimulated cells showed an increase of 4 U/I while medium from unstimulated macrophages showed an increase of 3.5 U/I (Figure 44.6). The intracellular enzyme content in CS- and TG-stimulated macrophages increased by 0.5 U/I while that of unstimulated macrophages remained constant or showed a slight decrease.

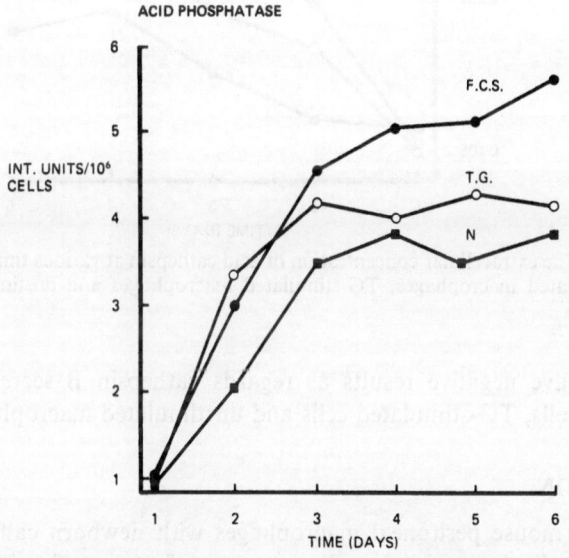

Figure 44.6 The extracellular concentration of acid phosphatase at various times after culture of FCS-stimulated macrophages, TG-stimulated macrophages and unstimulated macrophages

Cathepsin D (acid cathepsin)

The unit of enzymatic activity is calculated from the difference (Δ) in E 280 between test and blank filtrates. A E 280 of 0.10 results from the activity of 0.1 unit of enzyme from 1 h. Cells were cultured for 5 days during which the secretion of cathepsin D increased into the media. For CS-stimulated cells this increase was of the order of 3-fold the value on the 1st day of culture. TG-stimulated cells showed an approximately 2-fold increase while for unstimulated macrophages the corresponding value was about 1.5 (Figure 44.7).

Cathepsin B (neutral cathepsins)

As before optical density values ΔE 366 for azo casein (ΔE 520 for azo coll), were calculated by subtraction of blank values. A unit of proteolytic activity was defined as that amount which would have given a ΔE 366 of 1.0 in 30 min at 50 °C if response were linear to this value[9]. Both azo casein and azo coll

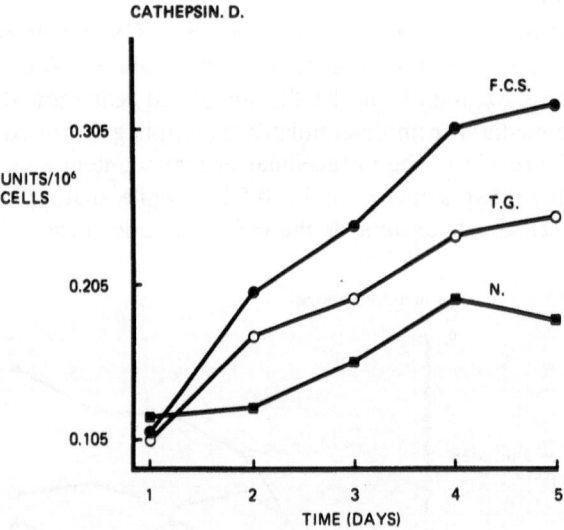

CATHEPSIN. D.

Figure 44.7 The extracellular concentration of acid cathepsin at various times after culture of FCS-stimulated macrophages, TG-stimulated macrophages and unstimulated macrophages

substrates gave negative results as regards cathepsin B secretion by CS-stimulated cells, TG-stimulated cells and unstimulated macrophages.

DISCUSSION

Stimulating mouse peritoneal macrophages with newborn calf serum (CS) allows the cells to attain the ultrastructural features of epithelioid cells. Subsequent culture *in vitro* enhances these features and leads to typical epithelioid cell contact via pseudopodia. The origin of epithelioid cells from macrophages is not in doubt and it has been suggested that epithelioid cells are macrophages specialized towards secretion of enzymes rather than phagocytosis and intracellular digestion. If it is accepted that macrophages elicited with newborn calf serum are comparable to epithelioid cells, on the basis of their ultrastructural similarities and tendency to close cell-to-cell contact, then this hypothesis now has some experimental basis.

Gordon *et al.*[10], showed that TG-stimulated cells as well as unstimulated macrophages synthesize and secrete large amounts of lysozyme *in vitro* and that this extracellular accumulation is continued for over 2 weeks in culture. The present experiments show that CS-stimulated macrophages are even more active as regards lysozyme production and secretion. The CS-stimulated macrophages also have a higher level of acid phosphatase secretion than TG-stimulated and unstimulated macrophages. It is of interest that macrophages appeared to actively synthesize GOT and secrete it extracellularly as shown by the increasing level of the enzyme both in the extracellular fluid and within the cells. This suggests that release of GOT from these cells may not, as usually thought, merely represent passive leakage of enzyme from damaged cells.

It is generally believed that secretion of lysozyme by macrophages is independent of stimulation while that of lysosomal cathepsins and phosphatases depends on stimulation of the cell, particularly by phagocytosis[11]. This is supported by the present study since the unstimulated macrophages had the lowest secretory activity of the three cell types studied. It would seem however that the relatively 'gentle' stimulation by newborn calf serum, inducing a special kind of cytoplasmic development is more effective than the high level of phagocytic and pinocytic activity induced by thioglycollate.

It may be therefore that the induction mechanism for extracellular secretion by macrophages is more complex than suggested and that one such pathway involves not phagocytic activity but epithelioid transformation.

SUMMARY

Mouse peritoneal macrophages elicited by injection of newborn calf serum had the ultrastructural characteristics of epithelioid cells. In culture, these cells synthesized and secreted more lysozyme, acid phosphatase, GOT, and acid cathepsin into the culture medium than did unstimulated macrophages or macrophages stimulated by thioglycollate which were active in phagocytosis. It is concluded that there is now some experimental suggestion that epithelioid cells have highly developed secretory activity.

References

1. Sutton, J. S. and Weiss, L. (1966). Transformation of monocytes in tissue culture into macrophages, epithelioid cells and multi-nucleated giant cells. *J. Cell Biol.*, **28**, 303
2. Papadimitriou, J. M. and Spector, W. G. (1971). The origin, properties and fate of epithelioid cells. *J. Pathol.*, **105**, 187
3. Argyris, B. F. (1967). Role of macrophages in antibody production. *J. Immunol.*, **99**, 744
4. Parry, R. M., Chandau, Jr., R. C. and Ehaham, R. M. (1965). A rapid and sensitive assay of neuramidase. *Proc. Soc. Exp. Med.*, **119**, 384
5. Reitman, S. and Frankel, S. (1957). A colorimetric method for the determination of serum glutamic oxalacetic and glutamic pyruric transaminase. *Am. J. Clin. Pathol.*, **28**, 56
6. Andersel, *et al.* (1947)
7. Fishman, W. H. and Lerner, F. (1953). A method for estimating serum acid phosphatase. *J. Biol. Chem.*, **200**, 89
8. Weissman, G., Spilberg, I. and Krakauer, K. (1969). Arthritis induced in rabbits by lysates of granulocyte lysosomes. *Arthritis Rheum.*, **12**, 103
9. Starkey, P. M. and Barrett, A. J. (1976). Neutral proteinases of human spleen. Purification and criteria for homogeneity of elastase and Cathepsin G. *Biochem. J.*, **155**, 255
10. Gordon, S., Todd, J. and Cohn, Z. A. (1974). *In vitro* synthesis and secretion of lysozyme by mononuclear phagocytosis. *J. Exp. Med.*, **139**, 1228
11. Davies, P., Page, R. C. and Allison, A. C. (1974). Changes in cellular enzyme levels and extracellular release of lysosomal acid hydrolases in macrophages exposed to group A Streptococcal cell wall substance. *J. Exp. Med.*, **139**, 1262

Discussion 44

C. da Rocha-Afodu: Would Dr. Mohktar correlate the short pseudopodia and the long
(Italy)   pseudopodia with the number of lysosomes in the macrophages? In
the experiment the number of lysosomes should be correlated with the
length of the pseudopodium in the experiments. There were some
macrophages which showed long pseudopodia, and others which
showed short pseudopodia. I think that this has a correlation with the
number of mitochondria.

Mohktar: The thioglycollate-stimulated macrophages, the phagocytosing macrophages that had the rather shorter pseudopodia showed a smaller
number of lysosomes, than the other cells with the long pseudopodia.

           The mitochondria were numerous, but they were smaller in size than
the mitochondria in the other cells that were more mature.

da Rocha-Afodu: Professor Vaes asked about the origin of macrophages. 'Macrophage'
is a bad term. Macrophages should be undifferentiated mesenchymal
cells. It appears that each tissue—e.g. bone—has its own macrophage
system. Cartilage has its own macrophage system, as does lung. Where
epithelioid cells are concerned, the particular tissue in which those
epithelioid cells are found has its own special macrophage system.
Macrophages can also migrate from other systems, in case of necessity.

45

Vascular changes during acute inflammatory responses in rat hindpaws

D. A. A. OWEN (UK)

In acute inflammatory responses, increased blood flow and vascular permeability are important events which largely determine the extent of tissue swelling. Although the vascular changes which follow the administration of many substances thought to be mediators of inflammation have been widely studied[1,2], simultaneous measurement of changes in blood flow and vascular permeability, and their relationship to the inflammatory response within discreet regions has not been clearly established.

A method has recently been developed in our laboratories to measure these vascular changes precisely and determine their relationship to swelling in rat hindpaws[3].

METHODS

Studies have been made in male rats, body weight 250 g. The measurements of swelling (increase in weight relative to the control paw), local blood flow (using radioactive microspheres, 25 μm diameter) and extravasation of albumin (using [^{125}I]human serum albumin) were made as described previously[3]. Inflammatory mediators were injected into the plantar surface of one hindpaw in a volume of 0.1 ml. The same volume of saline was injected into the other hindpaw to serve as control. Thermal injuries were elicited by immersion of the paw in water (for temperature see Results) for 30 s duration.

Animals were sacrificed 15 min after injection of the inflammatory mediators.

RESULTS

In uninjured rat hindpaws, mean blood flow was $0.4 \pm 0.06\%$ of cardiac output; albumin content was 0.05 ± 0.01 ml. Injection of saline, 0.1 ml, had no effect on blood flow, $0.38 \pm 0.05\%$ of cardiac output, but significantly increased albumin content to 0.17 ± 0.03 ml. Swelling in one paw did not change blood flow or albumin content of the other paw.

The injury-induced changes in paw blood flow are shown in Figure 45.1 and changes in extravasation of albumin are shown in Figure 45.2.

Thermal injury at 53 °C, 57 °C, 60 °C and 65 °C caused temperature dependent swelling, and increases in paw blood flow and extravasation of albumin.

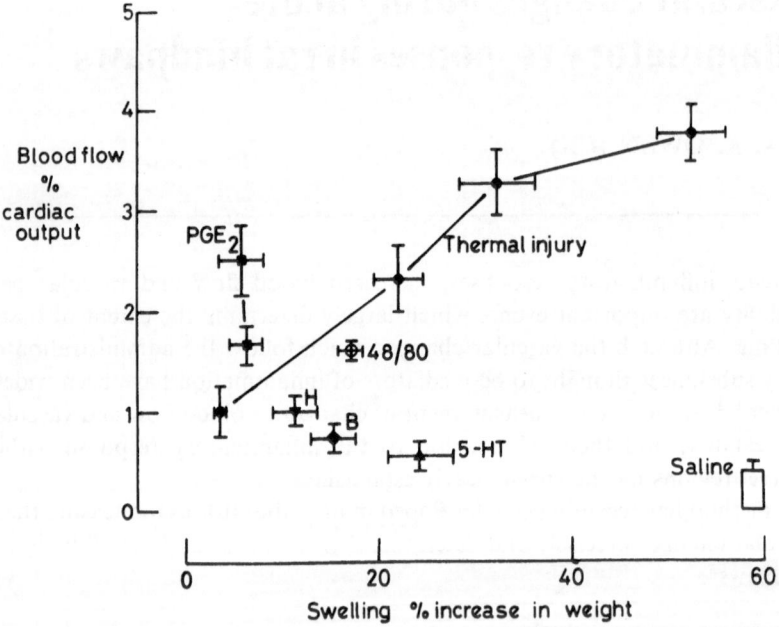

Figure 45.1 Swelling and changes in blood flow to rat hindpaws caused by inflammatory stimuli. Blood flow in untreated or saline injected paws was 0.4% of cardiac output (represented by histogram in lower right hand corner). Responses to various inflammatory stimuli are indicated as follows: Thermal injury (●), PGE₂ (■), 48/80 (○), histamine (▼, H), bradykinin (◆, B) and 5-hydroxytryptamine (▲ 5-HT)

5-hydroxytryptamine, 8 μg per paw, increased paw weight and caused marked extravasation of albumin with no significant change in local blood flow. In contrast, PGE_2, 25 and 50 ng caused large dose-dependent increases in blood flow to the paw although neither dose caused significant paw swelling.

48/80, 2.5 μg, caused substantial paw swelling with increases in both local blood flow and extravasation of albumin. Bradykinin, 2.5 μg, increased extravasation of albumin more effectively than blood flow. Histamine, 2.5 μg, caused small increases in paw weight, paw blood flow and extravasation of albumin.

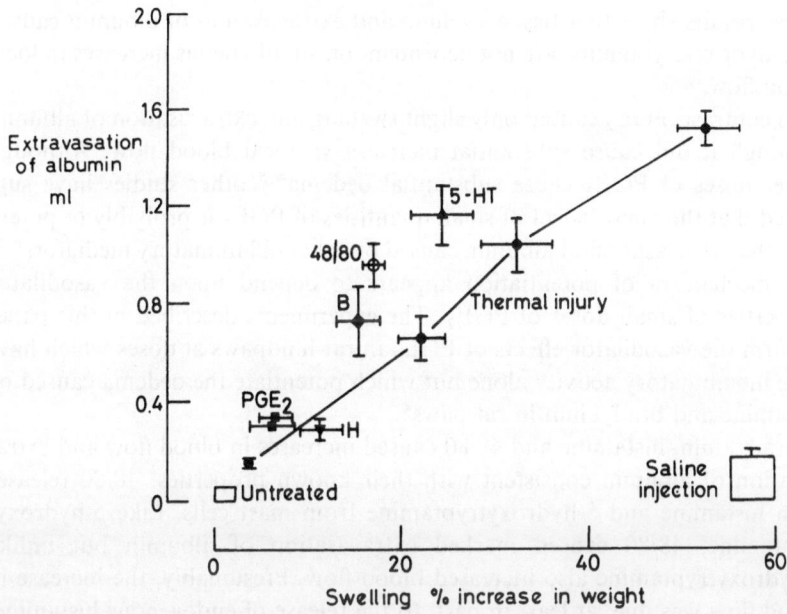

Figure 45.2 Swelling and extravasation of albumin in rat hindpaws caused by inflammatory stimuli. Albumin content in untreated paws was 0.05 ml (represented by histogram in lower left hand corner); saline injection increased albumin content to 0.17 ml (represented by histogram in lower right hand corner). Responses to various inflammatory stimuli are indicated as follows: Thermal injury (●), PGE$_2$ (■), 48/80 (○), histamine (▼, H), bradykinin (◆, B) and 5-hydroxytryptamine (△, 5-HT)

DISCUSSION

Tissue injury causes increases in local blood flow and extravasation of protein leading to tissue swelling. The mediators of acute inflammatory responses to tissue injury have been shown to be vasoactive and release of mediators in response to tissue injuries is thought to explain the acute vascular responses to injury[1,2]. The experiments described in this study were intended to quantify the vascular events due to mediator injections in rat hindpaws (a site used in many studies for acute and chronic inflammation studies) and to compare them with the response to thermal injury in the same tissue.

Thermal injury caused swelling accompanied by both increased local blood flow and extravasation of albumin, the classical profile of acute inflammatory responses. The changes in each parameter were temperature-dependent i.e. the more severe injury caused the largest swelling and the largest vascular responses.

Injection of mediators into the paw produced a variety of vascular responses associated with various degrees of tissue swelling.

5-hydroxytryptamine caused swelling associated with substantial extravasation of albumin without causing any significant increase in blood flow. 5-hydroxytryptamine is known to be a potent inflammatory agent in rats[2].

493

These results show that tissue swelling and extravasation of albumin caused by 5-hydroxytryptamine are not dependent on simultaneous increases in local blood flow.

In contrast, PGE_2 caused only slight swelling and extravasation of albumin although it did cause substantial increases in local blood flow. Although larger doses of PGE_2 cause substantial oedema[4,5] other studies have suggested that the major effect of small quantities of PGE_2 is probably to potentiate the extravasation of albumin caused by other inflammatory mediators[6,7]. The mechanism of potentiation appears to depend upon the vasodilator properties of small doses of PGE_2. The experiments described in this paper confirm the vasodilator effects of PGE_2 in rat hindpaws at doses which have little inflammatory activity alone but which potentiate the oedema caused by histamine and bradykinin in rat paws[4].

Bradykinin, histamine and 48/80 caused increases in blood flow and extravasation of albumin consistent with their known properties. 48/80 releases both histamine and 5-hydroxytryptamine from mast cells. Like 5-hydroxytryptamine, 48/80 caused marked extravasation of albumin but unlike 5-hydroxytryptamine also increased blood flow. Presumably, the increase in blood flow was due, at least in part, to the release of endogenous histamine.

These experiments characterize the vascular changes caused by different inflammatory mediators in the rat. Single doses only have been used for mediators except PGE_2 and a more comprehensive understanding of their effects would require a wide range of doses of each of the mediators. Nevertheless, the data described indicate that changes in blood flow and extravasation of protein are independent phenomena, both of which can contribute to tissue swelling.

Acknowledgement

I am grateful to Mrs. Helen Farrington for her skilled technical assistance throughout this study.

References

1. Wilhelm, D. L. (1973). Chemical mediators. In: *The Inflammatory Process* (B. W. Zweifach, L. Grant and R. T. McCluskey, eds.) (New York and London: Academic Press)
2. Willoughby, D. A. (1973). Mediation of increased vascular permeability in inflammation. In: *The Inflammatory Process* (B. W. Zweifach, L. Grant and R. T. McCluskey, eds.) (New York and London: Academic Press)
3. Owen, D. A. A. and Farrington, H. E. (1976). Inflammation and the vascular changes due to thermal injury in rat hindpaws. *Agents Actions*, 6, 622
4. Moncada, S., Ferreira, S. H. and Vane, J. R. (1973). Prostaglandins, aspirin-like drugs and oedema of inflammation. *Nature (London)*, 246, 217
5. Kuhn, D. C. and Willis, A. L. (1973). Prostaglandin E_2, inflammation and pain threshold in rat paws. *Br. J. Pharmacol.*, 49, 183P

6. Williams, T. J. and Morley, J. (1973). Prostaglandins as potentiators of increased vascular permeability in inflammation. *Nature (London)*, **246**, 215
7. Williams, T. J. (1976). The pro-inflammatory activity of E-, A-, D- and F-type prostaglandins and analogues of 16, 16-dimethyl-PGE_2 and (15S)-15-methyl PGE_2 in rabbit skin; the relationship between potentiation of plasma exudation and local blood flow changes. *Br. J. Pharmacol.*, **56**, 341 P

Section VI
Pharmacological Aspects: Animal/Man

CHAIRMAN: C. M. Pearson

46

Activators and inhibitors of fibrinolysis in rheumatoid joint inflammation

L. B. A. VAN DE PUTTE, C. KLUFT, V. NOORDHOEK HEGT, G. WIJNGAARDS, F. HAVERKATE AND A. CATS (The Netherlands)

INTRODUCTION

The presence of large amounts of fibrin-like material (FLM) in the synovial fluid and both in and on the synovial membrane is a conspicuous feature of rheumatoid joint inflammation[1]. Organization of FLM in these joints is a frequent finding[2], and it has been stated that this process may lead to fibrosis[3]. Therefore, the presence of FLM in rheumatoid joints may be related to a loss of compliance of the joint capsule and possibly to joint deformity. The fate of fibrin (in all probability one of the main constituents of FLM), once it is formed in the rheumatoid joint, is determined by the local fibrinolytic activity, and this activity is, in turn, the result of activator and inhibitor activity. The present communication is concerned with activators and inhibitors of the fibrinolytic system in rheumatoid as compared with non-rheumatoid synovial membranes and synovial fluids. We were especially interested in the question whether the presence of FLM in rheumatoid joints is accompanied by and related to a locally decreased fibrinolytic activity.

STUDIES ON SYNOVIAL MEMBRANES

A histochemical study on activators and inhibitors of fibrinolysis in rheumatoid and non-rheumatoid synovial membranes was reported recently from our laboratories[4]. In that study overall fibrinolytic activity was determined by Todds fibrin slide technique[5], which measures the result of local plasminogen activator-mediated fibrinolytic activity and inhibitor activity. Material inhibiting fibrinolysis was measured and localized in the tissue by the recently devised fibrin slide sandwich technique[6]. This technique is a two-stage procedure. First, inhibitor material is allowed to diffuse in a fibrin slide overlying the tissue section under study, and secondly, a section of gelatinous plasmin is placed on top of the fibrin slide. The plasmin digests any underlying fibrin lacking inhibitor material, but at sites where inhibiting material is present fibrin digestion is delayed. Semiquantitative measurements by both techniques were carried out according to Pandolfi[7].

Overall fibrinolytic activity of chronically inflamed rheumatoid synovial membranes was low compared with that in non-inflamed synovial tissues. Fibrinolytic activity in both rheumatoid and control specimens was related to blood vessels. In some rheumatoid synovial tissues exhibiting very low fibrinolytic activity, plasminogen activator-induced fibrinolysis by synovial lining cells was observed. The amount of material inhibiting fibrinolysis, as determined by the fibrin slide sandwich technique, was small or virtually nil in non-inflamed synovial membranes. In contrast, there was considerable inhibitory activity in inflamed rheumatoid tissues. Interestingly, this inhibitor activity was found predominantly at sites of chronic inflammatory infiltrates and deposits of FLM. Using Pandolfi's method of quantitation[7], we found that inhibitor activity in rheumatoid synovial tissues is inversely related to fibrinolytic activity, and therefore the low fibrinolytic activity of these specimens may be related to the presence of inhibitors of fibrinolysis. In addition, we conclude that inhibitors in FLM deposits are probably responsible for a prolonged persistence of these deposits in the rheumatoid joint[4].

STUDIES ON SYNOVIAL FLUIDS

Table 46.1 gives our results concerning paired synovial fluid and peripheral blood samples from patients with RA and osteoarthritis. It appears from these data that coagulation and fibrinolysis occur in synovial fluids of both groups. The virtual absence of fibrinogen and factor XIII in both groups of synovial fluids and the presence of FLM in rheumatoid synovial fluids are indicative for an active coagulation process, whereas high levels of fibrin degradation products indicate ongoing fibrinolysis. Apparently, fibrinolysis can lead to complete removal of fibrin in the osteoarthritic joint, but cannot keep up with fibrin formation in the rheumatoid joint.

Plasminogen activators cannot function unless plasminogen is present. Our data demonstrate that substantial amounts of plasminogen are indeed present in rheumatoid and osteoarthritic synovial fluids. The results obtained with the immunochemical method are in agreement with those obtained with plasminogen determination according to Brakman and Traas[12], thus indicating the presence of a functionally intact plasminogen.

Two important plasma protease inhibitors, i.e. a_2-macroglobulin and a_1-antitrypsin, were measured immunochemically. The concentration of a_1-antitrypsin was higher in rheumatoid than in osteoarthritic synovial fluids,

Table 46.1 Fibrinolytic data obtained in synovial fluid and plasma from patients with rheumatoid arthritis (RA) and osteoarthritis (OA)*

		Synovial fluid		Plasma		References
		RA	OA	RA	OA	for methods
Fibrinogen (mg%)	F	—	±	510⊕	330⊕	8
Fibrin-like material		+	—	—	—	
FDP (mg%)	I	40	25	n.d.	n.d.	9
Factor XIII	F+o	trace	trace	n.d.	n.d.	10
Plasminogen	I+	35	32	110	93	11
	F+	35	34	n.d.	n.d.	12
a_2-macroglobulin (mg%)	I	61	62	130△	220△	11
a_1-antitrypsin (mg%)	I	250△	160△	250	240	11
Plasmin inhibition	F+	50	50	n.d.	n.d.	13
Fibrinolytic activity	F	0	0	0	0	14
Euglobulin fibrinolytic activity (mm)	F	10.1△	6.4△	15.7	17.2	15

*Mean results; all patients older than 50 years, with classical RA (n = 5) (22) or OA (n = 5). n.d. = not determined; I = immunochemical; F = functional

△p < 0.05 for difference between RA and OA groups. °After addition of F XIII—free fibrin.

+ Expressed as % of pooled plasma

but interpretation of these findings in terms of differences in inhibitor activity requires caution since the results of immunochemical and functional measurements may differ within a given sample[16]. It is likely that the recently described antiplasmin[17] is also present in synovial fluids, and therefore plasmin inhibition was estimated in a small group (n = 6) representing both kinds of synovial fluids. A comparable degree of plasmin inhibition was found in rheumatoid and osteoarthritic synovial fluids. Determinations done on plasminogen-rich fibrin plates showed no fibrinolytic activity in either synovial fluid or plasma samples. The activity of the euglobulin fractions of the fluids was low in relation to the plasma values. However, these data too are difficult to interpret, because euglobulin fractionation may not be equally effective for plasma samples and synovial fluids.

Studies on plasma proteins in synovial fluids should take the plasma levels of these proteins into account. Correlation between plasma and synovial fluid concentrations has been shown for several proteins[18-20] and was also observed in our material. The plasma fibrinolytic activity of euglobulin fractions did not differ significantly between the RA and osteoarthritis group, which means that divergent plasma activities are not responsible for differences in fibrinolytic capacity between rheumatoid and osteoarthritic joint fluids. Of particular interest are the different plasma fibrinogen levels of the two groups. The higher fibrinogen levels in RA plasma samples may result in a higher input of fibrinogen into the rheumatoid synovial fluids than into the osteoarthritic fluids. This, in turn, could lead to the formation of larger amounts of fibrin in rheumatoid synovial fluids.

CONCLUSIONS

The present findings indicate that an active coagulation and fibrinolysis process occurs in the synovial fluids of both RA and osteoarthritis patients. However, appreciable amounts of fibrin-like material are present in rheumatoid synovial fluids but generally not in osteoarthritic fluids. This difference cannot be explained by clearcut differences between the two groups with respect to the fibrinolytic capacity of the synovial fluid. Some of the other findings may be relevant here. Firstly, larger amounts of fibrinogen are offered to the rheumatoid joint than to the osteoarthritic joint, and hence larger amounts of fibrin may be produced in the former type of joint disease. Secondly, rheumatoid synovial membranes have a lowered fibrinolytic activity, whereas osteoarthritic synovial tissues, which show less or no inflammatory changes, probably have a higher activity. Finally, the significance of the presence of inhibitors in fibrin-like material in the rheumatoid joint remains uncertain for the moment, but experimental data obtained by Kwaan et al.[21] suggest that the presence of inhibitors in fibrin clots results in delayed fibrin dissolution and enhanced formation of connective tissue.

References

1. Gardner, D. L. (1965). *Pathology of the Connective Tissue Disorders*, pp. 70–73, (London: Edward Arnold)
2. Fassbender, H. G. (1975). *Pathologie Rheumatischer Erkrankungen*, pp. 85–143. (Berlin, Heidelberg and New York: Springer Verlag)
3. Lack, C. H. (1959). Chondrolysis in arthritis. *J. Bone Jl. Surg.*, **41B**
4. van de Putte, L. B. A., Noordhoek Hegt, V. and Overbeek, T. E. (1977). Activators and inhibitors of fibrinolysis in rheumatoid and non-rheumatoid synovial fluids. *Arthritis Rheum.* (In press)
5. Todd, A. S. (1959). The histological localization of fibrinolysin activator. *J. Pathol. Bact.*, **78**, 281
6. Noordhoek Hegt, V. and Brakman, P. (1974). Histochemical study of an inhibitor of fibrinolysis in the human arterial wall. *Nature (London)*, **248**, 75
7. Pandolfi, M., Robertson, B., Isacson, S. *et al.* (1969). Fibrinolytic activity of human veins in arms and legs. *Thromb. Diath. Haemorrh.*, **20**, 247
8. Astrup, T., Brakman, P. and Nissen, U. (1965). The estimation of fibrinogen; a revision. *Scand. J. Clin. Lab. Invest.*, **17**, 57
9. Brittin, G. M., Rafinia, H., Raval, D., Werner, M. and Brown, B. (1972). Evaluation of single radial immunodiffusion for quantitation of plasma fibrinogen. *Am. J. Clin. Pathol.*, **57**, 89
10. Finlayson, J. S. and Morton, R. O. (1972). Gel electrophoresis for assessing fibrin crosslinking; a precaution. *Clin. Chim. Acta*, **36**, 254
11. Mancini, G., Carbonara, A. O. and Heremans, J. F. (1965). Immunochemical quantitation of antigens by single radial immunodiffusion. *Immunochemistry*, **2**, 235
12. Brakman, P. and Traas, D. W. (1976). Assay of plasminogen in blood on fibrin plates. In: *Progress in Chemical Fibrinolysis and Thrombolysis* (J. F. Davidson, M. M. Samama and P. C. Desnoyers, eds.) (New York: Raven Press) Vol. 2, pp. 79–82
13. Blix, S. (1964). The quantitative determination of fibrinolytic inhibitors in plasma or serum by means of the fibrin plate. *Scand. J. Clin. Lab. Invest.*, **16**, 403
14. Haverkate, F. and Brakman, P. (1975). Fibrin plate assay. In: *Progress in Chemical Fibrinolysis and Thrombolysis* (J. F. Davidson, M. M. Samama and P. C. Desnoyers, eds.) Vol. 1, pp. 151–159. (New York: Raven Press)

15. Kluft, C., Brakman, P. and Veldhuyzen-Stolk, E. C. (1976). Screening of fibrinolytic activity in plasma euglobulin fraction on the fibrin plate. In: *Progress in Chemical Fibrinolysis and Thrombolysis* (J. F. Davidson, M. M. Samama and P. C. Desnoyers, eds.) Vol. 2, pp. 57–65 (New York: Raven Press)
16. Shtacher, G., Maayan, R. and Feinstein, G. (1973). Proteinase inhibitors in human synovial fluid. *Biochim. Biophys. Acta*, **303**, 138
17. Collen, D., DeCock, F. and Verstraete, M. (1975). Immunochemical distinction between antiplasmin and alpha-1-antitrypsin. *Thromb. Res.*, **7**, 245
18. Pruzanski, W., Russell, M. L., Gordon, D. A. and Ogryzlo, M. A. (1973). Serum and synovial fluid proteins in rheumatoid arthritis and degenerative joint diseases. *Am. J. Med. Sci.*, **265**, 483
19. Willemsen, L. and Friis, J. (1975). A comparative study of the protein pattern in serum and synovial fluid. *Scand. J. Rheumat.*, **4**, 234
20. Ambanelli, U., Troise, W., Fadda, G. and Nervetti, A. (1975). Serum and synovial fluid concentrations of macroglobulin and $a_2$neuroaminoglycoprotein in rheumatoid arthritis. *Z. Rheumatol.*, **34**, 408
21. Kwaan, H. C. and Astrup, T. (1969). Tissue repair in presence of locally applied inhibitors of fibrinolysis. *Exp. Mol. Pathol.*, **11**, 82
22. Ropes, M. W., Bennett, G. A. Lobb, S., *et al.* (1959). Diagnostic criteria for rheumatoid arthritis, 1958 revision. *Ann. Rheum. Dis.*, **18**, 49

Discussion 46

W. Parish:
(UK)

In chronic cutaneous vasculitis there is also decreased fibrinolytic activity of the serum. Is the inhibitor activity that Dr. van de Putte and his colleagues have detected in joints due to an inhibitor that has infiltrated in with the fluid exudates or is it the result of local synthesis?

van de Putte:

We have no evidence for or against either possibility. We think that the inhibiting material somehow gets trapped into the fibrin clots and how that happens is being studied at the moment.

I. Ginsburg:
(Israel)

I recently read an extremely interesting publication which tried to explain the pathogenesis of the Shwartzman reaction on the basis of the interactions of fibrinogen degradation products with polyanionic substances released from polymorphs.

Is it possible that the polymorphs in the synovial membranes, of which there is an abundance, disintegrate and release the polyanionic substances which interact with fibrinogen degradation products to form a precipitate to fibrinolysin? In that case the persistence of precipitates may not be due to the presence of inhibitors but to the formation of new complexes which are then resistant to fibrinolysin.

van de Putte:

Of the clots which we got from the synovial fluid at least a part can be dissolved by plasmin. We have done that. Part of the story may be true as Dr. Ginsburg tells it, and part of it is as I have indicated.

There is a large amount of degradation product in the synovial fluid so that is a very real possibility.

M. Jasani:
(UK)

Many previous studies on the fibrinolytic activity or the potential of the synovial fluid have failed to reveal what Dr. van de Putte has demonstrated so well using the slide technique—and he is to be congratulated.

My colleagues and I have been looking at the possible origin of fibrin and we are therefore very much interested in the observation—obviously inferential in observation—that it may be the cellular infiltrate which may be responsible for the inhibitory activity that has been found. Investigations that we have carried out using rabbit-skin homografts suggest that the immune lymphocytes which are present in the synovium may be the source of fibrin-forming material, and in that context Dr. Ginsburg's observations that another type of inflammatory cell may be the source of inhibitory substances may be relevant.

van de Putte:

There is something I should stress. All we have done is to demonstrate localization of such substances. We do not have the origin of this kind of material.

T. L. Vischer:
(Switzerland)

Would Dr. van de Putte comment or speculate about the importance of the fibrinolytic activity he found around vessels in normal tissue. Why is there so much apparent fibrinolytic activity in normal tissue?

van de Putte:

I do not know. Probably it prevents a micro-thrombosis or something like that.

504

FIBRINOLYSIS IN SYNOVIAL MEMBRANES

P. Davies:
(USA)

I am a little concerned that the system may give some indication of substrate competition; in other words that the inhibition seen is due to consumption of endogenous fibrin-degrading activity by endogenous fibrin.

Has any attempt been made to directly extract inhibitors from the tissue and to show their activity in other exogenous systems?

van de Putte:

There have been some experiments, but I have not done any myself.

G. Vaes:
(Belgium)

An interesting Paper was recently published in the *Journal of Experimental Medicine* showing the preferential adsorption in the presence of a-2-macro-globulin on the surface of endothelial vascular cells—I do not remember in what tissue. If such a potent inhibitor of plasmin and of plasminogen activator is present, possibly this may explain some of Dr. van de Putte's data.

van de Putte:

I agree.

G. Loewi:
(UK)

Dr. van de Putte did some very beautiful stains with Lendrum's picro mallory.

If those are compared—as I have done—with a specific anti-fibrinogen with a peroxidase or fluorescence there is much less. That stain is a little misleading.

47

Relationships between increased vascular permeability, oedema, hyperalgesia and the effect of non-steroid anti-inflammatory drugs

S. H. FERREIRA, MARIA TERESINHA ZANIN AND
BERENICE B. LORENZETTI (Brazil)

The relationship between oedema, increased permeability and hyperalgesia has been a matter of debate for some time. On one side there are those who concluded that oedema formation and protein leakage are closely linked[1,2], but others have evidence indicating that the processes are independent[3,4,5]. A parallelism between the development of oedema and an increase in permeability during the development of inflammation induced by carrageenan was found in studies utilizing labelled protein[6,7]. However, Garcia Leme et al.[8] did not find this parallelism during the entire period of observation. When they measured the seepage of protein-bound Evans Blue into a perfusate (coaxial perfusion), they found that the major increase in permeability occurred in the early stages but that only a small residual increase in permeability was demonstrable at the time oedema was maximal (4th hour). These investigators also showed that non-steroid anti-inflammatory drugs, which are prostaglandin synthesis inhibitors, were only effective when given before administration of carrageenan. This observation is not consistent with the suggestion that prostaglandins are the mediators of the late phase of carrageenan oedema[6,9]. In addition, non-steroid anti-inflammatory drugs such as aspirin and phenylbutazone were shown to be effective in blocking oedema when given 2 h after carrageenan[10]. Hyperalgesia, on the other hand, had been shown to be more sensitive to curative treatment with aspirin-like drugs than oedema, and that oedema *per se* does not cause hyperalgesia (for discussion, see References 11 and 12).

In the present investigation, we have used the rat paw carrageenan oedema assay to re-investigate the interrelationships between increased vascular permeability, oedema and hyperalgesia. We shall also report the effect of non-steroid anti-inflammatory agents on these parameters and discuss the participation of inflammatory mediators in oedema, increased vascular permeability and hyperalgesia induced by carrageenan.

PERMEABILITY AND OEDEMA

Increased permeability was measured by determining the amount of Evans Blue extractable with formamide[13] for 24–48 h at 37 °C from rat paws which had been mechanically pulverized under liquid nitrogen. Since the dye binds strongly to plasma proteins after intravenous injection, the quantity of dye reflects the amount of protein leakage and thus is a measure of the increase in permeability. The values for the contralateral paw are subtracted from the experimental values as the reference control.

When Evans Blue (25 mg/kg) was injected intravenously at the same time as the intraplantar injection of 100 μg carrageenan, there was a parallel increase in oedema and accumulation of dye at 1, 2, 3 and 4 h after the phlogogenic stimuli. Comparison of oedema formation with permeability increase as a function of time (the dye is given at the beginning and the rat sacrificed at the end of the time interval) showed two distinctly different patterns (Figure 47.1). The lower dose of carrageenan (100 μg) caused a

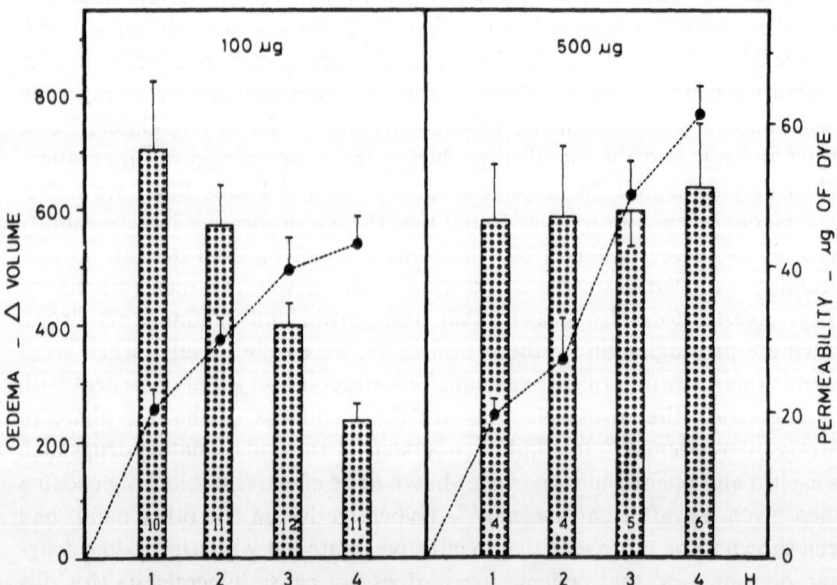

Figure 47.1 Comparison between permeability and oedema induced by low (100 μg) and high (500 μg) doses of carrageenan given into the rat paw. The oedema (filled circles) was measured pletsmographically and the permeability (bar) with Evans Blue. The number of animals is indicated within bars. The values represent mean ± EM

transitory increase in permeability which had its highest value in the first hour and decreased progressively. The permeability effect is relatively low at the time that the oedema is maximal (4th hour). When a second intraplantar injection of 100 μg of carrageenan is made at the 3rd hour, there is a marked enhancement of permeability without a significant effect on the oedema. These results indicate that the low dose of carrageenan (100 μg) loses its ability to increase permeability within a short time period, but that the vascular structures are still responsive. The data in Figure 47.1 (left panel) suggest that the increment in volume of the paw is correlated with the degree of permeability of the leg for the early time intervals. A statistically significant correlation was shown for the first two hours where the slopes are steepest.

The right panel of Figure 47.1 shows that the increase in permeability is maintained for 4 h while the oedema increases progressively. In fact, the 100 and 500 μg doses of carrageenan induced similar levels of changes in permeability and oedema during the first two hours. However, the oedema for the higher dose is much more intense at the later time.

Administration of indomethacin (2 mg, i.p.), $\frac{1}{2}$ h before, or 2 h after 100 μg of carrageenan, significantly ($P < 0.05$) inhibited the permeability increase (Figure 47.2), but the oedema was only significantly affected when this drug was given before carrageenan. The lower part of Figure 47.2 shows the

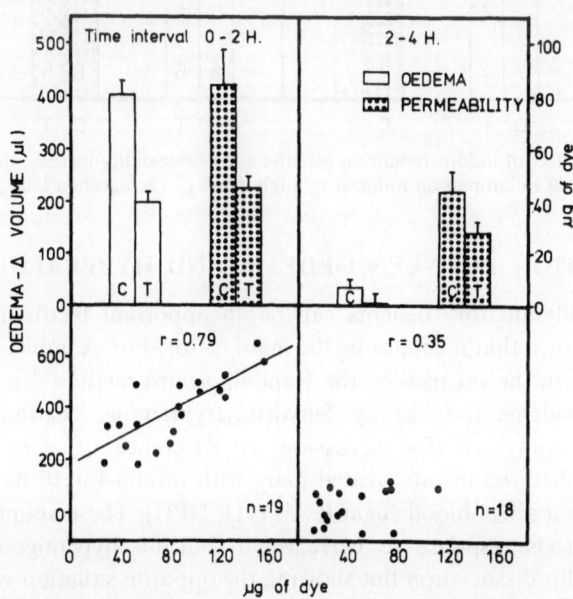

Figure 47.2 Effect of indomethacin on oedema and permeability increase during the early and late phase of inflammation induced by low doses of carrageenan (100 μg). The upper left panel give the results for the time interval 0–2 h for control (c) and rats treated with indomethacin, T, (2 mg/kg), i.p. The panel in the upper right gives the results for 2–4 h period. The lower panels show the relationship between oedema and permeability for the control rats

correlation between oedema and permeability during the early period which does not persist in the late period (2–4 h). Indomethacin given before or in the second hour after a high dose of carrageenan (500 µg) significantly inhibited the permeability increase and oedema at both intervals (0–2 and 2–4 h, see Fig. 47.3).

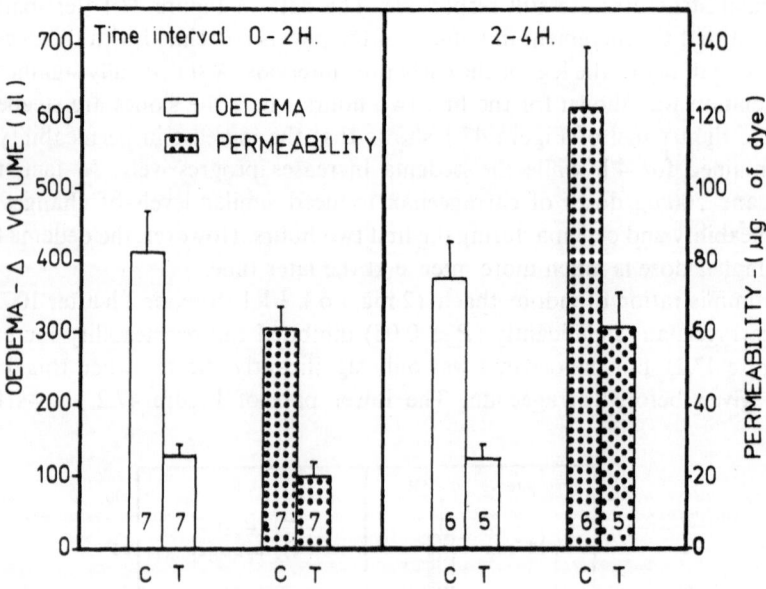

Figure 47.3 Effect of indomethacin on oedema and permeability increase during the early and late phase of inflammation induced by high doses of carrageenan (500 µg)

DISSOCIATION BETWEEN OEDEMA AND HYPERALGESIA

Although inflammatory oedema can be an important factor in promoting pain, it is known that it cannot be the main factor. For example, hyperalgesia as measured in the rat paw by the Randall–Selitto method[14] is not demonstrable in oedema induced by 5-hydroxytryptamine, dextran or passive cutaneous anaphylaxis (for discussion see Reference 12). One striking example was observed in rats treated daily with insulin for 10 days at a dose which does not affect blood sugar levels (1 U, NPH). These animals present a full oedematous response to carrageenan but no hyperalgesia. Another example of this dissociation but showing the opposite situation was observed in rats rendered leukopoenic (reduction of more than 60% in leukocyte count) by methrotexate treatment (3 daily doses of 2, 1, 1 mg/kg, respectively). These animals showed a reduction of more than 60% in the oedema induced by carrageenan, but still presented a clear hyperalgesic response as tested by the Randall–Selitto technique. The reduction of the oedema was of the same order as observed by treatment with indomethacin (2–4 mg/kg, i.p.), which displays full antialgic effect.

The final example of dissociation between oedema and hyperalgesia to be described is given by treating the rats with a non steroid anti-inflammatory agent 2 h after the intraplantar injection of a small amount of carrageenan (100 μg). Indomethacin (2 mg/kg, i.p.) produced an antialgic effect equal to that observed when given prior to carrageenan but had little or no effect on the oedema.

DISCUSSION

In this paper we have shown that the duration of the increase in vascular permeability in the rat paw depends on the dose of carrageenan. With a low dose (100 μg) the permeability effect of carrageenan is of short duration. This possibly reflects the loss of ability of carrageenan to generate mediators capable of increasing the permeability rather than the capacity of the system to respond, since a second injection of carrageenan is able to cause further increase in permeability. Recently, Garcia Leme et al.[14] demonstrated that histamine, 5-hydroxytryptamine, bradykinin and prostaglandins appear simultaneously in the lymph of rats after an intraplantar injection of a small dose of carrageenan (50 μg). The presence of those inflammatory mediators was transitory, occurring between $\frac{1}{2}$ and 3 h after carrageenan. If we consider the transit time (from the interstitial space to the cannula) it is probable that these mediators were released during the first two hours when the greatest increase in permeability was observed in experiments with a low dose of carrageenan.

It is interesting to note that with a low dose of carrageenan hyperalgesia reaches its maximum when the increase in permeability is minimal but that the oedema is still fully developed. We have shown in this communication, confirming previous observations[11,12,15], that oedema per se cannot account for hyperalgesia as measured by the Randall–Selitto method. This should be taken as an indication that, although with little effect on permeability, mediators responsible for hyperalgesia continue to be released. Prostaglandins seem to be the best candidates among the possible mediators of hyperalgesia in carrageenan inflammation. In several tests, prostaglandins cause hyperalgesia[12]. Among several mediators tested, only prostaglandin, when added to carrageenan, was able to cause hyperalgesia during the first hour when carrageenan itself did not cause this effect[16]. This experiment indicates that hyperalgesia in the rat paw depends on the combined action of prostaglandin and other mediator(s). The fact that indomethacin can significantly inhibit the permeability increase in the late period induced by high or low doses of carrageenan can be taken as circumstantial evidence for a prolonged release of prostaglandins.

At the moment there is not enough experimental evidence to identify the origin of the prostaglandin involved in the sensitization of pain receptors. Is it released from local cells, newly arrived polymorphs or from the sensory terminations themselves? The fact that prostaglandin synthetase inhibitors such as paracetamol display analgesic effects without conspicuous anti-inflammatory effects, seems to indicate a selective effect upon the nervous structure. The puzzling effect of insulin treatment in hyperalgesia induced by carrageenan without any action on the oedema supports the idea that one can block the pain associated with inflammation without interfering with the oedema. The effect was not of the type of morphine because control paws showed a normal hyperalgesic response which is much prolonged in the case of morphine treatment. However, it could be a central effect, since we recently observed that paracetamol injected into the cerebral ventricles displays an analgesic effect without affecting the threshold of normal paws. This central effect of paracetamol added to its local effect may explain the analgesic action of paracetamol[17]. It will be interesting to test the chronic insulin treatment in other models of experimental pain. It could be the basis for an auxiliary therapy in the inflammatory diseases in which pain is the prevalent symptom.

We have shown that with high doses of carrageenan the permeability effect continues for the period studied (4 h). Di Rosa et al.[6] have followed the development of oedema and permeability for 6 h. Their results obtained with high doses of carrageenan (1 mg) also showed that in a later phase (after the fourth hour) the increased permeability fell abruptly but the oedema persisted. Thus a late dissociation between oedema and increased permeability seems to be independent of the dose of carrageenan. The dissociation, however, is delayed for the higher doses.

The persistence of oedema has been interpreted to be due to the presence of leaking protein which maintains the water in the interstitial space[8]. Possibly the oncotic pressure in the interstitial space is also increased by the generation of large protein fragments which result from the increased enzymic hydrolytic activity as well as to extrusion of other large molecules by damaged cells. Thus one would expect parallelism between increased permeability and oedema during the period in which the factors which influence the maintenance of oedema are making a relatively small contribution. We have shown that with low doses of carrageenan there is a correlation between increment of the oedema and increased permeability which does not occur in the late phase. It is probable that with high doses of carrageenan this correlation would be demonstrable for longer times. Non steroid anti-inflammatory drugs such as indomethacin, which primarily inhibit the permeability increase, only affect oedema when the intervening factors in the maintenance of oedema are minimal, thus allowing oedema to be correlated to permeability increase. This is possibly the explanation for the little or no effect of indomethacin when given in the late phase of oedema induced by small doses of carrageenan. A similar situation may exist in rheumatoid arthritis, where non steroid anti-inflammatory agents are much more effective when given before rather than after the establishment of the 'morning stiffness' symptom.

Acknowledgement

We thank the Wellcome Foundation and Fundação de Amparo á Pesquisa do Estado de São Paulo (FAPESP-Grant 0296/75) for research support.

References

1. Parratt, J. R. and West, G. B. (1958). Inhibition by various substances of oedema formation in the hind-paw of the rat induced by 5-hydroxytryptamine, histamine, dextran, eggwhite and compound 48/80. *Br. J. Pharmacol.*, **13**, 65
2. Northover, B. J. and Subramanian, G. (1958). A study of possible mediators of inflammatory reactions in the mouse foot. *Br. J. Pharmacol.*, **18**, 346
3. Gözsy, B. and Kátó, L. (1957). Changes in permeability of the skin capillaries of rats after histamine depletion with 48/80, dextran or egg white. *J. Physiol.*, **139**, 1
4. Wilhelm, D. L. (1976). Chemical mediators. In: *The Inflammatory Process* (B. W. Zweifach, L. Grant and R. T. McCluskey, eds.), Vol. II, Chap. 8, p. 251. (New York, London: Academic Press Inc.)
5. Brown, D. M. and Robson, R. D. (1964). Effect of anti-inflammatory agents on capillary permeability and oedema formation. *Nature (London)*, **202**, May 23
6. Di Rosa, M., Giroud, J. P. and Willoughby, D. A. (1971). Studies of the mediators of the acute inflammatory response induced in rats in different sites by carrageenin and turpentine. *J. Pathol.*, **104**, 15
7. Doherty, N. S. and Robinson, B. V. (1975). The inflammatory response to carrageenin. *J. Pharm. Pharmacol.*, **27**, 701
8. Garcia Leme, J., Hamamura, L., Leite, M. P. and Rocha e Silva, M. (1973). Pharmacological analysis of the acute inflammatory process induced in the rat's paw by local injection of carrageenin and by heating. *Br. J. Pharmacol.*, **48**, 88
9. Willis, A. L. (1969). Parallel assay of prostaglandin-like activity in rat inflammatory exudate by means of cascade superfusion. *J. Pharm. Pharmac.*, **21**, 126
10. Levy, L. (1971). Anti-inflammatory drugs. *Biol. Sci. Tech. Rep.*, Riker Laboratories
11. van Arman, C. G., Carlson, R. P., Risley, E. A., Thomas, R. H. and Nuss, G. W. (1970). Inhibitory effects of indomethacin, aspirin and certain drugs on inflammation induced in rat and dog by carrageenin, sodium urate and ellagic acid. *J. Pharm. Exp. Therap.*, **175**, 459
12. Ferreira, S. H., Moncada, S. and Vane, J. R. (1974). Prostaglandins and the signs and symptoms of inflammation. In: *Prostaglandin synthetase inhibitors* (H. J. Robinson and J. R. Vane, eds.) (New York: Raven Press, p. 175)
13. Garcia Leme, J. and Wilhelm, D. L. (1975). The effects of adrenalectomy and corticosterone on vascular permeability responses in the skin of the rat. *Br. J. Exp. Pathol.*, **56**, 402
14. Souza, M. Z. A., Medeiros, M. C. e Garcia Leme, J. (1976). Detecção de fatores de permeabilidade na linfa de animais submetidos a estimulos inflamatórios. *XXVIII Reunião Anual da SBPC* (Brasilia), supl., p. 562
15. Gilfoil, T. and Klavins, J. (1965). 5-Hydroxytryptamine, bradykinid and histamine as mediators of inflammatory hyperesthesia. *Am. J. Physiol.*, **208**, 867
16. Ferreira, S. H., Harvey, E. A. and Vane, J. R. (1975). Hyperalgesia, inflammatory oedema and prostaglandin. In: *Proc. of Sixth Intern. Congr. Pharmacol.*, Abstract 1001, Helsinki, Finlandia
17. Ferreira, S. H., Lorenzetti, Berenice B., Castro, Maria Salete A. and Correa, F. M. A. (1977). Antialgic effect of aspirin-like drugs and the inhibition of prostaglandin synthesis. In: *Proc. of Symposium on Recognition of Anti-rheumatic Drugs*

Discussion 47

R. Vinegar: **(USA)**	It might be helpful in trying to explain Dr. Ferreira's experiments to realize that the oedema increases that occur in the carrageenan-treated foot are due to both oedematogenic action and inflammatory action. The inflammatory action is due to the inflammatory cells which are brought. Both of these actions produce hyperalgesia. Both have their independent rates of development and decay, and these take place simultaneously. The drugs which were studied only affect the inflammatory part, therefore one section is not affected by drugs whilst the other is affected. The inflammatory part is mostly affected by pretreatment with drugs. This would help to explain many of Dr. Ferreira's findings. I also reported recently that paracetamol is anti-inflammatory—which might also explain some of the things that have been found. Dr. Ferreira should explain how he measures the hyperalgesia so that we can perhaps go back and reproduce some of the work.
Ferreira:	The technique is modified slightly. However, I do not take Dr. Vinegar's main point. I believe that paracetamol in rats has a kind of anti-oedema effect, but I do not think that it blocks migration of cells inside the rat paw, which is a phenomenon which if it does occur occurs very early. If one tried to correlate cells and hyperalgesia—for the moment I do not think we can correlate it too well, at least in the dog joints. For example, where endotoxin is given in a joint, hyperalgesia occurs very early and when the cells are at a maximum, four to five hours later, the hyperalgesia is already finished. In a sense hyperalgesia cannot be strictly correlated to the oedema as well as to the presence of cells, but I think that they should be correlated to the presence of a mediator that has been somehow released from either the local or the migrating cells. I believe it is the local cells.
Vinegar:	If the action of paracetamol is studied in what we call carrageenan pleurisy where the cells that come in can be quantitatively measured one finds that paracetamol indeed inhibits the inflammatory cells from coming in, which is its mechanism of action. Unfortunately paracetamol does not work locally—which would really help out Dr. Ferreira. In our hands the local injection of paracetamol does not have any anti-inflammatory action, but it does work in the intact rat. We would definitely disagree here as to the local action.
Ferreira:	I have shown that put locally it causes hyperalgesia.
G. Haberland: **(Germany)**	I was extremely interested in the findings with regard to insulin and hyperalgesia. I should like to draw attention to the fact that insulin is a potent inhibitor of kininase too—which is identical with the actions in one converting enzyme and thus interferes with the mechanism of bradykinin directly, and of course indirectly with the metabolism of prostaglandins.

Ferreira: It could be. The only problem that I have is that if we are interfering in the kinin system, we should also have an effect on the oedema. There are indications that the bradykinin causes part of the oedema produced by carrageenan.

It could be. I have no explanation for it. I merely put it in because I thought it peculiar.

M. Jayson:
(UK) In discussing rheumatoid arthritis and the relationship with oedema it is important to recall that clinically we do see oedema quite commonly in rheumatoid disease and we are always trying to exclude all the better-known causes of oedema, e.g. hyperproteinaemia, obstruction to the blood vessels in the legs by cysts etc. Apart from that we are left with a residual number of cases who do have chronic persistent oedema of the legs, feet and ankles.

Some years ago we did a study (at Bristol) in which we measured capillary permeability in these people and found quite a good correlation between vascular permeability and the presence of a chronic oedema.

On the second point—the genesis of pain in the joints. When one thinks about this one should always give some thought to the location of the pain receptors that can be stimulated. There are no pain receptors in the synovium, and nor are there any in the intra-articular cartilage, but they are present in the joint capsule and apart from that in the periosteum and in blood vessels in bone. We measured the stiffness of the joint capsule, or the stiffness of the joints, on distending them, in patients with pain from a number of different causes and we were able to correlate quite closely the genesis of pain—the sensitivity to pain in joints—with the stiffness of the joint capsule.

I think it quite possible that oedema of the joint capsule could be the source of pain in such people.

Ferreira: I believe that in this situation the oedema happens. In fact in some situations taking some fluid from the patient leads to some improvement. If the same manoeuvres used to demonstrate pain in the arthritic patient were applied to a normal person the same type of pain would not present. The 'normal' person will not present pain, because in the lesions caused by arthritis there is probably a very small release of mediators which has sensitized the nerve endings to mechanical and chemical stimulation.

Jayson: It is a difficult point. We found a series of people who had had inflammatory joint disease, probably some time in the past, that was completely inactive at the time, and yet they still had chronic persistent pain on using their joints and there were no obvious pathological findings, or radiological findings, or haematological findings to explain it. The only objective changes were the increased stiffness of the capsule, presumably due to fibrosis of the capsule which had taken place in the past leading to mechanical deformation of the mechanoreceptors.

Ferreira: Did treatment with aspirin-like drugs improve the pain in such patients?

Jayson: No, not really.

Ferreira: Then we are not referring to the same case. This is a mechanical problem.

D. A. Willoughby:
(UK) Dr. Ferreira is to be congratulated on a masterly presentation. He has focussed attention on an important point, the question of oedema. For the benefit of those faced with the problem of looking for new anti-rheumatic or anti-inflammatory drugs could one suggest that instead of looking for these models that produce increased vascular permeability via the standard mediators, including Dr. Ferreira's favourites, the prostaglandins, perhaps they should be looking at the

other limb of the chronic inflammatory response. Possibly we should be seeking something that promotes lymphatic drainage.

There are a number of experts in the audience: Professor Lewis, Dr. Piller. Both of them have been working in this field for a number of years and they have concentrated on promoting the clearance of oedema rather than acting on the point of increased vascular permeability.

Would Dr. Ferreira himself suggest that this might be a good pathway to looking for new types of therapeutic agents?

Ferreira: I do not think so. We realize that the models we are using—shall we call them acute models of inflammation—are telling us that there is a group of symptoms which I would call 'immediate symptoms'. Why 'immediate symptoms'? Because once the trauma is there, something is generated, something may be a mediator, and then increased vascular permeability results. If that generation or the action of the mediator can be blocked, then the immediate events disappear. They may be in acute or in chronic models. These immediate events are a part of chronic inflammation as well as of acute inflammation: they include pain, hyperalgesia, etc.

We want to block the chronic events, the delayed events, some of them related to the destruction of bone, etc., which is far more important. It may be worth having a drug which increases the washing out of the interstitial space, but that may nonetheless be a kind of therapy that we more or less have in our hands—the prevention of symptoms, immediate symptoms.

I. L. Bonta:
(The Netherlands) Dr. Ferreira has shown us that the oedema components and the pain components can be separated, and I found that most interesting. He suggests that the important part of the pain component is the potentiating effect of the prostaglandin itself. Yesterday we heard Dr. Kuehl's most interesting talk on a new drug—possibly there are others too—when he showed us that there are certain compounds which may suppress the formation of PGG_2 and simultaneously, by a kind of a shunting effect, increase the production of PGE. I wonder whether such a compound may in fact enhance the pain component in Dr. Ferreira's model and whether there are any data on this. Dr. Kuehl may have done some work along these lines. There is the possibility that a drug that suppresses the pivotal inflammatory mediator such as PGG_2 might simultaneously increase the pain component.

My second question refers to dextran. As far as I know serotonin release is involved in dextran oedema. Dr. Ferreira has shown—and we know it already from his earlier work—that prostaglandin markedly enhances the effect of serotonin.

Ferreira: In the permeability increase.

Bonta: Does it not relate to all effects?

Ferreira: No. That is the beauty of the story. When the mediators are together the pool of mediators has one effect on permeability. Pain probably does not need the same pool, or—I think—needs another pool of mediators. That is the crucial point that we need to understand. Permeability depends on a group of mediators and they are not the same mediators as those that play a role in the generation of pain. It is up to us to demonstrate which are which. In permeability, particularly in the rat, 5-hydroxytryptamine is very important. It is important. The greater part of the dextran can be blocked by the antagonism of serotonin.

Bonta: But the prostaglandins—according to Dr. Ferreira's earlier studies—would very much sensitize to the pain-producing effect of serotonin or kinin. There is some confusion here with dextran.

Ferreira: In dextran it is the histamine and the 5-hydroxytryptamine that are

516

released, but very little prostaglandin. If prostaglandin is added to dextran a tremendous hyperalgesia results.

G. Nuss:
(USA)
Work done in 1965 showed a divergence of the activity of indomethacin. The algesia was more easily shown using yeast oedema. Does Dr. Ferreira feel that the mediators and the yeast-induced oedema in the rat's paw differ from those in carrageenan-paw oedema and in, for example, dextran-induced oedema?

Ferreira:
No. The relative proportions of the mediators will vary according to type. In a rat's paw, dextran will release one group of mediators and yeast will probably release the same group of mediators with the addition perhaps of bradykinin, more prostaglandin, and even other mediators deriving from the complement whose effects are not certain. The total effect would depend on the total sum of mediators released. They may have a direct vascular action. In that case I can say nothing. Burning, for example. For yeast oedema indomethacin can be given after two hours and the hyperalgesia can be blocked—different from the oedema also. One cannot change it.

Nuss:
The anti-inflammatory regression lines for indomethacin are considerably different—at least in my hands—between yeast-induced oedema and carrageenan oedema. I have repeated the work many times and I have found that the effects of indomethacin on carrageenan oedema are very different from the effects on yeast-induced oedema. I certainly feel that the mediation following Dr. Ferreira's plan is entirely different.

Ferreira:
Yes. There may be other mediators participating.

J.-P. Giroud:
(France)
Has Dr. Ferreira been using the full carrageenan, or a fraction? We have used fraction of carrageenan and produced some quite different answers.

Secondly, in acting on hyperalgesia with E_1 and E_2, have F_2alpha or the beta stimulants been tried?

Ferreira:
On the second point, no. On the first, I have used the marine colloid carrageenan.

Giroud:
The importance of these experiments is that they explain why we have different results. When we have a very sensitive rat, using 50 micrograms will give a prolonged effect and therefore this group of animals belongs to the large-dose group since these rats are releasing mediators over a long period of time, and then possibly we get the same group of phenomena as we see for very high doses. If very high doses are used, but the system is studied for only four hours, one will not see the same things as with a short experiment using very small doses.

D. Sofia:
(USA)
Have such substances as *dorivan*, propoxyphene or morphine been used and have they shown an effect on the hyperalgesia?

Ferreira:
Morphine.

Sofia:
Without an effect on the oedema?

Ferreira:
This is easy. If morphine is given intra-ventricularly into the rat—that was my positive control in these experiments although I have not shown it here because I must check the student who did the experiment. Rats that are absolutely mad have to be used. They have treated some animals with carrageenan, with morphine intraventricularly, and the oedema is perfect. Those rats have shown one thing. The response is increased for both legs—for the inflamed and the non-inflamed.

The method I am using, and the paracetamol doses I use produce no effect in the non-inflamed paw. It is an important point.

Sofia:
Have the relations between vascular permeability, hyperalgesia and oedema in the adjuvant rat been examined? Is there a similar-type correlation to that seen with carrageenan?

Ferreira:
Now that we more or less know what to do, we may go on to chronic models. I have considered using Nystatin models, because they are easy to produce.

PERSPECTIVES IN INFLAMMATION

A. Bryceson:
(UK)

The dissociation between pain and inflammation is interesting and is seen in other situations. For example, in South America there are some very nasty spiders and scorpions that produce extreme pain with practically no inflammation, and the pain there does not respond to anti-inflammatory drugs, but to such interesting compounds as, for example, emitine. This might provide a situation where the pain component could be looked at in greater separation from the inflammation component.

48

Two sites of action of steroids on the prostaglandin system

G. P. LEWIS AND P. J. PIPER (UK)

When fat cells are stimulated by a lipolytic agent such as ACTH, they are activated in such a way that a series of biochemical steps lead to activation of tissue lipase. The action of this enzyme on triglycerides causes the release of free fatty acids (FFA), among which is presumably arachidonic acid (AA). This is acted on by cyclo-oxygenase to produce endoperoxides, thromboxanes and prostaglandins (PGs). Prostaglandins, at least, have been shown to cause functional vasodilatation *in vivo* but perhaps some of the other products of the cyclo-oxygenase system also cause vasodilatation. In the experiments in which we examined subcutaneous adipose tissue in rabbits *in vivo*, FFA release was detected, the vasodilatation measured and the PG formation estimated in tissue extracts, obtained after activation of the adipose tissue by ACTH, and release of PGE_2 into the venous blood measured by radio-immunoassay[1,2]. In addition investigations were carried out in chopped fat and isolated fat cells *in vitro*. FFA and glycerol levels and PG formation during activation of chopped fat and in isolated fat cells *in vitro* were also measured[3].

After treatment with a non-steroid anti-inflammatory agent like indomethacin or aspirin before the ACTH, FFA release could still be demonstrated, but PG formation in the tissue and the vasodilatation were inhibited[4]. It is generally accepted that such agents act by preventing the conversion of arachidonic acid to PGs by inhibition of cyclo-oxygenase[5], and this action of aspirin-like drugs explains these results as shown diagrammatically in Figure 48.1.

When an anti-inflammatory steroid like hydrocortisone or betamethasone was given before activation with ACTH, a different pattern of changes was observed. It was still possible to detect release of FFA, indicating that lipolysis is not prevented. Formation of PG in the fat tissue occurred, indicating that the steroids do not affect the cyclo-oxygenase system. However, the release of the PG-like material into the venous blood and the vasodilatation were inhibited[6]. It was therefore suggested that the steroids might act at the membrane and in some way prevent the release of PG after its formation (see Figure 48.1).

Gryglewski et al.[7] have studied the action of anti-inflammatory steroids in different tissues and investigated the release of PGs from mesenteric blood vessels in response to injected noradrenaline and from perfused lungs in response to antigen challenge.

Stimulation of the appropriate cells (perhaps endothelial cells, or maybe some other cell type) by antigen or noradrenaline (in an analogous way to activation by ACTH) causes stimulation of biochemical pathways which lead to activation of phospholipase A. This enzyme has been shown to release arachidonic acid from membrane phospholipids[8]. As in the fat cells the arachidonic acid is converted to PGs which are released into the perfusing

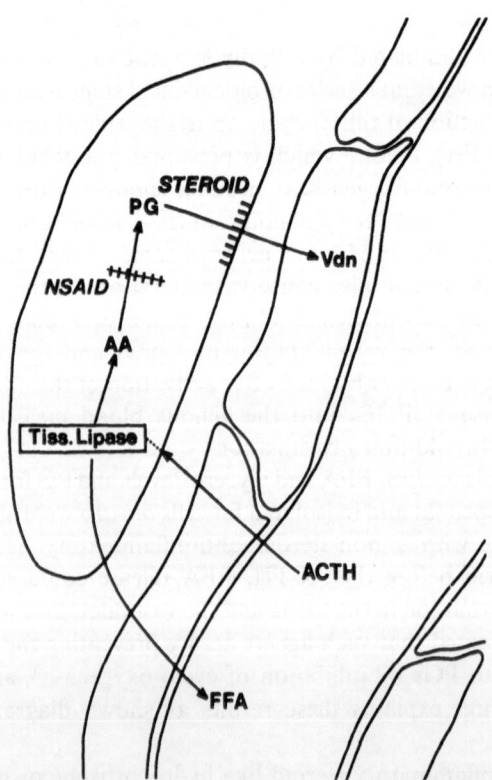

Figure 48.1 Diagrammatic representation of the formation of PGs from triglyceride-derived arachidonic acid in fat cells. The diagram indicates the possible sites of action of non-steroid anti-inflammatory drugs (NSAID +++++) and anti-inflammatory steroids (STEROID ⊔⊔⊔⊔⊔)

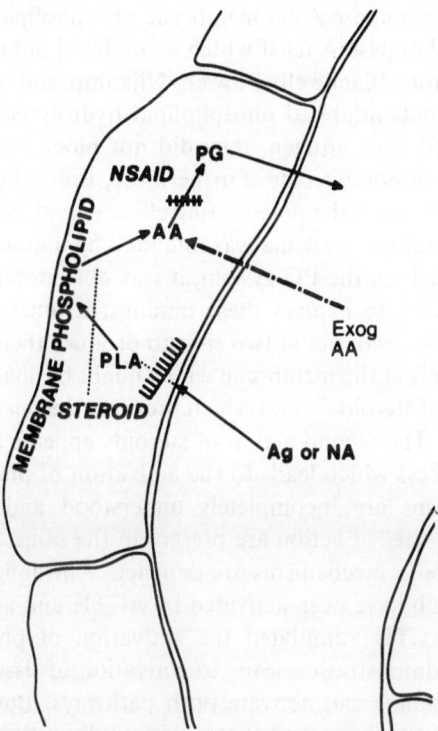

Figure 48.2 Diagrammatic representation of the formation of PGs from phospholipid-derived arachidonic acid in blood vessel or lung cells. The diagram indicates possible sites of action of non-steroid anti-inflammatory drugs (NSAID ┼┼┼┼┼┼) and the possible (STEROID . . . .) and more likely (STEROID ⊔⊔⊔⊔⊔⊔) site of action of anti-inflammatory steroids

fluid. This release of PGs is prevented by non-steroid anti-inflammatory agents (Figure 48.2).

Gryglewski and his colleagues also found that the release of PGs was prevented by anti-inflammatory steroids, as Lewis and Piper[2] had shown in adipose tissue. However, they also made an important finding which differed from those in adipose tissue. They showed that the steroid effect could be overcome by administering exogenous arachidonic acid, whereas the effect of indomethacin could not be reversed. These authors therefore suggested that steroids prevented the availability of the arachidonic acid, probably by inhibiting its release from membrane phospholipids and that the exogenous arachidonic acid entered the cell pool from which endogenous arachidonic acid had been excluded. This hypothesis could not be applied to adipose tissue since, in the above experiments, neither the non-steroid nor the steroid effect could be overcome by administration of arachidonic acid either in *in vivo* or *in vitro* experiments[3].

Recent studies by other authors support the view that steroids influence the action of phospholipase A on membrane phospholipids and suggest that it is not the phospholipase A itself which is inhibited but probably an earlier step in its activation. Blackwell, Flower, Nijkamp and Vane[9] have shown that although steroids inhibited phospholipid hydrolysis in perfused guinea pig lung challenged with antigen, they did not block the phospholipase A activity in a cell-free homogenate. Furthermore, Brain, Lewis and Whittle[10] have shown that although the potentiating effect of exogenous phospholipase A on carrageenan rat paw oedema was inhibited by indomethacin, indicating that it was mediated via the PG system, it was not inhibited by steroids.

Therefore, in order to explain these findings, it must be concluded that anti-inflammatory steroids act at two sites to produce their effects on the PG system. One action is at the membrane which might be analogous to the other membrane effects of steroids[11] and which prevents the release of PGs already formed in the cell. The second action of steroids appears to be inhibition of a biochemical process which leads to the activation of phospholipase A.

These mechanisms are incompletely understood and it is not known whether these two sites of action are present in the same cell.

In Figure 48.3 both mechanisms are depicted. Anti-inflammatory steroids act in systems which have been activated by ACTH and antigen but it is not known whether ACTH stimulated the activation of phospholipase A or whether antigen administration leads to activation of tissue lipase. Nor is it known if noradrenaline can activate both pathways. But it is known that ACTH activates tissue lipase and that noradrenaline stimulates tissue lipase to cause lipolysis via a β-adrenoceptor. In human adipose tissue we have already shown, in preliminary experiments, not only that noradrenaline causes PG formation but that release of this PG into the bathing medium is inhibited by steroids (Chang, Lewis & Piper, unpublished results). The

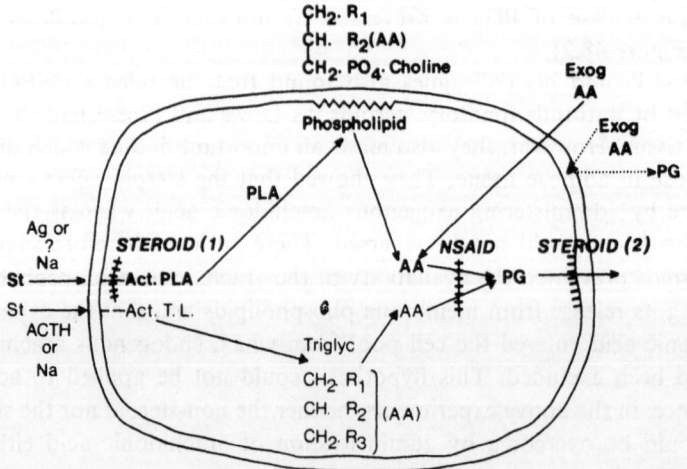

Figure 48.3 Diagrammatic representation of two possible pathways of synthesis of PGs and the possible sites of action of anti-inflammatory drugs

possibility therefore exists that in other tissue too, noradrenaline causes PG formation by releasing arachidonic acid from triglycerides.

Thus, in the presence of a non-steroid anti-inflammatory agent, stimulation of both pathways would lead to arachidonic acid release but no further. In the presence of an anti-inflammatory steroid the phospholipid pathway could be inhibited at site (1) while the triglyceride pathway would still lead to arachidonic acid release and PGs would be formed but held within the tissue by steroid action at site (2) as has been shown in adipose tissue.

Activation of the triglyceride pathway might well lead to some accumulation of PG in the tissue although the extent of this accumulation would depend on the availability of substrate and the PG metabolic activity of the particular cells. PG accumulation has been shown to occur in fat tissue when it is activated in the presence of steroids. In addition, PG metabolizing enzymes are virtually absent in this tissue[3]. In the presence of indomethacin there is no accumulation of PGs at all. In tissues other than adipose tissue, there is also evidence that PGs are present in cells treated with anti-inflammatory steroids. In mouse fibrosarcoma cells, for instance, those treated with hydrocortisone retained PGs while those treated with indomethacin contained only a small amount[12]. It is not yet known whether steroid treatment leads to the retention of PGs in the lungs following antigen challenge or in blood vessels stimulated by noradrenaline as in the experiments of Gryglewski[13].

Preliminary experiments have been carried out to analyse the triglyceride pathway leading to PG formation. In some experiments *in vivo* in which FFA release has been inhibited by nicotinic acid, PG formation has also been inhibited[4]. However, nicotinic acid is not an ideal inhibitor and there is need for further investigation of this pathway.

Finally, when considering the apparent reversal of the steroid effect by exogenous arachidonic acid, it must be concluded that where this is possible it is unlikely that there is a site (2) action of the steroid, since if the exogenous arachidonic acid entered into the normal cell pool, the PG formed should be held in the cell. When ^{14}C-labelled arachidonic acid was incubated with chopped adipose or lung tissue, at least 2 hours were necessary for uptake[3,14], whereas reversal of steroid action in the experiments of Gryglewski *et al.* was almost immediate. These findings raise the question of whether the arachidonic acid enters the normal pool for conversion to 'endogenous' PGs following stimulation by ACTH or antigen[14], or whether the exogenous AA might be converted to PG at the cell membrane or some other site or pool (see Figure 48.3). However, this does not happen in adipose tissue because there is no reversal of steroid action with arachidonic acid. Therefore, it seems that there are some differences between fat cells and other cells in respect of the action of steroids which might indicate that the two different sites of steroid action on the PG system might be present in different cell types. But both might occur in cells (other than fat cells) which contain a significant amount of triglyceride and the enzyme system which hydrolyses it.

Acknowledgements

This work was supported by the Medical Research Council and the Arthritis and Rheumatism Council.

References

1. Bowery, N. G., Lewis, G. P. and Matthews, J. (1970). The relationship between functional vasodilatation in adipose tissue and prostaglandin. *Br. J. Pharmacol.*, **40**, 437
2. Lewis, G. P. and Piper, P. J. (1975). Inhibition of release of prostaglandins as an explanation of some of the actions of anti-inflammatory corticosteroids. *Nature (London)*, **254**, 308
3. Chang, J., Lewis, G. P. and Piper, P. J. (1977). Inhibition by glucocorticoids of prostaglandin release from adipose tissue *in vitro*. *Br. J. Pharmacol.*, **59** (In press)
4. Bowery, B. and Lewis, G. P. (1973). Inhibition of functional vasodilatation and prostaglandin formation in rabbit adipose tissue by indomethacin and aspirin. *Br. J. Pharmacol.*, **47**, 305
5. Vane, J. R. (1971). Inhibition of prostaglandin synthesis as a mechanism of action for aspirin-like drugs. *Nature, New Biol.*, **231**, 232
6. Lewis, G. P. and Piper, P. J. (1976). The action of corticosteroids on the prostaglandin system. In: *The Role of Prostaglandins in Inflammation* (G. P. Lewis, ed.) pp. 148–160. (Bern: Hans Huber Publisher)
7. Gryglewski, R. J., Panczenko, Bogumila, Korbut, R., Grodzinska, L. and Ocetkiewicz, A. (1975). Corticosteroids inhibit prostaglandin release from perfused mesenteric blood vessels of rabbit and from perfused lungs of sensitized guinea-pig. *Prostaglandins*, **10**, 343
8. Kunze, H. and Vogt, W. (1971). Significance of phospholipase A for prostaglandin formation. *Ann. N.Y. Acad. Sci.*, **180**, 123
9. Blackwell, G. J., Flower, R. J., Nijkamp, F. P. and Vane, J. R. (1977). Phospholipase A_2 activity of guinea-pig perfused lungs: stimulation and inhibition by anti-inflammatory steroids. *Br. J. Pharmacol.* **59** (In press)
10. Brain, S., Lewis, G. P. and Whittle, B. J. R. (1977). Actions of phospholipase on mast-cell histamine release and paw oedema in the rat. *Br. J. Pharmacol.*, **59** (In press)
11. Weissman, G. (1973). Effect of corticosteroids on the stability and fusion of bio-membranes. In: *Asthma, Physiology, Immunopharmacology and Treatment* (K. F. Austen and L. M. Lichtenstein, eds.) pp. 221–230. (New York: Academic Press)
12. Tashjian, Jr., A. H., Voelkel, K. F., McDonough, J. and Levine, L. (1975). Hydrocortisone inhibits prostaglandin production by mouse fibrosarcoma cells. *Nature (London)*, **258**, 739
13. Gryglewski, R. J. (1976). Steroid hormones, anti-inflammatory steroids and prostaglandins. *Pharm. Res. Commun.*, **8**, 337
14. Crutchley, D. J., Piper, P. J. and Seale, J. P. (1977). Relationship between prostaglandin inactivation and release in challenged guinea-pig lungs. *J. Physiol. (London)* (In press)

Discussion 48

J. Sondergaard: (Denmark)	This was an interesting paper, and perhaps Professor Lewis might extend it. He referred to fibrosarcomatous tissue. Has he extended it at all to skin, human skin. We know that there is a significant production of prostaglandins in several inflammatory conditions and one of the still unknown actions of topical action of steroid. It would therefore be of interest to learn whether Professor Lewis has expanded his studies to this area too.
Lewis:	We are expanding our studies into human adipose—subcutaneous adipose tissue at the moment. The system seems to be the same there as we find in rabbits. The vasoconstrictor effect of topically applied steroids in humans might well be an inhibition of this system.
M. J. Parnham: (The Netherlands)	With regard to the theories about the second site of action of corticosteroids, the obvious field of controversy is whether or not prostaglandins are actually stored. There is evidence that corticosteroids acting on lymphocytes cause an accumulation of intracellular free fatty acids. If the corticosteroids are acting to prevent the release of prostaglandins, then I wonder whether it is not the release of prostaglandins that might be inhibited, but perhaps the release of arachidonic acid?
Lewis:	That could be a possibility. On the other hand, in practice we find an accumulation of prostaglandin.
Parnham:	But if the prostaglandin synthetase was on the inside of the membrane then if arachidonic acid was being accumulated inside the cell that would be converted to prostaglandins in any case.
Lewis:	Then prostaglandins would be accumulated!
Parnham:	Yes. Indirectly.
I. Ginsburg: (Israel)	I should like to report on some preliminary experiments which have been done at the Hadassah Medical School and at the Weizmann Institute showing that if chronic arthritis is induced in the knee joint of a rat by putting in soluble cell wall components of Group A streptococci, then the effect of prostaglandin E release can be inhibited by corticosteroids and this effect can be reversed by arachidonic acid. Arachidonic acid would enhance the secretion of prostaglandin from pieces of tissue in culture, and what is interesting is that the inhibitory effect of indomethacin on the release of prostaglandin E in this system could not be reversed by arachidonic acid. We obtained the same inhibition with dexamethasone and with prednisolone as with corticosteroids, which would corroborate some of Professor Lewis's results.
Lewis:	That would fit in with the steroids inhibiting phospholipase-A activation.

525

49

Studies on the clinical and laboratory pharmacology of drug formulations of bovine Cu–Zn superoxide dismutases (orgotein)

W. HUBER, K. B. MENANDER-HUBER, M. G. P. SAIFER
AND P. H-C. DANG (USA)

Orgotein is the generic name adopted by the USAN Council[1] for drug versions (Table 49.1) of superoxide dismutases which contain copper and zinc. Historically, the development of the therapeutic concept embodied in orgotein evolved from a search for a safe drug of mammalian tissue origin that would be suitable for chronic use in a wide variety of human and animal maladies with an inflammatory component. One of us discovered in 1964 that a metalloprotein preparation isolated from bovine liver was a potent anti-inflammatory agent[2]. Subsequent work established that it is a safe and effective drug in animals[3,4–7] and man[8–12] for the treatment of several inflammatory diseases. In 1969, five years after our basic discovery, McCord

Table 49.1 Properties of orgotein for injection

Form	freeze-dried solid
Excipient	sucrose, USP
Diluent	sodium chloride injection pH 6.5–7.0
Solubility	> 150 mg/ml
Shelf life	> 5 years at room temperature
Descriptive name	superoxide dismutase
Reaction catalysed	$2O_2^- + 2H^+ \rightarrow H_2O_2 + O_2$

The properties listed are those of orgotein prepared for pharmaceutical use in single-dose rubber-stoppered serum vials. Two milligrams of sucrose is present for each 1 mg protein. Vials contain 2, 4, 5 or 8 mg protein.

and Fridovich published their characterization of the enzyme superoxide dismutase (SOD)[13]. It soon became apparent to us that their SOD was the principal component in orgotein, which by that time we had obtained and characterized from ten species of mammals, birds and fish[14]. Orgotein is a new anti-inflammatory agent which is completely different from all other drugs presently used for the treatment of inflammatory disease, and is a protein which is unusually resistant to denaturants and to proteolytic enzymes near neutral pH[15]. Both the copper and zinc are so strongly chelated by the protein that even prolonged dialysis against millimolar EDTA at neutral pH will not remove them.

The structure of the molecule has been well characterized (Table 49.2). Its amino acid sequence and crystal structure have been determined recently by Hill *et al.*[16] and Richardson *et al.*[17], respectively. It is a compact globular molecule consisting of two identical subunits which are tightly but not covalently bound together. In nature, Cu-Zn SOD is an ubiquitous enzyme occurring in all cells of eukaryotic organisms studied to date. In all species the enzyme occurs intracellularly where it is a keystone defence against the superoxide radical which, as recent work has shown, is a commonplace intermediate in many biological oxidoreductions[18]. O_2^- is produced *in vivo* by aerobic actions of a number of enzymes, electron transport systems of organelles, and a host of autoxidations where O_2^- can act both as an oxidant and a reductant[18]. As a very active radical, O_2^- occurring extracellularly can be a threat to the integrity of living systems, since the concentration of Cu-Zn SOD in mammalian sera (about 10 ng/ml) is less than one-thousandth that of cytosol concentrations and less than one-tenth of that measurable following administration of a clinically effective dose of orgotein. That exogenous SOD *in vitro* inhibits such potential dangers of superoxide and its derivatives has been reported in numerous publications which have been recently reviewed[19]. In addition, McCord, Babior, Johnson, Karnovsky, Roos, and their colleagues have shown that phagocytic cells, both neutrophils and macrophages, when 'turned-on' by a variety of stimulants, generate significant amounts of superoxide anion into the surrounding medium[20]. This often leads to an

Table 49.2 Structural features of superoxide dismutase

Molecular weight	31 200
Number of subunits	2 (identical)
Metals content	XCu^{2+}, $2Zn^{2+}$
Amino acid sequence	151 amino acid per subunit; 1 Tyr, 4 Phe, 1 sh, 1 S–S, 0 try
Crystal structure at 3 Å	4 subunits/unit cell
Carbohydrate or lipid	none
Native conformation	protease resistant

The properties tabulated are those of beef erythrocyte SOD[16,17] which is identical to the beef liver Cu-Zn enzyme. Cu-Zn SOD of other animals are also dimers with similar structures and stability[2].

early death for the activated phagocytes. Lysis *in situ* at an inflamed site releases lysosomal inflammants which can reinitiate this cycle and maintain an inflammation *in perpetuo*. Exogenous SOD can delay this phagocytosis-induced premature death *in vitro*[21] without interfering with bacterial killing by phagocytes[22]. Oyanagui has shown intravenously administered SOD to suppress oedema formation during the 'prostaglandin' phase of carrageenan-induced inflammation in rats[23]. We have found that exogenous orgotein protects lysosomes against autolysis *in vitro* at 37 °C and it has been reported that orgotein inhibits naphthylamidase release from histamine-stimulated human skin cells[24]. In a histopathological comparison of antiserum-injected skin sites in a reversed Arthus model in the guinea pig after systemic treatment with prednisolone or orgotein, we found that in the orgotein-treated animals the PMNs around the injection sites were distributed differently, were more normal in appearance, and that the sites were strikingly free of cellular debris[25].

Here, we want to present some facts and speculations on the pharmacologic action mechanism of this molecule which is remarkable both for its physico-chemical and pharmacologic, as well as its clinically-observed properties.

The orgotein used in our studies was the commercial product* from bovine liver. Bioassay procedures and clinical protocols used are described in the text and the legends to figures and tables.

We have explored whether further insight into the *in vivo* action mechanism of orgotein and the role of the O_2^- related phenomena can be obtained in animal models of induced inflammation. The models used by us so far cover a variety of species and inflammants, both chemical and immunological in action (Table 49.3). Orgotein is active in the standard models, as well as in others which we have developed in response to US regulatory registration requirements, using blind trials against placebo, for demonstration of efficacy in horses and dogs. To demonstrate efficacy in an animal model of induced inflammation, methodology and dose regimens optimal for synthetic anti-inflammatories often do not work well with orgotein. With appropriate experimental conditions, however, inhibition can be reliably produced with doses above 0.5–3 mg/kg. In different model systems, effective dose ranges vary and the slopes of the dose–response curves range from about 10% to 70% per log dose (Table 49.4). The safety of orgotein allows experiments at doses of several hundred mg/kg to be performed without the complicating features of toxicity. In fact, an acute LD_{50} is reached only at doses above 4 g/kg and then only when administered intravenously.

Carrageenan-induced pleurisy in rats[26] provides a model of inflammation where both exudate volume and cellular infiltration can be quantitated

---

* Orgotein under the trade name Palosein® is available for use in horses and dogs from Diagnostic Data, Inc., Mountain View, Ca 94043. For human use, it is prepared by the same company under the trade name Ontosein® and is presently available in the USA only for investigational use.

Table 49.3 Orgotein in models of inflammation

Model	Test species	Effective dose (mg/kg)
Carrageenan-induced		
Foot oedema	rats; mice	$\geqslant 1.0$
Abscess	rats; mice	$\geqslant 0.5$
Pleurisy	rats	$\geqslant 1.0$
Adjuvant-induced		
Foot oedema	rats	$\geqslant 3.0$
	mice	$\geqslant 2.0$
Reversed Arthus reaction		
	rats	$\geqslant 0.5$
	guinea pigs	$\geqslant 0.08$
Autoimmune glomerulo-nephritis		
	mice (NZB × W)F_1	2.0
$ZnCl_2$ Necrosis	dogs	$\geqslant 0.5$
Counterirritant		
4% iodine, 10% ether in soybean oil	horse	$\geqslant 0.01$

Orgotein produced statistically significant suppression of the signs of inflammation measured in the listed models when administered at or above the cited dose rate. Dose-response relationships were observed in all models except autoimmune glomerulonephritis in which only one dose rate was tested. Administration was by subcutaneous injection in laboratory animals and intramuscularly in horses. The highest potencies were measured when orgotein administration was initiated prior to the time of induction of inflammation.

Table 49.4 Dose–response relationships in animal models

Assay	Species	Zero effect intercept (mg/kg)	Maximum slope %1/log (dose)	Maximum inhibition observed (%)
Carrageenan-induced				
Abscess	rat and mouse	0.01	10	35
Foot oedema	rat	—	—	50
	mouse	2.0	60	50
Pleurisy	rat			
Volume		0.01	15	65
Leukocytes		0.2	15	45
PMN (% × WBC)		0.03	20	60
Reverse Arthus reaction				
	rat	0.3	70	70
	guinea pig	0.02	18	50

Carrageenan-induced inflammation in these three models was more sensitive to orgotein when measured 18–30 h after induction than when measured at 3–6 h. The data shown are for 24 h responses to carrageenan, with orgotein administration in one or two doses given between 3 h before and 3 h after carrageenan injection. Antiserum-induced inflammation was quantitated by the gravimetric method of Ungar (30) 2 h after intradermal injection of rabbit antiserum. Orgotein was administered 1 or 2 h prior to antiserum in this model.

simultaneously. When assessed in blind experiments at 24 h after injection of 0.15 ml of a 1% solution of carrageenan into the pleural cavity, subcutaneous orgotein administration produced statistically significant decreases in all of the measured responses (Table 49.5). In the dose range studied, inhibition of leukocyte infiltration and exudate volume have parallel dose-

Table 49.5 Carrageenan-induced pleurisy in rats

Treatment	N	Volume (ml)	Total leukocytes ($\times 10^{-6}$)	% PMN
Saline control	34	0.9–1.4	127–173	68–82
Orgotein treated				
2–3 mg/kg	28	0.65–0.75*	101–118	60–72*
8 mg/kg	12	0.42–0.76*	92–109*	57–66**
27–32 mg/kg	28	0.36–0.56**	74–100**	50–66**

The ranges of results obtained in seven experiments with 4 to 5 rats per group are shown. The orgotein dose is the total dose given in two s.c. injections equally divided between 1 h before and 4 h after induction. The statistical significances shown are representative of those obtained in the individual experiments. * $= p < 0.05$; ** $p < 0.005$ by Student's t-test.

response curves (Figure 49.1). The diminution of leukocyte infiltration in orgotein recipients at 24 h is almost entirely due to a decreased influx of polymorphonuclear neutrophil leukocytes (PMNs) (Table 49.6). We have found that injection of orgotein into rats causes a mobilization of PMNs from tissue depots into the circulation, which peaks 4–6 h after orgotein administration. This phenomenon may be responsible for the fact that

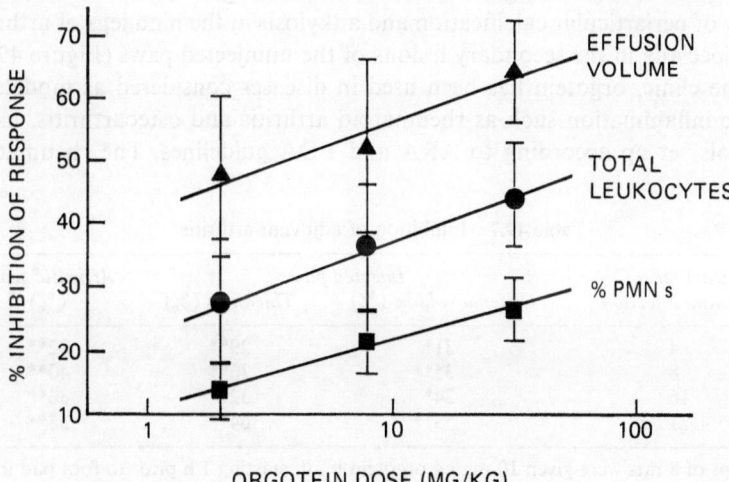

Figure 49.1 *Rat carrageenan pleurisy*. Results of three experiments with 4 rats per dosage group were pooled to produce the dose-response relationships shown. The methods used were the same as in Tables 49.5 and 49.6.

Table 49.6 Effects of orgotein on cellular responses in the carrageenan-pleurisy model

Response	Uninjected control	Pleurisy control	Pleurisy treated	% Inhibition
Total leukocytes	5×10^6	150×10^6	90×10^6	40*
% PMN	5	75	60	20*
Number of PMN	0.2×10^6	110×10^6	54×10^6	50*
Number of non-PMN	5×10^6	40×10^6	36×10^6	5

Details of the effect of a total of 30 mg/kg orgotein on cellular responses in a representative experiment summarized in Table 49.5 show that the decrease in pleurisy leukocytes induced by orgotein results almost exclusively from a reduction in the numbers of PMN present. PMN are still the predominant cell type in these exudates. * = $p <0.05$ by Student's t-test.

orgotein does not appear to inhibit PMNs in carrageenan pleurisy when scored 6 h after carrageenan injection. These observations show that orgotein can influence the PMN response which characterizes acute inflammatory events and distinguishes it from the usual non-steroidal anti-inflammatory agents[27].

Polyarthritis induced in the rat by injection of *M. tuberculosis* in perhydrosqualene, as proposed by Beck and Whitehouse[28], responds well to subcutaneously administered orgotein, which diminishes both primary and secondary immunological responses (Table 49.7, Figure 49.2 and 49.3). The inhibition of the arthritic changes persists through the treatment period and for at least 3 weeks beyond, representing a true inhibition of inflammation and not merely a delay in response to the adjuvant.

When given 5 days per week for 6 weeks, starting on the day of adjuvant injection, subcutaneous orgotein treatment caused significant inhibition in the density of periarticular calcification and ankylosis in the hind legs of arthritic rats, especially in the secondary lesions of the uninjected paws (Figure 49.4).

In the clinic, orgotein has been used in diseases considered as models of chronic inflammation such as rheumatoid arthritis and osteoarthritis, using protocols set up according to ARA and FDA guidelines. The rheumatoid

Table 49.7 Inhibition of adjuvant arthritis

Days since adjuvant injection	Injected paw Oedema volume (%)	Thickness (%)	Arthritic score (%)
4	31*	29**	32**
8	35**	36**	40**
16	34*	32*	36**
21	53**	64**	38**

Groups of 8 rats were given 10 mg/kg orgotein b.i.d. starting 1 h prior to foot pad injection of 0.05 ml of Perrigen PW. Oedema volume was measured by Archimedes' principle and paw thickness by micrometer caliper. Arthritic score included both injected and uninjected paws. Statistical significance was calculated versus the arthritis controls without correcting for normal growth of control paws. *$p \leqslant 0.05$; **$p \leqslant 0.005$ by Student's t-test.

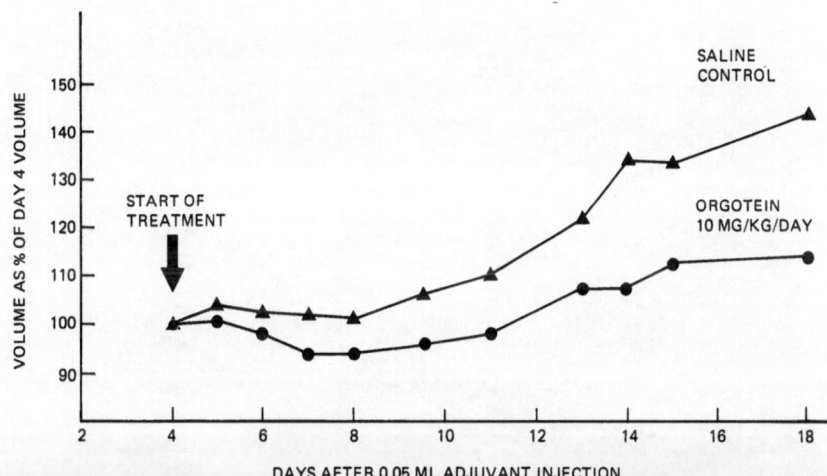

Figure 49.2 *Time course of arthritic development in adjuvant-injected hind paws.* Paw volumes were measured by mercury displacement at one or two day intervals after injection of 0.05 ml of Perrigen PW (Calibiochem) into one hind paw of Sprague-Dawley derived albino rats. Rats were assigned to the treated and untreated groups on day 4 so that the average volume increase for the two groups at the peak of the primary response (day 4) was identical. Orgotein was administered 5 days/week as a single daily s.c. dose of 10 mg/kg from day 4 until day 18

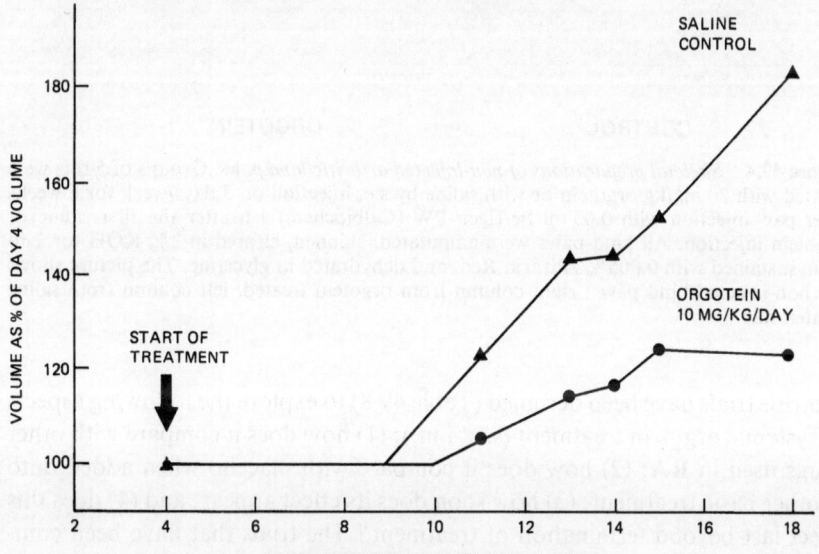

Figure 49.3 *Time course of arthritic development in non-injected hind paws.* The volumes of the uninjected paws of the rats in the experiment of Figure 49.2 were measured similarly. Secondary lesions of polyarthritis began to appear at day 10 to 11 in both groups. Orgotein treatment was the same as outlined in Figure 49.2

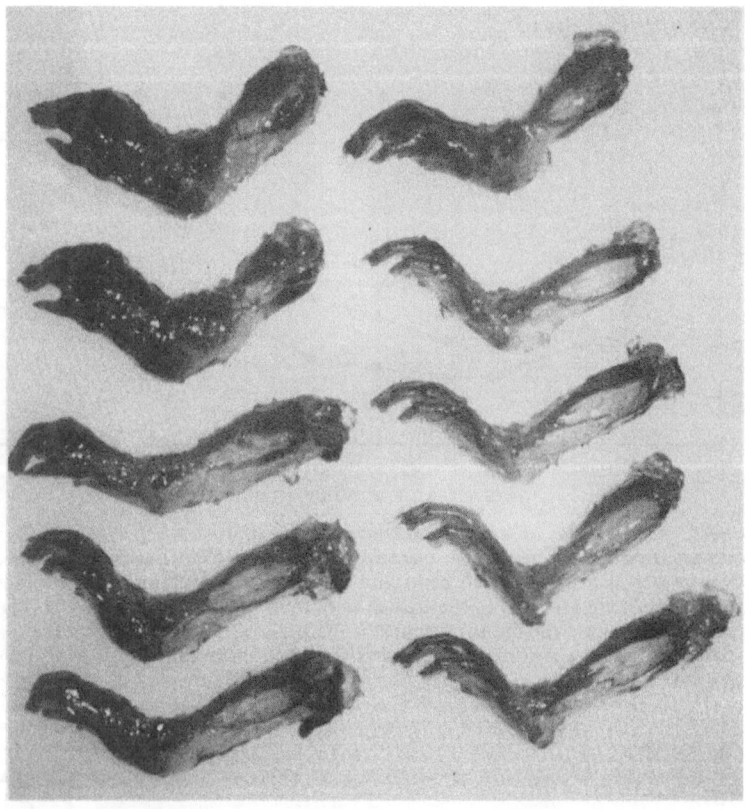

CONTROL   ORGOTEIN

Figure 49.4 *Skeletal preparations of non-injected arthritic hind paws.* Groups of 5 rats were treated with 20 mg/kg orgotein or with saline by s.c. injection on 5 days/week for 6 weeks after paw injection with 0.05 ml Perrigen PW (Calbiochem) 1 h after the first saline or orgotein injection. All hind paws were amputated, skinned, cleared in 2% KOH for 2 to 4 days, stained with 0.005% Alizarin Red, and dehydrated in glycerine. The picture shows the non-injected hind paws; right column from orgotein treated, left column from saline treated rats

arthritis trials have been designed (Table 49.8) to explore the following aspects of systemic orgotein treatment (s.c., i.m.): (1) how does it compare with other drugs used in RA; (2) how does it compare with placebo when added onto another basic treatment; (3) how soon does its effect appear; and (4) does this effect last beyond termination of treatment? The trials that have been completed so far support the observations in animals that orgotein is an effective, non-analgesic, and very safe anti-inflammatory drug. Its effects are seen within $\frac{1}{2}$–$1\frac{1}{2}$ months after start of treatment and last for more than 1 month after termination of treatment. Its benefit–risk ratio is far better than for gold. It produces a significant increase in improvement when used in conjunction

Table 49.8   Double-blind trials on orgotein efficacy in rheumatoid arthritis

| Country | No. of trials | No. of PTS/trial | Dose (mg) | | | Study time (wks) | Reference drug | Concomitant medication | |
			Per injection	Total				To be kept constant	To be used as needed
USA₁	4	24	8	320	16	Placebo	Cortico-steroid + ASA	Propoxyphene
USA₂	3	24	8	320	16	Placebo	ASA	Propoxyphene
USA₃	3	24	8	320	16	Placebo	Gold + ASA	Propoxyphene
England	1	24	12	652	26	Penicilla-mine	—	Other anti-inflammatories
France	1	31	4 or 12	214 or 652	26	Gold	—	Paracetamol; other anti-inflammatories*
Belgium	1	34	8	368	26	Gold	—	Other anti-inflammatories*

* Constant or reduced

Table 49.9   Controlled trials in rheumatoid arthritis

| Reference drug (dose) | Orgotein dose | | Duration of treatment (months) | Efficacy Orgotein vs. ref. drug | Safety Orgotein vs. ref. drug |
	mg/inj.	Total (mg)			
Placebo	8	320	3	Significantly better ($p < 0.05$–0.0005)	Comparable
Penicillamine*	12†	552	6	Same in morning stiffness, swelling, grip-strength	Much safer
Gold (75 mg/week)	4†	184	6	Same at $\geqslant 2$ inj./week of orgotein	Much safer
Gold (75 mg/week)	8†	368	6	Same at $\geqslant 2$ inj./week of orgotein	Much safer
Gold (75 mg/week)	12†	552	6	Same	Much safer

* 250 mg/day for 2 weeks, 500 mg/day for next 2 weeks, 750 mg/day for next 2 weeks etc. up to 2500 mg/day

† 3 inj./week for 4 weeks, 2 inj./week for 12 weeks, 1 inj./week for 10 weeks.

with corticosteroids and aspirin (Table 49.9). In active osteoarthritis, where the pathology is localized, the protocol called for orgotein (Table 49.10) to be given locally into the joint. The results of such a trial[10] show that orgotein is very effective when injected into and around the site of a chronic inflammation (Table 49.11).

Both the rheumatoid and the osteoarthritis trials confirm the animal data that orgotein does not act as an analgesic, as it has but minor effects in patients who are in pain because of morphological changes not related to

Table 49.10 Protocol parameters of double-blind placebo-controlled trial in osteoarthritis

	Protocol parameters
Patient selection	X-ray evidence of osteoarthritis of knee joints combined with active inflammation
No. of patients	44
Dosages of experimental drugs (orgotein, placebo)	2 mg injected into each knee joint every 2 weeks for 6 months
Parameters followed:	
Pain	Day pain, night pain, pain walking, use of analgesics
Function	Longest distance walked, limp, use of aids, stair climbing
Overall evaluation	Patient's evaluation, doctor's evaluation
Safety	Patients asked about possible side-effects

Table 49.11 Results of double-blind placebo-controlled trial in osteoarthritis

	Mean change	
Evaluated parameter	*Orgotein*	*Placebo*
Change in pain (%)	−80.0†	−31.3
Change in use of analgesics (%)	−60.7*	−30.0
Change in impairment of function (%)	−42.6*	−15.9
Doctor's evaluation (units)[a]	+120.0†	+57.0

[a] 0 = no change; 100 = improved; 200 = much improved
* $p < 0.05$ (Student's t-test)
† $p < 0.01$ (Student's t-test)

active inflammation. However, if the pain is caused by inflammation it subsides on orgotein treatment as the inflammation subsides.

The efficacy of orgotein in the amelioration of side-effects caused by high-energy irradiation in patients with bladder-tumours (Table 49.12) can be considered as an example of its effect on an acute inflammation. The results[11] show that 4 mg orgotein injected s.c. after each daily radiation treatment prevents or ameliorates to a significant degree the radiation-induced side-effects in the bladder and bowel (Table 49.13).

We are obtaining further information on the *in vivo* action mechanism by using animal models more sensitive to small differences in orgotein potency in anticipation that they will be sensitive to differences in its molecular structure. Carrageenan-induced foot oedema[29] in the mouse, modified for gravimetric quantitation, is an example of an assay in which the slope of the orgotein dose–response curve is steep, i.e., up to 60% per log dose (Figure 49.5). In our experience, this assay also measures the activity of subcutaneously administered orgotein much more reliably when quantitated 24 h after carrageenan injection rather than the more usual 3–6 h interval.

Table 49.12 Protocol parameters of double-blind placebo-controlled trial on orgotein efficacy in ameliorating side-effects due to radiation therapy of bladder tumours

	Protocol parameters
Patient selection	Patients with bladder tumours T2–T4
No. of patients	38
Orgotein or placebo dosage	4 mg subcutaneously after completion of daily radiation therapy
Radiation dosage	6400 or 8400 rad
Parameters evaluated	Maximal voiding volume, voiding frequency, pain, proctitis, medication used

Table 49.13 Results of double-blind trial on the efficacy of orgotein over placebo in ameliorating side-effects due to radiation therapy of bladder tumours

Improved parameters	*Level of statistical significance* (p)
Maximal voiding volume	<0.05[a]
Interval between voidings during day	<0.05[a]
Severity of signs and symptoms from bladder	<0.05[a]
Per cent visits with diarrhoea	<0.025[a]
Per cent of 'diarrhoea visits' requiring medication	<0.001[a]
Dose of antidiarrhoeal medication	<0.0025[b]

[a] Chi-square test
[b] Student's *t*-test

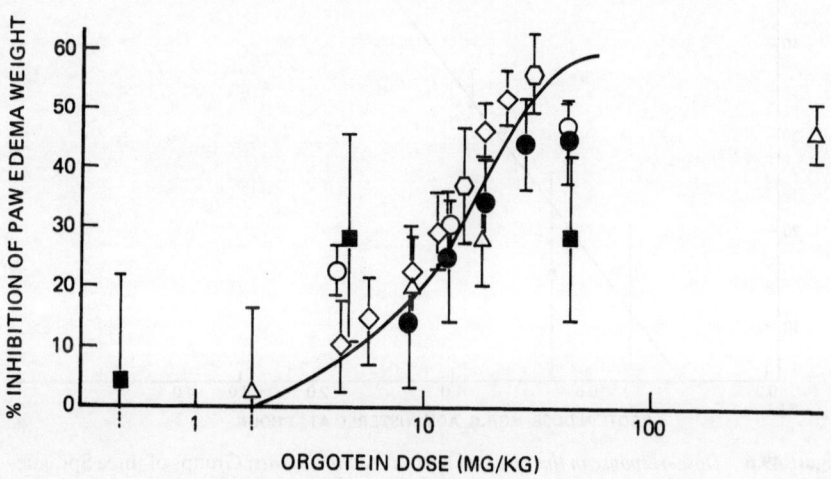

Figure 49.5 *Dose–response relation in the carrageenan paw/oedema model.* Groups of 10 mice per dose were injected in one hind foot pad with 0.03 ml of 1 % carrageenan to induce oedema which was measured after 24 h by weighing both amputated feet of each mouse. Plotted are the results of six experiments. The indicated orgotein doses were administered s.c., divided equally between 1 h prior to and 3 h after carrageenan injection

The reversed Arthus model in the rat, quantitated by the gravimetric method of Ungar[30], is an example of an immunologically-induced inflammation in which orgotein can produce up to 80% inhibition and also a slope of over 60% per log dose in the 0.5–5.0 mg/kg range (Figure 49.6).

By virtue of their steep slopes both these assays permit reliable determination of potency differences as small as 20% or less. This was demonstrated by blind runs comparing sets of 'standards' to sets of 'unknowns' with 80% potency (Table 49.14).

These assays, thus, can be used for exploration of the *in vivo* action mechanism of orgotein by comparing the assay potency of the native molecule to that of chemically modified preparations, some of which exhibit but slightly altered physicochemical properties, even though they have significantly reduced SOD activity[31]. Preliminary data show that SOD activity and bioassay activity need not always be correlated. This indicates that properties other than the SOD activity of orgotein may be important contributors to its

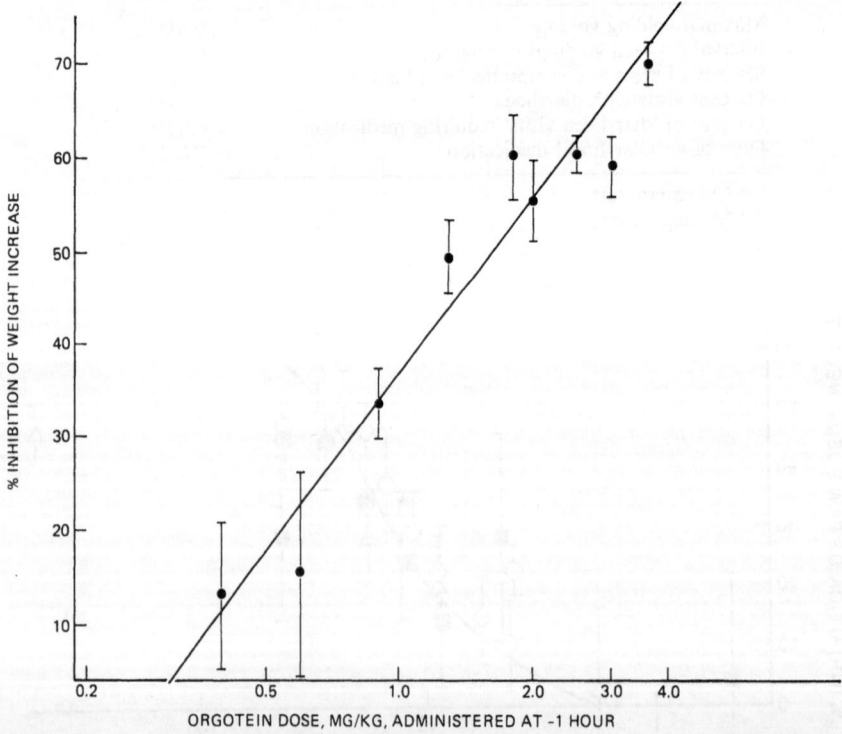

Figure 49.6 *Dose–response in the reversed Arthus reaction in rats.* Groups of three Sprague–Dawley rats per dose received the indicated dose of orgotein 1 h prior to intradermal injection of 0.05 ml of rabbit anti-rat serum at four dorsal sites and 0.05 ml saline at the four contralateral sites. 2 h after the intradermal injections, the rats were sacrificed and skinned and the skins punched at the i.d. sites. The 13 mm diameter skin punches were weighed to the nearest 1 mg and the oedema weight calculated as the difference between the weights of the saline-injected and the antiserum injected sites

Table 49.14   Mouse carrageenan footpad oedema

Orgotein concentration (mg/ml)	Day 1 Std = 100%	Day 1 Unk = 80%	Day 2 Std = 100%	Day 2 Unk = 80%	Day 3 Std = 100%	Day 3 Unk = 80%
			% Inhibition of weight increase			
0.63	12.5	11.4	14.1	9.8	16.8	9.7
1.25	35.0	26.0	25.9	20.4	27.9	22.0
2.5	54.4	46.4	49.8	45.2	53.0	47.9
Potoncy, unknown as % of standard $\pm$s.d.	83.6 ± 8.6		79.7 ± 10.7		75.7 ± 16.6	
Mean potency of unknown $\pm$s.d.			$79.7 \pm 4.0\%$			

Groups of 10 mice at each dose were treated s.c. with two equal doses of orgotein 1 h before and 3 h after carrageenan injection into one hind foot. Oedema was measured as the weight differences between the paired hind feet 24 h after carrageenan injection. The mice used were Swiss-Webster males and females over 6 weeks of age. The oedema weight in untreated mice was usually 40–50 mg per paw, and was measured to the nearest 1 mg

potency observed in bioassays, and perhaps in the clinic as well. Continued development of models of higher specificity, we think, will produce a clearer delineation between effects attributable to the enzymatic activity and to other properties of the protein. Such an understanding should permit a more goal-oriented use of orgotein and its derivatives in the clinic.

References

1. United States Adopted Names Council (1971). New Names List No. 106. *J. Am. Med. Assoc.*, **218**, 1936
2. Huber, W. and Saifer, M. G. P. (1977). Orgotein, the drug version of bovine Cu–Zn superoxide dismutase: I. A summary account of safety and pharmacology in laboratory animals. In: *Superoxide and Superoxide Dismutases* (A. M. Michelson, J. McCord and I. Fridovich, eds.) (London: Academic Press)
3. Carson, S., Vogin, E. E., Huber, W. and Schulte, T. L. (1973). Safety tests of orgotein, an antiinflammatory protein. *Toxicol. Appl. Pharmacol*, **26**, 184
4. Breshears, D. E., Brown, C. D., Riffel, D. M., Cobble, R. J. and Cheesman, S. F. (1974). Evaluation of orgotein in treatment of locomotor dysfunction in dogs. *Mod. Vet. Pract.*, **55**(2), 85
5. Cushing, L. S., Decker, W. E., Santos, F. K., Schulte, T. L. and Huber, W. (1973). Orgotein therapy for inflammation in horses. *Mod. Vet. Pract.*, **54**(7), 17
6. Linton, J. A. M. (1976). The use of orgotein in the treatment of soft tissue injuries of the horse. *Ir. Vet. J.* 30(4), 53
7. Faull, G. L., Baker, B. de B., v. d. Walt, H. S. and Hofmeyr, C. F. B. (1976). Clinical trials with orgotein (Palosein). *J. S. Afr. Vet. Assoc.*, **47**(1), 39
8. Marberger, H., Bartsch, G., Huber, W·, Menander, K. B. and Schulte, T. L. (1975). Orgotein: a new drug for the treatment of radiation cystitis. *Curr. Ther. Res.*, **18**(3), 466
9. Marberger, H., Huber, W., Bartsch, G., Schulte, T. L. and Swoboda, P. (1974). Orgotein: a new antiinflammatory metalloprotein drug: evaluation of clinical efficacy and safety in inflammatory conditions of the urinary tract. *Int. Urol. Nephrol.*, **6**(2), 61
10. Lund-Olesen, K. and Menander, K. B. (1974). Orgotein: a new antiinflammatory metalloprotein drug: preliminary evaluation of clinical efficacy and safety in degenerative joint disease. *Curr. Thera. Res.*, **16**(7), 706
11. Edsmyr, F., Huber, W. and Menander, K. B. (1976). Orgotein efficacy in ameliorating

side-effects due to radiation therapy: I. double-blind, placebo, controlled trial in patients with bladder tumors. *Curr. Thera. Res.*, 19(2), 198

12. Menander-Huber, K. B. and Huber, W. (1977). Orgotein, the drug version of bovine Cu–Zn superoxide dismutase: II. A summary account of clinical trials in man and animals. In: *Superoxide and Superoxide Dismutases* (A. M. Michelson, J. McCord and I. Fridovich, eds.) (London: Academic Press)

13. McCord, J. M. and Fridovich, I. (1969). Superoxide dismutase—an enzymic function for erythrocuprein (hemocuprein). *J. Biol. Chem.*, 244(22), 6049

14. Huber, W. and Schulte, T. L. (1972). Method of treating post-traumatic arthritis. US Patent No. 3, 637, 651

15. Huber, W., Chow, S. and Saifer, M. G. (1974). Enzymatic treatment of protein mixtures containing orgotein. US Patent No. 3, 806, 411

16. Steinman, H., Naik, V., Abernethy, J. and Hill, R. (1974). Bovine erythrocyte superoxide dismutase. Complete amino acid sequence. *J. Biol. Chem.*, 249(22), 7326

17. Richardson, J., Thomas, K., Rubin, B. and Richardson, D. (1975). Crystal structure of bovine Cu, Zn Superoxide dismutase at 3 Å resolution: chain tracing and metal ligands. *Proc. Natl. Acad. Sci. USA*, 72(4), 1349

18. Bors, W., Saran, M., Lengfelder, E., Spöttl, R. and Michel, C. (1974). The relevance of the superoxide anion radical in biological systems. *Curr. Top. Radiat. Res. Q.*, 9, 247

19. Fridovich, I. (1975). A free radical pathology: superoxide radical and superoxide dismutases, *Annu. Rep. Med. Chem.*, X, 257

20. Michelson, A. M., McCord, J. and Fridovich, I. (1977). *Superoxide and Superoxide Dismutases* (London: Academic Press)

21. Salin, M. L. and McCord, J. M. (1975). Free radicals and inflammation: protection of phagocytosing leukocytes by superoxide dismutase. *J. Clin. Invest.*, 56, 1319

22. Johnston Jr., R. B. *et al.* (1973). The role of superoxide anion generation in phagocytic bactericidal activity studies with normal and chronic granulomatous disease leukocytes. *J. Clin. Invest.*, 55, 1357

23. Oyanagui, Y. (1976). Participation of superoxide anions at the prostaglandin phase of carrageenan foot-oedema. *Biochem. Pharmacol.*, 25, 1465

24. Bitensky, L. Personal communication

25. Menander-Huber, K. B. and Gerstl, B. Unpublished observations

26. Vinegar, R., Traux, J. F. and Selph, J. L. (1973). Some quantitative temporal characteristics of carrageenan-induced pleurisy in the rat. *Proc. Soc. Ex. Biol. Med.*, 143, 711

27. DiRosa, M., Sorrentino, L. and Parente, L. (1972). Non-steroidal anti-inflammatory drugs and leukocyte emigration. *J. Pharm. Pharmacol.*, 24, 575

28. Beck, F. W. J. and Whitehouse, M. W. (1974). I. Drug sensitivity of rat adjuvant arthritis, induced with 'adjuvants' containing no mineral oil components. *Proc. Soc. Ex. Biol. Med.*, 146, 665

29. Winter, C. A., Risley, E. A. and Nuss, G. W. (1962). Carrageenan-induced edema in the hind paw of the rat as an assay for antiinflammatory drugs. *Proc. Soc. Ex. Biol. Med.*, 111, 544

30. Ungar, G., Kobrin, S. and Sezesny, B. R. (1959). Measurement of inflammation and evaluation of anti-inflammatory agents. *Arch. Int. Pharmacodyn.*, 123, 1–2, 71

31. Williams, L. D., Saifer, M. G. P. and Huber, W. (1977). Effects of chemical modification on the superoxide dismutase activity of the anti-inflammatory drug, orgotein. Abstracts, 173rd *National Meeting, American Chemical Society, New Orleans, LA*, March 1977

Discussion 49

R. Vinegar: (USA)	If orgotein inhibits the cells or the neutrophils from coming in in the carrageenan pleurisy, would that not provide a mechanism for its action in so far as inhibiting the prostaglandin phase is concerned, because the cells do not come in; they do not produce prostaglandins. To me this seems very reasonable.
Huber:	I would agree.
Vinegar:	Does the orgotein itself immobilize neutrophils? Is it itself an irritant?
Huber:	Yes. Time is limited, but we have done studies, upon injection, be it intraperitoneal, be it subcutaneous, be it intra-muscular, in animals, of orgotein itself. These are normal animals. There is a mobilization of PMNs which peaks at 4 hours and which returns to normal at about 24 hours. This is one of the reasons why we think it essential—in order to demonstrate the efficacy in an animal model—not to look at the inflamed sites at three or four hours, but to do so at 24 hours when the secondary mobilization involvements of PMNs are over.
D. Branceni: (France)	I was wondering about the route of administration in animals which seemed to be subcutaneous in one experiment. Was it always subcutaneous?
Huber:	In animal experiments we prefer, merely for reasons of methodology, to give it subcutaneously, usually into the scruff of the neck. Intramuscular injection is equally effective. In fact determinations of half-time concentration in the serum show just about the same for both routes.
Branceni:	It might be worth thinking about an eventual non-specific irritant action. Was inactivated enzyme perhaps used as a control?
Huber:	Inactivated enzyme? Yes. We have done that, and of course we have used placebo as a control. The commercial preparation is a lyophilized powder stabilized with two parts of sucrose per one part of protein.
M. Jayson: (UK)	Dr. Huber's experiments all showed efficacy in acute experiments against the various inflammatory mediators, whereas the clinical trials drew comparisons with gold and penicillamine which seemed to behave in quite a different way clinically and in which there are quite delayed effects against rheumatic disease with the benefits not developing for several weeks or for a couple of months. Would Dr. Huber comment?
Huber:	We did look at the adjuvant-induced polyarthritis, particularly where its immunological phases are considered a parallel to chronic inflammation, and there orgotein is effective. The effect is simply that the molecule appears to be as effective against chronic inflammatory events as against acute, and the radiation-induced side-effects on the bladder and the bowel are, of course, representative of an acute inflammatory event.
Jayson:	That seems quite different from the effects of gold and penicillamine.
Huber:	Yes. To be sure. But since the orgotein effects, at least in our hands, have been shown to be fairly long-lasting, we felt that it would be much

541

Jayson:

more representative to compare it against something like gold and penicillamine rather than, for example, aspirin. It was done deliberately. My second point concerns copper and zinc. I am not quite clear how much is contained in the molecule, but there is some evidence to suggest that copper may possess some anti-inflammatory properties. There has been some evidence from the USA that chelating it with various anti-inflammatory drugs will potentiate their anti-inflammatory action; that in experimental systems it will inhibit the formation of the prostaglandin E series—which until this meeting I thought were by and large inflammatory—and potentiate the PGF series, which I always thought of in the past as anti-inflammatory. In various forms of inflammatory diseases there are increases in the serum copper which it has been suggested may be a protective action in the body against inflammation. I wonder whether it might be a function of the copper itself.

Likewise there has been some experimental evidence to suggest that zinc preparations may have an anti-inflammatory effect in rheumatoid arthritis.

Huber:

We have considered the same thing. I can make two statements. Both the copper and the zinc in the native enzyme molecule are exceedingly tightly chelated at physiological pHs. In fact, dialysis against *millimolar* EDTA does not remove it.

The other thing we have done is to look at the effects of very high doses of orgotein. An LD_{50} can be found at doses of about 5500 mg/kg given intravenously, which is comparable to giving about 20 mg/kg copper. If parallel experiments are done with, for instance, copper glycinate, or copper EDTA, or zinc preparations, the toxicity of those preparations is higher by a factor of 5–10. From that can be drawn the working conclusion that the metals that sit in the protein molecules are probably functioning as a total rather than as a part.

F. A. Kuehl, Jr.
(USA)

Dr. Huber's findings are certainly consistent with the findings that I discussed very briefly yesterday. I did not discuss the nature of the free radical at all, but derived from the conversion of BGD to H and from oxidation of arachidonic acid. But the stability of the signal is very consistent with it being super-oxide and I should like to suggest the possibility that the superoxide we are dealing with is derived from oxidation of arachidonic acid—as I mentioned yesterday.

Huber:

Yes. I agree. Obviously where there are hydro-peroxide formations in the prostaglandin molecules, that seems a logical site for a super oxide dismutase to interact.

I. L. Bonta:
(The Netherlands)

I would also question this matter of the copper and the zinc. If orgotein or hepatocuprein are given simultaneously with a copper chelator, or, for example, with a thiol agent, is anything known about how the interaction would work, or is there any interaction? So far—and I must emphasize this—we have seen that under physiological pHs there is no interaction. This is one of the most stable chelates of which I am aware—probably by design. It fulfils, physiologically speaking, an enormously important defence mechanism in the body.

If one goes to a pH of the order of 5 or less, then the copper and the zinc start to come out, and then dialysis against EDTA or any other chelators will change it.

Huber:

It is well known that in certain local tissue damage the pH goes down, so that might have some influence.

Bonta:

If indeed these pHs go into the area of 4.5, then dialysis against 10th millimolar EDTA will remove all the copper, or eliminate the specific enzyme activity in a period of about $2\frac{1}{2}$–3 hours *in vitro*.

F. DeHalleux:
(Belgium)

I was interested to see that the product does not interfere—does not change intracellular killing of bacteria. Nor does it for phagocytosis.

In view of the role of peroxidase systems that produce free radicals

542

	in the cellular killing of some kinds of bacteria, including tuberculosis, I wondered whether Dr. Huber has tested this kind of exoplasmic phagocytosis of bacteria.
Huber:	Our work in this area is very limited, but Johnson and his group and McCord and his associates have looked at these phenomena quite extensively and their data are published in the literature. They show that as long as the superoxide dismutase is extracellular, it does not interfere with the intracellular processes. Of course if there is SOD in the medium and there is invagination into a lysosomal vacuole, a very small amount of superoxide may go in, but it does not seem in any way to interfere with the bactericidal or the phagocytosing phenomena of the PMN's neutrophils and macrophages.
D. Sofia: (USA)	Does orgotein display anti-inflammatory activity in animals that have been adrenalectomized or hypophysectomized?
Huber:	Yes. It does. Adrenalectomized animals behave equally to non-adrenalectomized animals.
M. Jasani: (UK)	From that last remark, as well as from many of Dr. Huber's remarks during the course of his presentation, the implication would seem to be that orgotein may be working in the extravascular or interstitial space. What is its molecular weight and are there any studies on its passage from the vessels into the interstitial space?
Huber:	Its molecular weight is 31 600. Its amino acid sequence was determined by Hill and his co-workers at Duke University.

We have looked at the transition from the vessels into the interstitial space and the metabolism is most intriguing. Upon intravenous administration, the half time of disappearance in the rat and the dog is 6–10 minutes, and it is selectively accumulated in the cortex of the kidney. It is probably redistributed from the cortex into the tissue because from looking at the urine, or the faeces, it appears but in minute quantities. For clinical purposes we prefer, therefore, apart from methodological considerations, a subcutaneous or intramuscular injection.

K. Fehr: (Switzerland)	The turnover of the polymorphs in rheumatoid arthritis in the joint is very high. The decay of those polymorphs is very fast and very pronounced. Has Dr. Huber studied this phenomenon, and does orgotein prevent this decay? Has he any data on the turnover when the orgotein is given in rheumatoids?

Secondly, in osteo-arthritis, as well as in rheumatoid arthritis, what was observed in regard to cartilage destruction?

Huber:	Referring to the first question, there is extensive work by Johnson, by McCord and by Babian—we have done it too—showing that *in vitro* PMNs that phagocytose are in a way self-programmed for destruction. This can be inhibited *in vitro* by extracellular SOD or orgotein. We have, because we are interested in the clinical use of the molecule, concentrated on *in vivo* situations, and we have indications that in synovial fluid orgotein stabilizes the PMNs, by which I mean that it extends the time necessary for *in situ* lysis, and therefore for the release of lysosomal inflammates.

The second, and perhaps more persuasive evidence is that we have looked in the reverse Arthus model of induced inflammation at the injection site and we have compared that against prednisilone and we find that with orgotein the distribution of the PMNs is different. It is much more uniform—this is at 90 minutes. They may in fact have already disappeared from the site. What is even more impressive is that where the prednisilone PMNs are surrounded by debris, are breaking open, are clustered around the inflamed vessels, the orgotein PMNs look nice and round yet they are phagocytosing clearly because they are full of stuff inside.

It may indeed be that the stabilization of the PMNs, and perhaps

543

the phagocytosing neutrophils and macrophages later on, is one way that this drug works in both chronic and acute inflammation.

Z. Bacq:
(Belgium)

May I ask what is the origin of the enzymes? Is it a pure enzyme, or are there any iso-enzymes, and when they are injected do they give birth to antibodies?

Huber:

In answer to the first question, we prepare it from bovine liver. The mammalian liver is the richest source of this enzyme. Wet liver contains about 0.03% superoxide dismutase. Our orgotein preparation as we use it for clinical trials is in excess of 96% pure. It is as pure a protein preparation as one can reasonably expect to produce. It is a very weak antigen—that is one of its nice things as far as its use in humans and animals is concerned.

There are several reasons why we think that that is so. It is highly soluble. It is an extremely compact molecule and it has a very low concentration of antigenicity-inducing amino acids. It has no tryptophan. It has about two tyrosines. Of course if it is used with adjuvant in the rabbit antibodies can be produced. We have produced them, we have purified them, and we have used them for studies of immunological cross-reaction—which incidentally is quite pronounced. The advantage for the clinical use is that the immune system of one species does not necessarily recognize the orgotein derived from another species as a foreign body protein, so that works quite well.

There are a number of patients where one can, and will, after orgotein administration, find positive titres of antibodies, but the interesting thing is that these patients do not show any immunological events. By the same token, once in a while in clinical trials one finds delayed hypersensitivity at the injection sites, and if one then looks at the antibody titres in the serum, they are very often negative.

R. Turner:
(USA)

I understand how it works, or may work, in rheumatoid arthritis, where there is a lot of inflammation and polymorphonuclear leukocytes. I have a little difficulty in conceptualizing an agent which also works in osteoarthritis where there is less inflammation.

In his clinical trials did Dr. Huber see any correlation in osteoarthritis with the amount of inflammation that was found?

Huber:

The protocol by definition required inflammation to be present. It is inflammatory osteoarthritis. As I tried to point out, in the osteoarthritic where all that there is is a morphological change, the drug is not effective, and, further, it is not effective on the pain parameters at all.

50

Humoral control of monocytopoiesis (*Abstract*)

D. VAN WAARDE AND E. HULSING-HESSELINK (The Netherlands)

Ed: Unfortunately the complete manuscript was not received in time for publication.

During inflammatory reactions induced in mice by an intraperitoneal injection of particulate substances the number of peritoneal macrophages increases and a monocytosis occurs. The regulation of this increase of mononuclear phagocytes in the tissues and circulation has been investigated. It has been demonstrated that serum of these mice contains a factor increasing monocytopoiesis (FIM). FIM could be demonstrated during the early phase of an acute or chronic inflammatory reaction. The highest level was always reached before the highest number of peripheral blood monocytes was attained, indicating that this factor acts on monocyte precursors. FIM has been shown to increase monocyte production by reducing the cell–cycle time of the promonocytes and increasing the number of these cells; there is evidence that FIM also affects the mitotic rate of the monoblasts.

FIM is a protein, lacking carbohydrate moieties essential for its function, and has a molecular weight between 18 000 and 24 000 Daltons. FIM is not a clotting factor nor a biologically active fragment of a complement factor. It has no chemotactic activity towards macrophages.

FIM activity could be demonstrated in extracts of normal peritoneal cells. After induction of a sterile peritonitis, the FIM activity of peritoneal cell extracts decreased and returned to normal values when the inflammation subsided.

These findings lead us to postulate a scheme for the humoral control of monocytopoiesis during acute inflammatory reactions in which the increase of monocyte production is regulated by FIM and a counter-regulatory effect is exerted by a monocytopoiesis inhibitor (MPI).

Discussion 50

S. Normann: I should like to ask about the specificity of this factor. Dr. van Waarde
(USA) has demonstrated that it elevates the monocytic series, but is there any
elevation of other leukocytes such as PMNs or lymphocytes, or is this
specific for this series?

van Waarde: It is a specific event. The number of polymorphonuclear leukocytes
or lymphocytes is not increased, or shows only a moderate increase
which in general is not significant, following injection of any of these
sera.

However, in the primary reaction to silica or latex neutrophilic
granulocytes are found.

Normann: Dr. van Waarde has emphasized the particulate nature of the stimulus
and I therefore presume that where other types of stimuli are used—
inflammatory stimuli that are not particulate—this response would
not be seen.

van Waarde: Yes. We used newborn calf serum at the commencement of the study
but newborn calf serum diffuses into the serum and one then has to
prove that the newborn calf serum components that are present in
the mouse serum are not the cause of the inflammation or of the
monocytosis found after the injection of these mice sera. It can be
proved and work has been published in *Cell Tissue Kinetics* (1976)—
January 1976.

P. Davies: Has any attempt been made to produce FIM *in vitro* by exposure of
(USA) macrophages to any of the inciting stimuli, or for that matter to any
other stimuli?

van Waarde: No. That has not yet been tried. Extracts of macrophages have been
produced—as was shown—and they are fresh macrophages, but when
they are cultured the results are not clearcut and we cannot claim to
have activity in the supernatant or in the cells.

W. E. Parish: First, a point on the first question. We have done the same sort of test
(UK) using silica and if serum is injected there is a biphasic reaction in which
polymorphs come first, with the mononuclear cells later. These two
things can be separated on gel filtration so that more than one factor
is released in a whole serum with the acute inflammatory response.

Has Dr. van Waarde any evidence that the increased maturation in
the bone marrow is a response to something acting directly on the
bone marrow or to cells being drawn out of the bone marrow in a
feedback mechanism?

van Waarde: The last point remains possible, but in our opinion it is not very likely
because the increase in monocyte production and the increase in the
mitotic activity of the promonocytes precedes the monocytosis. After
6–12 h the production of monocytes is increased and it is only after
12–24 h that monocytosis can be seen to develop in these animals.

Parish: So that the increased cell division occurs before the release?

van Waarde: I believe so.

HUMORAL CONTROL OF MONOCYTOPOIESIS

Parish: We tried rather a silly experiment. We injected the serum, plus a mass of normal monocytes in the hope that we might show a depression. In fact normal monocytes alone cause increased maturation of monocytes in the bone marrow.

J.-P. Giroud:
(France) When the silicate is injected, how long is it before the phenomena can be seen?

van Waarde: We have tested from 18 to 192 h. At 192 h we no longer find FIM, or rather we can no longer demonstrate it. It may be apparent earlier than 18 h. I would not know since we have not tested. But it is at least 18–144 or 168 h.

G. Vaes:
(Belgium) Referring back to Dr. Davies's question, we have developed a nice system of development of macrophages from rabbit bone marrow in culture. The advantage of the system is that it works without the addition of any conditioned medium.

Having recently been visited by Dr. van Furth, and having heard about the FIM factor, we are now wondering whether some cells differentiating at the initial phases of the cultures together with the macrophages could produce something like FIM that would allow the differentiation of the macrophages, which might explain why we did not need any conditioned medium.

For a proper differentiation a very peculiar medium, very high in serum, is needed. We have done some experiments, and we have looked at the medium of cultures where macrophages had been fully differentiated to see whether there was anything that would favour the differentiation of macrophages in cultures in a medium that would not allow a proper differentiation. The cultures are all negative so far and we have been unable to find anything, but of course these are negative experiments and they mean what they mean.

General Discussion

Chairman: C. M. Pearson

R. Vinegar:
(USA)

Referring back to Dr. Ferreira's work, if we are to make some sense from that type of study—not only Dr. Ferreira, but also the others—we must realize that the oedema that is produced, or the fluid that is produced—this type of foot oedema, or carrageenan pleurisy—that the fluid comes into two sources. One is a quick, very rapid accumulation which has nothing to do with inflammation and has to do with whatever mediators are there. There is another part which is due to inflammation, and the drugs only work against the inflammatory part, but not the initial part, the other mediators. In the rat foot the most likely mediator is serotonin and the anti-inflammatory agents will not work there.

Coming back to the development of hyperalgesia, this can be due to both parts, both accumulations of fluid, plus the mediators that may be released by the inflammatory cells that produce pain itself. All these hyperalgesias that do develop have their own individual rate of decay, so any amount of hyperalgesia measured at any function of time is, needless to say, a highly complex sum. In trying to explain it in terms of Dr. Ferreira's findings, this has to be related to his times. Unfortunately so far as my own work is concerned he has picked the wrong times because he has picked 2 h and four. The first phase is gone in 20 min. If he had done his measurements within 20 min that would have taken care of the immediate mediators in that part, and then to study it at 3 h would show what has now come to be termed the prostaglandin-like mediators responsible for that type of inflammation and that type of hyperalgesia.

Ferreira:

Dr. Vinegar's method of measuring hyperalgesia is completely different from mine. That is the main problem.

Vinegar:

We have different methods. I give a known force for a certain amount of time. It gives slightly different results, but at least we know what we are giving and that we are giving it for a known time.

Also we get no local analgesia with paracetamol. That is for sure.

D. Freed:
(UK)

Dr. van Waarde said that the monocytopoietic agent liberated from macrophages was not a complement component. That is the point on which I have doubts. I may be revealing my ignorance and I only know about complement what I read in the books, but it seems to me that this would do very well for one of the classical components, one of the classical pathways, C142. If I got it right, Dr. van Waarde treated his serum in such a way that it would remove components C_3 and subsequently by the alternative pathway but it would not remove the classical pathway components. Also, the stuff was protected by aminocaproic acid, which would protect C_1.

Would Dr. van Waarde comment?

GENERAL DISCUSSION

van Waarde: We have excluded the complement origin of the factor FIM in three ways:

(1) treating the animals *in vivo* with cobra venom factor which is supposed to remove the complement components from C_3 on;

(2) *in vivo* we tried to generate FIM from normal mouse serum by 'the addition of zymosan which again activates C_3 and on, and by activating the complement with aggregated IgG.

In the cobra venom factor treated mice, the factor could be generated as in normal mice, and it was not possible to generate FIM *in vivo* by one of the mentioned methods.

There is a further point, but it does not exclude Dr. Freed's point. We have used C_5 deficient mice, and these also generate FIM.

Freed: None of these would enable the possibility of C_1 to be excluded.

van Waarde: No, but it makes it highly unlikely.

Chairman's Summing-up and Future Trends

C. M. Pearson (USA)

I am expected, during the next few minutes, to summarize this morning's proceedings, but I feel that that is almost impossible to do. There have been so many questions, comments and discussion about the very nice papers that were given this morning, and I think I shall forgo that exercise.

I have had the privilege of attending all of the three sessions of this Congress; the first in Verona, the second in Paris, and the third here in London; and I have seen progressively increasing amounts of activity, information and results that make for an interesting amount of sense in relation to inflammatory mechanisms, although I think that we would all admit that we are still far from having all of the answers which are present in these complicated systems. Even though some of my main interests are in immunology, I shall forgo discussing much of immunology at this present time and during this meeting.

I was particularly interested in Professor Vischer's discussions a day or two ago about the neutral proteases. I believe personally that as we project into the future we shall pay a great deal of attention to the neutral proteases and that they will probably have more and more effect on bodily mechanisms, homeostasis, etc. They well may be a major mechanism in controlling inflammatory reactions. In such a sense they may function as biological modulators or regulators. Cathepsin-D, pronase, the elastases, the collagenases and the other neutral enzymes that function at or near normal body pH probably are responsible for maintaining homeostasis, maintaining a fair amount of the housekeeping of the body, and bringing things back to normal after an inflammatory event or some other kind of insult to the individual.

Some interesting points have come on the scene within the past year or two, not recorded here in this meeting, but have relevance to it. For instance, some new observations in tissue culture of striated muscle. There is now evidence in muscle, in tissue culture that after a few days even under the best of circumstances, the muscle fibres will spontaneously begin to show deterioration. Several Japanese workers have reported a number of very small peptides (5–10 amino acids, each from bacterial origins) that are inhibitors of neutral proteases, and to a lesser extent of some of the acid and alkaline proteases. These are pepstatin, leupeptin and anti-pain. They are very small peptides and they seem to have the ability of delaying or retarding the spontaneous deterioration of muscle in culture. When placed, for example, in a solution of DMSO so that they can permeate the cell membrane they will retard the breakdown of contractile proteins, myofibrils and other intracellular materials. These may well have some interesting applications when we all meet three years from now (in a location yet to be decided).

I am continuously amazed at the ingenuity of those who have worked with adjuvant arthritis. When I first saw adjuvant arthritis a number of years ago in our laboratory, I felt that it was a nice interesting model, I took it only so far by histology etc. and more recently our attempts to induce adjuvant arthritis with the small bacterial cell wall preparations have been met with a good deal of success. On the other hand, many of you have described a variety of alterations such as an increase in platelets, in acute phase reactant proteins, in prostaglandins, in the inhibition of the diseases by exogenous interferon (in small amounts). These observations are intriguing and in preventing this disease provide significant challenges, as well as possibilities that an understanding of some disease processes, such as lupus erythematosus and rheumatoid arthritis in the human, may be gained by studying this and similar models.

I was very interested, as all of us were, in the newer observations about the central role of the macrophage in a number of the reactions that involve the inflammatory circuit. Macrophages, or monocytes, it seems, were until fairly recently relatively rejected as important cells. They were considered generally to be cells that come in at the end of an inflammatory circuit and do the 'cleaning-up' process. But since it has now been shown that they can secrete C_3 which is then cleaved into a C_3 *a* and *b*, that they possess interactive properties with lymphocytes so to stimulate lymphokine formation as well as to produce a number of the other materials, including antibodies, that they possess antigen-processing and delivery (to lymphocytes) properties, as well as secreting acid hydrolases, prostaglandins, plasminogen activators and so forth they now become terribly interesting cells. These are new and important findings that were not known about in Verona and were only briefly speculated on in Paris.

Dr. Glynn mentioned that we need to know a great deal more about cell surface receptors and that we know very little about them. I believe that the first priority of the challenges for all of us—not only those of us in this room, but for biology in general—is to learn more about cell surface receptors because in the future I predict that they will provide a great deal of information about mechanisms, stimulation of cells, finding drugs etc.—cymetedine has just been discovered as a small polypeptide which blocks the histamine receptor site in the gastric mucosa, and therefore retards HCl secretion and seems to be successful in treating peptic ulcers. Many other rather simple agents will be forthcoming when we know more of the location of cell surface receptors, their configuration and their reactive sites, so that they can be blocked or stimulated as the case may be in order to try to prevent some of the adverse inflammatory events that have been discussed here.

One interesting point that has been made in addition to the histamine receptor matter just mentioned is something that many of you may not have heard of. It is a story about acetylcholine receptors and it provides us with some information that is extremely practical now—in 1977. There is a material, a-bungerotoxin, derived from snake venom, that has specificity for acetylcholine receptors. These receptors have now been shown to have a molecular weight of about 6000 and they contain both carbohydrate and protein. After applying this toxin, especially in the electric eel organ end-plate where they are concentrated in very large numbers, it is possible to then remove the receptors and the toxin, cleave those two and come out with a pure receptor site.

What has been the outcome of studies of the acetylcholine receptors? Ach. receptors are not only located in the electric eel organ (in order to generate a very high voltage there) but they are also present at motor end-plates in muscle in significant quantities, and in addition are located along the surface of muscle fibre membranes. By taking small quantities of these purified Ach. receptors, inoculating them in Freund's adjuvant into a rabbit, classical myasthenia gravis has been produced; a startling event indeed! The animals will develop profound weakness and myasthenia during the time of development of antibody to the Ach. receptors, and the animals must be preserved by artificial means—respiratory support, neostigmine, or whatever, in order to allow them to live long enough so as to make sufficient quantities of antibodies in order to label them so as to localize the Ach. receptor sites or muscle by fluorescent means, etc. These are very exciting events.

One other point that is pertinent to some discussion about the future is a development that was reported just a few weeks before this meeting. It has been known for some time that in the central nervous system there are receptor sites for opiates, morphine and its derivatives. Why in the world would there be receptors for morphine and morphine-like agents in the nervous system for alkaloids obtained from certain poppy flowers? In fact, these receptors are located on CNS cells, primarily in the pain pathways of the brain. The discovery, made many years ago, lay fallow for a number of years and then it occurred to some that perhaps there were materials that had a tertiary structure resembling the opiates that occur naturally in the human brain, or in the animal mammalian brain, and that were subserving a function of some type or another. As long ago as 1964, Dr. Li[1] who was at that time in Berkeley attempting to synthesize growth hormone from the pituitary, as he successfully did, also found another peptide that he called a-lipotropin.

Here was a substance that he sequenced with 91 amino acids for which there was *no* known biological activity. It was present in the pituitary, and in the neuro-hypophysis. So, since 1964 that material has been around and its amino acid sequence has been fully known about. It was also known that if an animal was given morphine, and developed the effects of the morphine dose, that brain homogenates when given to the animal or placed in contact with the opiate the morphine effects could be rapidly dispersed within a matter of a minute or two.

Recently Dr. Hughes and his group in Scotland[2], and Dr. Roger Guillemin, Dr. Ling and others in Southern California[3,4] have described two very interesting compounds or agents which they call the *enkephalins* (these are pentapeptides that seem to be derived from the β-lipotropin), or the *endorphins*. Guillemin, especially, has described the endorphins in four categories. From the 91 amino acids in β-lipotropin he has found four separate preparations by placing the purified compound in contact with brain extracts. His co-workers have termed these fractions alpha, beta, gamma, etc. and they contain from 15 to 26 amino acids in the different fractions. He has done studies on these to demonstrate that the a-endorphin when injected i.v. or into the brain ventricle produces in the rat transient analgesia on the side of the face and neck especially when injected intracysternally. This effect subsides after a short period of time. The most important of these small molecular weight 'mini-hormones' appears to be the beta-fraction, or the so-called C fragment, which has some 20 amino acids from number 61 to 81 of β-lipotropin. This compound has 5–10 times the activity as does pure morphine itself. It has been isolated from the pituitary and from the neuron hypophysis per se.

The point I am getting to in part is that the β-lipotropin found more than a decade ago by Li, and for which he could find no biological effect, is very probably a *pro-hormone* that is excreted by dendrites, neurones and so forth, and that cleavage (probably by local enzymes) occurs in the immediate location of those cells so as to give rise to their focal action, likely at receptor sites on the nervous system, that may well be influencing behaviour in some fashion or another. We are beginning to have a better understanding of the chemical effects of what makes us tick, and so forth.

Is it possible that some of the inhibitors, some of the stimulators, the antagonists and the others that we discuss at these meetings could well fit into the same category, that it is not only possible that these materials that I have discussed occur in the nervous system, but it is also possible that mesenchymal cells such as fibroblasts, osteoblasts, etc. could be producing in the local environment similar types of agents which then could be cleaved and have local activity; not only agents we already know about such as prostaglandins, histamine, 5-hydroxytryptamine, and various others assume importance to us, but also *pro-hormones* then could be broken down, or cleaved, locally and exert their effects to stimulate, for instance, collagen production, to stimulate an inflammatory reaction, to attract motile cells, to control local cell responses, etc. are very likely.

To come back for a moment a little closer to our field of inflammation and immune response, Bach and Carnaud[5] have some preliminary data to suggest that thymosin, as isolated, may itself be a precursor or one of several precursors for the potent thymic factors that are known to possess profound effects on lymphocyte (T-cell) differentiation and biological functions. I personally believe that there is a significant analogy between these areas. Moving from the nervous system to the mesenchymal system and to the monocyte and the circulating cells that come from the bone marrow and the spleen and the liver is really not too remote. It has been known for some time, for instance, that for no 'apparent' reason whatsoever material such as gastrin, usually thought to be a small peptide in the stomach, is also found in the central nervous system. Vaso-active intestinal peptides are also found in the central nervous system—in small quantities, as is somatostatin. Why are these agents in the CNS? It is very likely that they have no function in the nervous system—although I cannot say so for certain, and no one can at present—but obviously the nervous system has extensions, cells in the intestinal mucosa and so forth, that could equally be producing these small peptides that have direct action, inducing histamine release and other actions biologically that we now know about in human biology.

To come back briefly to the endorphins, I might mention one or two matters that I find extremely intriguing and to point out their significance and the potential significance of other pro-hormones that we may well be discussing in 1980 and beyond. When some of the aforementioned small peptides+20-amino-acids are inoculated into a rat, intracysternally or into the ventricle, they will produce a transient state in the rat that in the human resembles schizophrenia, especially the variety in which there is profound rigidity or the catatonic state. This will last for some 4 hours or so and then subside, and can be reversed almost immediately by some of the morphine antagonists such as naloxone. It is logical to think that perhaps some of the mental disorders that are present in a number of humans in the world in our mental institutions could theoretically be treated by a morphine antagonist or opiate antagonists with significant beneficial results. There are already (within the past 3 or 4 weeks) some reports (isolated reports, with some conflicting results) with the use of naloxone and other of these compounds in mentally-ill patients. These morphine antagonists are said to relieve a state of agitation, hallucinations and catatonia in a few people that have been tested with naloxone. Such effects are said to last for a period of 3 or 4 hours and then the condition returns as though there is a re-accumulation of the chemical agents which may well be affecting behaviour. These are very exciting results, very exciting times, and I believe also that the effects of the pro-hormones, small peptides, the locally acting compounds about cells, whether they be fibroblasts, monocytes or some of the other connective tissue cells, endothelial cells or synovial lining cells will play a significant role in our future meetings and in our further understanding of the mechanisms involved in the inflammatory reaction and in our ability to generate drugs and compounds to counteract these specific types of reactions in a more effective way that has so far not been possible, even by effecting the so-called pro-hormone, the inhibitor or the stimulator or whatever else.

Those happen to be my predictions for the next three years. We shall see how they turn out.

References

1. Li, C. H. (1964). Lipotropin, a new active peptide from pituitary glands. *Nature (London)*, **201**, 924
2. Hughes, J., Smith, T. W., Kosterlitz, H. W. *et al.* (1975). Identification of two related penta-peptides from the brain with potent opiate agonist activity. *Nature (London)*, **258**, 577
3. Ling, N., Burgus, R. and Guillemin, R. (1976). Isolation, primary structure and synthesis of a-endorphin, and γ-endorphin, two peptides of hypothalamic-hypophysial origin with morphinomimetic activity. *Proc. Nat. Acad. Sci. (USA)*, **73**, 3942
4. Guillemin, R. (1977). Endorphins, brain peptides that act like opiates. *N. Eng. J. Med.*, **296**, 226
5. Bach, J.-F. and Carnaud, C. (1976). Thymic factors. *Prog. Allergy*, **21**, 372

Section VII
Pharmacological Aspects: Man/Animal

CHAIRMAN: D. A. Willoughby

CO-CHAIRMAN: P. Franchimont

Co-Chairman's Opening Remarks

P. FRANCHIMONT AND G. HEYNEN

One of the most critical points in the study of anti-inflammatory drugs is the assessment of the clinical and biological activity due to inflammation. Most studies in man and animals are related to the human disease called rheumatoid arthritis. In this case we are faced with the assessment of the activity of a disease whose etiology is unknown, physiopathology unclear and whose course is unpredictable and variable from one case to another.

With these limitations, we have to choose criteria, which must be reliable and reproducible. For practical purposes (clinical evolution of anti-inflammatory drugs) these criteria should also be as simple as possible.

Let us review and discuss these criteria, which can be separated into two groups.

CLINICAL CRITERIA

As long as so many unknown variables are present in rheumatoid arthritis, the clinical criteria predominate over the biological ones and must be taken into account in the evaluation of the disease.

These are subjective and objective, and are listed in Table 1.

Table 1

Clinical criteria

---

1. *Subjective*
    A. Quantitative evaluation of articular pain
    B. Length of morning stiffness
    C. Time for appearance of pain after motion
    D. Daily analgesic consumption
2. *Objective*
    A. Ring test
    B. Local temperature
    C. Number of involved joints
    D. Changes in tenderness as scored by Ritchie's index
3. *Functional*
    A. Grip strength
    B. Time to walk a constant distance

BIOLOGICAL CRITERIA

The biological criteria are listed in Table 2.

Table 2

Biological criteria

1. Inflammatory tests
   Sedimentation rate
   Fibrinogen
   Haptoglobin
   CRP
   a_2-globulin
2. Immunological tests
   Immunoglobulins
   Rheumatoid factors
   Lymphocyte functions
   Complement
   Immune complexes

CONCLUSIONS

1. Clinical assessment is an end point.

2. The duration of the study must take into account the proposed goal of the clinical trial. For instance, if we look at the anti-inflammatory component, a short term study may be sufficient, but if we look at the anti-rheumatoid activity, long term study is mandatory.

3. The variable spontaneous course of rheumatoid arthritis, especially during the few first years of the disease, and the semi-quantitative or totally subjective feature of some criteria makes double blind studies essential.

4. The classical non steroid anti-inflammatory drugs acting on the acute phase of the inflammation (vasodilatation, inhibition of PG synthesis, etc.) have never been proved to fundamentally modify the course of the disease. We urgently need more basic perpetuating compounds truly affecting the major processes which are responsible for the self perpetuating activity of the disease. Among these processes, circulating immune complexes and disturbed lymphocyte function have recently received more attention, but remain under investigation. Penicillamine, gold salts and the recently introduced drug lévamisole have clinical effects. It will be most interesting to compare the clinical activity of these drugs with their assessment by these new immunological criteria.

51

Difficulties in the clinical evaluation of new anti-inflammatory drugs

G. KATONA (Mexico)

The experimental evaluation of new drugs with a supposed potential or expected beneficial effect on some pathological processes is, from the clinical point of view, an ancient activity of man who is trying to help sick people. Throughout the centuries there have been an enormous number of 'researchers' looking always for new possibilities in order to fight illness. Some of them are well-known personalities of the History of Medicine, but the majority are unknown soldiers of the eternal war.

The enhancement of our knowledge in pathology and clinic, as well as in biochemistry and pharmacology in the last hundred and fifty years, is the real source of the oncoming flow of new drugs; for which there is an absolute and imperative need to determine their real value, advantages or disadvantages, and even to assess the proper use of these new substances in clinical practice. Clinical pharmacology, or simply clinical trials, are reaching more and more importance; a reason why a large amount of people of different disciplines are looking for the best, more accurate and objective methods to determine the real therapeutic value of new drugs.

These trials, of course, are increasingly obtaining more importance within the pharmaceutical science, because very often the future of the new compound depends on the results of the first clinical experiences.

We have been working in this fascinating field for about 18 years and during this period we have had the opportunity to study 78 new anti-inflammatory drugs in rheumatic patients and performed about 134 different trials (Table 51.1). For this reason, a few months ago, I proposed to Professor Willoughby as a possible topic for this meeting the necessity to discuss the field experiences of a clinical investigator, and mainly, to talk about the difficulties in the clinical evaluation of new compounds which surged during this quite

Table 51.1 Clinical trials performed during the years 1959–1976 with different anti-inflammatory compounds*

I. NON HORMONAL ANTI-INFLAMMATORY COMPOUNDS

Name of compound	Trials performed	Double blind	Open	Objective methods
Aladione (diftalone)	5	4	1	
Alclofenac	1	1		
AL-0559 (5 amino-1 phenyl tetrazole)	1	1		
AY-23289 (prodolic acid)	2	2		
AY-21367 (αoxo 2 dibenzofuran butyric acid)	1	1		
Azathioprine	1	—	1	1
Clopirac (BRL-13856)	1	1		
Cetophenylbutazone	—	—	1	
Dantrolene†	1	1		
Droxaryl (P-butoxyphenyl-aceto hydroxamic acid)	1	1		
Diclofenac sodium	1	1		
DMSO (Dimethyl-sulfoxide)	1	—	1	
DF-55272 (aluminium flufenamate)	1	—	1	
ENM-19166	1	1		
EMD 26 644 (mercapto oxazolic-carbonic acid)	2	1	1	
Flufenamic acid	1	—	1	
Febuzine (tomanol)	1	—	1	
Fenoprofen calcium	3	3		
Fenbufen (Cl 82204)	2	2		
Indomethacin	10	4	5	1
Ibuprofen	5	4	1	
ICI 54-450 (4Chloro phenyl thiazol 4-acetic acid)	1	1		
Jonctum (N-acetyl hydroxyproline)	1	—	1	
Ketoprofen	4	2	1	1
K 4277 (indoprofen)	4	4		
Litial (hydroxyphenylbutazone)	1	—	1	
LH-150	1	—	1	
MK-231 (clinoril)	4	—	4	
MK 615	1	1		
Naproxen	14	8	4	2
Niflumic acid	3	2	1	
Phenylbutazone	1	—	1	
R-760 (flumefenine)	1	1		
Ro-4-5000	1	—	1	
Ro-2o-5700	2	1	1	
Rp 16091 (soripal)	1	1		
Sch 10304 (clonixin)	4	4		
Thiocolchicoside	1	—	1	
Tolectin	1	—	1	
Trimethylglycoside esther of the phenyl butazone	1	—	1	
Total of compounds	39			
No. of trials	89			

* Alphabetical order

† Muscle relaxant principally

EVALUATION OF NEW ANTI-INFLAMMATORY DRUGS

II. CORTICOSTEROIDS

Name of compound	Trials performed	Double blind	Open	Objective methods
Triamcinolone acetonide	1	—	1	
Steaoril glycolate of prednisone	1	—	1	
16βmethyl prednisolone	1	1		
6αmethyl prednisolone	1	1		
Triamcinolone	1	1		
Paramethasone	8	5	2	1
Ultralan (fluocortolone)	1	—	1	1
Dihydroparamethasone	1	1		
Flumethasone	4	2	2	
Paramethasone phosphate	2	1	1	
Fluocinolone acetonide (inj. intrart)	1	1		
Dexamethasone	2	2		
Cloprednol	5	2	2	1
15 different halogenated corticosteroids	15	—	1	
Alcohol of bethamethasone	1	1		

Number of compounds 29
Number of trials 45

long period. I will only try to point out some of these well-known problems that we have to face during our experimental work and also in our daily practice.

One of the main problems is how to transfer, how to extrapolate the biological and pharmacological findings in animals into human clinic. A thousand years ago, Avicena recommended that drugs should be tried, but he stressed out that 'testing drugs on a lion or on a horse might not prove anything about its effect on man'. This problem is nowadays still the same.

Today, when we take in our hands a new drug to be evaluated in human beings, there is always available an enormous amount of data, the results of many long years of careful investigations in the laboratories using all kinds of animals. The main target for the clinical investigator is still the efficacy and tolerance, expecting always something really different, something with additional and better characteristics of the already known compounds. In these new drug information pamphlets, one can find the results of hundreds of trials in thousands and thousands of animals like rats, dogs, cats, guinea pigs and some other exotic animals, and—not very often—in monkeys too. The results are generally very promising, and we can be sure that the new compound in the left back leg of the guinea pig proved to have 150 times more anti-inflammatory activity than aspirin; and now?—what does it mean in practice?—sincerely, not too much (!); as we can see in Tables 51.2 and 51.3, where I took only as an example the results of some biological assays performed, using differing methods in different animals with two relatively new anti-inflammatory compounds such as Tolectin and Fenbufen, comparing their well-known activity in clinical practice, taking as effective anti-

Table 51.2 Comparison of tolmetin with other anti-inflammatory compounds in protecting rats against oedema in animal/man

Inducing agent	ED_{30} (mg/kg)				
	Tolmetin	Indo-methacin	Phenyl-butazone	Aspirin	Flufenamic acid
Carrageenan	33	19	420	122	38
Relation: (dose, mg/kg)	1	0.57	12.73	3.7	1.15
Kaolin	7.8	2.2	21	67	43
Relation: (dose, mg/kg)	1	0.28	2.69	8.59	5.5
Recommended daily useful dose (mg) in man	1200	75	300	3000	1500
Dose (mg/kg)	17	1	4.3	43	21.2
Relation (dose, mg/kg)	1	0.06	0.25	2.5	1.46

inflammatory activity of each drug the average used daily maintenance dose (Table 51.2). As we can see, there is no relationship between the efficacy measurement in the biological experiments compared with the clinical; not even in the proportion of relative activity reported in the different trials and different animals (Table 51.3). Even in the case of the adjuvant arthritis, considering it as the more similar model to the inflammatory process observed in rheumatoid arthritis.

No doubt there are many factors which influence the activity of a drug, such as its absorption, excretion, transportation, protein binding, metabolism, plasma half-life, etc., which evidently determine their activity. Table 51.4, taken from Djerassi, illustrates the important differences found with one compound in different species of animals. The next table (Table 51.5) shows that the same compound can be found in a very variable concentration in different tissues and this can be another reason for the differences observed in the biological and clinical activity of the same compound. Resuming, I think that the results of the animal trials are only a guide, and they could give us only information about the possible anti-inflammatory effect of the drug, as well as of its toxicity. Tolerance can be observed only in clinical practice, this parameter being really an exclusive property of the human organism (headache, heartburn, dizziness, nausea, etc.).

The importance of absorption, metabolism and pharmacokinetic studies in the development of a new drug has grown considerably in the last 10–15 years and made us clear a lot of the mystery related to its efficacy and tolerance.

A quite new and very important chapter of clinical pharmacology is the increased knowledge on possible interactions of the new compound with other drugs, or even with some other substances, to explain sometimes the therapeutic problems or intolerance. Clinicians expect today a precise and accurate study on this topic.

The trial designs for testing drugs with anti-inflammatory activity are getting always more and more difficult with the increase of our knowledge and the need to have accurate, precise and objective methods.

The numerous and different methods which have been used in an attempt to assess objectively the value of the antirheumatic drugs, are, by itself, a statement of their inadequacy.

The universally accepted model to test anti-inflammatory effect in humans is rheumatoid arthritis; a chronic inflammatory process with constant activity; the main changes caused by the disease have objective and measurable manifestations at joint level (swelling, tenderness, local temperature, limitation of movements).

Table 51.3 Comparison of Cl 82204* effective dose and the reference drugs in various anti-inflammatory, analgesic and antypiretic tests—and in the human clinic

	Cl 82204	Aspirin	Indo-methacin	Phenyl-butazone
ANTI-INFLAMMATORY EFFECT				
Carrageenan-induced oedema (rat)	90	133	15	47
Relation: (dose, mg/kg)	1	4.8	0.17	0.5
Adjuvant induced arthritis (rat)	9.8	165	0.62	9.8
Relation: (dose, mg/kg)	1	16.84	0.06	1
Ultraviolet light-induced erythema (guinea pig)	7.0	44.0	4.8	8.0
Relation: (dose, mg/kg)	1	6.29	0.68	1.14
Sodium urate-induced synovitis (dog)	3.5	—	2.4	—
Relation: (dose, mg/kg)	1	—	0.69	—
ANALGESIC EFFECT				
Phenylquinone writhing (mouse)	7.7	28.6	0.24	35.5
Relation: (dose, mg/kg)	1	2.71	0.03	0.46
Yeast-induced paw pain (rat)	20	200	10	20
Relation: (dose, mg/kg)	1	10	0.5	1
ANTI-PYRETIC EFFECT				
Yeast-induced pyresis (rat)	135	78	10	90
Relation: (dose, mg/kg)	1	0.53	0.07	0.67
HUMAN				
Daily recommended useful dose (mg)	600	3000	75	300
Relation (dose, mg/kg)	8.58	43	1	4.3
Relation (dose, mg/kg)	1	5	0.12	0.5

* Fenbufen

Table 51.4 Excretion pattern and plasma half-life of a synthetic drug in various species*

Species	Excretion Urine (%)	Faeces (%)	Plasma half-life (h)
Man	94	1–2	14
Rat	90	2	4–6
Guinea pig	90	5	9
Dog	29	50	23–35
Rhesus monkey†	90	2	2–3
Capuchin monkey	45	54	20
Stump-tail monkey†	40	60	1
Minipig	86	1–2	4–7

* Adapted from Djerassi, C.: *Science*, **169**, 941–951, Sept. 4, 1970.

† These two species belong to the same genus (Macaca).

Table 51.5 Radioactivity levels in tissues of a rat 24 h after oral administration of 3 mg/kg of ^{3}H-labelled naproxen

Tissue	d.p.m./Total tissue	d.p.m./g tissue	Per cent of administered dose
Spleen	1050	1390	0.01
Heart	890	680	0.01
Lung	10 010	2910	0.03
Liver	36 770	2000	0.12
Kidney	9160	2510	0.03
Digestive system	168 500	8100	0.50
Faeces	478 000	168 280	1.50

On the other hand, RA has a lot of disadvantages; it varies widely. It can start at a very early age or in the late sixties or seventies; last a few days or weeks, or 40–50 years; it can involve a few joints, or 50, or it can sometimes have important irreversible deformities; it can be only articular or systemic, and being a chronic process, it can be accompanied by an important psychological component. So, it is quite difficult to get together a carefully matched and really comparable group for controlled trials and it is very true what Hart and Huskisson have several times stated: 'it is easy to have a negative result by choosing the wrong patients'; I should add that even erroneous positive results could come out for the same reason.

In Table 51.6 we can see the generally accepted or known and used parameters to assess the anti-inflammatory activity of a compound.

Some of them, such as swelling, local hyperthermia, limitation of motion, are really objective and measurable symptoms. There are a good number of different methods which I prefer to name as *apparently objective*, as objective observation often contains features which have a subjective factor in their appreciation, as morning stiffness, intensity of pain, etc. or mood and psycho-

Table 51.6 Clinical evaluation of the anti-inflammatory effect

Subjective data	Clinical symptoms	Apparently objective method	Objective methods
Pain (+−)	(Usual method)	Number of painful joints (+)	(Special non-habitual methods)
Morning stiffness (+−)	Swelling	Number of swelling joints (+)	
Fatigue in the evening (+)	Local hyperthermia	Number of tender joints (+)	Arthroscopy
General condition (+−)	Limitation in the degree	Duration of morning stiffness (+−)*	Biopsy
Side-effects	of motion	Grip strength (−)†	Histopathology
		Time required to walk 50 feet (−)†	Electronmicroscopy
		Circumference of joints (+−)*	Joint scintigraphy
		Range motion degree (+−)*	Biochemical methods
		Laboratory changes in:	Thermometry
		(a) erythrosedimentation rate†	Thermography
		(b) rheumatoid factor titre	
		(c) C-reactive protein‡	

* Altered by several factors.
† Inaccurate method.
‡ Unspecific tests.

logical state can influence them, as is the case for walking time or time needed to perform various simple tasks. Even when we take as an example the grip strength, I feel that the psychological features, as well as the time of performing the test, the possible deformation or limitation on the correspondent joints, have an important influence on the results. Unfortunately, the circumference of joints, even the interphalangeals, can be reduced only in a small proportion of patients with RA, although this parameter is included in almost all trials. Sedimentation rate and C-reactive protein are not specific and the titres of rheumatoid factor generally are not in accordance with the clinical activity.

One of the important effects of the antirheumatic drugs today is the relief of joint pain which is generally the most important problem for the patient suffering from RA, but it is also one of the most difficult problems how to measure, in a real objective way, its intensity. The information given by the patient is very subjective and depends upon many different factors in a positive as well as in a negative form. A good number of different methods to measure the intensity of pain, have been proposed, but not one of them was accepted as an absolutely useful one. When we are asking the patient about his pain, we are expecting in his answer a comparative value too; better? or worse?—but what does it mean really if he says better, or even much better?—does it have the same meaning if the patient has no pain any more, instead of the mild pain that he had before; or if he relates that he has now only mild pain as compared with the strong one that he had previously; or does it have the same value 'the severe pain' of an upset, nervous patient, or the same information from a calm and objective person?

The relationship between patient and physician has undoubtedly an important influence in our experience; sometimes we can observe a 'positive' tendency from the patients willing to help the investigator, expressing relatively 'good' results(!).

Looking for tolerance in the clinical trials is not so easy either; being subjective, some of the more frequent undesirable effects as headache, dizziness, nausea, etc.; but the use of some laboratory parameters can help us to detect renal and hepatic toxicity, occult intestinal bleeding, etc.

In recent years, a variety of methods have been suggested and used to assess more objectively the anti-inflammatory effect. This objective method allows us to observe and measure more accurately changes in the inflammatory process.

After many years we have been specially interested to look for and to use this kind of procedure, trying to confirm the real efficacy and sometimes obtain data even in the possible mechanism of action.

The joint scintigraphy with radioisotopes of short half life, such as 99 mTc Technetium in the form of pertecnatate is accepted as a useful objective method to measure the anti-inflammatory effect, performing the test before starting the administration of the drug and repeated some time later. The change in the density of the concentration of radioisotopes shows the improvement in an objective form.

Arthroscopy is an endoscopic procedure which we have used for about 10 years in the evaluation of different anti-inflammatory compounds such as: indomethacin, naproxen, ibuprofen, fenbufen, etc. It allows direct visualization of the synovial membrane and the observation of the inflammatory changes, and at the same time permits us to take biopsies under direct visual control from the most involved areas; assuming in this way the most accurate and specific diagnoses. Arthroscopy and biopsies are also performed by our group, before starting with the drug and then 3, 6 or more months later to observe the changes due to the treatment.

This method helped us in the investigation of some new anti-inflammatory drugs and different steroids with systemic or local effect and recently with azathioprine, obtaining always very important and interesting data.

The development of a new drug in clinical pharmacology from the phase I studies through the phase II comparative trials to the different safety and efficacy studies, is a fascinating experience but it also has its difficulties. The trial design, the selection of groups, looking for different models such as osteoarthritis, non-articular rheumatic processes, or finally, other acute or chronic inflammatory conditions.

In this generally long period of different experiments, the investigator has plenty of rewards and some difficulties too. If the clinician occasionally has some particular observation related to the efficacy, dosage or side-effects of the new drug and he tries to communicate with people who know the compound, but only from the laboratory experiments, very often will be rejected, only because in the laboratory they have found different data. Specifically, when we studied naproxen, we observed that in some cases, for example in the acute gouty attack or in cases of very active rheumatoid arthritis patients, we had to give higher doses of the compound than the generally recommended average maintenance doses to control the activity. They tried to explain to us that there was no reason to give higher doses because the drug would be eliminated anyway in the urine. Very nice curves about the naproxen plasma levels and its urinary excretion after the administration of different doses were shown to us as arguments. Runkel *et al.* recently published a paper on the 'Pharmacokinetics of naproxen overdoses', where they revised previous conclusions because they found that the plasma areas showed a further increase with increased dose up to 4 g and they did not plateau in the 900 mg dose region in a non-linear fashion, probably because of an increase in the renal clearance of the drug, mostly of its free non-protein-bound fraction through the active secretion by the renal tubules (Figure 51.1). These pharmacokinetic findings suggest that naproxen is a relatively safe drug and its accumulation, because of this observation, practically is not probable. We are very satisfied with this information which confirmed our clinical impression, observing in some more active cases better results with higher doses.

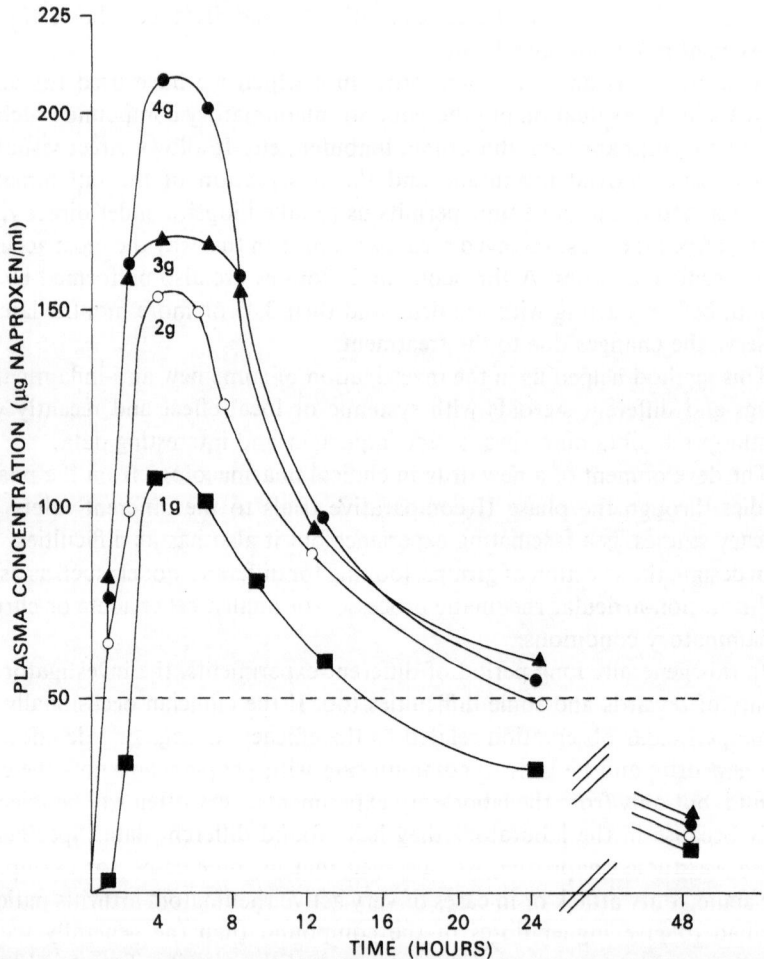

Figure 51.1 Naproxen plasma profiles following single oral doses of 1, 2, 3, and 4 g

To have a really objective and complete analysis of a drug about its efficacy and tolerance, one should have a long-term experience with a good number of patients observed for many years taking the same drug, the short time trials can give us only partial information on the efficacy of the product, but not really on its tolerance.

One of the most important sources of error in a clinical trial may be the differences and variations between the assessments made by different physicians and this is one of the reasons why we are against the so-called multicentric studies, in which the results of the observations of different groups and centres belonging to different communities, habits and standards, performed by different observers, investigators or, 'who knows who', are mixed together in a commune pool and usually evaluated by a computer. I mean, the 'promotional' trials developed by different pharmaceutical firms and not the well-prepared, scrupulously performed and organized studies by the most-recognized centres and societies in the UK and USA.

In this brief communication, I wanted to show some of the difficulties which are present in relation with any clinical trial. Most of them are well known by anybody who ever tried to develop a clinical study and probably these problems and difficulties make the research of the new drug more fascinating, besides the eternal challenge and attraction of the new and unknown.

CONCLUSIONS

'Do not believe' the data of the biological tests, take them only as basic orientation to controlled studies, but taking care with placebo. Take into account the different factors to evaluate effects and tolerance. Recognize the limitations of the usual model (RA). Match the groups as well as possible. Use objective methods, and look for new ones. Run long-term studies to determine chronic tolerance.

References

Cosh, J. A. (1974). Antiinflammatory drugs in rheumatic diseases. *Practitioner*, **213**, 1276, 519

Hart, A. D. and Huskisson, E. C. (1972). Measurements in rheumatoid arthritis. *Lancet*, **i**, 28

Huskisson, E. C. *et al.* (1976). Four new antiinflammatory drugs: responses and variations. *Br. Med. J.*, **1**, 1048

Katona, G. (1976). Objective methods to assess the antiinflammatory activity of anti-rheumatic compounds. *Agents Actions*, **6**, 346

Katona, G. (1973). Four years of clinical experience with naproxen—and objective methods of evaluation. *Scand. J. Rheum.*, **2**, Suppl., 101

Lee, P. and Webb, J. *et al.* (1973). Method for assessing therapeutic potential of anti-inflammatory antirheumatic drugs in rheumatoid arthritis. *Br. Med. J.*, **2**, 685

Runkel, R. and Chaplin, M. D. *et al.* (1976). Pharmacokinetic of naproxen overdoses. *Clin. Pharmacol. Ther.*, **20**, 269

Shridhar, D. D., Carson, W., Dick, R., Hodgkinson and Buchanan, W. W. (1973). Measurement of clinical response to antiinflammatory drug therapy in R.A. *Q. J. Med.*, **2**, 166, 287

Discussion 51

M. Jayson:
(UK)

I should like to talk about the use of arthroscopy and biopsy in the assessment of degree of inflammatory activity. Our group has had quite extensive experience of the use of arthroscopy and biopsy and I am unhappy about using it to try and assess the degree of inflammation. When using an arthroscope it is very easy to alter the appearances of the synovial membrane for several reasons. One is that it is very difficult when one arthroscopes a patient on one occasion and one comes back some time later to return to exactly the same site to make comparative observations.

A second problem is that the distance from the tip of the telescope to the synovial surface is absolutely critical, because as one is within a few millimetres of the surface, and as the intensity of the light falls off according to the distance away, any small deviation or alteration of the distance will cause a tremendous difference in the colour of the synovial surface and it is quite easy, simply by looking at the surface which appears dead white or which goes a deep red at the other extreme.

The third difference problem is that when one irrigates the joint and one has fluid flowing through it, and according to the pressure of the fluid that is driving the irrigating fluid through, so one can again squeeze blood or allow blood into the synovial membrane, and again alter the appearance of erythema.

The fourth problem is the actual temperature of the irrigating fluid. By altering temperature one can considerably alter the appearances.

The other problem is the problem of assessing biopsies. We all know that the appearances of the synovial membrane differ considerably in different parts of the joint. A biopsy from one part of the joint will show quite gross inflammatory change whereas another part of the joint might show very little. Even adjacent biopsies can show quite gross differences. To evaluate this problem we did a careful study two or three years ago, published in the *Annals of Rheumatic Diseases*, in which we independently correlated the clinical appearances, the radiological appearances, the arthroscopic appearances, and the histological appearances, and we classified all these features and looked for correlations, and found it extremely difficult to draw any real comparisons and to get meaningful data in trying to interpret one in terms of the other.

Katona:

Dr. Jayson has posed several problems: too many! We started to use arthroscopy 12 or 13 years ago and we have performed around 800 arthroscopies. When we first began to use arthroscopy for these special investigations we had had some experience and all of Dr. Jayson's comments are correct, but anyone who begins a serious trial will try to put the situation on to a standard basis. We therefore try to perform arthroscopy in the same situation in all patients, to the same standards, with the fluid at the same temperature and at the same pressure, always looking at the same place of the synovial membrane, and we always try to take biopsies from the same section of the anatomy. We understand the problems. We have met the same problems and we are trying to standardize our procedures since that is the only way that we can defend our findings.

Dr. Jayson's comment is correct and he shows how difficult it is to find a standard basis. However, after several years of doing it we can defend our methods and our findings.

Chairman: There are many people involved in multi-centre trials, to which Dr. Katona seems to object. Are there any supporters of multi-centre trials?

W. Lyle:
(UK) There are multi-centre trials and multi-centre trials. Dr. Katona was talking about the collections of vast numbers of case records from almost equally vast numbers of observers, but most people here would hardly regard that as a multi-centre trial—just a sort of porridge!

The multi-centre trial in which the various observers number perhaps not more than three, four or five centres, and meet repeatedly in designing the protocol, and perhaps do the same tests in a kind of trial run before, and so forth, is not only justifiable but might be the only way to do these things properly, and I would plead for some discretion in the use of the term 'multi-centre trial'.

Katona: I dealt with it in the last part (of the Paper). I mentioned that I was referring to multi-centre trials on the basis of collecting data and cases, and on the basis of screening by the pharmaceutical firms merely to have more and more experience. I was not referring to those good multi-centre trials, properly prepared, run on a serious basis, and organized by serious people.

Lyle: In fact I was replying to Professor Willoughby (the chairman) who was being provoking.

52

Is the mechanism of action during treatment of rheumatoid arthritis with penicillamine and gold thiomalate the same?

EGIL JELLUM AND EIMAR MUNTHE (Norway)

INTRODUCTION

1977 is the World Rheumatism Year, as well as the 50th anniversary of the introduction of gold treatment for rheumatoid arthritis. Fifty years ago, Landé[1] and Pick[2] made independent reports on the use of gold salts in the treatment of a few cases of polyarthritis. However, the father of gold treatment in rheumatoid arthritis is said to be Forestier, who published the first results on a large series of cases in 1929[3]. Forestier's decision to use gold compounds in treating rheumatoid arthritis was based upon the assumed tuberculostatic effect of gold, and on the mistaken assumption that a relationship existed between rheumatoid arthritis and tuberculosis. Forestier found good effect of gold on arthritis and his work was later confirmed by a large number of European investigators. However, after 50 years, the rationale of gold treatment for RA is still empiric. Despite its often serious side effects, it still holds its position as an effective and worth-while therapy in many cases, also when the risk/benefit relationship is taken into account.

However, after 50 years, the significance of the gold part of the compounds for the clinical effect is still unclear. It is frequently observed, however, that during treatment of rheumatoid arthritis with gold thiomalate and penicillamine, the clinical responses, clinical courses and side effects are rather similar, despite there also being definite differences. The question to be considered is whether there may be similarities in the mechanism of action of these two drugs.

575

CHEMISTRY

Figure 52.1 shows the formula of penicillamine and of gold thiomalate. The former is an amino acid which contains a free thiol group. Gold thiomalate also contains a thiol group, which, however, is not free, but blocked by mercaptide formation with gold (I) ion. The thiomalate moiety is a dicarboxylic acid and not an amino acid.

From metal-chelation chemistry[4] it is well known that different thiols have a different ability to bind heavy metal ions, depending upon the stability constants of the various complexes[5].

In the human body there is an abundance of free thiol groups, both in the extracellular fluids (mainly protein-SH) and in the intracellular compartments (mainly protein-SH and glutathione-SH). Immediately after injection of gold thiomalate the equilibrium shown in Figure 52.2 will therefore exist. If the protein-thiol groups have a much higher affinity for the gold ions than the thiomalate, the metal ions will become protein bound with a concomitant liberation of free thiomalate.

$$
\begin{array}{ll}
\text{SH} & \text{S-Au} \\
| & | \\
\text{CH}_3\text{-C-CH}_3 & \text{CH-COOH} \\
| & | \\
\text{CH-NH}_2 & \text{CH}_2 \\
| & | \\
\text{COOH} & \text{COOH}
\end{array}
$$

Penicillamine   Gold - thiomalate

Figure 52.1 Formula of the penicillamine and gold thiomalate molecules

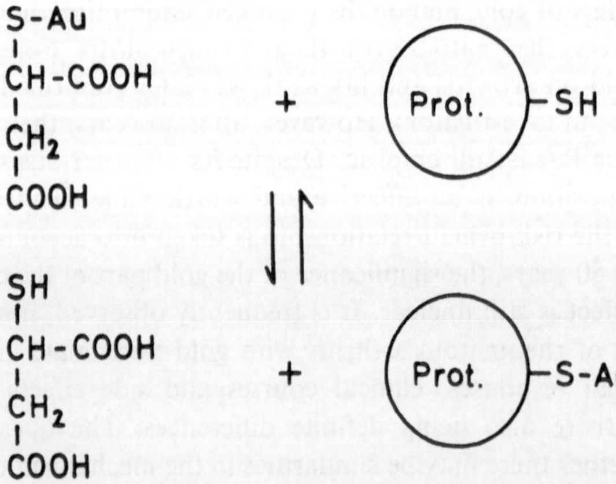

$$
\begin{array}{l}
\text{S-Au} \\
| \\
\text{CH-COOH} \\
| \\
\text{CH}_2 \\
| \\
\text{COOH}
\end{array}
\quad + \quad \text{(Prot.)} \text{-SH}
$$

$$
\Updownarrow
$$

$$
\begin{array}{l}
\text{SH} \\
| \\
\text{CH-COOH} \\
| \\
\text{CH}_2 \\
| \\
\text{COOH}
\end{array}
\quad + \quad \text{(Prot.)} \text{-S-Au}
$$

Figure 52.2 Interaction of gold thiomalate with protein-SH

MATERIALS AND METHODS

Human serum and labelled gold thiomalate were used to throw light on the problem of the relative affinity of gold ions for thiomalate and protein-SH. Radioactive gold [S^{35}]-thiomalate was synthesized in the following way: Equivalent amounts of labelled sodium sulphide ($Na_2[S^{35}]$, Radiochemical Centre, Amersham, England) was mixed with maleic acid, the pH was adjusted to 7.5 and the mixture was left at 20 °C for 2 h. Addition across the double bond occurred and yielded [S^{35}]-thiomalate. After acidification with dilute hydrochloric acid any unreacted sulphide was removed (as H_2S) by bubbling nitrogen through the solution. The labelled thiomalate was purified by preparative thin layer chromatography using Butanol/acetic acid/water (80/20/20) as solvent. In this system thiomalate had an Rf-value of 0.58. The identity of the product was checked by means of combined gas chromatography (GC) and mass spectrometry (MS) which confirmed the structure. (The thiomalate was converted into the S-methyl-dimethylester with diazomethane before GC-MS.)

In order to prepare radioactive gold thiomalate with the label in the thiomalate moiety, gold-sodium thiomalate (Myocrisin®) was allowed to equilibrate with a small amount of [S^{35}]-thiomalate synthesized as above. Gold [S^{35}]thiomalate was also prepared by mixing labelled thiomalate with sodium auric chloride; reduction of auric ions to auro ions then took place before the gold thiomalate complex was formed.

The gold [S^{35}]-thiomalate was mixed with human serum and allowed to stand for about 1 minute at 20 °C before gelfiltration on a column of Sephadex G-25. Fractions were collected, radioactivity (S^{35}) was counted and gold was determined by atomic absorption and protein was measured by the biuret reaction.

RESULTS

The results are shown in Figure 52.3. The figure shows that all the gold has rapidly become protein-bound, with a concomitant release of free thiomalate. Only a small fraction of the latter was protein-bound, possibly due to mixed disulphide formation with disulphide linkages in the protein and/or due to unspecific adsorption.

In a simple dialysis experiment shown in Figure 52.4 it was shown that upon mixing of human serum and gold thiomalate, all the gold becomes protein-bound. In a control experiment serum was omitted. Equal concentrations of gold were then found outside and inside the dialysis bag.

DISCUSSION

On the basis of these experiments and from the results of other investigators[6] it may thus be postulated that very soon, and most probably immediately, after injection of gold-thiomalate into a patient, two chemical forms will dominate, protein-bound gold and free thiomalate. This explains the findings reported by other workers that the circulating form of gold in patients on Myocrisin treatment is mainly albumin-bound gold[7,8]. It seems to us that the question should be raised as to which of the two chemical forms, free

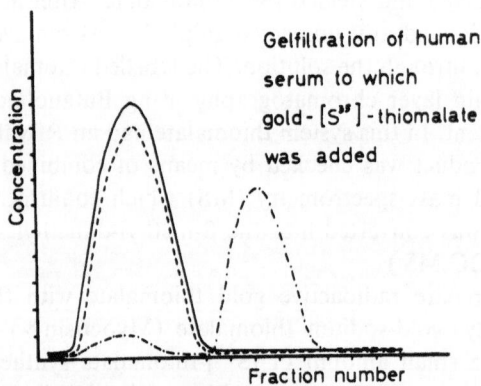

Figure 52.3 Interaction of gold thiomalate with human serum proteins. Human serum (2 ml) was mixed with gold [S^{35}] thiomalate (10 mg, 500 000 counts per min) and after 1 min at 20 °C gel filtration on a column (20 cm × 1.5 cm) of Sephadex G-25 (coarse grade) was carried out. Fractions were collected and analysed for the following 3 components: ——— protein; - - - - - - - - gold; –.–.–.–.–. S^{35} radioactivity (thiomalate)

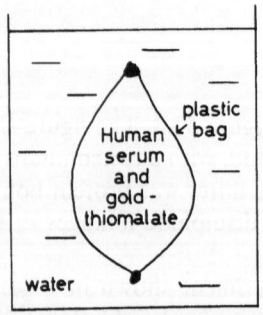

After 20 hours :

Concentration of gold outside bag : 0,002 Mg/ml

"   "   inside   "   : 560.- "

Figure 52.4 Principle and results of a dialysis experiment. In a control experiment the serum was omitted. Equal concentrations of gold were then found outside and inside the dialysis bag

578

thiomalate or albumin-bound gold, is responsible for the beneficial effect in rheumatoid arthritis.

Since free thiomalate most probably is present *in vivo* after injection of gold thiomalate, this question is relevant. Most cited papers claim that thiomalate has no beneficial effect. In the most widely cited work by Preston *et al.* from 1942[9], they used an animal model of PPLO-induced arthritis in mice with 20 days observation period in the experiments to prove that thiomalate was ineffective. However, it is equally certain that had penicillamine been similarly tested and observed using the same model, this thiol would also have given a negative result. Thiomalate should therefore be studied in animal models of arthritis where Myocrisin and penicillamine are known to work.

SIMILARITIES AND DIFFERENCES BETWEEN PENICILLAMINE AND THIOMALATE

Comparison of the properties of thiomalate and penicillamine shows that the two compounds have much in common[10]: Both contain a free thiol group; both can be oxidized to the corresponding disulphide, although penicillamine more slowly due to the steric hindrance of the methyl-groups; both can undergo thiol/disulphide exchange reactions with protein-SH and protein-SS; both compounds in the disulphide forms are substrates for the four known disulphide reductions system operating *in vivo* (provided that the drugs penetrate into the cells); both thiols penetrate poorly the erythrocyte membrane[11]; both compounds may cause profound alterations in the metabolism of a cell (effect on CoA-SH dependent reactions, uncoupling of oxidative phosphorylation, stimulation of glutathione peroxidase etc.[10]); both may chelate metal ions although the stability constants of the complexes may vary considerably; both thiols may interact with double bonds, e.g. in fumaric acid (a citric acid cycle intermediate); both are likely to form mixed di-sulphides with histone F3 of the chromosomes[10]; both are likely to disturb SH/SS-proteins involved in the mitotic processes and both may disturb biosyntheses of the nucleic acids.

The biochemical *differences* of penicillamine and thiomalate are mainly due to lack of an amino group in the latter molecule. Interaction of the two drugs with aldehyde-groups, e.g. in crosslinking of collagen, will be different: both penicillamine and thiomalate will form hemithioacetals with aldehydes, but only penicillamine will cyclize to form the thiazolidine ring. Penicillamine and its disulphide can become reversibly bound to DNA (see Figure 52.5). Thiomalate which does not contain the positively charged amino-group cannot interact with the negatively charged phosphate-groups of the DNA molecules. Finally it is highly probable that the transport mechanism of the amino acid penicillamine will be different from that of thiomalate, a dicar-boxylic acid. Also the metabolic degradation of the two compounds will probably be different.

579

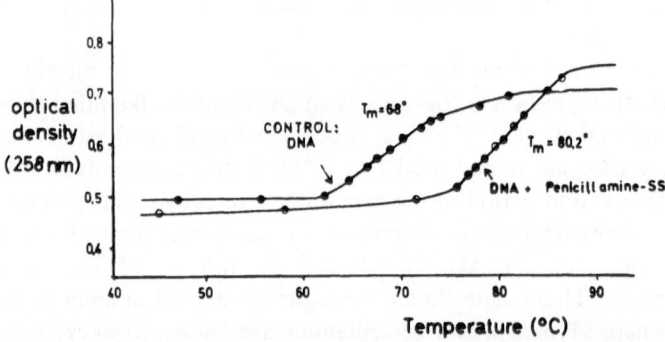

Figure 52.5 Experimental evidence for the binding of penicillamine disulphide to DNA. Penicillamine disulphide (final concentration 3×10^{-2} M) dissolved in saline-citrate (0.015 M NaCl — 0.0015 M Na-citrate) and DNA (3 mg, from calf thymus) were mixed and transferred to an electrically heated cuvette. This was placed in a Zeiss RPQ 20 A recording spectrophotometer. Changes in optical density (258 nm) were noted and the transition midpoints (Tm) were calculated. In the control experiment the penicillamine disulphide was omitted. The increased stability of the DNA-helix is due to binding of the diamino—disulphide to the phosphate groups of the nucleic acid[12]

PROPOSALS

Since there are many biochemical similarities between thiomalate and penicillamine, one would like to establish with certainty whether or not thiomalate has an effect on rheumatoid arthritis in man. Tests on animal models seem difficult and results must be used with caution as recently emphasized by Willoughby and Dieppe[13]. Maybe a controlled clinical trial in man should be carried out. Irrespective of the outcome of such a trial, the results will be equally interesting. Should thiomalate be without effect, one should consider to eliminate this, potential toxic, thiol from the drug Myocrisin, and perhaps instead use albumin-bound gold. Should thiomalate have effects in man similar to that of penicillamine, the toxic heavy metal gold could be avoided and one should examine which of the two thiols, penicillamine or thiomalate is best tolerated. Should *both* gold and thiomalate be of importance, the gold (III)-penicillamine complex could also be investigated for effect and tolerance. And perhaps a search for other, more effective thiols or with fewer side effects, should be started.

ACKNOWLEDGEMENT

The skilful technical assistance of Elisiv Rogge Wang is gratefully acknowledged.

References

1. Landé, K. (1927). *Münch. Med. Wochenschr.*, **74**, 1132
2. Pick, E. (1927). *Wien Klin. Wochenschr.*, **40**, 1175

3. Forestier, J. (1929). *Bull. et. Mem. Soc. med. hop. Paris*, **53**, 323
4. Catch, A. (1964). *Radioactive Metal Mobilization in Medicine*. (Springfield, Illinois: Charles C. Thomas Publishing Co.)
5. Jellum, E., Aaseth, J. and Eldjarn, L. (1973). Mercaptodextran, a metal-chelating and disulphide-reducing polythiol of high molecular weight. *Biochem. Pharmacol.*, **22**, 1179
6. Danpure, C. J. (1976). The interaction of aurothiomalate and cysteine. *Biochem. Pharmacol.*, **25**, 2343
7. Queen, E. G. and Dykes, P. W. (1969). Transport of gold in the body. *Ann. Rheumat. Dis.*, **28**, 437
8. Lorber, A., Bovy, R. A. and Chang, Chin C. (1972). Relationship between serum gold content and distribution to serum immunoglobulins and complement. *Nature New Biol.*, **236**, 250
9. Preston, W. S., Block, W. D. and Freyberg, C. (1942). Chemotherapy of chronic progressive arthritis in mice. 1. Role of sulphur in gold-containing compounds. *Proceed. Soc. Exp. Biol. Med.*, **50**, 253
10. Jellum, E. and Skrede, S. (1976). Biological aspects of thiol-disulphide reactions during treatment with penicillamine. In: *Penicillamine Research in Rheumatoid Disease. Proceedings of an International Symposium on Penicillamine, Norway, 1976*. (E. Munthe, ed.). pp. 68–77. (Oslo: Fabritius)
11. Aaseth, J. (1976b). Discussion. In: *Penicillamine Research in Rheumatoid Disease. Proceedings of an International Symposium on Penicillamine, Norway, 1976*. (E. Munthe, ed.), pp. 150–151. (Oslo: Fabritius)
12. Jellum, E. (1965). Interaction of cystamine and cystamine derivatives with nucleic acids and nucleoproteins. *Internat. J. Radiat. Biol.*, **9**, 185
13. Willoughby, D. A. and Dieppe, P. A. (1976). The effects of D-penicillamine in animal models. In: *Penicillamine Research in Rheumatoid Disease. Proceedings of an International Symposium on Penicillamine, Norway 1976*. (E. Munthe, ed.). pp. 45–48. (Oslo: Fabritius)
14. Aaseth, J. (1976). Mobilization of methyl mercury in vivo and in vitro using *N*-acetyl-DL-penicillamine and other complexing agents. *Acta pharmacol. (Copenhagen)*, **39**, 289

Discussion 52

A. Lewis: (UK)	First a comment. We have shown in a very simple model of inflammation, the guinea pig UV erythema test, that both penicillamine and gold thiomalate do suppress the erythema. However, thiomalic acid is inactive in this model.
	Then a question. If so much emphasis is placed on thiomalate, is it suggested that perhaps thio-glucose, and perhaps triethyl phosphine, the other moieties in gold therapies in addition to the gold, are the important parts of the molecules, or not?
	Would Dr. Munthe be prepared to speculate on those compounds?
Munthe:	It is quite striking that most of the gold complexes that have been found to work on rheumatoid disease have been thiol components.
D. Walz: (USA)	We have tested the substructure of oranofin—a triethyl phosphine. The substructure has had no effect in the animal models, whereas the total gold-containing compound has activity. We have separated out the thiol glucose molecule from the phosphine oxide molecule compared to the activity seen with the total molecule.
	One other point. If the sulphydryl is used by sulphide interchange, both of these moieties are inactive, whereas the compound oranofin is inactive also, but gold sodium thiomalate inhibits, so that there are differences even in the thiol compound. Gold chloride is active in the animal models which have no thiol moiety, so there is much investigation based on Dr. Munthe's concept.
Munthe:	We know that gold chloride, for instance, inhibits in the complement system, but the question is whether the animal models that are used are reliable in relationship to the effect in the human disease.
N. Svartz: (Sweden)	It was an interesting paper and I share Dr. Munthe's opinion that thiols have to be studied further. They have a strong effect on the metabolism. They split the rheumatoid factor, and when patients are treated with thiols the rheumatoid factor diminishes.
	Thiols have a strong effect on the metabolism. Does Dr. Munthe think that they also have a pronounced effect therapeutically?
Munthe:	I do not know whether thiols have an effect on rheumatoid arthritis, but it is important to know whether they have. The only way to test them would be to do a clinical trial. If we can show with certainty that when Myocrisin is injected into a human being then immediately after the injection thiomalate operates as a free molecule, it would not be unethical to perform trials using thiomalate alone, which would give us some information.
Z. Bacq: (Belgium)	Dr. Munthe comes from a city where thiols—disulphides—are very well-known for other reasons, i.e. chemical protection against ionizing radiation. I would recall that mixed disulphide formation is a very rapid non-enzymatic process and that the gluthathione reductase system will very rapidly put the system back to its original condition.
	I should also mention that we have seen that simpler cysteamine—

glutathione also, but cysteamine mainly, which is a very good protection against ionizing radiation, has some anti-inflammatory influence, but that it does not last long, because the substance is metabolized erratically in the body. One reason why penicillamine and thiomalate are more active when used in chronic therapy may be that they are not so rapidly metabolized within the body.

Recently we have seen that gold salts in the *in vitro* system of bull seminal vesicle extract is an extremely effective inhibitor, in the same way as silver salts, whereas copper, by contrast, increases the yields of prostaglandin in this particular *in vitro* system.

J.-P. Giroud:
(France)
Does Dr. Munthe think there would be any correlation between the side effects of gold and penicillamine?

Secondly, could the metabolism of penicillamine be different for polyarthritis, where many more side effects are seen?

Munthe:
On the first question, it is quite likely that some of the side effects which are similar for penicillamine and thiolamate, e.g. the nephropathy, the immune complex kidney disease, where we have noted several taking the same course, could be due to the formation of mixed disulphides with kidney basement membrane proteins and it may be that both drugs alter the antigenicity of the renal proteins—perhaps by mixed disulphide formation in the kidney. This is an hypothesis.

Gold itself has not been demonstrated in the glomeruli, in the immune complex nephritis that occurs during gold treatment. This could support the argument.

On metabolism—it may be that the metabolisms of the drugs are different in different diseases.

Giroud:
But we do not yet know anything about the metabolism in man with polyarthritis with penicillamine.

W. H. Lyle:
(UK)
We know a little bit about it. There is mixed disulphide with penicillamine very quickly after absorption. This has been shown, and there seems to be a correlation between clinical response in arthritis and the serum levels of the mixed disulphide. I do not know what it means.

There are some other very elementary studies in which there seems to be much the same sort of excretion in urine of mixed disulphide, internal dimer, and a fair amount of poor absorption.

I hope to go into this later.

I do not think that there is any real difference in metabolism. I suspect that the rheumatoid patient is very much more susceptible to the toxic effects of these drugs than other patients.

I. Ginsburg:
(Israel)
If we believe that the cells in the advancing pannus are those which secrete the enzymes of all evil—the elastases, collagenases, neutroproteases, which destroy cartilage, and then bone, then has Dr. Munthe any experience on the selective inhibition of all these enzymes by gold thiomalate, and of whether there is a good exchange between the albumin-bound gold and perhaps the surface of the advancing cells. As Professor Vaes showed us, serum may inhibit collagenase activity and so would thiols or cysteine, and there is a possibility that there is a direct transfer of some of the enzymes from the advancing pannus over the target cells on the cartilage and bone.

I believe that we probably have to localize, or to determine quantitatively the amount of the available gold thiolamate at the advancing pannus.

Has Dr. Munthe any comment?

Munthe:
No, although such studies should be extremely interesting to do. We have not looked at it.

We have looked at the ability of thiolamate to form mixed disulphides and they do form them, although to a lesser extent than penicillamine.

583

53

About immunological anomalies in treated and non-treated rheumatoid arthritis: rosette test and immunofluorescence of B-cells

H. ROUX, P. MERCIER, Y. JEANDEL,
M. T. GABRIEL-BROUILLET AND G. SERRATRICE (France)

There is a large amount of recent data about the differentiation of T- and B-lymphocytes in the blood. But as concerns patients with rheumatoid arthritis, sometimes contradictory results are published. A small increase in B-cells is found by Papamichail et al.[1], but in a subsequent study, with similar techniques the increase is no longer present. Using the same technique on surface immunoglobulins Mellbye et al.[2] observed a small decrease in B-lymphocytes in blood, which is confirmed by the study of B-cells detected by rosette formation with C_3; but which is not found later[3]. Clements[4] et al. observed a small decrease of absolute values of B-cells. Rosenthal and Muller[5] show that this decrease is not significant.

A number of studies with normal values of B-cells of blood have been published[3,6-12].

Increased values of T-lymphocytes are found in a report by Frøland et al.[6], and later in 1975[12]. But in these publications normal levels for T-lymphocytes (E-rosette test) are 14.8%. Normal values of T-lymphocytes appear in the publication of Williams et al.[3], Micheli and Bron[10], Winchester et al.[11] (1974), Holborrow et al.[13], Scheinberg et al.[14].

Increased values of B-cells in active rheumatoid arthritis has been observed by Clements et al.[4], with absolute values only, and by Rosenthal and Muller[5] without any statistical significance. A decrease of T-lymphocytes is only possible in active disease[3].

High values of null cells are sometimes observed[3,6], perhaps only in the active diseases.

MATERIAL AND METHODS

We have retained in this study 89 cases of rheumatoid arthritis (RA): without any treatment, 30 cases; with cortisone treatment (5–10 mg of prednisone per day), 10 cases; with chloroquine or hydroxy-chloroquine treatment, 8 cases; with gold therapy, 11 cases; with penicillamine therapy, 21 cases and with levamisole therapy, 9 cases.

Correlation between the activity of the disease, blood haemoglobin level, fibrinaemia, a_2- and γ-globulins, erythrocyte sedimentation rate, serum iron and rheumatoid factors (Waaler Rose and Latex) has been instigated.

Enumeration of T- and B-cells was made by immunofluorescent staining for the presence of surface immunoglobulins (B-cells) and spontaneous rosette formation with sheep red blood cells (E-rosette: T-cells).

Normal values of the B-cells (surface immunoglobulins) is 15% or with absolute values:

$|165| <$ B lymphocytes $< |525|$ mm³ and for T-cells (E rosette) 70 $\pm$ 7% at the risk of 1%, or with absolute values $|945| <$ T lymphocytes $< |1925|$ mm³.

RESULTS

RA without treatment (30 cases)

Very different values of T- and B-lymphocytes are observed and it is possible to separate two groups of RA. The first one with normal values of T-cells (absolute values): 17 cases, the second one with lowering of T-cells (13 cases) Table 53.1.

In the group with normal values of T-cells there is no anomaly for total lymphocytes and relative and absolute values of T- and B-cells. In the group

Table 53.1

	Total lympho-cytes	T-cells (%)	T-cells absolute values	B-cells (%)	B-cells absolute values	Null cells (%)
Rheumatoid arthritis with normal levels of T-cells, $n = 17$	2532 1600–6500	70.7	1666	16.18	534	13.12
Rheumatoid arthritis with decrease of T-cells $n = 13$	1071	53	636.7	23.4	239.5	18
Rheumatoid arthritis without treatment Total: $n = 30$	1899 500–6500	65.78	1220	15.89	347	15.23

with decreased values of T-cells, lymphopenia is present in every case. Lymphopenia can be considered as dependent of the decrease of T-cells. Mean values of T- and B-cells are normal and there is no correlation with blood haemoglobin, fibrinaemia, a_2 and γ-globulins, erythrocyte sedimentation rate and serum iron. In the seropositive RA, a decrease of T-cells is present in 38% of cases versus 36% in the seronegative forms. Numerous null cells are observed in six cases, and numerous fluorescent cells in three cases with the possibility of a contamination by monocytes.

Treated RA

21 patients have been treated with penicillamine for more than 3 months. A decrease of T-lymphocytes is present in relative values six times, and in absolute values eight times, a decrease of B-lymphocytes in five of 15 cases (relative values) and four of ten cases (absolute values).

With chloroquine or hydroxychloroquine therapy (eight cases) a decrease of T-cells is observed in three of eight cases (relative values), and in two of seven cases (absolute values), a decrease of B-cells in one of six cases (relative values) and in one of five cases (absolute values).

In cortisone treated RA a decrease of T-cells is observed in two of ten cases (relative values) and in four of ten cases (absolute values) and a decrease of B-lymphocytes in one of ten cases (relative values) and in two of ten cases (absolute values).

With gold treatment a decrease of T-lymphocytes is present in seven of eleven cases (relative values) and in four of nine cases (absolute values). B-cells values are always normal.

With levamisole treatments (nine cases) a decrease of T-cells appears in two of nine cases (relative values) and in three of eight cases (absolute values) without decrease of B-cells in every case. After a treatment for more than 4 months in six cases T- and B-cells values are not modified, an increase of T-cells (absolute and relative) appears in two cases only (after nine and 6 months of treatment) without any modifications of B-cells (Table 53.2).

Table 53.2

	Decrease of T-cells		Decrease of B-cells	
	Relative values	Absolute values	Relative values	Absolute values
Penicillamine	6/21	8/21	5/15	4/10
Chloroquine and hydroxychloroquine	2/8	2/7	1/6	1/5
Cortisone	2/10	4/10	1/10	2/10
Gold	7/11	4/9	0/9	0/7
Levamisole	2/9	3/8	0/9	0/9

DISCUSSION

The data presented here do not show any modifications of the mean number of B- and T-cells in blood in RA patients. But as it was said by Williams et al.[3], two groups of patients appear, the first one with normal values of T-cells, and the other one with a decrease of T-cells and lymphocytes.

In our cases the decrease of T-cells does not correlate with the activity of the disease. In treated RA the two groups are also present with the same frequency. A decrease of T-cells is present in 40% of 59 treated RA versus 43% of non-treated RA.

Enumeration of B and T does not appear as an evolutive test and gives no help to control a treatment. With cortisone treatment the mean number of B- and T-cells is normal: it was lowered in the papers by Yu et al.[15] and Fauci and Dale[16]. With levamisole treatment T-cells increase in a few cases (2/9). Decrease of T-cells in about 40% of RA remains difficult to explain. It is possible to consider a central phenomenon, perhaps genetic, or a peripheric captation. It is known that T-cells are more numerous in synovial fluid[6,17]. But an haematopoietic phenomenon remains a possibility perhaps by the mean of fragilizing anti-T antibody. The phenomenon being close to what happens in systemic lupus erythematosus, where blood T-lymphocytes are decreased[14].

CONCLUSION

The data presented here are a study of 89 cases of RA by the means of the technique of immunofluorescent staining for the presence of surface immunoglobulins (B-cells) and spontaneous rosette formation with sheep red blood cells (E-rosette: T-cells).

In 30 cases of untreated RA, two groups appear; the first one with normal values of T-cells, the other one with a decrease of T-cells and lymphocytes. In treated RA (cortisone: ten cases, penicillamine 21 cases, gold therapy 11 cases, levamisole nine cases) the same differences are present at the same rate.

In the levamisole treated group an increase of T-cells is present in two of nine cases. There is no relation with a parameter of activity in every group.

References

1. Papamichail, M., Brown, J. C. and Holborrow, E. J. (1971). Immunoglobulins on the surface of human lymphocytes. *Lancet*, ii, 850
2. Mellbye, O. J., Messner, R. P., Deboard, J. R. and Williams, R. C. (1972). Immunoglobulin and receptors for C3 on lymphocytes from patients with rheumatoid arthritis. *Arth. Rheum.*, 15, 371
3. Williams, Jr., R. C., Board, J. R. de, Mellbye, O. J., Messner, R. P. and Lindstrom, F. D. (1973). Studies of T and B lymphocytes in patients with connective tissue disease. *J. Clin. Invest.*, 52, 283
4. Clements, P. J., Yu, D. T., Leoy, J., Paulus, H. E. and Barnett, E. U. (1974). Effects

of cyclophosphamide on B and T lymphocytes in rheumatoid arthritis. *Arthritis Rheum.*, **17**, 347

5. Rosenthal, M. and Muller, W. (1975). Lymphocyte subpopulations in normals and patients with rheumatoid arthritis and ankylosing spondylitis. *J. Rheum.*, **2**, 4, 355

6. Frøland, S. A., Natvig, J. B. and Husby, G. (1973). Immunological characterization of lymphocytes in synovial fluid from patients with rheumatoid arthritis. *Scand. J. Immunol.*, **2**, 67

7. Keith, H. O. and Currey, H. J. F. (1973). Rosette formation by peripheral blood lymphocytes in rheumatoid arthritis. *Ann. Rheum. Dis.*, **321**, 202

8. Winchester, R. J., Siegal, F. P., Bentwich, Z. H. and Kunkel, H. G. Alteration in the proportion of B and T lymphocytes in rheumatoid arthritis joint fluids with low complement and increased complexes. *Arthritis Rheum.*, **16**, 138

9. Yu, D. T., Clements, P. J., Peter, J. B., Levy, J., Paulus, H., and Barnett, E. V. (1974). Lymphocyte characteristics in rheumatic patients and the effect of azathioprine therapy. *Arthritis Rheum.*, **13**, 37

10. Micheli, A. and Bron, J. (1974). Studies on blood T and B lymphocytes in rheumatoid arthritis. *Ann. Rheum. Dis.*, **33**, 435

11. Winchester, R. J., Winfield, J. B., Siegal, F., Wernet, P., Bentwich, Z. and Kinkel, H. G. (1974). Analysis of lymphocytes from patients with rheumatoid arthritis and systemic lupus erythematosus. *J. Clin. Invest.*, **54**, 1082

12. Frøland, S. S., Natvig, J. B. and Wisloff, F. (1975). Lymphocytes subpopulations in rheumatoid arthritis. In: *Immunological Aspects of Rheumatoid Arthritis. Rheumatology*, (Clot., Sany and Rothstein, eds.) Vol. 6, pp. 231–241. (Basel: S. Karger)

13. Holborrow, E. J., Sheldon, P. J. and Papamichail, M. (1975). Studies on synovial fluid lymphocytes in rheumatoid arthritis. *Immunological Aspects of Rheumatoid Arthritis. Rheumatology* (Clot, Sany and Rothstein, eds.) Vol. 6, pp. 215–218. (Basel: S. Karger)

14. Scheinberg, M. A., Mendes, N. F., Koperstych, S. and Cathcart, E. S. (1976). Clinical applications of T, B and K cell determinations in rheumatic diseases: a review. *Sem. Arth. Rheum.*, **6**, 1

15. Yu, D. T., Clements, P. J., Paulus, H. E., Peter, J. B., Levy, J. and Barnett, E. V. (1974). Human lymphocyte subpopulations. Effect of corticosteroids. *J. Clin. Invest.*, **53**, 565

16. Fauci, A. S. and Dale, D. C. (1974). The effect of *in vivo* hydrocortisone on subpopulations of human lymphocytes. *J. Clin. Invest.*, **53**, 240

17. Vernon-Roberts, B., Currey, H. L. F. and Perrin, J. (1974). T and B cells in the blood and synovial fluid of rheumatoid patients. *Ann. Rheum. Dis.*, **33**, 430

Discussion 53

M. J. Parnham: (The Netherlands)	Seeing as there appears to be no real correlation with anything at all with any of the symptoms—at one time it goes up and another time it goes down, and another time it does not change at all—would Dr. Roux comment or speculate on the possibility that—in fact so far as I am aware nobody at the meeting has said—everybody is looking for a possible common mode of action in rheumatoid arthritis, but in fact what is happening is that there are many different aetiologies, and the fact that such varied results have been obtained is an indication of this.
Roux:	That is what we suppose, but we have absolutely no proof. We are now studying peculiar liver groups where these cells are decreased. We are studying them with HLA and also with various peripheral phenomena we are searching for the existence of anti-T-cell antibodies.
D. A. Willoughby: (UK)	In view of the fact that in the majority of cases shown a lowering of the T-cells has been observed, would Dr. Roux speculate on the suggestion that rheumatoid arthritis is an immune deficiency disease?
Roux:	That is difficult to answer.
M. Jasani: (UK)	I was much stimulated by Professor Willoughby's remark. In the case of the homo-transplant patients, data are already available that show that during the time of rejection there is a lowering of circulating T-cells. If these patients are given steroid treatment, the level of T-cells rises quite significantly. A static blood count level could therefore be interpreted as indicating utilization of T-cells as much as a possible deficiency.
J. Symoens: (Belgium)	We have followed patients during several months of levasimole treatment and we have seen a dynamic movement in the T-cell numbers. At the beginning there is often the tendency to decrease, then after two or three months' treatment there is a tendency towards restoration.
	Had the patients shown, who had been treated with levasimole, originally low T-cell numbers—all of them? If they were not low at the beginning, then I should expect increases and decreases within the normal range. If they were below normal at the beginning, then I should expect a restoration. Was this correlation seen?
Roux:	They were on four months of treatment, and they had a low level of T-cells at the beginning of treatment. They were treated with 150 mg/day.

54

Should penicillamine be prescribed for rheumatoid arthritis?

W. H. LYLE (UK)

It is a dismal truism that rheumatoid arthritis is less of a threat to life than are some of the drugs prescribed for its treatment. Those drugs which are able to reduce ESR or C-reactive and other acute phase proteins and which may therefore affect the progress of erosive disease[1], are all potentially lethal even when prescribed in an orthodox manner. Penicillamine is one such drug. Since February 1973, when the Licensing Authority permitted rheumatoid arthritis to be added to the indications for the use of penicillamine, more has been written about its adverse than about its beneficial effects, and at meetings where the drug is discussed, almost invariably the chief topic is its toxicity. Four years is not long enough for one to define the place of penicillamine in the treatment of rheumatoid arthritis, but many rheumatologists here have now gained a good deal of experience with this drug and, on the basis of their data, published and otherwise, it is possible to give at least a provisional, interim, answer to the question—'should penicillamine be prescribed for rheumatoid arthritis?'

WILSON'S DISEASE AND CYSTINURIA

D-penicillamine, 3,3 dimethylcysteine, was introduced by Walshe[2] for the treatment of Wilson's disease and has long been the therapeutic mainstay in this rare disorder of copper metabolism. Walshe's first patient is still on the drug, after 21 years, in good health and having borne three normal children. None of his series of about 100 patients has died from the effects of penicillamine but 10 have had to be given alternative treatment (Trien) because of drug intolerance. This withdrawal rate is much lower than any reported for penicillamine in rheumatoid arthritis, despite the fact that Walshe's standard starting dose is 1500 mg daily[3]. Scheinberg[4] has reported that only 4 of the 400 patients he and Sternlieb have treated with penicillamine for Wilson's disease have had to be taken off it because of serious toxic reactions. Three of these died from a drug-induced Goodpasture-like syndrome after 2–3 years on 1 g to 3.5 g daily of penicillamine[5].

In cystinuria also, doses of about 2 g daily are prescribed long term. Rash and proteinuria, though occurring frequently, are not often regarded as indicating withdrawal.

Stephens[6], reviewing 34 cystinuric patients treated with penicillamine over the past 13 years found that only four had discontinued the drug because of nephrosis (three patients) and severe anorexia and nausea (one patient).

Thus, in these two metabolic diseases large doses of penicillamine are tolerated by 90% or more of patients, long term. In particular contrast with its record in rheumatoid arthritis, penicillamine has so rarely caused thrombocytopenia that the routine of frequent and regular blood counts so familiar to rheumatologists is not employed by those treating Wilson's disease or cystinuria.

RHEUMATOID ARTHRITIS

Jaffe[7], not unreasonably, began in 1962 to give his rheumatoid patients doses of penicillamine of the order of those used in Wilson's disease and found that 30% of them developed taste loss or nephrosis, neither of which had been recorded among patients with Wilson's disease at that time. Rash, fever, thrombocytopenia, nausea, vomiting and anorexia also occurred as early reactions and were much reduced in incidence by a more gradual introduction of the drug, starting with 250 mg daily and increasing at 14 day intervals by the same amount to 1500 mg, and occasionally to 2000 mg[8]. This regimen was used in the multi-centre trial which confirmed Jaffe's observations both with respect to the benefits and hazards of penicillamine therapy[9], and in comparisons with gold[10] and azathioprine[11] in which the performance of penicillamine was similar to that of the other drugs.

It is not on grounds of general inefficacy that objections to its use in rheumatoid arthritis may be based, but on its unpredictability, toxicity and cost.

It is impossible to predict whether a particular patient with active rheumatoid arthritis will benefit (if he can tolerate the drug), or whether and when he will react with a rash, proteinuria or thrombocytopenia—all three being common events. This uncertainty has engendered wide differences in usage at different clinics with, so far, no clear indication of which gives the best results.

Since proteinuria occurs in 30% of patients with rheumatoid arthritis (or cystinuria) taking more than 500 mg daily for more than six months, and significant thrombocytopenia in about 10% (with the possibility of subsequent aplasia which may be fatal), the need for frequent follow-up examination is evident and generally recognized. It is in this that the main cost of penicillamine therapy lies and which has limited some clinics to 30–50 patients on the drug. Beyond that number a special weekly clinic seems to be necessary, except in the larger units. This seems unavoidable because the adverse effects of penicillamine are only partly dose-related, and thrombocytopenia and nephrosis occur among patients taking less than 500 mg daily, though less often than among those taking more[12].

Reduction of the maintenance dose from 1200 mg to 600 mg daily[13], or from 1500 mg to 750 mg[14], reduced the incidence of adverse reactions, other than proteinuria, but not therapeutic efficacy. Only when the dosage falls below 500 mg daily does the incidence of proteinuria fall to below 10%; but this is at the cost of a poorer response. Golding and his colleagues treated 127 patients with Steinbroker stage 2 or 3 disease with maintenance doses of 125 to 500 mg daily, and, of these, 18 withdrew because their arthritis worsened, but only 15 of the 30 with adverse reactions. The remainder after one year had improved in varying degrees[15].

Others have confirmed the effectiveness of 250 mg doses for some patients[16,17], so that it is probably worth maintaining that dose for 8 weeks before adding increments of 125 mg at not less than monthly intervals[18]. It now seems likely that the 'standard' maintenance dose will, except for patients with late or recalcitrant disease, fall to below 500 mg. No dose brings about much improvement within 8 weeks and there is therefore no point in pushing up the dose more quickly.

This development undoubtedly puts the drug in a better light. So far the number of patients treated in this way has been too small to demonstrate whether the less common adverse reactions, such as myasthenia, pemphigus foliaceus, Goodpasture syndrome, alveolitis and lupus will become rarities.

Until quite recently most rheumatoid patients were maintained on doses of about 1000 mg, and it is worth bearing in mind that the deaths reported to the C.S.M. between March 1964 and December 1975 as attributable to penicillamine numbered 4. Not all will have been reported and others have occurred since, but may still be below double figures. If this is the case it is because prescribers hitherto have exercised due caution.

Further exploration of the use of penicillamine in rheumatoid arthritis is clearly necessary. If 125 mg or 250 mg of penicillamine can, even in a few patients, halt an active rheumatoid process, this must mean that quite minute amounts are required at the site of action, for although penicillamine is well absorbed from the gut if taken fasting, its absorption is impaired by iron[19], and almost certainly by food.

The pharmacodynamics of penicillamine have not been studied in detail in man but it is clear that 30% or more of a given oral dose remains (as the disulphide) in the faeces, and that about 40% is excreted in the urine within 8 hours, either as mixed or internal disulphide, with a little S-methyl penicillamine[20]. Presumably it is the 30% remaining which is important in rheumatoid arthritis. If this is so then much of the individual variation in response to the drug may ultimately be attributable to variations in absorption, distribution and excretion. This offers the possibility of improvement in formulation of the drug, and further dose reduction.

On present evidence, further investigation of penicillamine in rheumatoid arthritis is indicated and the drug should continue to be prescribed, cautiously.

References

1. Amos, R. S., Constable, T. J., Crockson, R. A., Crockson, A. P. and McConkey, B. (1977). Rheumatoid arthritis: relation of serum C-reactive protein and e.s.r. rates to radiographic changes. *Br. Med. J.*, **1**, 195
2. Walshe, J. M. (1956). Wilson's disease. New oral therapy. *Lancet*, **i**, 25
3. Walshe, J. M. (1977). Brief observations on the management of Wilson's disease. *Proc. R. Soc. Med.* (In press)
4. Scheinberg, I. H. (1975). Uses and usefulness of penicillamine. *N. Engl. J. Med.*, **292**, 1080
5. Sternlieb, I., Bennett, B., and Scheinberg, I. H. (1975). D-penicillamine induced Goodpasture's syndrome in Wilson's disease. *Ann. Intern. Med.*, **82**, 673
6. Stephens, A. D. (1977). The management of cystinuria in 1976. *Proc. R. Soc. Med.* (In press)
7. Jaffe, I. A. (1968). Effects of penicillamine on the kidney and on taste. Symposium on penicillamine. *Postgrad. Med. J.* Suppl. **44**, 15
8. Jaffe, I. A. (1968). Penicillamine in rheumatoid disease with particular reference to rheumatoid factor. Symposium on penicillamine. *Postgrad. Med. J.* Suppl. **44**, 34
9. Multicentre Trial Group (1973). Controlled trial of D-penicillamine in severe rheumatoid arthritis. *Lancet*, **i**, 275
10. Gibson, T., Huskisson, E. C., Wojtulewski, J. A., Scott, P. J., Balme, H. W., Burry, H. C., Grahame, R. and Hart, F. D. (1976). Evidence that D-penicillamine alters the course of rheumatoid arthritis. *Rheumatol. Rehabil.*, **15**, 211
11. Berry, H., Liyanage, S., Durance, R., Barnes, C. G. and Berger, L. (1976). Trial comparing azathioprine and penicillamine in treatment of rheumatoid arthritis. *Ann. Rheum. Dis.*, **35**, 542
12. Day, A. T., Golding, J. R., Lee, P. N. and Butterworth, A. D. (1974). Penicillamine in rheumatoid disease: a long-term study. *Br. Med. J.*, **1**, 180
13. Dixon, A. St. J., Davies, J., Dormandy, T. L., Hamilton, E. B. D., Holt, P. J. L., Mason, R. M., Zutshi, D. W., Thompson, M. and Weber, J. C. P. (1975). Synthetic penicillamine in rheumatoid arthritis. Comparison of high and low dose regimens. A double blind controlled trial. *Scand. J. Rheumatol.*, **4**. Suppl. 8, Abstr. 21
14. Hill, A. G. S. and Hill, H. F. H. (1976). Penicillamine in rheumatoid arthritis: comparison of two dose schedules. *Ann. Rheum. Dis.*, **35**, 541
15. Golding, J. R., Day, A. T., Tomlinson, M. R., Brown, R. M., Hassan, M. O. and Langstaff, S. R. (1977). Rheumatoid arthritis treated with small doses of penicillamine. *Proc. R. Soc. Med.* (In press)
16. McKenzie, J. M. M. (1975). Dosage and toxic reactions of penicillamine in the treatment of rheumatic disorders. *Scand. J. Rheumatol.*, **4**, Suppl. 8, Abstr. 21
17. Jaffe, I. A. (1977). Penicillamine treatment of rheumatoid arthritis with a single daily dose of 250 mg. *Proc. R. Soc. Med.* (In press)
18. White, A. G. (1976). Marrow aplasia and penicillamine. *Lancet*, **ii**, 683
19. Lyle, W. H., Pearcey, D. F. and Hui, M. (1977). Inhibition of penicillamine-induced cupruresis by oral iron. *Proc. R. Soc. Med.* (In press)
20. Perrett, D. (1977). An outline of D-penicillamine metabolism. *Proc. R. Soc. Med.* (In press)

Discussion 54

D. A. Willoughby: Would Dr. Lyle speculate on the mode of action of penicillamine?
(UK)

Lyle: There are many more skilled speculators in the audience than I. One hobbyhorse that I have had for a long time is that somewhere it will be a matter for chelation—the original reason for introducing the stuff—at some very elementary level. It is probably an extra-cellular function because penicillamine does not cross cell membranes. It may attach itself to the surface, but it does not get inside. Copper possibly may be something to do with it. We know that this proteinurea has excited a great deal of interest. 30% is a large number of patients. That might almost be a good success rate for a treatment—a 30% response. Here there is a glomerular lesion with a gross protein leak and nothing much else, and nobody has ever shown that the penicillamine is in fact the hapten. I wonder whether ultimately this might not be the effect of penicillamine shifting stores of cadmium from tissue into the renal tubule where it does damage, and the tubular protein acts as an antigen, and immune complex diseases are arising as a result of that.

I have slides that demonstrate that cadmium renal damage can be produced by giving penicillamine at the same time in rats; gross tubular damage. This is by an uptake by the kidney of cadmium without any increase in excretion, so that balance studies tell one nothing at all about it. The metal is merely shifted from one compartment to another, where it does some injury.

I suspect—to come back to the question—that something of the sort may be happening, but we cannot see it, with some metal, therapeutically, rather than in the way of toxicity.

It must be—I suspect—a very small amount of stuff, and the dynamics will be extremely important—how it is carried about.

W. Brocklehurst: Dr. Lyle mentioned chelation, and brushed it off. Is he assuming that
(UK) the copper should be got rid of, or that it should be chelated in order to make it more bio-available?

There has been speculation recently that combination between copper and some of the anti-inflammatory compounds may be more effective. In some preliminary animal studies that we have done we cannot show it. We cannot indeed repeat the experiments which were quoted in the literature. But, leaving that aside, people do wear copper bracelets, and it could well be that the manner in which the body reacts to the combination between penicillamine and copper, in Wilson's disease, where one is getting rid of an excess, is entirely different from what happens in rheumatoid or other comparable diseases.

Lyle: Yes. The excretion curve—as shown by my last slide—is of a rapid and in a slow phase in urine. I believe that it is the rapid phase which is

595

important in Wilson's disease and cysteinurea, where it is just picking up, exchanging with cysteine, and taking up excess copper and flinging it out in the urine. That is what is wanted for that disease.

But the slow rate—one can find the stuff in the plasma days and days afterwards, some percentage. This, I suspect, is having an effect which one cannot detect in balanced studies. This is probably at enzymatic level in rheumatoid arthritis; quite different from the Wilson's disease.

C. M. Pearson:
(USA)
Referring to Professor Willoughby's comments on mechanisms of action there is some unpublished work by Dr. Whitehouse, when he was with us in Los Angeles, that seems to show that if penicillamine is placed in physiologic contact with lymphocytes for an hour or so and incubated, and then those lymphocytes were removed and washed and so forth, that they were unresponsive to mitogens and so forth. It is possible that utilizing this type of technique in small doses may be one of the modes of action.

Willoughby:
One of the problems when dealing with the penicillamine-like substances *in vitro* is that if one is dealing with a chelating agent and one puts it into any culture system one will immediately have the problem that one is upsetting the balance of the culture medium. This is one of the major hazards with *in vitro* studies of penicillamine.

Lyle:
And not only that, but as Kendall showed very clearly, the ready formation of the mixed disulphide with cysteine in the culture medium will instantly interfere with the cells' health.

J. Arnold:
(UK)
What effect do the dimethyl groups adjacent to the sulphydroxyl group on the side chain have in relation to this mode of action? Would the variation of putting, for example, an ethyl group, or yet another possible chelating amino-ethyl group on the side chain instead of the methyl group have any beneficial effect?

What is the effect on hyaluronic acid concentrations and chondroitin sulphate concentrations in synovial joint fluid?

Lyle:
I do not know the answer to the second question.

In answer to the first, the function of the methyl group is to prevent metabolic degeneration of penicillamine. These things disappear very fast otherwise.

Questions about replacing one methyl group with another should be asked of a chemist. I cannot answer that either.

Arnold:
Would utilization of benzylpenicillin (or some readily breakdownable penicillin) as a result of its metabolic breakdown, have any effect in relation to some possible arthritic achievements.

Lyle:
Benzylpenicillin breaks down to penicillamine to some extent in the body. That is how it was described in the first instance. One does get penicillamine if one is given penicillin.

Arnold:
I was wondering if penicillin-G itself is at all useful in arthritic therapy, as a result of its metabolic breakdown.

Lyle:
Conceivably. I do not know. Has anyone tried penicillin-G as a treatment for rheumatoid arthritis? Wilder things have happened.

Chairman:
Perhaps Dr. Munthe would comment.

E. Munthe:
(Norway)
There have been some scattered reports on the effect of some antibiotics—the beneficial effect of certain antibiotics in rheumatoid disease, and we have observed it in quite a few patients undergoing surgery who had prophylactic antibiotic treatment. However, single observations of this nature would not hold in a controlled trial. Some years ago we held a controlled trial with penicillin but we did not obtain any definite results.

Arnold:
If one considers that penicillamine is a metabolic breakdown product of some penicillins *in vivo*, then has anyone tried any cephalosporin breakdown products which are similar, and have they any effect on arthritics?

PENICILLAMINE AND RHEUMATOID ARTHRITIS

Z. Bacq:
(Belgium)
I am not exactly up to the point, but in Liege and Louvain there have been investigations of the metabolism of penicillin in relation to its mode of action, and apparently within this mechanism, which has now been recently published.

Penicillamine does not appear as a metabolite of penicillin, or at 'least an active one.

Lyle:
That is most interesting. The original discovery of the stuff was as much a hydrolysase of penicillin, by Erun, Chain and co-workers at Oxford. Then when Walsh was looking after a patient with cirrhosis of the liver who happened to be given penicillin for an infection, he found that the copper in the urine had increased, and he then went back to look at the known breakdown products, the metabolites of penicillin, and saw that this particular structure was in the literature, and got it made. It again looks as if medicine has made another giant stride forward by mistake!

However, penicillin cannot exist for very long in the free state in body fluids. It is bound to be picked up by some metal, or else form a disulphide of some sort.

This may be a possibility. This is probably the answer.

A. Doble:
(UK)
On the question of the cephalosporin possibly acting in the same way as the penicillin, giving rise to something useful like penicillin, giving rise to something useful like penicillamine—as far as I can remember it is a mistake to think that the structure of cephalosporin is anything like penicillin. I do not think that that is really a possibility.

55

Long-term evaluation of intermittent levamisole treatment in rheumatoid arthritis

E. M. VEYS AND H. MIELANTS (Belgium)

INTRODUCTION

Some recent studies have indicated that humoral and cellular immunity could be impaired in RA[1-5]. It would therefore seem reasonable to assume that an agent capable of restoring impaired cellular immunity might be of value in treatment of the disease.

In 1973, we consequently decided to examine the effect of levamisole on the evolution of RA patients.

The preliminary results have already been reported elsewhere[6,7]. Our patients were all treated discontinuously from the beginning of the study (150 mg/day, four days per week). Since the onset of the present study interesting results have been reported by Schuermans[8] and by Huskisson et al.[9], who administered the drug continuously (150 mg/day).

MATERIAL AND METHODS

Seventy patients with definite or classical RA, according to the ARA criteria, were selected for this open study. All patients received levamisole at a dosage of 150 mg once daily or 50 mg thrice daily for four consecutive days per week.

Patient groups

Group I: 47 patients stabilized on an optimal anti-inflammatory regimen which remained virtually constant for the duration of the study. Decrease of dosage of anti-inflammatory drugs was permitted. No patient received other basic treatments such as chrysotherapy or D-penicillamine. Fourteen dropped out of the trial after one or two weeks because of immediate toxicodermia, anorexia or nausea. The remaining 33 patients, constituting this report on drug activity, all had active disease. Assessments were made before onset of the treatment and again after 6, 12, 18, 24, 30 and 36 months. They included duration of morning stiffness, articular index[10], grip strength (right and left hand in mm Hg), proximal interphalangeal joint circumference, erythrocyte sedimentation rate (ESR), rheumatoid factor titre and immunoglobulin levels.

The classification of the 33 patients according to the anatomical stage of Steinbrocker[11] was as follows: stage I—7 patients; stage II—10 patients; stage III—7 patients and stage IV—9 patients. Twenty-nine patients were found to be seropositive at the start of the study and four were seronegative. All were treated with levamisole for at least six months, twenty-four patients were followed during 12 months, 16 during 18 months, seven 24 months, three 30 months and one 36 months.

Statistical methods: Wilcoxon's matched-pairs signed-ranks test for paired differences, two-tailed, was used to compare the differences between the successive periods of treatment. Initial values were compared with those obtained after 6, 12, 18 and 24 months of treatment. The differences between values observed after 6 and 12 months were also evaluated. The group of patients with more than two years' treatment was too small for statistical evaluation.

Group II: Eleven patients were treated simultaneously with gold-salts and with levamisole. Both treatment regimens were started at the same moment. This group was not used to evaluate the activity of levamisole but furnished data about toxicity.

Group III: Twelve patients, not completely cleared after chrysotherapy received a further maintenance treatment of 50 mg gold each month in addition to 150 mg levamisole 4 days per week. This group gave important indications about toxicity. No evaluation of activity was possible since the patients received two different basic drugs.

RESULTS

Activity

Evolution of the morning stiffness is shown on Figure 55.1, of Ritchie index on Figure 55.2, of grip strength on Figure 55.3 and of ESR on Figure 55.4. Table 55.1 gives the statistical evaluation of the results. After a 6-month treatment, a statistically significant improvement was recorded in morning stiffness, Ritchie index, grip-strength and ESR. No decrease in rheumatoid factor titre was observed. After 12 and 18 months of treatment, morning

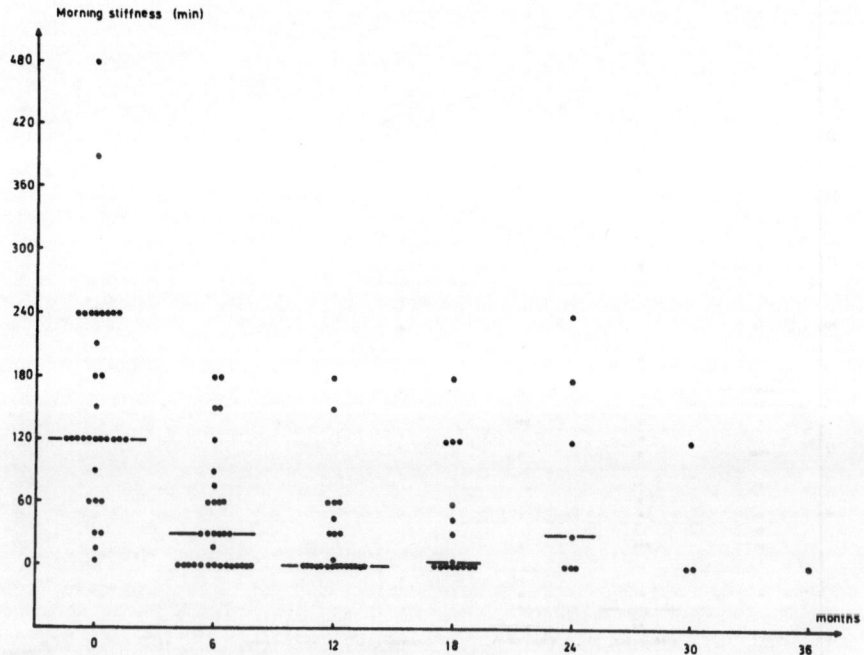

Figure 55.1 Evolution of morning stiffness during levamisole treatment. The medium value is indicated by a line

Table 55.1 Statistical evaluation of the parameters during levamisole treatment ($n =$ number of patients)

| Parameters | Statistical evaluation* between | | | | |
	0 and 6 mo	0 and 12 mo	0 and 18 mo	0 and 24 mo	6 and 12 mo
Morning stiffness	$n = \cdot 33$	$n = 24$	$n = 16$	$n = 7$	$n = 24$
	$2a < 0.01^+$	$2a < 0.01^+$	$2a < 0.01^+$	$2a > 0.10$	$2a > 0.10$
Ritchie index	$n = 33$	$n = 24$	$n = 16$	$n = 7$	$n = 24$
	$2a < 0.01^+$	$2a < 0.01^+$	$2a < 0.01^+$	$2a > 0.10$	$2a > 0.10$
Grip strength	$n = 31$	$n = 21$	$n = 16$	$n = 7$	$n = 21$
	$2a < 0.01^+$	$2a < 0.01^+$	$2a < 0.01^+$	$2a > 0.10$	$2a < 0.01^+$
PIP index	$n = 24$	$n = 17$	$n = 13$	$n = 7$	$n = 17$
	$2a > 0.10$	$2a > 0.10$	$2a > 0.10$	$2a > 0.10$	$2a > 0.10$
Sedimentation rate	$n = 33$	$n = 24$	$n = 16$	$n = 7$	$n = 24$
	$2a < 0.01^+$	$2a < 0.01^+$	$2a < 0.01^+$	$2a < 0.05^+$	$2a > 0.10$

* Wilcoxon matched-pairs signed-ranks test for paired differences, two-tailed (Siegel, S.: *Nonparametric Statistics*, McGraw-Hill Book Company, New York (1956), pp. 75–83).
  $^+$ Statistically significant improvement

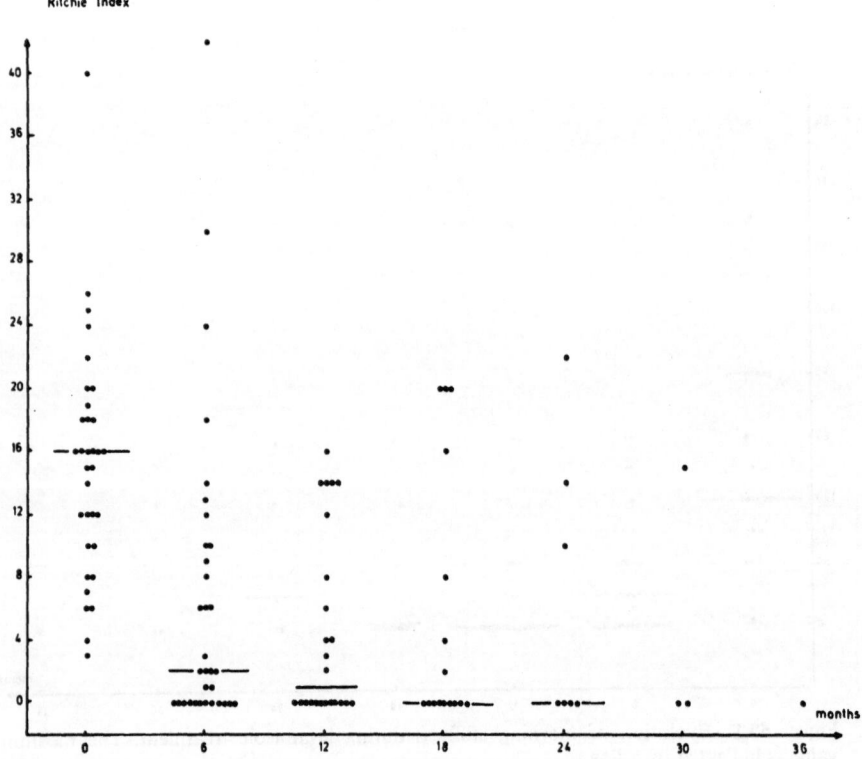

Figure 55.2 Evolution of the Rítchie index during levamisole treatment. The mean value is indicated by a line

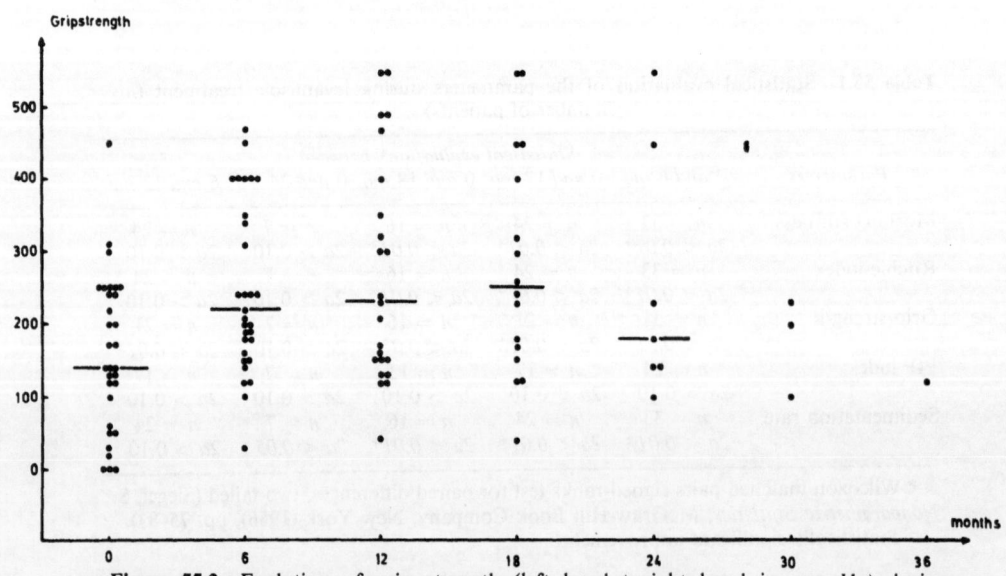

Figure 55.3 Evolution of grip strength (left hand + right hand in mm Hg) during levamisole treatment

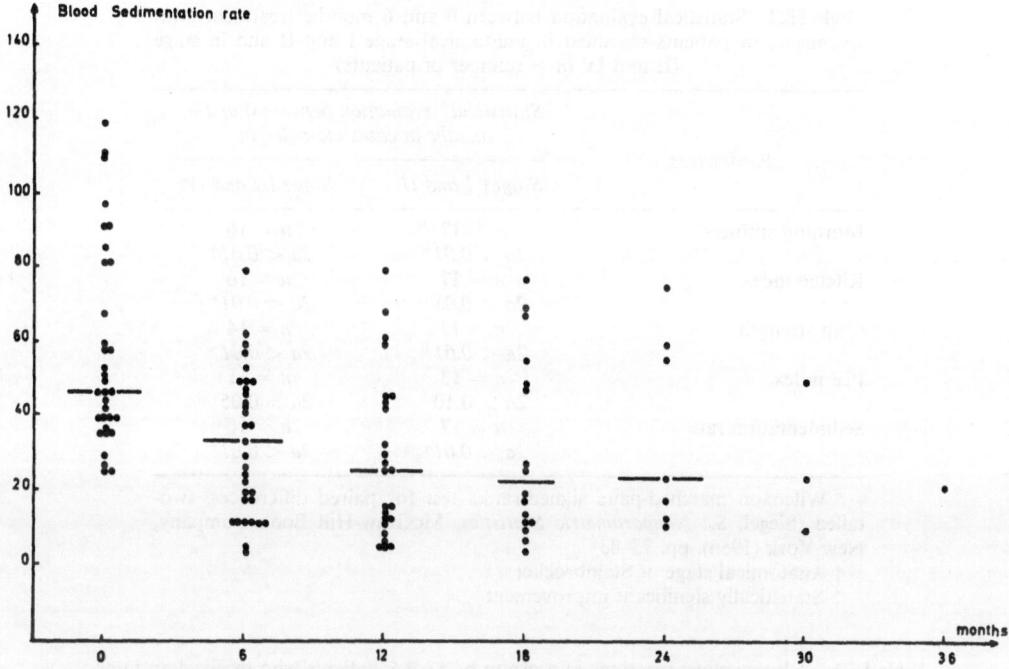

Figure 55.4 Evolution of the e.s.r. during levamisole treatment

stiffness, Ritchie index, grip strength and ESR had improved significantly. After 24 months of treatment, no variables had improved any further, when compared with the initial situation. But we must stress that the number of cases in the class of 24 months is small and that definite conclusions cannot be made. Comparison of values observed after 6 and 12 months revealed no significant difference for any variable.

Classification according to the stage of the disease allowed us to evaluate the response of patients in stages I and II and in stages III and IV. The results observed during the first six months of treatment are presented in Table 55.2. In stages III and IV, as well as in stages I and II, there was improvement in morning stiffness, Ritchie index, grip strength and ESR.

Toxicity (Table 55.3)

Fourteen patients of group I showed early signs of toxicodermia with pruritus (eight patients) or nausea and anorexia (six patients) during the first month of treatment so that further evaluation of these patients was impossible. Later on side-effects occurred in 12 of the 33 patients. Mild toxicodermia was observed in seven patients, allergic vasculitis in two patients, granulocyto-penia in one case, ulcerative stomatitis in six patients, neurosensory irritability in two patients, transient gastralgia in four patients and hypergeuses-thesia in four patients. Consequently a total of 26 side-effects was noticed

Table 55.2 Statistical evaluation between 0 and 6 months treatment with levamisole in patients classified in anatomical stage I and II and in stage III and IV (n = number of patients)

Parameters	Statistical* evaluation between 0 and 6 months in cases classified in	
	Stage† I and II	Stage III and IV
Morning stiffness	$n = 17$	$n = 16$
	$2a < 0.01^+$	$2a < 0.01^+$
Ritchie index	$n = 17$	$n = 16$
	$2a < 0.05^+$	$2a < 0.01^+$
Grip strength	$n = 17$	$n = 14$
	$2a < 0.01^+$	$2a < 0.01^+$
PIP index	$n = 13$	$n = 11$
	$2a > 0.10$	$2a > 0.05$
Sedimentation rate	$n = 17$	$n = 16$
	$2a < 0.01^+$	$2a < 0.01^+$

* Wilcoxon matched-pairs signed-ranks test for paired differences, two-tailed (Siegel, S.: *Nonparametric Statistics*, McGraw-Hill Book Company, New York (1956), pp. 75–83)
† Anatomical stage of Steinbrocker
+ Statistically significant improvement

Table 55.3 Adverse clinic reactions in a group of 47 RA patients who received an intermittent levamisole treatment

Group I (47 patients)		
Early Toxicity:	—toxicodermia with pruritus	8 patients
(14 patients)	—nausea and anorexia	6 patients
Late Toxicity:	—toxicodermia	7 patients
(12 patients)	—allergic vasculitis	2 patients
	—granulocytopenia	1 patient
	—ulcerative stomatitis	6 patients
	—neurosensory irritability	2 patients
	—transient gastralgia	4 patients
	—hypergeusesthesia	4 patients

in this group; some patients suffering from more than one side-effect (toxicodermia and stomatitis frequently occurred simultaneously).

After a longer period administration of levamisole was interrupted in 6 patients because of toxicodermia with persistent pruritus: case 1 after 9 months, case 4 after 12 months, case 9 after 6 months, case 10 after 10 months, case 12 after 18 months and case 27 after 6 months. In one patient (case 30) the treatment was dicontinued after 6 months because of ulcerative stomatitis. In two cases, levamisole treatment was stopped because of allergic vasculitis: case 21 after 12 months and case 23 after 6 months. In one case (case 32), administration of the drug was interrupted after 13 months because of granulocytopenia (white blood cell count: 3300 per mm^3 and 28% polymorphonuclear cells on 11.12.1976), spontaneous reversion was observed.

All side-effects observed in Group I were reversible and disappeared completely one month after interruption of the treatment. In Group II the frequency of adverse clinical experiences was the same as in Group I, but in Group III three cases of agranulocytosis, of the same type as described by other authors[12] were observed. Fortunately our patients recovered completely.

DISCUSSION

In this open trial morning stiffness, Ritchie index and sedimentation rate improved on levamisole and grip strength in patients with RA increased. The proximal interphalangeal joint size was not influenced by the drug. These results suggest that levamisole is effective in RA.

Considering all variables, the overall assessment in the 33 patients was as follows: at the 6-month evaluation, the disease was completely suppressed in 18 patients, markedly improved in eight patients and unchanged in seven patients on levamisole treatment. At the 12-month evaluation (including 24 patients), the disease was completely suppressed in 12 patients, markedly improved in five patients and remained unchanged in the same seven patients who had not improved at the 6-month evaluation. At the 18-month evaluation (including 16 patients), the disease was entirely suppressed in nine patients and improved in three patients, while four patients had deteriorated slightly.

It would thus appear that levamisole is a drug of slow action in this disease, achieving maximum benefit in about 6 months. Further on the response of levamisole in RA seems to be controlled by an all-or-nothing law. However, it should be noticed that in some patients presenting persisting side-effects after 10 and 12 months of treatment, to such an extent that administration of the drug was interrupted after this period, the improvement continued for more than 18 months after discontinuation of therapy. This would suggest that it might be better to discontinue the drug after symptoms have been controlled, and possibly institute treatment again after occurrence of an exacerbation.

In a previous study[8] we did not observe any significant decrease in rheumatoid factor titre or in IgG levels. However IgM and IgA levels were significantly decreased after 6 months of treatment. We have no definite explanation for these data. The results presented in this study indicate that levamisole is effective in patients with severe radiological lesions (stages III and IV) as well as in early cases (stages I and II). Our results with intermittent levamisole administration seem comparable with those of other investigators using continuous treatment[8,9].

Minor side-effects (toxicodermia, ulcerative stomatitis, gastralgia, hypergeusesthesia and neurosensory irritability) and major adverse reactions (allergic vasculitis, granulocytopenia) occurred as frequently with intermittent levamisole administration as with continuous treatment.

As to the leucopenia it should be noticed that in Group III, the white blood cell count was determined only once each month at the instant of gold salts injection. In Groups I and II the white blood cell count was effected weekly or fortnightly and the single case of granulocytopenia was detected earlier than those observed in Group III, where a total lack of polymorphonuclear cells was observed in three cases. But we do not know if a more frequent determination of white blood cell count would permit to detect at time cases with evolution to agranulocytosis. We believe there are two groups of side-effects on the white blood cells. A first one: a slow fall in the total white blood cell count which is easily reversible by stopping the drug and which can be detected by previous regular white blood cell count. A second: with a dramatic fall in the percentage of granulocytes which occurs in the time of a few days. Only the chance permits us to detect these cases at time (thus more determinations will detect earlier cases). So we feel that a white blood cell count must be performed each week in patients of levamisole treatment. The fact that we observed three cases of granulocytopenia in the group of patients receiving simultaneously levamisole and gold salts suggests a possible cumulative toxic effect of both drugs on the granulocytes.

Our beneficial results, obtained through immunostimulation as opposed to immunosuppression, require substantiation in controlled trials on a larger number of patients. They further suggest that intermittent levamisole therapy is as effective as continuous treatment in RA.

Actually we can conclude that levamisole is active in treatment of RA. But the place of levamisole on the arsenal of the basic treatment of the disease is not yet clear.

With a better knowledge of the mode of action of the drug, we hope to find some parameters which can indicate if a case will answer to this immunomodulating therapy.

References

1. Veys, E. M. and Claessens, H. (1968). Serum levels of IgG, IgM and IgA in rheumatoid arthritis. *Ann. Rheum. Dis.*, **27**, 431
2. Veys, E., Loore, J. de and Mielants, H. (1971). Dosage des immunoglobulines G, M et A dans le liquide synovial. *Rev. Rheum.*, **38**, 289
3. Veys, E. M. (1974). Comparative investigation of protein concentration in serum and synovial fluid. *Scand. J. Rheumatol.*, **3**, 1
4. Reynolds, M. D. and Abdou, N. I. (1973). Comparative study of the *in vitro* proliferative responses of blood and synovial fluid leucocytes of rheumatoid arthritis patients. *J. Clin. Invest.*, **52**, 1627
5. Mowat, A. G. and Baum, J. (1971). Chemotaxis of polymorphonuclear leucocytes from patients with rheumatoid arthritis. *J. Clin. Invest.*, **50**, 2541
6. Veys, E. M., Mielants, H., de Bussere, A., Decrans, L. and Gabriel, P. (1976). Levamisole in rheumatoid arthritis. *Lancet*, i, 808
7. Veys, E. M. and Mielants, H. (1977). Long term evaluation of intermittent levamisole treatment in rheumatoid arthritis. *J. Rheumatol.* (In press)

INTERMITTENT LEVAMISOLE TREATMENT

8. Schuermans, Y. (1975). Levamisole in rheumatoid arthritis. *Lancet*, **i**, 111
9. Huskisson, E. C., Dieppe, P. A., Scott, J., Trapnell, J., Balme, H. W. and Willoughby, D. A. (1976). Immunostimulant therapy with levamisole for rheumatoid arthritis. *Lancet*, **i**, 393
10. Ritchie, D., Boyle, J. A., McInnes, J. M., Jasani, M. K., Dalakos, T. G., Grieveson, P. G. and Buchanan, W. W. (1968). Clinical studies with an articular index for the assessment of joint tenderness in patients with rheumatoid arthritis. *Q. J. Med.*, **37**, 393
11. Steinbrocker, O., Traeger, C. H. and Batterman, R. C. (1949). Therapeutic criteria in rheumatoid arthritis. *J. Am. Med. Assoc.*, **140**, 659
12. Trabert, U., Rosenthal, M. and Muller, W. (1976). Therapie entzündlich-rheumatischer Krankheiten mit Levamisol, einer immunomodulierenden Substanz. *Schweiz. Med. Woschenchr.*, **106**, 1293

Discussion 55

R. Numo: (Italy)	Could Professor Veys list the criteria by which patients were included in the trial? If the drug is really an immuno-stimulant, was it possible to separate or to identify the patient who needed to be immuno-suppressed or to be immuno-stimulated? It is a critical point since I would speculate about one of the cases presented on slide—the allergic vasculitis. In some cases the drugs could worsen the natural progress of the disease. May we also hear something about the granular cytopenia cases? Finally, could this drug replace other drugs normally used in the disease?
Veys:	On the question of basis for selection, I have already said that the study started four years ago and the sole basis for putting a patient on to levasimole treatment is the presence of active disease. We did not look for the cell immunity in these patients. Next, allergic vasculitis. One of the three cases with allergic vasculitis was most interesting. The patient was a woman who presented allergic vasculitis after two months of treatment with levamisole. We thought then that it was a natural evolution of the disease, perhaps increased in this case, so we stopped the levamisole, and the allergic vasculitis had completely disappeared within a month. Six months later we again started the patient on levamisole, and the allergic vasculitis again appeared—within 3 weeks. When the levamisole was stopped, that stopped too. Perhaps in this case the levamisole had worsened the situation in this particular patient. The third question dealt with granular cytopenia. This is an important point since this is the most important of the drug's toxic effects. There are many reports of granulocytosis in rhuematoid arthritis treated with levamisole, and most authors are in agreement on one point. When a granulocytosis occurs one should do nothing. The patient should be put in a sterile room, given no antibiotics, no trans-fusions, no therapy, and complete recovery will occur within two or three days. Unfortunately we had a granulocytosis which we treated with antibiotics and the granulocytosis lasted for two or three weeks, and in one case presented severe infection. Fortunately all the cases recovered completely. There is no definite solution. White blood cell counts have to be done as frequently as possible because there are some dramatically presenting granulocytoses. I agree that it is an important point.
M. Lequesne: (France) Veys:	What about the bone marrow in Professor Vey's cases? Was it some-times normal, or sometimes poor? Bone marrow studies in cases of granulocytosis are not too interesting. They show a stopping of maturation, but that is because of an allergic reaction.

608

	These patients also recover completely within several days, with no treatment being given.
E. Munthe: (Norway)	Were there any relapses after withdrawal, and if there were, then how long after the withdrawal did the relapse occur?
	How long should treatment continue to avoid relapses? What is the lowest possible maintenance dose?
Veys:	That is an important question. Since we have observed a granulocytosis after a short time, we have decided to stop all the patients when they are in remission after a minimum of six months of treatment. We then wait for symptoms of relapse. There were two cases treated for six or more months that were stopped because of toxicity, and these two cases are now in remission; one for over a year and the other for more than two years—with no treatment. This is important data on relapses in patients in whom treatment was stopped.
	I can also report on another case; not from my own series. A patient was treated with levamisole discontinuously, and under treatment symptoms *relapsed*. Then a colleague started to treat the patient daily, and he was again in remission—but that is an isolated case.
M. Jasani: (UK)	One way to find out something about the patients under study would be to get some idea of the average Ritchie Index at the commencement of the study. Could Professor Veys recollect what the average Ritchie Index of those patients was?
Veys:	I showed this on the slides. They all had active disease.
Jasani:	There are so many drugs available today which can shift the Ritchie Index by 7–10 points at the most between initial value and final value. When a new remedy is described, then we need to know if the observed difference between initial and six-months value is greater than that kind of level. That is what I am after. Statistical values certainly help, but they do not give that part of the picture.
Veys:	It is certain that rheumatoid arthritis when it is classified in stage 3 or 4, even where there is no more inflammation, the Ritchie Index will always read more than 0. Once there is a deformed joint, the Ritchie Index will remain positive, and when the joint is mobilized, then pain is created.
	Morning stiffness might perhaps be a good parameter. The slides showed that it no longer existed in all the cases in which there was complete remission—median value was under 20 min (*from slide*).
	The evolution of the Ritchie Index was shown on another of the slides (accompanying the Paper). We started with a median of 15% with a Ritchie Index of 2 (after 6 months) and 1 (after 12 months). That is hardly a small decrease. It is an important decrease.
Jasani:	I am not very keen on stiffness. What happened to the joint swellings?
Veys:	Joint swellings decreased, but I did not include numbers of joint swellings in my parameters. A current double-blind study shows that the Ritchie Index falls faster than joint swelling.
Jasani:	Was there any difference that impressed Professor Veys as a clinician, either on the basis of the clinical picture, or on the basis of laboratory data, which distinguished those who responded from those who did not?
Veys:	I have no parameters other than the sedimentation rate and the fall in acute phase proteins. The question of which patients will respond to treatment cannot be determined in a laboratory.

609

General Discussion

Chairman: D. A. Willoughby (UK)

N. Piller:
(Australia)

I have a number of comments on Dr. Ferreira's paper (Thursday).

As a lymphologist I am always concerned about the absence of information relating to the functioning of the lymphatic system during all of the events that we have discussed. One particular case was the lack of correlation between vascular permeability and oedema following carrageenin-induced oedema. The lymphatic system can only handle a certain volume of protein and fluid, and above this level protein and fluid will begin to accumulate in the tissues, and then we find a very good correlation between oedema formation and vascular permeability. But the lymphatic system eventually can remove this protein, and at that stage, when the lymphatic system is functioning maximally, no correlation, or very little correlation will be found between oedema formation and the vascular permeability.

Secondly, we have been working with what we call anti-inflammatory drugs. This is somewhat outside the field since I am a lymphologist and this is a den of biochemists and I must admit to feeling a little insecure. However, Dr. Davies mentioned zymosan and he said that this caused the release of acid hydrolases from macrophages. For the inflammatory agents, he, like others, measures the extent of inflammation by the extent by which the release of proteases is caused, thereby causing a disruption to the functioning of the tissues as a whole.

Working with some benzpyrenes, we have found a very strong correlation between enzyme release and acid protease release, neutral protease release, and the oedema reducing ability of a number of drugs, including venolot and the components of venolot, coumarin, *Troxerutin*, reparol, and levamisole—but levamisole, as is well known, has very little effect on oedema formation. We are interested because we have been finding a very strong correlation—in the region of 90% or 95% between the release of proteases, active at acid and neutral pHs, and the extent of oedema reduction. This is suggesting that maybe these types of drugs should be considered as being useful in the treatment of rheumatoid arthritis and related conditions.

We are using drug-induced proteolysis as a measure of a restoration of the disorder of the tissues caused by inflammatory agents, so we are going one more step up the scale.

Chairman:

So that whereas there are several people trying to inhibit proteases, Mr. Piller is suggesting the novel approach of increasing protease activation in the lymphatics.

Piller:

These increases are found in the extra-cellular compartments of the skin and the muscle. We are talking about a model of thermal oedema. Also, in the acute and chronic phase of an experimental model of

610

	lymphoedema, orderly increases in proteases, active at neutral and acid pH, are found in the extra-cellular compartment of the skin, particularly in thermal and lymphoedema, and to a lesser extent in the extra-cellular compartment of the muscle.
	In dealing with thermal oedema and lymphoedema there is an extremely good correlation between the protease levels in the oedema fluid and the effectiveness of the drug in reducing the oedema.
G. Velo: (Italy)	I should like to come back to the problem of gold thiomalate and penicillamine and to have Dr. Munthe comment on the possibility that gold thiomalate could chelate copper. Has he any knowledge or experience of this problem?
E. Munthe: (Norway)	From a theoretical point of view it could well be that thiomalate could chelate copper. We are currently measuring copper values in patients treated with Myocrisin to see whether there are any changes. The results of the study are not yet available, but we have seen some copper depression in penicillamine treated patients.
Chairman:	Mr. Cashin might comment—about SOD.
C. Cashin: (UK)	There are two observations in the literature which to my mind show a paradox—an apparent paradox—following the papers here today and yesterday—that is that D-penicillamine has been reported in both man and rats to reduce superoxide dismutase levels. From Thursday's papers it would appear that the free radicals produced during inflammation and during prostaglandin synthesis are rather nasty things and the action of orgotein in inhibiting these radicals appears beneficial. Yet apparently with penicillamine there is the opposite effect.
D. Freed: (UK)	Is it possible that superoxide dismutases are reduced by using them up?
Cashin:	That might be so in the case of penicillamine. Superoxide dismutase is a copper and zinc containing enzyme, and it might be that the chelating properties of penicillamine which are known to be important in its action in Wilson's disease, and it is also known to chelate zinc to a lesser extent. This might be its action.
F. W. Kuehl: (USA)	I am happy to hear of this interest in superoxide, but we have no data about the free radical other than what I have given out.
Chairman:	We do not need data at this point in the meeting, we are interested in speculation and future trends.
W. Brocklehurst: (UK)	May I throw out another possibility in relation to what Mr. Cashin has said. Since we know that cysteine mops up free radicals, why should penicillamine not do the same?
	I am toying with the idea of throwing out further challenges. Changes in the rheumatoid factor could result from alterations in the tertiary structure of the immune globulins. If immune globulins are to be altered, then that will also alter the response of those cells which react as a consequence of their ability to recognize other events in their milieu which are mediated through the immune globulins on their surface. If the activity of enzymes is dependent on their tertiary structure—and everyone knows that it is—then if the thiol links are altered within the protein the tertiary structure will be altered again.
	These are a couple of examples of the way in which something as active as penicillamine can be interfering in a whole lot of biological processes, so let us not cramp our sights on this and think of only one action.
Chairman:	No one would consider that there was just one action with any of these drugs. If only there were.
Kuehl:	I can at least say that cysteine does not scavenge the free radical derived from the oxygenation of arachidonic acid.
Chairman:	Would Dr. Brocklehurst explain the mode of action of penicillamine.
Brocklehurst:	I do not know how penicillamine works. I have steadfastly refused to try and do studies on it in the lab because I do not know how it works,

and therefore I do not know how to do tests which relate to its mode of action.

There are so many activities in relation to protein structure which are crucial to the biological function of tissue which can be changed by penicillamine that any of those modes of action may be the one which really matters.

C. da Rocha-Afodu: The site of action of penicillin on bacteria is known to be the cell wall.
(Italy) The breakdown product of penicillin is known to be penicillamine. From the work of Dr. Svartz we know that following the injection of streptococcus Group B into joints the rheumatoid factor is produced. If penicillamine is a metabolite of penicillin, this means that penicillin acts by changing the structure of the cell wall in which the antigens are located. If these antigens are destroyed then there will be no rheumatoid factor and therefore this would be the mode of action of penicillamine.

I have a question for Professor Veys, which refers to some of the measurements that he directed to the treatment with levamisole—grip strength, morning stiffness, Ritchie Index, PIP Index, and sedimentation rate. How does he measure grip strength and morning stiffness? Are the data empirical, or is there any basis behind them?

E. M. Veys: Determination of morning stiffness was done by asking the patient.
(Belgium) I used no other method. The patient was asked to say how long he was stiff that morning.

Grip strength was measured with a manometer.

da Rocha-Afodu: So it is not quantitative! Before these things can be produced, and before anything can be deduced from these measurements they have to be quantitative.

Veys: I think we all know that, but there are no better parameters.
Z. Bacq: I should like to come back on some basic effects of thiols. When
(Belgium) reducing the disulphide bonds of proteins, two effects may be observed. Certain macroglobins are really S–S polymers so that if there is a sufficient concentration of an active thiol, the molecular weight of these macroglobulins may be reduced and some clinically favourable effects result.

The second physico-chemical effects of reducing the disulphide bonds in the protein is to increase the number of available sites in the molecule to the binding of free fatty acids and free unsaturated acids like arachidonic acid. The site where this arachidonic acid is bound to the protein is not exactly the SH function, but it is very near the sulphydryl function. Therefore if the number of sulphydryl functions in a protein is increased by a thiol, then the binding of arachidonic acid may be increased, and that of these acids which are the precursors to prostaglandin; this mechanism may be reducing the synthesis of prostaglandin and improving some at least of the inflammatory actions.

J. Arnold: Somebody asked about the chelation of copper in gold-thiomalate and
(UK) the relation of this to penicillamine. Looking at the structure of gold-thiomalate, one can note two carboxyl groups separated by two carbon atoms between them. Perhaps this possibly chelates to Cu^{++} in solution via COO^-, whereas with penicillamine there is only one carboxyl group, with an amino group attached on the same carbon atom, and a sulphydryl group at a distance of two carbon atoms. Possibly this would account for the difference there.

Possibly one can get a clearer picture of the modes of action by drawing three dimensional structural models—e.g. on a blackboard—which also show the unbonded electron pairs. For example, in sulphydryl there is a tetrahedryl structure with an SH group and two tetrahedrally bonded electron pairs. Obviously these play important parts in any ionic or hydrogen bonding processes.

GENERAL DISCUSSION

For example, a lot of arthritis will appear to be due to variations in viscosity in synovial fluid in joints owing to variations on protein carbohydrate structure in hyaluronic acid and chondroitin sulphate. As someone mentioned previously, the breakdown of long-chain proteins, long-chain helical polypeptides in solution may obviously vary the viscosity of these solutions. Perhaps some of the arthritis is due either to the absence of hyaluronic acid, or of chondroitin sulphate, and therefore a lot of increased joint friction, or to an increase in viscosity in the hyaluronic acid chondroitin sulphate which would also cause problematics in that area.

If we look at the structure of penicillamine, we can see a sulphydryl group which is very similar to acetyl cysteine in bronchial therapy whereby by cleaving the S–S bonds in muco-protein with an SH group of acetyl-cysteine, or cysteine-type products, the viscosity is reduced, and perhaps the sulphydryl group there plays a very similar role.

Obviously there is a very close amino group on a virtually adjacent carbon atom and presumably this does something in the rupture of CONH polypeptide bonds, attaches itself there, and then possibly ruptures the sulphydryl group and thus varies viscosity.

There is also a carboxyl group. This will obviously have a totally different effect because there will be a COO$^-$ ion with a free electron pair which will obviously incorporate itself, with pH variations, into the CONH bond of various polypeptides. Most of these polypeptides are helical-type structures with hydrogen bonding between the CO and NH groups and the globulins there—pleated polypeptides producing what appears to be an oval-type structure. But basically these structures are always the same.

A molecule, such as penicillamine, with these three key groups—SH, NH and COO$^-$ will also have a massive interference effect in all these processes just by virtue of having these groups.

For gold thiomalate there will be a slightly different effect because there are two COO$^-$ groups and an SH group—again all fairly close—producing what effectively is like a central point with three groups, COO$^-$, SH and COO$^-$ coming out from the centre, producing some kind of tetrahedral spike effect. Lots of groups can join in on to these groups.

What conclusions can be drawn for synthetic methods, or synthetic possibilities from these two molecules? Obviously they must be molecules which contain SH, NH$_2$ and COO$^-$ groups, at reasonably close range. If one fiddles around with molecules in that sort of way possibly one can get a lot of interesting effects.

R. Numo:
(Italy)
Could we come back for a moment to the problem levamisole.

In any particular evaluation which has parameters—mainly immunological parameters—it is possible to monitor when starting which results might be expected in some patients: e.g. immune response, delayed hypersensitivity immune response, immune complex detectability; vasculitis, etc.

In a critical evaluation, are those who work with levamisole able to forecast or to predict which patients would be likely to have positive results?

Veys:
The first question was whether levamisole works in rheumatoid arthritis. We think that it does. We have serum stored from all these cases and we are waiting for better knowledge of the mechanism of action of the drug to do something with this. Perhaps in time we shall be able to draw up parameters as to whether a patient will respond to treatment, but we have nothing yet. Dr. Roux's paper would seem to bear this out. He did not find any difference or any variation in T-lymphocytes before or after and he had good results in patients with low T- and with high T-lymphocyte counts.

613

We cannot draw up parameters.

D. A. Willoughby:
(UK)
When lists of patients with side effects are written up, it can be very misleading if one patient happens to have all of the side effects, or one patient shows only one of the side effects. So many of these are allergic-type phenomena. It would be very interesting to know how widely diffused the side effects are throughout the whole population.

Veys:
The number of patients is too small for this, but those patients in whom an allergic vasculitis develops—I showed slides—who are treated with penicillamine almost always develop a proteinurea immediately. Perhaps this is important.

I. Ginsburg:
(Israel)
This session is an appropriate session in which to make some very wide speculations. I read something about future trends and about the possible topics for the next meeting in the series. I should like to speculate on the inflammatory response in general and on what I personally see as some important avenues of research to be pursued in order to understand the mechanism of tissue destruction that we see in such debilitating diseases as rheumatoid arthritis and other similar phenomena.

We know very well that the matrix of the connective tissue has a very high percentage of sulphated mucopolysaccharides and that these may be generated or released by enzymes of both polymorphs and macrophages, as well as enzymes coming from other sources.

It is well-known and established among biochemists that many lysosomal enzymes may be strongly inhibited by excess glycosaminoglycans, such as chondroitin sulphate, heparin sulphate, keratin sulphate and other materials.

On the other hand, we have to take into consideration that during the breakdown of tissues, histones and other cationic substances may be released from either nuclei or from polymorphs, and then form complexes with the anionic poly-electrolytes. These may precipitate and do all kinds of tricky things to the tissues.

I want to raise a general question to which I do not know the answer. It is possible that when the evolution of an inflammatory response is followed, that in normal cases a healing process can be seen in which the polymorphs come first, the monocytes come second, and then there are probably some colony-stimulating factors that enhance fibroblast proliferation, the position of collagen, elastic fibres and so forth? Is it possible that the cessation of inflammation under normal conditions reaches a point where there are excess inhibitors of lysosomal enzymes that are concentrating in the tissues, thus preventing the deleterious effect of lysosomal enzymes?

However, what do we know about balances between cationic and anionic poly-electrolytes in tissues? I should like to suggest the following. Since we know that many lysosomal enzymes can be inhibited, at least *in vitro*, in the test tube by anionic poly-electrolytes, and if we believe that when chondroitin sulphate is released from the mucopolysaccharides it is just washed away because it depolymerizes, then would it be possible to form artificial complexes or artificial substances coupled to chondroitin sulphates that make them insoluble and leave the N-groups of the sulphates out to capture the lysosomal enzymes, and then thus prevent the neutralization of the anionic polyelectrolytes by the counterparts, cationic material which accumulates in an inflammatory site?

I have another general question. Is it possible that the cessation of inflammation is due to the accumulation of enzyme inhibitors?

Willoughby:
Dr. Ginsburg and I are old friends and I know that when he poses a question and says that he does not know the answer, it probably means that not even God knows the answer!

The question has been posed!

H. Jones:
(UK)

One interesting feature of penicillamine therapy in patients is that as well as reducing the symptoms of the disease it reduces the RF titre and the ESR. Dr. Huskisson has said that this indicates that the penicillamine is aborting the fundamental in the logical error in that patient. Can anybody suggest how penicillamine does this? Does it operate to prevent the production of ongoing antibody, or does it destroy the immune complexes and macroglobulins that are in the pool, or does it perhaps cause precipitation of immune complexes circulating in the patient? The last possibility could be responsible for some of the toxic effects of penicillamine.

I would be interested in any information on these points.

Willoughby:

The paper to which Dr. Jones refers was not confined to penicillamine but included levamisole. The paper was published in *Rheumatology and Rehabilitation* during 1976. In fairness to Dr. Huskisson, he was postulating a modification of the immunological pathway. It was not really intended as a bald statement of fact. Since then, over many late nights and cups of coffee, his theory has probably gone around 360 degrees.

Jones:

I did not ask for an appreciation of Dr. Huskisson's view. I asked for information on the way in which penicillamine might affect the immune complex pool.

W. Lyle:
(UK)

It is extremely variable. The effects on various immunoglobulins have been studied by Stamworth and co-workers in Birmingham and they found that the only consistent change is an initial rise in IgE—in patients with rheumatoid arthritis—followed usually by a fall which can be sustained, and of various degrees. Just occasionally IgA is virtually eliminated—but very occasionally, changes in IgM and IgG are relatively slight; from high levels they would be reduced, but the reductions are not very great.

The disulphide polymers of these salts tend to decline after there has been a clinical response. It's late—things like ESR and clinical effects, like morning stiffness and so forth decline before there is a decline in rheumatoid factor. This was probably what Dr. Huskisson was getting at when he said that there was a common cause. This was not a chain of circumstance, but separate things which were happening as a result of something else—which he did not know.

Jones:

I appreciate the point, but I wonder whether we know the biodynamics of these changes.

Willoughby:

The short answer to that is 'No'.

Closing Remarks

D. A. WILLOUGHBY (UK)

It is most important to realize that only by a close integration between the study of therapeutic agents, in both man and animal, can we hope to achieve advances in this difficult field of the arthropathies. It is for that reason that I will not restrict my closing remarks to this session but also refer to the previous session.

Logically one can pose a series of well-defined questions. Dr. Katona outlined the problems of relating animal data and the problems of assessment of inflammation in man. In the past few years we have progressed a long way in assessment in man from the basic question, 'Do you feel better?' Slowly thermography, arthroscopy, isotopic clearance were added to the parameters being measured. Yet the visual analogue scale still gives good reliable results despite the credulity of the basic scientific people in the audience. Nevertheless we are faced with the basic question number one, namely, the problem of better methods of evaluation in man. Certainly the interesting results shown by Professor Roux and his colleagues showed that with some of the anti-rheumatic drugs, laboratory measurements are fruitless. For myself, his paper contained a fascinating aspect, namely that of lowered populations of lymphocytes. Are we dealing with an immunodeficiency disease? Certainly the most specific agents for the treatment of rheumatoid are the 'immunomodulators' or enhancers of the immunological response. We have heard from Professor Veys of the usefulness of levamisole. Thus we can pose a further question, do we suppress or enhance the immune response in the treatment of rheumatoid arthritis?

One thing that has emerged from these sessions is that we have heard a lot about novel approaches to therapy, thus we learned about drugs acting via the superoxide dismutase 'orgotein'. There was the interesting point raised regarding the drugs acting to clear the exudate which had arrived in the tissues. Possibly by elevating interstitial proteases. Such an approach with the rutin derivatives could resolve the dilemma of oedema and increased vascular permeability.

Once again the prostaglandins have been resuscitated by the elegant experiments of Professor Lewis who has proposed their implication in the mode of action of steroids.

One must then pose the question of how can we detect this whole variety of drugs ranging from penicillamine, levamisole, orgotein, rutin derivatives, etc.? Are the existing animal models adequate? The answer must be no, nevertheless these drugs are on the scene and we must as medical scientists find ways of detecting them and developing further compounds. The future is exciting from a therapeutic point of view.

What does the future hold in terms of advances in therapeutics? Already we are witnessing the usual pattern of a change, in the approach to treatment coming not from the laboratory but from the clinic. Now we urgently need new ways of detecting these drugs but without their potentially dangerous side effects. Dr. Lyle drew attention to the hazards of certain of the new compounds.

In an attempt at crystal ball gazing, I would predict that new models will be developed in the next few years. I suspect that we will find populations of patients with rheumatoid arthritis who need a certain specific form of therapy and other populations who require yet another type. Certainly during the course of this meeting, it has been made very clear that with the distribution of 'responders' and 'non-responders' to any new therapy, inevitably we need a simple method, to determine differences in these populations prior to treatment. This allows me to end these remarks with a final question: how do we pre-select 'responders' and 'non-responders'?

Finally, may I take this opportunity of thanking you all for attending this meeting, and for all those people who have helped us in the preparation and organisation. Particularly I would like to thank the publishers and printers for the speedy publication.

Poster Sessions

The Culturing of Inflammatory Cells with Helminths *in vitro*: A Model of Parasitic Inflammation

Most tissues reactions to helminths involve many types of inflammatory cells, particularly eosinophils, mast cells and macrophages. The interactions between these cell types, and between various cell types and parasites, is poorly understood.

An *in vitro* model, using cells from normal and parasitized rats, allows a temporal and morphological study of these interactions in the presence or absence of humoral factors such as antibody and complement. The trematode, *Schistosoma mansoni*, and the nematodes, *Nippostrongylus brasiliensis* and *Trichinella spiralis*, have been investigated in this system. In culture, mast cells quickly attach to worms that have been coated with specific antibody and will slowly release some of their granules. Similarly, eosinophils very rapidly attach to the surface of the parasites flattening out along the worm's surface as the culture proceeds. A series of ultra-structural changes is seen in these latter cells, particularly the loss of granules and the development of large vacuoles in the cytoplasm. The contents of these vacuoles may be released onto the surface of the worms, possibly causing damage to the parasite. Macrophages are seen to be intimately involved in the later stages of culture when they are seen to ingest eosinophil granules and other cellular and parasite-derived remnants.

A degree of correlation exists between these *in vitro* findings and the inflammation induced in the skin by the invasion of *S. mansoni* and *N. brasiliensis* larvae, particularly in terms of the sequence that cells appear in these reactions. Correlation exists between cell adherence *in vitro* and the killing of some forms of these parasites, and also with the release of radioactive markers from labelled worms.

It is thought that this model assists greatly in the investigations into the cellular components of parasitic inflammation.

C. D. Mackenzie, National Institute of Medical Research, Mill Hill, London NW7 1AA, UK.

Development of Chronic Cicatrising Ocular Inflammation in Guinea Pigs Repeatedly Infected with Guinea Pig Inclusion Conjunctivitis Agent: an Animal Model for the Study of Human Trachoma

Guinea pig inclusion conjunctivitis (GPIC), caused by a member of *Chlamydia psittaci*, is an acute but benign conjunctivitis. The disease is short-lived and resolves spontaneously within 30 days. A chronic and more severe conjunctivitis, lasting for several months, is produced by repeated infections. Pannus and scarring develop. The clinical and pathological features of the chronic disease are similar to those of trachoma in man. This model is being used to determine the immunological basis of the adverse modulation of the host responses, induced by programmed reinfection, which appears to be the critical factor leading to blinding disease in hyperendemic trachoma.

Marjorie A. Monnickendam and S. Darougar, Department of Clinical Ophthalmology, Institute of Ophthalmology, Judd Street, St. Pancras, London, WC1H 9QS.

Cat as a Model for Studying the Immunopathogenesis and Chemotherapy of Chlamydial Ocular and Genital Tract Infections

A model of the cat infection of the eye and genital tract by a member of *Chlamydia psittaci* is described. This is a close analogue to human chlamydial infections including trachoma and chlamydial urethritis (NSU).

This model is being used to study the efficacy of chemotherapy by various agents of direct relevance to human disease.

It also offers the opportunity to study the immunopathogenesis of an animal disease analogous of trachoma and NSU and is being used to investigate the apparent synergistic pathogenesis of inflammatory disease resulting from mixed bacterial and chlamydial infections as compared with either alone.

H. El-Sheikh, R. Woodland and C. Squire, Department of Clinical Ophthalmology, Institute of Ophthalmology, Judd Street, St. Pancras, London, WC1H 9QS.

Effect of Antirheumatic Drugs on Cathepsin B$_1$ from Bovine Spleen

The inhibitory effect on cathepsin B$_1$ of 39 antirheumatic and other agents has been studied. The enzyme was purified from bovine spleen (specific activity 2.8 units/E_{280} unit) and the effect of the drugs measured by determining the decrease of enzyme activity towards BANA as substrate. Analgesics, antimalarials, cytostatic agents, steroids as well as D-penicillamine, colchicine, allopurinol, chlorzoxazone and chlorpromazine either had no effect on cathepsin B$_1$ or inhibited it to a very small extent. Typical anti-inflammatory and antirheumatic agents like gold and pyrazolone derivates (with the exception of sulfinpyrazone) suppressed the activity of the enzyme at a concentration of 10^{-6}M. Two others, indomethacin and diclofenac, suppressed it at a concentration of 10^{-5}M. Two sulphonated polysaccharides, arteparon and pentosan polysulphate (SP54), were also potent inhibitors. Salicylates, however, inhibited cathepsin B_1 only at much higher concentrations (10^{-2}M). Higher concentrations of cysteine (2mM) decreased the inhibitory effect of some otherwise effective drugs. Inhibition of cathepsin B_1 may be one way in which some of the drugs tested exercise their therapeutic effect in rheumatic diseases.

K. Fehr, D. Kruze and A. Böni, University Department of Rheumatology, Cantonal Hospital, Zurich, Switzerland.

Inflammatory Reaction into Rabbit: Serum Anti-Proteases Behaviour

Rabbit a1M and a2M labelling was carried out *in vitro* with ^{131}I in order to determine their half-life in rabbits. We also studied the half-life of these proteins when obtained from rabbits exhibiting an inflammatory reaction.

When radioactivity decrease curves were linear, inflammatory reactions were induced with subcutaneous turpentine injection.

a2M catabolism is faster than the a1M one in every case. When inflammatory reactions were induced during the half-life study, we noted an increased catabolism for normal a1M, acute phase a1M, normal a2M but no modifications were noted for acute phase a2M.

C. Versavel, B. Jousset-Stevenet, T. Lebreton de Vonne, J. C. Besnard and H. Mouray. Laboratoire de Biochimie, Faculté de Médecine, 2 bis Boulevard Tonnelle F 37032, Tours, Cedex.

Interaction of Carrageenan Inflammation and Platelets

The numerous similarities that exist between different aspects of the inflammatory process and the changes occurring in platelets during aggregation have led to the suggestion that platelets may play a role in inflammation.

The experiments described here were designed to investigate whether an accumulation of platelets could be observed in the inflamed area. The properties of the platelets during the inflammation were also determined.

Rat platelets, labelled with ^{51}Cr, were injected into the tail vein of rats with a carrageenan-induced oedema in one of the hind paws. The radioactivity of the injected paw was measured and compared to the control one. It was found that an accumulation of platelets occurred during the first 3–4 h, which diminished later. The peak of the radioactivity did not coincide with the maximal increase in weight.

During the inflammation, the aggregability of the platelets changed. The lag time between the addition of collagen and the beginning of the aggregation was increased and reached the highest value after 4 h.

These data indicate that platelets first are retained in the inflamed area and then released. It was investigated whether the changes in the properties of the platelets are due to differences in the amounts of mediators present. A possible contribution of the platelets to the inflammatory response is discussed.

J. E. Vincent and F. J. Zijlstra, Department of Pharmacology, Erasmus University, Rotterdam, P.O. Box 1738, Rotterdam, The Netherlands.

Interactions of Macrophages and Complement Components in the Pathogenesis of Chronic Inflammation

Several agents able to elicit chronic inflammatory reactions *in vivo*, e.g. dextran sulphate, carrageenan and cell walls of certain bacteria and fungi, are activators of complement by the alternative pathway. As a result of complement activation there is generation of C3b, which is a potent macrophage stimulator. Macrophage cultures exposed to C3b secrete hydrolases, including proteinases. Enzymes secreted from activated macrophages cleave C3. In this way a self-amplifying system is generated. Activation of the complement system can produce factors chemotactic for macrophages. Hence materials which initiate complement activation by the alternative pathway can produce granulomatous reactions.

A. C. Allison and H. U. Schorlemmer, Clinical Research Centre, Harrow, Middlesex HA1 3UJ, and Institut für Med. Mikrobiologie, Johannes-Gutenburg-Universität, 6500 Mainz, Germany.

Autologous Fab₂ Fragments as Mediators of Articular Inflammation

Intra-articularly injected autologous Fab_2 produced from IgG with homologous cathepsin D induces acute synovitis after 1 and 3 injections, subacute synovitis after 6 injections and chronic destructive synovitis after 12 and more injections. Serologically a high percentage of animals become Rf-positive and develop an increase in titre of homoreactants against cathepsin D Fab_2. In the synovial exudate and synovial membrane, phagocytosis of homoreactants and Rf-like antibodies can readily be demonstrated. Both types of antibodies are synthesized by synovial plasma cells. An established chronic auto-immune synovitis of this type will persist at least during six months after cessation of the intra-articular injections, although the intensity of inflammation will gradually decrease. Phagocytosis and synthesis of anti-IgG antibodies was demonstrable up to 6 months after cessation of the injections, suggesting that autoimmune processes might, at least in part, prolong the chronicity of the synovitis. The synovitis tends to project into other joints which are not injected with Fab_2 fragments.

Kurt A. Fehr, Magda Velvart and Albert Böni, University Department of Rheumatology, 8091 Zurich, Switzerland.

Thrombocytosis and Platelet Aggregates in the Circulation of Adjuvant Arthritic Rats

Platelet count was determined at different times after injection of adjuvant. Platelet count was significantly elevated compared to controls from the time when the first signs of arthritic swellings were observable. Thrombocytosis is persistent, it was still significant 3 months after the inoculation of adjuvant. An association appeared to exist between thrombocytosis and severity of arthritic disease. Treatment of severe arthritis rats with aspirin (1 week) has normalized the platelet count. Numbers of large platelets (megathrombocytes) were significantly increased in the stained blood film of arthritic rats and platelet-size distribution curve of rats with adjuvant disease differed significantly from the controls. By the use of the platelet count ratio technique, circulating platelet aggregates were demonstrated in the blood of severe arthritic rats. Acute aspirin treatment was ineffective while prolonged treatment normalized the decreased platelet count ratio (means circulating platelet aggregates) in the blood of arthritic rats. These findings together with our previous observations (decreased bleeding time, increased tendency to thrombus formation in the microcirculation of adjuvant arthritic rats) indicate a distinct tendency to shift the haemostatic equilibrium in favour of thrombosis in severe arthritic disease. These data give some new aspects to the pathomechanism of vascular complications of connective tissue disorders and further supports the therapeutic use of anti-platelet drugs in rheumatoid arthritis.

P. Görög and Iren B. Kovacs, EGYT Pharmacochemical Works, Budapest, and Korvin Otto Hospital, Budapest, Hungary.

Counter-irritant Effects and Influence of Serum Complement Activity by Carrageenan in Carrageenan Oedema as well as in Primary and Secondary Inflammation of Adjuvant Arthritis Rats

Single i.p. administration of carrageenan (10–15 mg/kg) inhibited the carrageenan-induced oedema of the rat paw by 50–60% but was without significant effect on total haemolytic serum complement activity. The inhibitory effect of i.p. carrageenan remained unaffected by simultaneous i.p. administration of 0.5 mg of phenylbutazone, a dose being effective only at the site of injection and having no systemic anti-inflammatory activity. The complement level was elevated by about 50–80% in both phases of adjuvant arthritis. I.p. carrageenan once daily, three times repeated during the 1st to 3rd or 12th to 14th day of adjuvant arthritis was followed by a decrease of complement activity beyond the normal level whereas paw swelling was significantly inhibited in the primary phase but was nearly unaffected in the secondary one. The results are discussed with regard to the mechanism of counter-irritant activity of carrageenan and to the role of the complement system in inflammatory processes.

Rolf Hirschelmann, Heinz Bekemeier and Axel Stelzner, Department of Pharmacology, Section of Pharmacy, Martin Luther University of Halle-Wittenberg, Halle, and Institute of Medical Microbiology, Friedrich Schiller University of Jena, Jena, GDR.

Inflammatory T-Lymphocytes in Mice with Delayed Type Hypersensitivity (DTH) to Sheep Red Blood Cells (SRBC)

We are able to show that T-cells which mediate DTH reactions to SRBC in mice enter into inflammatory exudates from where they can be recovered and, after passive transfer to normal recipients, express DTH. Such T-cell-containing exudates need not contain specific antigen for inducement of T-lymphocyte immigration. The production of exudate seeking T-cells is enhanced by the use of adjuvants such as BCG vaccine or by cyclophosphamide treatment of donors previously to immunization. The exudate seeking property is a distinguishing feature of T-lymphocytes formed early in the immune response. Later on, this property is lost, as is shown by the difference in vinblastine sensitivity of DTH-transferring cells recovered on the 4th day after sensitization and cells recovered 7 days after sensitization. It is concluded that the majority of exudate seeking T-lymphocytes in this system are recently formed blast cells.

In this way, the immunized host creates a system of mobile cells able to initiate inflammatory reactions at any tissue site which has been altered by an inflammatory stimulus.

Supported by DFG grant Ha 598/6

H. Hahn (Ruhr-Universitat, P.O.B. 102148, D-4630 Bochum, Germany), T. E. Miller, G. B. Mackaness (Trudeau-Institute, Saranac Lake, N.Y. 12983, USA).

T-Lymphocyte Stimulating and Antimetastatic Activity of 3-(p-Chlorophenyl-2,3-Dihydro-3-Hydroxythiazolo[3,2-a]-Benzimidazole-2-Acetic Acid (Wy-13,876)

The antitumour and antimetastatic activity of Wy-13,876 in mice and its stimulatory effect on rat T-lymphocytes have been reported by Fenichel, Gregory and Alburn (*Br. J. Cancer*, **33**, 329, 1976). Further experiments have shown that the T-lymphocyte stimulation can be sustained for 2 or 3 consecutive days in normal rats by daily single dose oral administration of 50, 75 or 100 mg/kg. Delayed hypersensitivity was significantly increased in normal guinea pigs by the compound as measured by the dinitrochlorobenzene technique.

Metastases were increased when drug treated BDF_1 mice with transplanted Lewis Lung or B-16 tumours were given anti-T-lymphocyte serum (1 ml anti-theta serum 1:30). Therefore it is believed that the antimetastatic action of Wy-13,876 is due to the T-cell stimulation.

R. L. Fenichel, H. E. Alburn, and F. J. Gregory, Research Division, Wyeth Laboratories, P.O. 8299, Philadelphia, Pennsylvania, 19101 USA.

DNA Synthesis of Rat Peritoneal Macrophages in Culture Induced by a Pleural Inflammatory Exudate: Influence of Anti-inflammatory and Immunosuppressive Agents

As previously reported, the acute inflammatory exudate obtained 4 h after intrapleural injection of dextran in rats was able to induce DNA synthesis and division of normal rat macrophages in culture. This has been found to be a general property of a variety of pleural, provoked by immunological and non-immunological, stimuli.

The influences of two types of pretreatment of rats with anti-inflammatory or immunosuppressive agents were investigated.

Exudates of rats treated with indomethacin or methylprednisolone have no effect on the DNA synthesis of untreated rat macrophages. On the contrary, exudates of rats treated with dexamethasone and cyclophosphamide decrease the DNA synthesis; exudates of rats treated with methotrexate increase this phenomenon.

In rat macrophages treated with indomethacin, methylprednisolone, dexamethasone or cyclophosphamide, the DNA synthesis induced by untreated rat exudates was increased; on the contrary in rat macrophages treated with methotrexate the DNA synthesis was increased.

M. Pelletier (Department de Pharmacologie, ERA 629, Faculté de Médecine Cochin Port-Royal, 24 rue du Faubourg Saint-Jacques, 75014, Paris), J. Fontagne, M. Loizeau, M. Adolphe, and P. Lechat (Institut de Pharmacologie, 21 rue de l'Ecole de Médecine, 75006, Paris, France).

Antiproteinuric Effect of Indomethacin in Experimental Extra-Membranous (Heymann-Type) Nephritis in Rats

Indomethacin is known to have an immediate and reversible anti-proteinuric effect in human nephrotic syndromes; the purpose of this work was to study whether this effect could likewise be realized in an animal experimental model.

The disease was induced in inbred male PVG/C rats by repeated intra-peritoneal immunization with diazotized Wistar rat kidney antigen. The glomerulopathy is associated with proteinuria (400–900 mg/rat/day) and hypalbuminaemia (26% of healthy control); there is no impairment of GFR, no oedema occurs and natriuresis is normal.

Indomethacin (daily doses of 2×0.15 to 2×0.60 mg/rat) fails to reduce protein excretion in animals receiving standard-feed (sodium content 191 μEq/g feed). When animals on salt-restricted diet (5μEq/g) are given the drug (2×0.60 mg daily), an immediate decrease of the proteinuria to about 60% of controls is observed. The effect is very similar to the short-term indomethacin effects in humans. This model affords possibilities for analysis of pharmacological and pathogenetic aspects of human disease and its treatment.

Starting from the observed obligatory salt restriction and from the drug's being a prostaglandin synthetase inhibitor, one may conclude that apparently in the rat inhibition of prostaglandin synthesis causes a reduction of protein-uria only if hypovolaemia is achieved by superimposing salt restriction on hypalbuminaemia, or if low proximal rejection of sodium or tubular urine is present. Possibly an enhanced activity of the renin–angiotensin system is a pre-requisite of prostaglandin synthesis inhibition implying an antiproteinuric effect.

F. W. J. Gribnau, H. L. Y. Siero, G. J. Fleuren, P. J. J. van Munster, Ph. J. Hoedemaker and P. G. A. B. Wijdeveld, Medical Faculty, University of Nijmegen; and Department of Pathology, University of Groningen, The Netherlands.

Effects of Indomethacin on the Course of Extramembranous (Heymann-Type) Glomerulonephritis in Rats

Opinions differ as regards the question whether indomethacin favourably influences the course of human glomerulonephritis. This prompted us to study the effect of the drug on the course of an experimental glomerulo-nephritis in rats.

Nephritis was induced in inbred male PVG/C rats by immunization (12 injections intraperitoneally in 6 weeks) with diazotized Wistar rat kidney antigen, and for periods up to 500 days proteinuria, endogenous creatinine clearance (ECC) and renal morphology were studied. The disease is associated with proteinuria (400–900 mg/rat/day), hypalbuminaemia (about 26% of controls) and hypercholesteraemia (10 mmol/l). ECC remains normal, as to renal capacities for sodium excretion and retention. In animals on standard feed (191 μEq Na/g feed) no oedema occurs. From week 4 on a non-prolifera-tive glomerulonephritis starts, with characteristic 'spikes', granular pattern of immunofluorescence (IgC and C3), subepithelial electrondense deposits increasing in size and irregularity with thickening of the glomerular basement membrane (GBM). From week 33 on electron-microscopically empty spaces develop around the deposits in the GBM and later on even holes. About week 75 these holes have been filled with newly formed GBM substance.

The drug reduces proteinuria only if given during the phase of immuniza-tion; reduction is dose-dependent by 26% (dose 0.30 mg/rat/day) to 45% (dose 0.60 mg/rat/day). ECC is not influenced. Change of morphological features is only seen in electron microscopy, and the differences seem to be of minor importance; in the first 22 weeks the EM characteristics seem to be accelerated, in the later phase fewer empty spaces develop. The reported results—with all reserve—lend no support to the expectation of benefit from long-term indomethacin treatment in chronic glomerulonephritis.

F. W. J. Gribnau, et al., *Pharmacological Institute and Division of Nephrology, Department of Medicine, University of Nijmegen; Department of Pathology, University of Gronigen, The Netherlands.*

The Influence of Phenylbutazone, Indomethacin and Dexamethasone on the Prostaglandin E Content in the Paw of the Adjuvant Arthritis Rat

Adjuvant arthritis was investigated up to the 32nd day after injection of the complete Freund's adjuvant. The prostaglandin E content of the paw of adjuvant arthritic rats was enhanced, especially in acute stages of the inflammatory process. This applies to the injected paw as well as to the non-injected one. The increase of prostaglandin content preceded the increase of paw swelling. Oral administration of phenylbutazone (50 mg/kg), indomethacin (1 mg/kg) or dexamethasone (0.3 mg/kg) once daily inhibited significantly the paw swelling but did not inhibit (or only weakly inhibited) the increase of the prostaglandin content in the paw.

H. Bekemeier, A.-J. Giessler, R. Hirschelmann and Karin Schrank. Department of Pharmacology, Section of Pharmacy, Martin Luther University of Halle-Wittenberg, Halle, GDR.

Vascular Changes During Acute Inflammatory Responses in Rat Hindpaws

In acute inflammatory responses, increased blood flow and vascular permeability are important events which determine the extent of tissue swelling. A method has recently been developed in our laboratories to measure these changes precisely during inflammatory responses in rat hindpaws (Owen & Farrington, *Agents & Actions* (1976), **6**, 622–626).

The vascular responses and oedema caused by injection of some inflammatory mediators into the plantar surface of the rat hindpaw have been measured and compared with the effect of inflammatory responses due to tissue injury (immersion in water at 57° C for 30 s).

The results indicate a different profile of vascular responses to different inflammatory stimuli.

Tissue injury caused oedema associated with an increase in both blood flow and vascular permeability in the injured paw. Histamine and bradykinin also increased blood flow and vascular permeability. 5-hydroxytryptamine caused a very large increase in vascular permeability with little change in blood flow, whereas PGE_2 caused the largest increase in blood flow but was less effective in increasing vascular permeability.

D. A. A. Owen, Department of Pharmacology, The Research Institute, Smith Kline and French Laboratories Limited, Welwyn Garden City, Hertfordshire.

Prostaglandin Endoperoxides and Inflammation: the Microvascular Changes Induced by Prostaglandin G_2

Prostaglandin (PG) G_2 is an unstable intermediate in arachidonic acid metabolism and is released by platelets and possibly other cells. The microvascular effects of PGG_2 in the hamster cheek pouch (HCP) and rabbit skin have been examined using microscopic and isotopic techniques.

In the HCP, arterioles having a low vascular tone, produced a short-lasting vasoconstriction (maximum at 30–60 s) in response to topically applied PGG_2. Repeated doses of PGG_2 rapidly induced tachyphylaxis which was not observed on isolated vascular strips. Doses of noradrenaline equiactive with PGG_2 were of longer duration and were not tachyphylactic. On vessels having a high tone induced by a continuous superfusion of noradrenaline, PGG_2 produced a much smaller vasoconstriction followed by a protracted phase of strong vasodilatation. In these concentrations of PGG_2, white body formation was not observed.

When PGG_2 mixed with ^{133}Xe in saline was injected into the dorsal skin of the rabbit and ^{133}Xe washout monitored using a γ-detector, reduced blood flow was apparent for the first 70 s, which was followed by a protracted phase of increased flow.

Because of the protracted phase of vasodilatation produced by PGG_2, a pro-inflammatory effect on bradykinin-induced exudation would be expected. Using a method for measuring exudation and blood flow changes simultaneously in rabbit skin using ^{131}I-albumin and ^{133}Xe, PGG_2 was found to have a strong potentiating effect on bradykinin-induced exudation.

G. P. Lewis, J. Westwick and T. J. Williams, Department of Pharmacology, Institute of Basic Medical Sciences, Royal College of Surgeons of England, Lincoln's Inn Fields, London WC2A 3PN.

Potentiation of Inflammatory Exudation by Endogenous Factors: New Evidence for the Release and Action of Prostaglandins in Inflammatory Reactions

A method has been developed in order to measure plasma exudation and blood flow changes simultaneously in rabbit skin, using ^{131}I-albumin and ^{133}Xe. Intradermal injection of *Bordetella pertussis* (killed vaccine, 2.5×10^8 organisms/site) produces minimal plasma exudation. If, however, a following injection of bradykinin ($0.5 \ \mu g$) is given into the same site, a potentiation of the exudation response to bradykinin is observed. Other particles (e.g. zymosan, antigen–antibody complexes) and colloids (e.g. carrageenan) produce the same effect. This potentiation is maximal when the interval between the two injections is 1 h; no significant potentiation is observed with bradykinin/particle mixtures. This suggests that an accumulation of haematogenous cells is a prerequisite. In support of this, intradermal injection of PMN-leukocytes followed 1 h later by injection of bradykinin also results in potentiation. Further, depletion of PMN-leukocytes using nitrogen mustard suppresses the potentiation produced by particles.

The potentiation is similar to that observed with prostaglandin (PG)/ bradykinin mixtures, which appears to be dependent on the vasodilator activity of PGs. In addition, the particle potentiation effect is abolished by the addition to the first injection of indomethacin (1 μg/site) or dexamethasone (1 μg/site).

These results suggest that PGs are released in response to the introduction of particulate or colloidal matter into tissues. The source of the PG appears to be the PMN-leukocyte. These observations correlate some of the *in vitro* and *in vivo* observations of PG release and action, and emphasize the importance of mediator interactions in inflammatory responses.

T. J. Williams, Department of Pharmacology, Institute of Basic Medical Sciences, Royal College of Surgeons of England, Lincoln's Inn Fields, London WC2A 3PN.

The Inflammatory Response to Paraffin in the Peritoneal Cavity of the Rat

The mediators and products of inflammatory reactions influence more than local vasculature; we are concerned with their effects on overlying epithelia. By choosing various periods of stimulation it may be possible to produce inflammatory exudates of variable biochemical and cellular composition which, when added to mucosa in organ culture, may simulate effects seen in man. This report describes the characteristics of the inflammatory response in the rat to intraperitoneal paraffin.

60 adult rats were injected with 5 ml paraffin and killed at intervals up to 120 h. The paraffin and resultant exudate were aspirated after washing the peritoneal cavity with a fixed volume of tissue culture medium containing Evans Blue. The paraffin and cells were separated by centrifugation, total and differential cell counts performed and the exudate volume calculated by dilution of the dye measured spectrophotometrically. At 0 h the mean total cell count per animal was 10.5×10^6 with 16% polymorphs (PMN), 50% monocytes (M), 18% lymphocytes and 16% mast cells. Exudate volume was 0.6 ml. Cellular influx reached a peak at 24 h when total cell numbers had increased 6 times; it then declined slowly so that at 120 h numbers were 3 times those in control animals. PMN and M predominated throughout the experimental period. The PMN's showed a 3-fold increase to 6×10^6 cells

per animal at 4 h reaching a peak of 28 × 10^6 at 72 h; cells appearing at 4 h were predominantly of mature type, whilst those at 72 h were mainly immature. M response was biphasic with peak numbers of 34 × 10^6 and 25 × 10^6 at 24 h and 96 h respectively. Exudate volume increased up to 4 h but rose only slightly thereafter to a maximum of 2 ml at 120 h. These findings contrast with published results in rabbits and guinea pigs in which paraffin-induced peritoneal lesions show a prolonged monocyte response.

It is concluded that intra-peritoneal paraffin in rats can be used to produce exudates with different compositions but in no case is there a predominant cell type.

Supported by grants from the Medical Research Council and Wellcome Foundation. Patricia M. Hancock, M. W. Hill and N. W. Johnson, Department of Oral Pathology, The London Hospital Medical College, London, E1.

An Assessment of the Anti-inflammatory Activity of Gold Salts in Three Models of Inflammation

Chrysotherapy has been an important tool in the treatment of rheumatoid arthritis for many years. However, few and sometimes conflicting studies describing the anti-inflammatory activity of gold compounds have been reported. We have consequently investigated the effects of gold sodium thiomalate (GTM; Myocrisin) in 3 models of inflammation using a variety of dosage regimens, in attempts to quantitate the activity of gold compounds.

Male Wistar rats (CE/CFHB strain) or female Dunkin Hartley guinea pigs were used in the following experiments. In the kaolin-induced rat paw oedema GTM (10–30 mg/kg, i.m.) did not affect the response when administered at 1 h, 1 day, 3 days, 7 days or 14 days prior to the irritant. Administration of single doses of GTM (30 mg/kg) to rats 21 days, but not 28 days, 14 days or 7 days prior to adjuvant (*M. butyricum* in liquid paraffin) significantly suppressed the 24 h primary swelling. Dividing the 30 mg/kg dose over this 28 days period failed to inhibit the primary swelling.

Neither the primary nor secondary lesion of adjuvant-induced arthritis examined over 21 days was affected by daily administration or administration on alternate days of GTM (30 mg/kg i.m.).

However, in the guinea pig u.v. erythema model GTM (10–100 mg/kg) administered i.m. 1 h prior to irradiation significantly suppressed the erythema from 3 h to 24 h. Triethylphosphine gold chloride (10–100 mg/kg), but not GTM possessed oral anti-erythemic activity also administered 1 h prior to irradiation.

From these data it would appear that only the guinea pig u.v. model of the models examined provided a reproducible model for quantitation of the anti-inflammatory activity of gold salts *in vivo*.

A. J. Lewis, J. Cottney D. J. Nelson and M. McArthur, Organon Laboratories Limited, Newhouse, Lanarkshire ML1 5SH, Scotland.

Inhibition of Anaphylactic and Compound 48/80 Induced Reactions in Rat by Tiaramide Hydrochloride (THC)

Tiaramide hydrochloride is a basic molecule which is endowed with anti-inflammatory properties. Its anti-anaphylactic action was investigated using rat mast cells. It was found that THC exerts a strong inhibitory action on antigen-induced and Compound 48/80-induced histamine release from isolated rat peritoneal mast cells in a fluorometric assay. The inhibition of *in vitro* anaphylactic histamine release is 90% with 10^{-3} M THC, and 20% with 10^{-3} M THC. Using Compound 48/80 (0.5 μg/ml), the inhibition of histamine release is 52 % with 10^{-3} M THC and 21% with 10^{-5} M THC.

Compound 48/80-induced vasodilatation in rat skin is inhibited by prior intradermal injection of THC, as measured by blueing of skin due to intravascular Evans Blue dye. The percentage of inhibition ranges from 92.3 $\pm$ 10.1 (10^{-2} M THC) to 8.3 $\pm$ 4.3 (10^{-6} M THC).

THC inhibits radio-labelled serotonin release from Compound 48/80 challenged rat mast cells. The percentage of inhibition ranges from 80 (10^{-2} M THC) to 30% (10^{-3} M THC).

In these experimental systems, a similar action was exerted by disodium chromoglycate, but higher drug concentrations were needed.

It is concluded that THC exhibits experimentally an anti-anaphylactic action. Further studies are needed to determine its exact mode of action and eventual clinical use in the field of allergic diseases. In any case, the demonstration of the inhibition of mast cell degranulation contributes to the understanding of its action as an anti-inflammatory drug.

M. L. Renoux, B. Weill and D. Wallach, Laboratoire de Médecine Expérimentale et Immunologie Générale. Faculté de Médecine Cochin-Port-Royal. 75674, Paris, Cedex 14 (France).

Are Immune Complexes Essential for the Development of Rat Adjuvant Disease?

The pathogenesis of adjuvant disease in rats is generally thought to be due to cell-mediated immune mechanisms because of the histological appearance of the lesions and the ability to transfer the disease with lymphoid cells but not with serum. However, the fact that neonatal thymectomy increases the susceptibility of rats to the disease suggests that this view may be an oversimplification. Furthermore the onset and severity of disease do not correlate well with delayed hypersensitivity (DH) to PPD; neither is a correlation between antimycobacterial antibody and disease evident although a degree of complement dependence has been observed.

In the present work male PVG/c rats were dosed i.p. with 100 mg/kg cyclophosphamide (Cy) to deplete them of rapidly dividing cells. Three days later each rat received 300 μg of heat-killed mycobacteria in 0.05 ml of liquid paraffin given intradermally into one hind paw. Rats receiving Cy failed to develop the secondary lesions normally seen 12–14 days after adjuvant. The response of Cy-treated rats to adjuvant was restored by normal spleen cells given 2 h before adjuvant. Rats treated with Cy and given adjuvant showed enhanced and prolonged DH to PPD.

The most likely explanation of these results is that immune complexes are of considerably more importance in the pathogenesis of adjuvant disease than was previously supposed (at least in the initiation of the joint lesions), although cell-mediated processes clearly play an equally important role in determining the final form of the disease.

Alternatively, suppressor B-lymphocytes may prevent the development of strong cell-mediated immunity capable of efficient elimination of the mycobacterial antigen. The response which does develop is relatively weak and may result in slow elimination of antigen and a prolonged inflammation.

A. R. MacKenzie, C. R. Pick, P. Sibley and B. White, Departments of Biochemistry and Pathology, Allen and Hanburys Research Ltd., Ware, Hertfordshire, England.

Immune Deposits in Arthritic Cartilages

Immunohistochemical studies were carried out in cartilage specimens obtained at synovectomy or autopsy from 40 patients with various joint and/or connective tissue diseases. Antisera against IgG, IgA, IgM, C3 and C1q were prepared as described elsewhere (van de Putte *et al.*, *N. Engl. J. Med.* **290**, 1165, 1974). Both immunoglobulins (Ig) and complement components (C) were found in specimens from patients with rheumatoid arthritis (17 out of 21), unclassified arthritis (1/2), coxarthrosis (2/7), osteochondritis dissecans (1/2), and in a cartilage specimen obtained at autopsy from a non-inflamed joint of a SLE patient. In these specimens Ig and C generally occurred in the same location, suggesting the presence of immune complexes. Although usually present in the superficial layers of the cartilage, fluorescent deposits were occasionally seen just below the superficial layer or even deeper in the cartilage. Neither Ig nor C could be detected in some patients with rheumatoid arthritis (2/21) ankylosing spondylitis (1/2), unclassified arthritis (1/2) or coxarthrosis (3/7), or patients with avascular necrosis of bone, slipped capital femoral epiphysis or scleroderma. Few specimens contained only Ig or C. Control studies indicated that positive staining was not merely the result of rheumatoid factor activity of the immunoglobuline deposited in the cartilage. We conclude that immune deposits in articular cartilage occur in a variety of arthritic disorders. Their occasional non-association with arthritis and their absence in some forms of chronic arthritis make the significance of these deposits uncertain.

L. B. A. van de Putte, T. E. Overbeek, G. J. M. Lafeber. Department of Rheumatology, University Hospital Leiden.

In vitro Handling of DNA–Anti-DNA Complexes by Human Blood Phagocytes

In order to study phagocyte function in SLE patients, we have studied the uptake of DNA–anti-DNA complexes of well-defined composition. ^{3}H-labelled PM_2-DNA, a circular DNA with a M.W. of 5.9×10^6, was incubated with anti-DNA serum (from SLE patients with a high anti-DNA titre as measured with the Farr assay) for 1 h at 37 °C. Human PMN or monocytes were incubated with the complexes thus obtained, spun down at 4 °C, treated with DNAse to remove non-ingested complexes, and washed twice. The radioactivity in the cell pellet was counted.

The uptake of DNA–anti-DNA complexes depends on cell and complex concentration and on the time of incubation, but also on the size and the composition of the complexes. When the size of the complexes was increased by overnight settling at 4 °C (presumably as a result of Fc aggregation) or by raising the Ab:Ag ratio, ingestion also increased. For optimal phagocytosis, about 4 times as much IgG anti-DNA was needed per mole of DNA as IgM anti-DNA.

Several indications were found that IgM–anti-DNA complexes were ingested exclusively via a C3 receptor-mediated process, while IgG–anti-DNA complexes were phagocytosed by an Fc receptor-mediated process which was increased in the presence of complement. Uptake of IgM-anti-DNA complexes required fresh serum in a concentration dependent way. Treatment of this serum with EDTA or Cobra venom factor inhibited the complex phagocytosis, illustrating that activation of C3 is needed for this process. No inhibition was observed when C4-deficient serum or Mg EDTA was used. Thus, this activation of C3 may proceed via the alternative pathway. In contrast, uptake of IgG–anti-DNA complexes was independent of complement activation because complexes made from heat-inactivated anti-DNA serum were internalized without addition of a complement source. Moreover, trypsin treatment of the cells completely abolished the phagocytosis of IgM–anti-DNA complexes, but hardly affected the uptake of IgG–anti-DNA complexes. Taken together, these findings strongly suggest that IgG-containing complexes are phagocytosed after binding to Fc receptors on the cells, while IgM-containing complexes bind to C3 receptors. Thus, the contribution of both receptors to the process of phagocytosis may now be measured separately and in a quantitative way.

D. Roos, R. S. Weening, M. De Boer and L. A. Aarden, Central Laboratory, Netherlands, Red Cross Blood Transfusion Service, P.O. Box 9190, Amsterdam, Netherlands.

Destruction of IgG-sensitized Human Erythrocytes by Human Blood Monocytes

It is generally assumed that in man the destruction of erythrocytes sensitized with non-complement binding IgG antibodies, which predominantly occurs in the spleen, is mediated by mononuclear phagocytes located in that organ. However, the mechanism(s) of destruction are not exactly known. For this reason we decided to study in what way human erythrocytes sensitized with non-complement binding IgG alloantibodies were destroyed by human blood monocytes *in vitro* (blood monocytes are the precursor cells of tissue macrophages). We found that when monocytes were incubated with a relatively low number of IgG-sensitized erythrocytes (EAIgG) destruction of EAIgG mainly occurred by way of extracellular cytotoxic lysis, but, when the number of EAIgG per monocyte was increased it was found that phagocytosis became quantitatively as important as cytotoxic lysis. However, it was found that a considerable number of IgG sensitized red cells that were neither lysed nor phagocytosed had an increased osmotic fragility. Unsensitized cells did not show this phenomenon. The number of red cells 'osmotically' damaged even greatly exceeded the number of cells lysed or phagocytosed. There was experimental evidence indicating that the mechanisms of 'osmotic' damage and cytotoxic lysis of the red cell by the monocyte are very similar and that 'osmotic' damage precedes lysis. The increase in osmotic fragility of EAIgG after contact with monocytes *in vitro* correlates strikingly with the fact that *in vivo* in the peripheral blood of patients with autoimmune haemolytic anaemia due to non-complement binding IgG autoantibodies an increased osmotic fragility of the red cells is a characteristic finding. This suggests that the mechanisms of destruction *in vivo* are similar to those operating *in vitro* and thus possibly also mediated by mononuclear phagocytes. A problem which remained was that the interaction between monocytes and EAIgG *in vitro* is easily inhibited by low concentrations of normal IgG which makes it difficult to understand how these mechanisms might work *in vivo* in the presence of far higher concentrations of IgG. The following experimental conditions decreased inhibition by IgG *in vitro*: (1) An increase in the number of EAIgG per monocyte; (2) An increase in the number of antibody molecules per EAIgG; (3) *In vitro* culture of monocytes (maturation to macrophages). This possibly explains why red cell destruction occurs in the spleen as *in vivo* the above mentioned conditions are effectuated in this organ.

A. Fleer, F. W. van der Meulen, A. E. G. Kr. von dem Borne, and C. P. Engelfriet, Central Laboratory, Netherlands Red Cross Blood Transfusion Service, P.O. Box 9190, Amsterdam, Netherlands.

The Kinetics of Opsonization, Phagocytosis and Intracellular Killing by Granulocytes

Granulocytes perform their function mainly in the tissues. At that site it is virtually impossible to investigate the functions of these cells quantitatively.

Since phagocytic cells in inflamed tissues are derived from circulating cells, the study of peripheral blood granulocytes should give adequate information about their functional capacities. Techniques have been developed for quantitative measurement of phagocytosis and intracellular killing of live microorganisms by phagocytic cells. The phagocytic assay also provides a means to measure opsonization of bacteria.

It has shown that the rate of phagocytosis, measured as the decrease in number of extra-cellular bacteria, is temperature-dependent and that the concentration of opsonins can be rate-limiting.

The attachment and ingestion of bacteria requires the presence of immunoglobulins, but immunoglobulins alone opsonize poorly; most of the opsonizing activity of serum was shown to be due to complement.

The phagocytosis of *Staphylococcus aureus* or *Escherichia coli* measured at various bacteria-to-cell ratios follows first order kinetics.

The rate of intracellular killing was assessed independently of the rate of phagocytosis. Cells were permitted to phagocytose pre-opsonized bacteria for 3 min and then washed. The rate of killing was followed by viable counting of bacteria released from lysed cells.

P. C. J. Leijh, M.Th. v.d. Barselaar and Th. van Zwet, Department of Infectious Diseases, University Hospital, Leiden, The Netherlands.

Storage of Monocytes in Liquid Nitrogen

The activity in various functional test systems of the peripheral blood monocytes (PBM) of different individuals appears to differ quite strongly. Therefore it would be of great advantage to have at one's disposal a pool of monocytes that can be stored and remain unchanged for a long period of time to study the *in vitro* behaviour of human peripheral blood monocytes. We investigated the effect of programmed freezing and thawing (V. P. Eijsvoogel *et al.*, Cryopreserved lymphocytes: Functional properties *in vitro*. In: *Cryoconservation des cellules normales et neoplasiques* (Ed. Weiner, Oldham and Schwarzenberg) Inserm, Paris, 1973) on EA rosette formation and the cytotoxic lysis of IgG sensitized target cells as parameter for the quality of the PBM, Monocytes were isolated from human peripheral blood by means of Ficoll-Isopaque density gradient centrifugation and plastic adherence. Suspensions containing 70–90% monocytes were thus obtained. The overall recovery after freezing and thawing was 62% whereas the percentage of monocytes in the suspension remained the same. Over 90% of the cells excluded Trypan Blue. The percentage of cells forming EA rosettes was the same before and after freezing and thawing (70–80%). The inhibition by free IgG of EA rosettes formation by monocytes that were kept frozen overnight was slightly but significantly increased when compared with freshly prepared monocytes. However, there was no difference in EA rosette formation between monocytes kept frozen overnight and monocytes stored in the frozen state for 3 months.

In preliminary experiments, cytotoxicity of IgG-sensitized red cells by monocytes remained about constant using either freshly prepared monocytes, monocytes kept frozen overnight and monocytes stored frozen for 2 weeks. These results suggest that by storing monocytes in liquid nitrogen one can have cells at one's disposal which, once frozen, remain constant in the activity of EA rosetting and antibody mediated cytotoxicity.

F. W. van der Meulen, A. E. G. Kr. von dem Borne, and C. P. Engelfriet, Central Laboratory, The Netherlands Red Cross Blood Transfusion Service, P.O. Box 9190, Amsterdam, The Netherlands.

Lymphoendothelial Dysfunction in the Pathophysiology of Inflammatory Rheumatic Disease

Immunopathogenetic concepts of rheumatoid arthritis and allied diseases are conveniently illustrated by reference to experimental immunological models of rheumatoid vasculitis, subcutaneous nodules, hyperplastic lymph-adenitis and lymphocytic synovitis produced by intense and persistent lymphokine-mediated stimulation to local lymphocytic emigration and activation in otherwise (genetically) normal laboratory animals. However, the consistent failure to identify extrinsic antigens at sites of chronic rheumatic inflammation in Man raises a conceptual paradox in applying classical immunopathological mechanisms to the understanding of inflammatory rheumatic disease. The 'rheumatoid' response, which these experimental models mimic closely, may be viewed as involving a host failure to restrain recirculatory lymphocyte activation and lymphokine production following systemic stimuli which would otherwise elicit transient or subclinical local 'connective tissue' responses in the normal subject. A new concept is proposed of a 'lymphoendothelial' system (LES) whose physiology and pathology would include the participation of lymphokines active upon microvascular endothelium and other cell types in connective tissue. In this discussion, rheumatoid disease is viewed as an example of reactive LES pathology, precipitated by microbial and other stimuli, acting at a distance from sites of rheumatic pathology, which may reveal an underlying disorder of lymphocyte:endothelial interactions.

Dudley C. Dumonde, Kennedy Institute of Rheumatology, London W6 7DW.

A Role for L-lymphocytes in the Pathogenesis of Chronic Inflammation

L-lymphocytes are a newly described population of human blood lymphocytes which generally comprise 10–20% of the total population. They have high avidity Fc receptors capable of binding small aggregates of IgG present in normal human serum and were accordingly named L-lymphocytes because of membrane-*labile* IgG determinants. L-lymphocytes do not form rosettes with sheep erythrocytes, lack membrane-incorporated Ig markers and lack receptors for mouse complement. They can be isolated by negative selection with rosetting techniques and are the only lymphocyte population capable of killing human lymphocytes coated with IgG antibodies. L-lymphocytes then have K-cell activity. Purified L-lymphocytes cannot proliferate in response to mitogens and antigens, do not develop surface Ig when cultured *in vitro* and cannot be induced to develop cytoplasmic Ig by pokeweed mitogen. In subjects with connective tissue diseases they are decreased in the blood. In contrast, in subjects with infections L-lymphocytes are increased in proportion to T- and B-cells.

One may speculate that L-lymphocytes have a major role in perpetuating tissue injury in chronic inflammatory states by the following mechanisms. Host cells are injured by an exogenous agent (virus) which also alters self antigens, thus provoking an immune response by T-cells and B-cells. The resulting IgG auto-antibodies attach to surface antigens on uninjured host cells and prime them for non-specific killing by L-lymphocytes. Alternatively immune complexes in antibody excess can arm L-lymphocytes and enable them to specifically kill target cells. Macrophage removal and degradation of injured cells make available more antigen to perpetuate the immune response and the inflammatory cycle. It is likely that an increased understanding of the modulating role of L-lymphocytes in the immune response will lead to new insights in the mechanism of chronic inflammation.

David A. Horwitz, M.D., University of Virginia School of Medicine, Charlottesville, Virginia 22901, USA.

Cartilage Degradation by Macrophages, Fibroblasts and Synovial Cells in Culture

To investigate the mechanisms of destruction of articular tissues in rheumatoid arthritis we are developing *in vitro* models in which cells are cultivated in contact with ^{35}S-labelled devitalized cartilage. The degradation of cartilage proteoglycans (CPG) and collagen is monitored by the release of ^{35}S-soluble material and hydroxyproline. Rabbit bone marrow macrophages and fibroblasts as well as synovial cells from rabbits or humans are studied. Macrophages degraded completely the CPG over 3 days culture. This effect was inhibited by cycloheximide or serum and linked to the synthesis and secretion of a CPG-degrading protease that accumulated linearly in the medium over 6 days. This secretion was parallel to that of collagenase but levelled off sooner than that of lysozyme or β-glucuronidase. The protease did not accumulate within the cells. It had optimal activity at pH 7.5 and was inhibited by EDTA, cysteine and serum (but not by Dip-F). It degraded CPG into fragments larger than those obtained by papain, presumably by splitting the protein core of their subunits. The conditions under which the cartilage collagen is being degraded by the macrophages are investigated. Fibroblasts from various origins (carcass, synovium, skin) and 'ages' were tested. A limited number of cultures only resulted in the degradation of the CPG as well as in the accumulation of collagenase in the medium. However, primo-cultures of synovial cells from arthritic (Dumonde-Glynn) rabbits or rheumatoid patients degraded extensively both the PG and the collagen of the cartilage. This *in vitro* model is thus suited for the study of the factors controlling tissue degradation in arthritis as well as for the testing of anti-rheumatic drugs.

G. Vaes, P. Hauser, G. Huybrechts-Godin and Ch. Peeters-Joris. Laboratoire de Chimie Physiologique, Université de Louvain and Institute of Cellular Pathology, Av. Hippocrate, 75, 1200 Brussels, Belgium.